Internal Medicine
Essentials
for
Clerkship Students
— 2 —

Patrick C. Alguire, MD, FACP
DIRECTOR
EDUCATION AND CAREER DEVELOPMENT
AMERICAN COLLEGE OF PHYSICIANS
EDITOR-IN-CHIEF

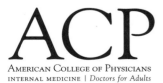

AMERICAN COLLEGE OF PHYSICIANS
INTERNAL MEDICINE | *Doctors for Adults*

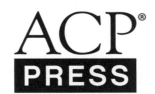

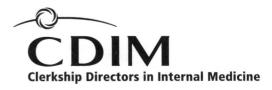

Clerkship Directors in Internal Medicine

Associate Publisher and Manager, Books Publishing: Tom Hartman
Production Supervisor: Allan S. Kleinberg
Senior Production Editor: Karen C. Nolan
Editorial Coordinator: Angela Gabella
Design: Michael E. Ripca

Copyright © 2009 by the American College of Physicians. All rights reserved. No part of this publication may be reproduced in any form by any means (electronic, mechanical, xerographic, or other) or held in any information storage or retrieval systems without written permission from the College.

Printed in the United States of America
Printed by Sheridan Books
Composition by Scribe, Inc. (www.scribenet.com)

ISBN: 978-1-934465-13-4

The authors and publisher have exerted every effort to ensure that the drug selection and dosages set forth in this book are in accordance with current recommendations and practice at the time of publication. In view of ongoing research, occasional changes in government regulations, and the constant flow of information relating to drug therapy and drug reactions, however, the reader is urged to check the package insert for each drug for any change in indications and dosage and for added warnings and precautions. This care is particularly important when the recommended agent is a new or infrequently used drug.

09 10 11 12 13 / 10 9 8 7 6 5 4 3 2 1

Section Editors

Thomas M. DeFer, MD, FACP
Clerkship Director
Division of Medical Education
Department of Internal Medicine
Washington University School of Medicine
St Louis, Missouri

D. Michael Elnicki, MD, FACP
Director, Ambulatory Medicine Clerkship
Director, Section of General Internal Medicine
University of Pittsburgh School of Medicine
UPMC Shadyside
Pittsburgh, Pennsylvania

Mark J. Fagan, MD
Clerkship Director
Department of Medicine
Alpert Medical School of Brown University
Providence, Rhode Island

Sara B. Fazio, MD
Assistant Professor, Harvard Medical School
Director, Core I Medicine Clerkship
Division of General Internal Medicine
Beth Israel Deaconess Medical Center
Boston, Massachusetts

James L. Sebastian, MD, FACP
Director of Student Teaching Programs
Department of Medicine
Medical College of Wisconsin
Clement J. Zablocki Veterans Affairs Medical Center
Milwaukee, Wisconsin

Contributors

Arlina Ahluwalia, MD
Clinical Assistant Professor of Medicine
Stanford University School of Medicine
Clerkship Site Director
Palo Alto VAHCS
Palo Alto, California

Eyad Al-Hihi, MD, FACP
Associate Professor of Medicine
Clerkship Director, Ambulatory Medicine
Section Chief, Division of General Internal Medicine
Medical Director, Internal Medicine Clinics
Truman Medical Center-Hospital Hill
University of Missouri-Kansas City School of
    Medicine
Kansas City, Missouri

Erik K. Alexander, MD, FACP
Director, Medical Student Education
Brigham & Women's Hospital
Assistant Professor of Medicine
Harvard Medical School
Boston, Massachusetts

Irene Alexandraki, MD, FACP
Assistant Professor of Medicine
University of Florida College of Medicine
Jacksonville, Florida

Mark R. Allee, MD, FACP
Assistant Professor of Medicine
Department of Internal Medicine
University of Oklahoma College of Medicine
Oklahoma City, Oklahoma

Hugo A. Alvarez, MD, FACP
Associate Professor of Medicine
Sub-Internship Director
Clerkship Site Director, Department of Medicine
Rosalind Franklin University of Medicine and Science
Mount Sinai Hospital
Chicago, Illinois

Alpesh N. Amin, MD, MBA, FACP
Medicine Clerkship Director
Associate Program Director, IM Residency
University of California, Irvine
Irvine, California

Mary Jane Barchman, MD, FACP, FASN
Associate Professor of Medicine
Section of Nephrology and Hypertension
Director, Introduction to Medicine Course
Clerkship Director, Internal Medicine
Brody School of Medicine at East Carolina University
Greenville, North Carolina

Seth Mark Berney, MD, FACP
Professor of Medicine
Chief, Section of Rheumatology
Director, Center of Excellence for Arthritis and
    Rheumatology
Health Sciences Center
Louisiana State University School of Medicine
Shreveport, Louisiana

Cynthia A. Burns, MD
Assistant Professor
Clerkship Director, Inpatient Internal Medicine
Section of Endocrinology and Metabolism
Department of Internal Medicine
Wake Forest University School of Medicine
Winston-Salem, North Carolina

Amanda Cooper, MD
Assistant Professor of Medicine
University of Pittsburgh School of Medicine
University of Pittsburgh Medical Center
Pittsburgh, Pennsylvania

Nicole M. Cotter, MD
Fellow, Section of Rheumatology
Center of Excellence for Arthritis and Rheumatology
Health Sciences Center
Louisiana State University School of Medicine
Shreveport, Louisiana

Reed E. Drews, MD, FACP
Program Director
Hematology-Oncology Fellowship
Co-Director, Core Medicine 1 Clerkship
Beth Israel Deaconess Medical Center
Harvard Medical School
Boston, Massachusetts

Steven J. Durning, MD, FACP
Major, Medical Corps, US Air Force
Associate Professor of Medicine
Co-Director, Intro to Clinical Reasoning Course
Uniformed Services University of the Health Sciences
Bethesda, Maryland

Richard S. Eisenstaedt, MD, FACP
Chair, Department of Medicine
Abington Memorial Hospital
Professor of Medicine
Temple University School of Medicine
Philadelphia, Pennsylvania

J. Michael Finley, DO, FACP, FACOI
Associate Professor and Chair of Medicine
Department of Medicine
Western University College of Osteopathic Medicine
Pomona, California

Janine M. Frank, MD
Assistant Professor of Medicine
University of Pittsburgh Medical Center
University of Pittsburgh School of Medicine
Pittsburgh, Pennsylvania

Jane P. Gagliardi, MD
Assistant Clinical Professor
Department of Internal Medicine
Department of Psychiatry and Behavioral Sciences
Duke University School of Medicine
Durham, North Carolina

Peter Gliatto, MD
Assistant Professor of Medicine
Director, Medical Clerkships
Mount Sinai School of Medicine
New York, New York

Eric H. Green, MD, MSc
Course Director, Patients, Doctors, and Communities
Assistant Professor of Medicine
Montefiore Medical Center
Albert Einstein College of Medicine
Bronx, New York

Mark C. Haigney, MD
Professor of Medicine
Director of Cardiology
Uniformed Services University of the Health Sciences
Bethesda, Maryland

Charin L. Hanlon, MD, FACP
Assistant Professor of Internal Medicine
Clerkship Director, Internal Medicine
West Virginia University-Charleston Division
Charleston, West Virginia

Warren Y. Hershman, MD
Director of Student Education
Department of Medicine
Boston University School of Medicine
Boston, Massachusetts

Mark D. Holden, MD, FACP
Eagle's Trace Medical Director
Erickson Retirement Communities
Houston, Texas

Ivonne Z. Jiménez-Velázquez, MD, FACP
Professor and Vice-Chair for Education
Geriatrics Program Director
Clerkship Director, Internal Medicine Department
University of Puerto Rico School of Medicine
San Juan, Puerto Rico

Lawrence I. Kaplan, MD, FACP
Professor of Medicine
Section Chief, General Internal Medicine
Internal Medicine Clerkship Director
Temple University School of Medicine
Philadelphia, Pennsylvania

Asra R. Khan, MD
Assistant Professor of Clinical Medicine
Associate Program Director, Internal Medicine
    Residency
Medicine Clerkship Director
University of Illinois College of Medicine
Chicago, Illinois

Sarang Kim, MD
Assistant Professor of Medicine
Division of General Internal Medicine
University of Medicine and Dentistry of New Jersey
Robert Wood Johnson Medical School
New Brunswick, New Jersey

Christopher A. Klipstein, MD
Clerkship Director of Internal Medicine
Associate Professor
Department of Medicine
University of North Carolina School of Medicine
Chapel Hill, North Carolina

Cynthia H. Ledford, MD
Clerkship Director of Internal Medicine
Ohio State University College of Medicine
Columbus, Ohio

Bruce Leff, MD, FACP
Associate Professor of Medicine
Medicine Clerkship Director
Johns Hopkins University School of Medicine
Baltimore, Maryland

Fred A. Lopez, MD, FACP
Associate Professor and Vice Chair
Department of Medicine
Louisiana State University Health Sciences Center
Assistant Dean for Student Affairs
LSU School of Medicine
New Orleans, Louisiana

Anna C. Maio, MD, FACP
Division Chief and Associate Professor
Division of General Internal Medicine
Department of Internal Medicine
Creighton University School of Medicine
Omaha, Nebraska

Brown J. McCallum, MD, FACP
Assistant Professor
Co-Clerkship Director
Department of Internal Medicine
University of South Carolina School of Medicine
Columbia, South Carolina

Kevin M. McKown, MD, FACP
Associate Professor of Medicine
Co-Chief, Section of Rheumatology
Program Director, Rheumatology Fellowship
Co-Clerkship Director
Department of Medicine
University of Wisconsin School of Medicine and
    Public Health
Madison, Wisconsin

Melissa A. McNeil, MD, MPH
Professor of Medicine and Obstetrics, Gynecology &
    Reproductive Sciences
Chief, Section of Women's Health
Division of General Medicine
University of Pittsburgh
Pittsburgh, Pennsylvania

Janet N. Myers, MD, FACP, FCCP
Associate Professor of Medicine
Deputy Clerkship Director, Department of Medicine
Uniformed Services University of the Health Sciences
Bethesda, Maryland

Kathryn A. Naus, MD
Chief Fellow, Section of Rheumatology
Center of Excellence for Arthritis and Rheumatology
Health Sciences Center
Louisiana State University School of Medicine
Shreveport, Louisiana

Robert W. Neilson Jr., MD
Assistant Professor
Clerkship Director
Department of Internal Medicine
Division of General Internal Medicine
Texas Tech University Health Sciences Center
Lubbock, Texas

Katherine Nickerson, MD
Vice Chair
Department of Medicine
Associate Professor of Clinical Medicine
Clerkship Director
Columbia University, P & S
New York, New York

L. James Nixon, MD
Clerkship Director
Division of General Internal Medicine
University of Minnesota Medical School
University of Minnesota Medical Center, Fairview
Minneapolis, Minnesota

Carlos Palacio, MD, MPH, FACP
Clerkship Director
Assistant Professor of Medicine
University of Florida College of Medicine
Jacksonville, Florida

Hanah Polotsky, MD
Assistant Professor of Medicine
Clerkship Director
Montefiore Medical Center
Albert Einstein College of Medicine
Bronx, New York

Nora L. Porter, MD
Co-Director, Internal Medicine Clerkship
St. Louis University School of Medicine
St. Louis, Missouri

Priya Radhakrishnan, MD
Clinical Assistant Professor
University of Arizona College of Medicine
Clerkship Director and Associate Program Director
Department of Internal Medicine
St. Joseph Hospital & Medical Center
Phoenix, Arizona

Joseph Rencic, MD, FACP
Assistant Professor of Medicine
Clerkship Site Director, Associate Program Director
Department of Internal Medicine
Tufts-New England Medical Center
Boston, Massachusetts

Kathleen F. Ryan, MD
Associate Professor of Medicine
Clerkship Director
Division of General Internal Medicine
Department of Internal Medicine
Drexel University College of Medicine
Philadelphia, Pennsylvania

Brijen J. Shah, MD
Chief Medical Resident, Department of Medicine
Beth Israel Deaconess Medical Center
Harvard Medical School
Boston, Massachusetts

Patricia Short, MD
Major, Medical Corps, US Army
Associate Professor and Associate Clerkship Director
Department of Medicine
Uniformed Services University of the Health Sciences
Bethesda, Maryland
Madigan Army Medical Center
Tacoma, Washington

Diane C. Sliwka, MD
Instructor of Medicine
Beth Israel Deaconess Medical Center
Harvard Medical School
Boston, Massachusetts

Harold M. Szerlip, MD, FACP, FCCP
Professor and Vice-Chairman
Department of Medicine
Medical College of Georgia
Augusta, Georgia

Gary Tabas, MD, FACP
Associate Professor of Medicine
University of Pittsburgh School of Medicine
Pittsburgh, Pennsylvania

Tomoko Tanabe, MD, FACP
Assistant Professor of Medicine
Associate Clerkship Director
University of California, San Diego
San Diego, California

David C. Tompkins, MD
Associate Chair
Department of Medicine
SUNY Stony Brook Health Sciences Center
Stony Brook, New York

Dario M. Torre, MD, MPH, FACP
Clerkship Director
Department of Medicine
Medical College of Wisconsin
Milwaukee, Wisconsin

Mark M. Udden, MD, FACP
Professor of Medicine
Department of Internal Medicine
Baylor College of Medicine
Houston, Texas

H. Douglas Walden, MD, MPH, FACP
Co-Director, Internal Medicine Clerkship
St. Louis University School of Medicine
St. Louis, Missouri

Joseph T. Wayne, MD, MPH, FACP
Associate Professor of Medicine
Associate Professor of Pediatrics
Clerkship Director, Internal Medicine
Albany Medical College
Albany, New York

John Jason White, MD
Assistant Professor of Medicine
Nephrology Section
Department of Medicine
Medical College of Georgia
Augusta, Georgia

Kevin D. Whittle, MD
Assistant Professor
Third Year Clerkship Director, Internal Medicine
Sanford Medical School of the University of South
    Dakota
Sioux Falls, South Dakota

Contents

V   Hematology

VI   Infectious Disease Medicine

VII   Nephrology

VIII   Neurology

IX   Oncology

X   Pulmonary Medicine

XI   Rheumatology

Foreword

Internal Medicine Essentials for Clerkship Students is a collaborative project of the American College of Physicians (ACP) and the Clerkship Directors in Internal Medicine (CDIM), the organization of individuals responsible for teaching internal medicine to medical students. The purpose of IM Essentials is to provide medical students with an authoritative educational resource that can be used to augment learning during the third year internal medicine clerkship. Much of the content is based upon two evidence-based resources of ACP: the Medical Knowledge Self-Assessment Program (MKSAP) and the Physician Information and Education Resource (PIER); other sources include recently published practice guidelines and review articles. IM Essentials is updated every two years with the best available evidence and is designed to be read cover-to-cover during the clerkship.

Based upon student feedback, IM Essentials 2 contains twice as many color plates and algorithms as its predecessor and more than 100 extra tables to enhance learning (and passing tests!). An index now provides fuller subject access. The most exciting addition is the Book Enhancement section found at the end of each chapter. This section directs the reader to a book-related Web site that contains nearly 500 links to additional tables, algorithms, color plates, and patient care tools. The Book Enhancement section also identifies specific chapter-related self-assessment questions published in a separate companion book, MKSAP for Students 4.

MKSAP for Students 4 consists of a printed and electronic collection of patient-centered self-assessment questions and answers. The questions begin with a clinical vignette, just as in the medicine clerkship examination and the USMLE Step 2 licensing examination. The questions are organized into eleven sections that match the eleven sections found in IM Essentials. Each of the more than 450 questions has been specifically edited by a group of clerkship directors to meet the learning needs of students participating in the medicine clerkship. Each question comes with an answer critique that supplies the correct answer, an explanation of why that answer is correct and the incorrect options are not, and a short bibliography. We recommend that students first read the appropriate chapter in IM Essentials, then assess their understanding by answering the designated questions in MKSAP for Students 4.

The content of IM Essentials is based upon The Core Medicine Clerkship Curriculum Guide (available at www.im.org/CDIM), a nationally recognized curriculum for the required third-year internal medicine clerkship, created and published by the CDIM and the Society for General Internal Medicine. A collaboration of 66 authors, all of whom are either internal medicine clerkship directors or clerkship faculty, representing 45 different medical schools, IM Essentials 2 is unique in that it is created by faculty who helped design the internal medicine curriculum and who are actively involved in teaching and advising students on the internal medicine clerkship.

*   *   *   *   *

Founded in 1915, the American College of Physicians is the nation's largest medical specialty society. Its mission is to enhance the quality and effectiveness of health care by fostering excellence and professionalism in the practice of medicine. ACP's 124,000 members include allied health professionals, medical students, medical residents, and practicing physicians. Physician members practice general internal medicine and related subspecialties, including cardiology, gastroenterology, nephrology, endocrinology, hematology, rheumatology, neurology, pulmonary disease, oncology, infectious diseases, allergy and immunology, and geriatrics.

The Clerkship Directors in Internal Medicine is the national organization of individuals responsible for teaching internal medicine to medical students. Founded in 1989, CDIM promotes excellence in the education of medical students in internal medicine. CDIM serves internal medicine faculty and staff by: providing a forum to share ideas, generate solutions to common problems, and create opportunities for career development; participating in the development and dissemination of innovations for curriculum, evaluation, and faculty development; encouraging research and collaborative initiatives among medical educators; and advocating for issues concerning undergraduate medical education.

*　　　*　　　*　　　*　　　*

Publication of *Internal Medicine Essentials for Clerkship Students 2* would not have been possible without the invaluable and entirely voluntary contributions of many individuals, only some of whom are listed in the Acknowledgments. Others, not specifically named, were representatives from a wide spectrum of constituencies and organizations such as the Executive and Educational Committees of the Clerkship Directors in Internal Medicine and the Education Committee and the Council of Student Members of the American College of Physicians.

Patrick C. Alguire, MD, FACP
Editor-in-Chief

Acknowledgments

The American College of Physicians and the Clerkship Directors in Internal Medicine gratefully acknowledge the special contributions to Internal Medicine Essentials for Clerkship Students 2 of Nicole V. Baptista, CDIM Policy Coordinator, Clerkship Directors in Internal Medicine; Sheila T. Costa, Director of Meetings and Communications, Clerkship Directors in Internal Medicine; Rosemarie Houton, Administrative Representative, American College of Physicians; Lisa Rockey, Education and Career Development Coordinator, American College of Physicians; and Helen Kitzmiller, Patient Education Project Administrator, American College of Physicians. We also thank the many others, too numerous to mention, who have contributed to this project. Without the dedicated efforts of them all, publication of this volume would not have been possible.

Section I
Cardiovascular Medicine

Chapter 1

Approach to Chest Pain

Dario M. Torre, MD

Chest pain is one of the most common complaints in internal medicine. In outpatients, the most common cause is musculoskeletal chest pain; in emergency settings, approximately 50% of patients have acute coronary syndrome (i.e., myocardial infarction or unstable angina). Differential diagnosis of chest pain can be approached as cardiac, pulmonary, gastrointestinal, musculoskeletal, and psychiatric causes (Table 1).

Cardiac Causes

Acute coronary syndrome is an important cause of chest pain. Ischemic chest pain classically presents as substernal pressure, tightness, or heaviness with radiation to the jaw, shoulders, back, or arms. The pain is typically related to exertion and relieved by rest or nitroglycerin, and may be accompanied by dyspnea, diaphoresis, and nausea. Recent onset or increasing symptoms of chest discomfort occurring at rest without elevation of biomarkers (e.g., creatine kinase and troponin) is consistent with unstable angina. Patients with diabetes, women, or the elderly may present with atypical symptoms, such as dyspnea without chest pain. Ischemic chest pain typically lasts <20 minutes; pain of longer duration suggests myocardial infarction or an alternative diagnosis. The most powerful clinical features that increase the probability of myocardial infarction include chest pain that simultaneously radiates to

both arms (positive likelihood ratio = 7.1), an S_3 (positive likelihood ratio = 3.2), and hypotension (positive likelihood ratio = 3.1). In contrast, a normal electrocardiogram result (negative likelihood ratio = 0.1-0.3), chest pain that is positional (negative likelihood ratio = 0.3), chest pain reproduced by palpation (negative likelihood ratio = 0.2-0.4), or chest pain that is sharp or stabbing (negative likelihood ratio = 0.3) makes ischemic etiology less likely. Patients suspected of having acute coronary syndrome are hospitalized and evaluated with serial electrocardiograms and cardiac biomarkers, chest x-ray, and often echo- cardiography (Table 2). Low-risk patients without evidence of myocardial infarction are evaluated with an exercise or pharmacologic stress test.

Coronary artery vasospasm (Prinzmetal's angina) classically presents as rest pain, similar to angina, and may be associated with ST-segment elevation on the resting electrocardiogram. Cocaine use can cause chest pain and ST segment changes due to ischemia or secondary to vasospasm without evidence of direct myocardial injury.

Acute pericarditis (viral or bacterial) may be preceded or accompanied by symptoms of an upper respiratory tract infection and fever. Pericarditis is characterized by sudden onset of sharp, stabbing substernal chest pain with radiation along the trapezius ridge; the pain is often worse with inspiration and lying flat, and is frequently alleviated with sitting and leaning forward. A pericardial

Table 1. Differential Diagnosis of Chest Pain

Disease	Notes
Acute coronary syndrome (see Chapter 3)	Chest pain, nausea, or dyspnea. Associated with specific ECG and echocardiographic changes. Cardiac enzymes help establish diagnosis of myocardial infarction.
Aortic dissection	Substernal chest pain with radiation to the back, mid-scapular region. Often described as "tearing" or "ripping" type pain. Chest x-ray may show a widened mediastinal silhouette, a pleural effusion, or both.
Aortic stenosis (see Chapter 7)	Chest pain with exertion, heart failure, syncope. Typical systolic murmur at the base of the heart radiating to the neck.
Esophagitis (see Chapter 17)	Burning-type chest discomfort, usually precipitated by meals, and not related to exertion. Often worse lying down, improved with sitting.
Musculoskeletal pain	Typically more reproducible chest pain. Includes muscle strain, costochondritis, and fracture. Should be a diagnosis of exclusion.
Panic attack	May be indistinguishable from angina. Often diagnosed after a negative evaluation for ischemic heart disease. Often associated with palpitations, sweating, and anxiety.
Pericarditis	Substernal chest discomfort that can be sharp, dull, or pressure-like in nature, often relieved with sitting forward. Usually pleuritic. ECG changes may include ST-segment elevation (usually diffuse) or more specifically (but less common) PR segment depression.
Pneumothorax (see Chapter 74)	Sudden onset of pleuritic chest pain and dyspnea. Chest x-ray or CT confirms the diagnosis.
Pulmonary embolism (see Chapter 80)	Commonly presents with dyspnea. Pleuritic chest pain is present in approximately 30% of patients. Look for risk factors (immobilization, recent surgery, stroke, cancer, previous VTE disease).

CT = computed tomography; ECG = electrocardiography; VTE = venous thromboembolism.

Table 2. Laboratory and Other Studies for Chest Pain

Test	Notes
Electrocardiogram	More than 50% of patients with CAD have normal resting ECGs. The presence of pathologic Q waves or ST-T wave abnormalities consistent with ischemia increases the likelihood of CAD. Approximately 50% of patients with CAD will have some abnormality on an ECG obtained during an episode of chest pain. ST elevations and other abnormalities are present in approximately 90% of patients with pericarditis. Abnormalities are present in 70% of patients with pulmonary embolism. Most common abnormalities are nonspecific ST segment and T wave changes. P pulmonale, right axis deviation, right bundle branch block, and right ventricular hypertrophy occur less frequently.
Arterial blood gasses	Distributions of PaO_2 and alveolar-arterial oxygen gradient are similar in patients with and without pulmonary embolism.
Chest radiograph	There are no randomized controlled studies in which any symptom or diagnosis is evaluated with a control arm of no chest x-ray to truly evaluate its clinical significance. Will make diagnosis of pneumothorax, and widened mediastinum may suggest aortic dissection.
Cardiac enzymes	Creatine phosphokinase, MB isoenzyme of creatine phosphokinase, and cardiac troponin I are obtained as indicated by clinical history with elevations signifying active myocardial ischemia or injury.
Echocardiography	Improves diagnostic accuracy in patients with chest discomfort when diagnosis is uncertain. May help differentiate ACS and aortic dissection. Transthoracic or transesophageal echocardiography may rarely identify central pulmonary artery emboli or intracardiac thrombi. Echocardiography can detect very small pericardial effusions that may help with the diagnosis of pericarditis.
Exercise ECG	For patients considered low-risk for an ACS (i.e., atypical chest pain, normal cardiac markers, normal ECG), can be used as an early, rapid diagnostic tool for CAD.
D-dimer (ELISA)	Helpful to exclude PE in patients with low pretest clinical probability or nondiagnostic lung scan.
Contrast enhanced spiral CT scan	Often preferred test for PE. An advantage of CT is the diagnosis of other pulmonary parenchymal, pleural, or cardiovascular processes causing or contributing to symptoms (dissection, aneurysms, malignancy).

ACS = acute coronary syndrome; CAD = coronary artery disease; ELISA = enzyme-linked immunosorbent assay; PE = pulmonary embolism.

friction rub is present in 85%-100% of cases at some time during its course. The classic rub consists of three components: atrial systole, ventricular systole, and diastole. A confirmatory electrocardiogram will show diffuse ST-segment elevation and PR-segment depression, findings that are specific but not sensitive (Figure 1). An echocardiogram may be helpful if there is suspicion of significant pericardial effusion or pericardial tamponade.

Patients with dissection of the thoracic aorta typically present with abrupt onset of severe, sharp, or "tearing" chest pain often radiating to the abdomen, or back pain. Aortic dissection can be associated with syncope due to decreased cardiac output, stroke, and myocardial infarction caused by carotid and coronary artery occlusion/dissection, cardiac tamponade, and sudden death due to rupture of the aorta. Hypertension is present in 50% of patients and is not helpful diagnostically. A pulse differential (diminished pulse compared with contralateral side) on palpation of the carotid, radial, or femoral arteries is one of the most useful findings (sensitivity = 30%; positive likelihood ratio = 5.7). An early diastolic murmur due to acute aortic insufficiency may be heard, particularly if the dissection involves the ascending aorta, but the presence or absence of a diastolic murmur is not useful in ruling in or ruling out dissection. Focal deficits on neurological exam can be present in a minority of patients but are highly suggestive in the proper clinical context (positive likelihood ratio = 6.6-33).

A wide mediastinum on a chest radiograph is the most common initial finding (sensitivity = 85%) and the absence of this finding helps rule out dissection (negative likelihood ratio = 0.3). When aortic dissection is suspected, imaging the aorta is indicated. Computed tomography of the chest, MRI, transesophageal echocardiography, and aortic root angiography all have a high sensitivity and specificity for detection of a dissection flap; the specific diagnostic modality chosen depends on the rapidity with which the examination can be performed and the stability of the patient.

Aortic stenosis is a cause of exertional chest pain and may be also accompanied by dyspnea, palpitations, and exertional syncope due to a diminished cardiac output. Physical examination reveals a systolic, crescendo-decrescendo murmur best heard at the second right intercostal space with radiation to the carotids. A transthoracic echocardiogram is the diagnostic test of choice for suspected aortic stenosis.

Syndrome X is a cause of angina-like chest pain in young women. It is characterized by anginal symptoms, ST-segment depression on exercise testing, and normal coronary arteries on angiography. The etiology of the pain is unknown, but there is a strong correlation with psychiatric disorders.

Pulmonary Causes

Pulmonary embolism may present with acute pleuritic chest pain, dyspnea, and, less often, cough and hemoptysis. The presence of risk factors for pulmonary embolism such as recent surgery, immobilization, history of previous venous thromboembolism and malignancy may suggest the diagnosis. Physical examination findings are nonspecific but may include tachycardia, tachypnea, and wheezing; a right-sided S_3 and a right ventricular heave may be present if there is acute right heart failure secondary to pulmonary hypertension.

Pleuritic chest pain can also be a manifestation of pneumonia and often is associated with fever, chills, cough, purulent sputum, and dyspnea. The physical examination may show wheezing or crackles and signs of consolidation such as dullness to percussion, egophony, and bronchophony.

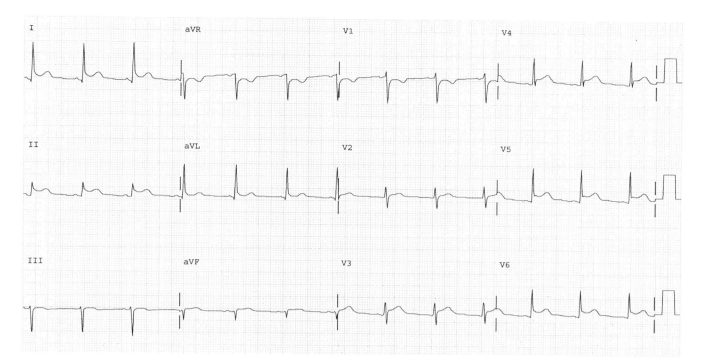

Figure 1 Electrocardiogram showing sinus rhythm with diffuse ST-segment elevation consistent with acute pericarditis. Note also the PR-segment depression in leads I, II, and V_4-V_6.

Pneumothorax should be considered in any patient with sudden onset of pleuritic chest pain and dyspnea. The physical examination may show decreased breath sounds on the affected side; if a tension pneumothorax is present, hypotension and tracheal deviation to the opposite side of the pneumothorax can be seen.

Pulmonary causes of chest pain are initially evaluated with a chest x-ray. In patients with dyspnea, pulse oximetry or an arterial blood gas analysis is indicated. In the setting of moderate to high suspicion for pulmonary embolism, a helical CT scan of the chest or a ventilation/perfusion lung scan with or without duplex Doppler examination of lower extremities is an appropriate initial approach. A negative D-dimer helps exclude the diagnosis of pulmonary embolism and is most helpful when the clinical suspicion is low.

Gastrointestinal Causes

Gastroesophageal reflux disease can mimic ischemic chest pain. Important distinctions include pain lasting minutes to hours and resolving either spontaneously or with antacids. Discomfort associated with reflux is often positional, worse when lying down and after meals, or awakens patients from sleep. Other symptoms may include heartburn, regurgitation, chronic cough, sore throat, and hoarseness. On physical examination, patients may exhibit wheezing, halitosis, dental erosions, and pharyngeal erythema. In unclear cases it is most appropriate to exclude cardiac causes of chest pain before evaluating gastrointestinal etiologies. For patients with a high probability of gastroesophageal reflux disease, empiric treatment with a proton pump inhibitor for 4 to 6 weeks is an appropriate initial diagnostic and therapeutic approach.

Musculoskeletal Causes

Musculoskeletal causes of chest pain are more common in women than men; common causes include costochondritis, arthritis, and fibromyalgia. Musculoskeletal chest pain has an insidious onset and may last for hours to weeks. It is most recognizable when sharp and localized to a specific area of the chest; however, it can also be poorly localized. The pain may be worsened by turning, deep breathing, or arm movement. Chest pain may or may not be reproducible by chest palpation (pain reproduced by palpation does not exclude ischemic heart disease), and the cardiovascular exam is often normal. The presence of tender points in the upper chest increases the likelihood of fibromyalgia. For musculoskeletal chest pain, the history and physical examination are keys to the diagnosis; selected x-rays and laboratory tests may be indicated depending upon the clinical circumstances.

Psychiatric Causes

Chest pain can also be a manifestation of severe anxiety and panic attack. Patients may complain of sweating, trembling, or shaking, sensations of choking, shortness of breath or smothering, nausea or abdominal distress, or feeling dizzy, unsteady, or lightheaded. On physical examination, tachycardia and tachypnea may be present, but the remainder of the cardiovascular and pulmonary exam is unremarkable. Psychosomatic chest pain is a clinical diagnosis; other causes of chest pain are usually excluded by careful history and physical examination.

Book Enhancement

Go to www.acponline.org/essentials/cardiovascular-section.html to estimate the pretest probability of coronary artery disease, access an electrocardiogram interpretation tutorial, and see examples of mediastinal widening, pneumothorax, and the ECG manifestations of an acute myocardial infarction. In *MKSAP for Students 4*, assess yourself with items 7-9 in the **Cardiovascular Medicine** section.

Bibliography

American College of Physicians. Medical Knowledge Self-Assessment Program 14. Philadelphia: American College of Physicians; 2006.

Klompas M. Does this patient have an acute thoracic aortic dissection? JAMA. 2002;287:2262-72. [PMID: 11980527]

Lee TH, Goldman L. Evaluation of the patient with acute chest pain. N Engl J Med. 2000;342:1187-95. [PMID: 10770985]

Panju AA, Hemmelgarn BR, Guyatt GH, Simel DL. The rational clinical examination. Is this patient having a myocardial infarction? JAMA. 1998;280:1256-63. [PMID: 9786377]

Chapter 2

Chronic Stable Angina

Anna C. Maio, MD

Angina pectoris means "strangling or suffocation in the chest." Ischemic conditions that provoke angina do so by increasing myocardial oxygen demand, decreasing myocardial oxygen supply, or both. Myocardial oxygen demand is determined by the heart rate, systolic blood pressure (afterload), myocardial contractility, and left ventricular wall stress which is proportional to left ventricular end-diastolic volume (preload) and myocardial mass. Myocardial oxygen supply is dependent upon coronary blood flow and perfusion pressure. The subendocardium, at greatest risk for ischemia, receives most of its blood supply during diastole; tachycardia, which shortens diastole, may cause ischemia. Some patients report dyspnea on exertion as a manifestation of ischemia. This is known as an anginal equivalent and is difficult to differentiate from heart failure or pulmonary disease. The pathogenesis is an elevated left ventricular filling pressure induced by ischemia that leads to vascular congestion. Angina also may be present in the absence of coronary artery obstruction. Some of these patients have coronary vasospasm, and some have increased left ventricular mass (hypertrophy) due to aortic stenosis, hypertrophic cardiomyopathy, or systemic arterial hypertension.

Prevention

Identify and modify cardiovascular risk factors, focusing efforts on patients at highest risk. Encourage smoking cessation in all patients who smoke. Assess all adults ≥20 years old periodically for dyslipidemia. Measure blood pressure at each office visit to identify and treat hypertension. Risk factors for coronary artery disease need to be treated particularly aggressively in persons with diabetes because strict blood pressure and lipid control appears to provide additional benefits to patients with diabetes above those seen in the general population. The Framingham risk score allows estimation of the 10-year risk of coronary artery disease using age, gender, and other risk factors (see Book Enhancement section).

Stop hormone replacement therapy in women when prescribed solely for cardioprotection. Consider primary prevention with aspirin (75-325 mg) in asymptomatic patients with multiple risk factors, or with diabetes, barring contraindication. Encourage all patients to engage in regular physical activity, such as brisk walking for 30 minutes or more, 5 to 7 times per week. Advise all patients to limit cholesterol and fat, particularly saturated fats, and refined sugars in their diets; recommend a diet rich in fruits, vegetables, fiber, and whole grains. Do not recommend antioxidant vitamins for risk reduction. Inadequate data exist to recommend testing or treating homocysteine and/or lipoprotein (a).

Screening

Do not routinely screen for coronary artery disease in asymptomatic persons without cardiovascular risk factors. Although exercise testing may identify persons with coronary artery disease, two factors limit the utility of routine stress testing in asymptomatic adults: false-positive results are common, and abnormalities of exercise testing do not accurately predict major cardiac events. Electron-beam CT is an evolving technology. In 2007, the American College of Cardiology concluded that it may be reasonable to use electron-beam CT in patients with an estimated 10%-20% 10-year risk of coronary events based on the possibility that such patients might be reclassified to a higher risk status and offered more aggressive risk management interventions.

Diagnosis

The type of chest pain (typical angina, atypical angina, or noncardiac chest pain) and presence of cardiac risk factors (age, gender, smoking history, hyperlipidemia, diabetes mellitus, hypertension, physical inactivity, and family history) allows estimation of the pretest probability for coronary artery disease. Exercise treadmill tests or other noninvasive tests provide the most diagnostic information about persons with intermediate probability of coronary artery disease (e.g., 20%-80%). Physical examination findings suggesting peripheral vascular or cerebrovascular disease increase the likelihood of coronary artery disease. Look for conditions that increase myocardial oxygen demand (e.g., aortic stenosis, hypertrophic cardiomyopathy, uncontrolled hypertension, tachyarrhythmias, hyperthyroidism, cocaine use), diminish tissue oxygenation (anemia and hypoxemia), or cause hyperviscosity (polycythemia or hypergammaglobulinemia) that may precipitate angina in the setting of nonsignificant coronary artery disease. Obtain a complete blood count, thyroid-stimulating hormone, or a drug screen as indicated by the clinical situation.

Obtain a resting electrocardiogram in all patients without an obvious noncardiac cause of chest pain. Obtain a chest x-ray in all patients with signs or symptoms of heart failure, valvular heart disease, pericardial disease, aortic dissection, or aneurysm.

Standard echocardiography is obtained in patients with possible valvular disease, signs or symptoms of heart failure, or history of myocardial infarction. In patients with stable angina, reduced left ventricular function is associated with a worse prognosis.

Patients who are able to exercise for 6 to 12 minutes and do not have baseline resting electrocardiogram abnormalities are evaluated with exercise electrocardiography (Table 1). Exercise electrocardiography has a sensitivity of 40% and a specificity of 96% when diagnosing coronary artery disease in men. Myocardial perfusion imaging or stress echocardiography is preferred in settings where exercise electrocardiography alone is difficult to interpret (e.g., baseline electrocardiographic abnormalities). Pharmacologic stress tests are preferred in patients who cannot exercise.

Patients with coronary artery disease may be categorized according to short-term risk of cardiac death and nonfatal myocardial infarction on the basis of clinical parameters and the results of noninvasive functional testing. Patients with low-risk exercise treadmill results have an estimated cardiac mortality rate of <1% annually and do not require further risk stratification. Patients with high-risk exercise treadmill results have an estimated cardiac mortality rate of ≥3% annually and are referred for coronary angiography and possible revascularization. Patients with intermediate exercise treadmill results are stratified into low-risk (appropriate for medical management) and high-risk (consider revascularization) groups.

Refer patients for coronary angiography who have an uncertain diagnosis after noninvasive testing or probable high-risk coronary artery disease. Coronary angiography is also recommended in patients with suspected left main or three-vessel disease, survivors of sudden cardiac death, those with probable coronary artery spasm, and those with an occupational requirement for diagnosis, such as pilots. In patients with a high pretest probability of severe coronary artery disease (e.g., abnormalities on the resting electrocardiogram associated with chest pain), direct referral for coronary angiography is more cost-effective than an initial noninvasive study followed by coronary angiography.

Always consider potentially life-threatening causes of chest pain, such as myocardial ischemia, pericardial tamponade, aortic dissection, pulmonary embolism, and pneumothorax (Table 2). Although chest pain may have a benign cause, initially exclude a life-threatening cause.

Table 1. Choice of Diagnostic Stress Test

Exercise ECG without imaging	Obtain in patients with an intermediate probability of CAD who are able to exercise, including patients with <1 mm ST depression or complete right bundle-branch block on a resting ECG. Left ventricular hypertrophy with repolarization abnormality on the resting ECG reduces the specificity of exercise treadmill testing.
Exercise ECG with myocardial perfusion imaging or exercise echocardiography	Obtain in patients with an intermediate probability of CAD and who are able to exercise and have one of the following ECG abnormalities: pre-excitation (Wolff-Parkinson-White) syndrome or >1 mm ST depression. Also appropriate in patients with an intermediate pretest probability of CAD and a history of previous revascularization (PTCA or CABG). Exercise echocardiography is an acceptable choice in patients with left bundle-branch block on resting ECG. Stress imaging is recommended to further stratify patients with intermediate-risk exercise treadmill tests.
Pharmacologic stress myocardial perfusion imaging or dobutamine echocardiography	Obtain in patients with an intermediate pretest probability of CAD and an electronically paced ventricular rhythm or left bundle-branch block. Also appropriate in patients with an intermediate pretest probability of CAD who are unable to exercise.

CABG = coronary artery bypass grafting; CAD = coronary artery disease; ECG = electrocardiography; PTCA = percutaneous transluminal coronary angiography.

Table 2. Differential Diagnosis of Angina

Test	Notes
Acute coronary syndrome (see Chapter 3)	Associated with specific echocardiographic and electrocardiographic changes. Cardiac enzymes help establish diagnosis of myocardial infarction.
Anxiety disorders	May be indistinguishable from angina; often associated with palpitations, sweating, and anxiety. Often diagnosed after a negative evaluation for ischemic heart disease
Aortic dissection (see Chapter 1)	Classically described as a tearing pain of abrupt onset that may radiate to the back. Blood pressure measured in both arms may show differences >10 mm Hg. Chest x-ray may show a widened mediastinum or abnormal aortic contour in approximately 80% of patients.
Arrhythmias (see Chapter 4)	May cause typical angina related to increased myocardial oxygen demand and/or diminished diastolic filling of the coronary arteries.
Chest wall (see Chapter 1)	Characteristically reproduced with palpation or movement. Reproduction with palpation does not exclude angina.
Esophageal (see Chapter 17)	May be indistinguishable from angina. Often diagnosed after a negative work-up for ischemic heart disease. Response to empiric proton pump inhibitor helps establish diagnosis.
Pericarditis (see Chapter 1)	Pain is often pleuritic but may resemble angina. Classically relieved by sitting up and leaning forward. May be associated with a friction rub on auscultation and diffuse ST-segment elevation on electrocardiogram (or PR-segment depression).
Pulmonary embolus (see Chapter 80)	Pain is often sharp and pleuritic and associated with dyspnea. Syncope, hypotension, elevated neck veins, and characteristic findings on electrocardiogram are more commonly seen with large, central pulmonary emboli.
Valvular heart disease (see Chapter 7)	May cause typical angina related to left ventricular outflow obstruction and increased myocardial wall stress. Auscultation typically shows a long, late-peaking systolic murmur at the base of the heart. Aortic stenosis commonly radiates to the carotids and is associated with a weak and delayed carotid upstroke. Murmurs of hypertrophic cardiomyopathy (with outlet obstruction) increase with the Valsalva maneuver.

Table 3. Drug Treatment for Chronic Stable Angina

Agent	Notes
β-blockers	Inhibition of β-adrenergic receptors. Reduce heart rate, contractility, and arterial pressure, resulting in diminished myocardial oxygen demand. First-line agent in patients with stable angina. All β-blockers appear equally effective in treating angina.
Dihydropyridine calcium channel blockers	Inhibits vascular smooth muscle and myocardial voltage-gated calcium channels. Reduction of blood pressure. Second-line agent for stable angina. Use in addition to β-blockers if symptoms persist, or instead of β-blockers if unacceptable side effects supervene. Avoid short-acting nifedipine.
Non-dihydropyridine calcium channel blockers	Inhibits vascular smooth muscle and myocardial voltage-gated calcium channels. Reduction of blood pressure. Negative chronotropy and inotropy reduce myocardial oxygen demand. Second-line agent for stable angina. Use in addition to β-blockers if symptoms persist, or instead of β-blockers if unacceptable side effects supervene.
Angiotensin-converting enzyme inhibitors	ACE inhibition results in reduced levels of angiotensin II and reduced degradation of bradykinin. Reduction of blood pressure and afterload by reduction in angiotensin II levels. Reduction of ventricular remodeling and fibrosis after infarction. Improved long-term survival in patients with LVEF ≤ 40% and in patients with high cardiovascular risk. Improved short-term survival in subsets of patients with acute MI.
Long-acting nitrates	Nitrates are metabolized to nitric oxide, resulting in vasodilation (reduces preload and dilates coronary arteries). Third-line agent for stable angina. Use in addition to β-blockers and/or calcium-channel blockers if symptoms persist, or instead of β-blockers and/or calcium-channel blockers if unacceptable side effects supervene. Tachyphylaxis with continued use; requires 8-12 hr nitrate-free period.
Short-acting nitrates	Dilates coronary arteries and reduces preload. Should be given to all patients with chronic stable angina for use on an as needed basis.
Piperazine derivative (ranolazine)	Mechanism of action is unknown. Indicated for patients not responding to standard therapy; used in combination with a nitrate, β-blocker, or calcium-channel blocker.
Aspirin	Antithrombotic effect by inhibiting cyclooxygenase and synthesis of platelet thromboxane A_2. Treat all patients with stable angina barring contraindication; reduces major cardiovascular events by 33%.
Thienopyridine derivatives	Antithrombotic effect by inhibiting ADP-dependent platelet aggregation. Clopidogrel is a reasonable alternative to aspirin, although significantly more expensive. Among high-risk subjects, clopidogrel results in a greater reduction in the risk for major cardiovascular events than aspirin, although the incremental benefit is small. Ticlopidine has not been shown to reduce coronary events.
HMG-CoA reductase inhibitors	Inhibition of the commitment step in the synthesis of LDL cholesterol. In mild-moderate elevations in total and LDL cholesterol, and a history of MI, statins are associated with a 24% risk reduction for fatal and nonfatal MI.

ACE = angiotensin-converting enzyme; ADP = adenosine diphosphate; CAD = coronary artery disease; LDL = low-density lipoprotein; LVEF = left ventricular ejection fraction; MI = myocardial infarction.

Therapy

Encourage patients with chronic stable angina to stop smoking and incorporate regular aerobic exercise and dietary modification into their lifestyle.

Drug therapy for chronic stable angina is directed at reducing the incidence of myocardial infarction and death and relieving symptoms. β-blockers are first-line therapy in most patients. They reduce angina severity and frequency by reducing heart rate and contractility. Titrate the β-blocker dose to achieve a resting heart rate of approximately 55-60 bpm and approximately 75% of the heart rate that produces angina with exertion (based upon exercise electrocardiography results).

Calcium-channel blockers are indicated for patients unable to tolerate β-blockers or if symptoms are inadequately controlled with β-blockers. Calcium-channel blockers produce vasodilatation, increase coronary blood flow, and reduce myocardial contractility. Nondihydropyridine agents have a greater effect on myocardial contractility and conduction; dihydropyridine agents exert relatively more effect on vasodilatation. Short-acting calcium-channel blockers are contraindicated because of their association with increased risk of myocardial infarction, and perhaps mortality.

Long-acting nitrates, in combination with or instead of β-blockers or calcium-channel antagonists (if these agents are contraindicated or are not tolerated), are used for chronic stable angina. Nitrates alleviate angina symptoms by dilation of epicardial coronary vessels and increasing capacitance of the venous system, resulting in diminished cardiac preload and myocardial oxygen demand. Patients are taken off their nitrates at night to mitigate nitrate tolerance.

Ranolazine, a piperazine derivative, is available for patients who have not received an adequate response to standard antianginal therapy. Its mechanism of action is unknown, but it might reduce intracellular calcium concentration and improve left ventricular function.

Aspirin (or other antiplatelet therapy) is prescribed unless there is a history of significant gastrointestinal bleeding or aspirin allergy. Aspirin reduces platelet aggregation and acute coronary events and decreases the risk of myocardial infarction and death.

Use a statin to reduce the LDL cholesterol <100 mg/dL to improve survival and reduce the risk of major coronary events. An optional LDL goal of <70 mg/dL is recommended for patients at high risk. Patients who have angina, low HDL cholesterol, and relatively normal levels of LDL cholesterol and triglycerides benefit from gemfibrozil.

Treatment with an angiotensin-converting enzyme inhibitor reduces mortality in patients with heart failure and reduced left ventricular function (ejection fraction <35%) and reduces mortality, myocardial infarction, and stroke in patients with vascular disease or diabetes and at least one additional cardiovascular risk factor. Table 3 summarizes drug treatment options for chronic stable angina.

Follow-Up

Address angina symptoms, medication use, and modifiable risk factors during regular follow-up visits that can be anywhere from 4 to 12 months apart depending on patient stability. Do not obtain routine resting electrocardiograms when there have been no changes in symptoms, examination, or medications. A repeat stress test is indicated if there is a change in symptoms.

Book Enhancement

Go to www.acponline.org/essentials/cardiovascular-section.html to access tools to determine the best noninvasive test for your patient, to estimate likelihood of coronary artery disease following an exercise stress test, to estimate mortality rates, and to review indications for revascularization. In *MKSAP for Students 4*, assess yourself with items 10-11 in the **Cardiovascular Medicine** section.

Bibliography

Snow V, Barry P, Fihn SD, et al. Primary care management of chronic stable angina and asymptomatic suspected or known coronary artery disease: a clinical practice guideline from the American College of Physicians. Ann Intern Med. 2004;141:562-7. [Erratum in: Ann Intern Med. 2005;142:79.] [PMID: 15466774]

Sutton PR, Fihn SD. Chronic Stable Angina. http://pier.acponline.org/physicians/diseases/d032. [Date accessed: 2008 Jan 9] In: PIER [online database]. Philadelphia: American College of Physicians; 2008.

Chapter 3

Acute Coronary Syndrome

Patrick C. Alguire, MD

The term *acute coronary syndrome* (ACS) refers to any component of the clinical syndromes caused by acute myocardial ischemia. It encompasses unstable angina, non–ST-segment elevation myocardial infarction (non-STEMI), and ST-segment elevation myocardial infarction (STEMI). STEMI has a clinical presentation consistent with acute myocardial infarction (MI) and electrocardiographic evidence of ST-segment elevation. Unstable angina and non-STEMI are closely related and differ only in the severity of ischemia. Non-STEMI is associated with elevated biomarkers of myocardial injury and unstable angina is not; the principles of risk stratification and therapy are identical for both.

The pathophysiology of ACS is characterized by atherosclerotic plaque rupture, formation of a platelet and fibrin thrombi, and local release of vasoactive substances. Unstable angina and non-STEMI are most commonly caused by a nonocclusive thrombus. Rare causes of unstable angina and non-STEMI include vasospasm of an epicardial coronary artery (Prinzmetal's angina) and secondary angina (e.g., hypoxemia, anemia, tachycardia, or thyrotoxicosis). The most common cause of STEMI is an occlusive thrombus.

Prevention

All patients who smoke should be encouraged to stop. Asymptomatic adults ≥20 years old should be periodically screened for dyslipidemia. All patients should be routinely screened for hypertension. All patients with coronary artery disease (CAD) and high-risk individuals should be screened for diabetes. Moderate strenuous exercise and a high-fiber diet rich in fresh fruits and vegetables and low in cholesterol, saturated fats, and refined sugars may reduce risk.

Aspirin reduces the risk of cardiovascular events by inhibiting platelet activation and is most effective in patients with multiple risk factors. Hormone replacement therapy is not indicated in the prevention of CAD in postmenopausal women and may increase the incidence of nonfatal MI.

Screening

Routine screening for CAD in asymptomatic persons without cardiovascular risk factors is not recommended. Although exercise testing may identify persons with CAD, its usefulness is limited by the low prevalence of CAD in asymptomatic adults, thus reducing the predictive value of a positive test. Calcification of coronary arteries that is detected by electron-beam CT scanning appears to predict nonfatal MI. In 2007, the American College of Cardiology concluded that it may be reasonable to use electron-beam CT in patients with an estimated 10%-20% 10-year risk of coronary events based on the possibility that such patients might be reclassified to a higher risk status and offered more aggressive risk management interventions.

Diagnosis

A strong clinical predictor of angiographic CAD is the character of the chest discomfort. Typical angina, characterized by substernal discomfort, exertional onset, and prompt relief with nitroglycerin or rest, is associated with a 94% probability of CAD in certain patients. The most common reason for failure to diagnose acute MI is that the patient has either "noncardiac" or "atypical" symptoms of dyspnea, fatigue, nausea, abdominal discomfort, or syncope, which is why any of these symptoms, with or without chest discomfort, should always prompt consideration of ACS. Up to 25% of ACS patients have atypical symptoms, especially women, diabetics, and the elderly. Chest pain that is pleuritic, sharp, stabbing, or positional significantly decreases the likelihood of acute coronary syndrome.

Although physical findings alone are not used to exclude the diagnosis of ACS, a thorough physical exam can aid diagnosis and prognosis. A new murmur may suggest valvular incompetence caused by papillary muscle dysfunction or rupture. A new S_4 gallop can represent decreased diastolic compliance. Heart failure may be present if ischemia results in left ventricular diastolic or systolic dysfunction or valvular incompetence and is a high-risk feature for death. Look for physical examination signs most predictive of MI: elevated central venous pressure, hypotension, bibasilar crackles, and an S_3.

Obtain an electrocardiogram (ECG) immediately in suspected ACS to help guide the initial management. New ST-segment elevation and Q waves are the most powerful predictive findings for MI. The initial ECG may be nondiagnostic in half of patients; therefore, serial ECGs are recommended (e.g., every 20 minutes for 2 hours). The diagnostic yield of the ECG is improved if a tracing can be recorded during an episode of chest discomfort. STEMI is characterized by chest pain and ST elevations >1 mm in two or more contiguous leads (Figure 1), new left bundle-branch block, or evidence of true posterior infarction on electrocardiography. Non-STEMI is defined by elevated cardiac biomarkers and absence of ST-segment elevation. A persistently normal ECG decreases the probability of MI.

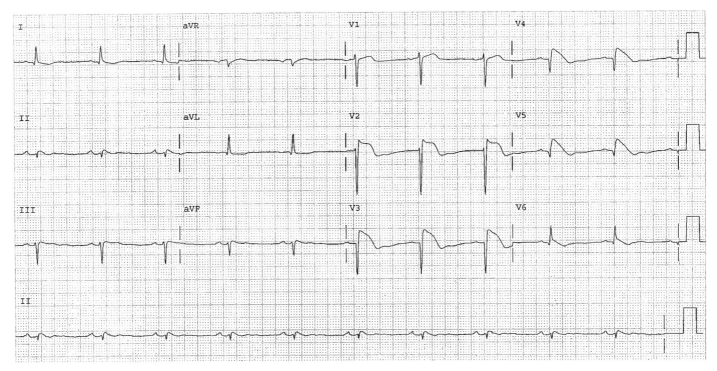

Figure 1 Electrocardiogram showing abnormal Q waves in leads V_3-V_5 and ST-segment elevation in leads V_2-V_5. The T waves are beginning to invert in leads V_3-V_6. This pattern is most consistent with a recent anterolateral myocardial infarction.

During MI, the cardiac myocytes lose membrane integrity and leak proteins (e.g., creatine kinase, myoglobin, cardiac troponin) into the serum; by serially measuring cardiac marker proteins evidence of myocardial damage within the last 24 hours can be detected. Repeat the measurements at 6 and 12 hours after onset of symptoms. In patients with acute ST elevations, do not delay further management pending return of the biomarkers.

Obtain an echocardiogram to detect regional wall motion abnormalities before serum marker results are known in any patient with a nondiagnostic electrocardiogram in whom non-STEMI or unstable angina is suspected. Echocardiography can show the progressive course from hypokinesis to akinesis during ischemia, as well as show impaired myocardial relaxation during diastole. An echocardiogram demonstrating normal wall motion excludes extensive myocardial damage but does not rule out non-STEMI. The differential diagnosis of acute chest pain is broad (Table 1). Use echocardiography to identify nonischemic conditions that cause chest pain, such as myocarditis; aortic stenosis; aortic dissection; pulmonary embolism; and mechanical complications of acute infarction, such as papillary muscle dysfunction or rupture; and ventricular septal defect.

Coronary angiography provides detailed information about the coronary anatomy and facilitates invasive management of occluded coronary arteries. It is most often considered in the setting of ACS in patients with STEMI or new left bundle branch block in whom immediate angioplasty is an option; unstable angina/non-STEMI and high-risk features (e.g., hypotension, heart failure, mitral regurgitation); or repeated episodes of ACS despite optimal therapy.

Mechanical complications occur in 0.1% of post-MI patients between days 2 and 7. These complications include ventricular septal defect, papillary muscle rupture leading to acute mitral valve regurgitation, and left ventricular free wall rupture leading to cardiac tamponade. Ventricular septal defect and papillary muscle rupture usually lead to a new, loud systolic murmur and acute pulmonary edema or hypotension. Diagnosis is critical because the 24-hour survival rate is approximately 25% with medical therapy alone but increases to 50% with emergency surgical intervention. Pericardial tamponade from free wall rupture usually leads to sudden hypotension, pulseless electrical activity on electrocardiography, and death.

Therapy

Effective analgesia early in the course of ACS is an important therapeutic intervention. Morphine sulfate reduces sympathetic tone through a centrally mediated anxiolytic affect. Morphine also reduces myocardial oxygen demand by reducing pre-load and by a vagally mediated reduction in heart rate.

The vasodilating action of nitroglycerin results in combined preload and afterload reduction, decreased cardiac work, and lower myocardial oxygen requirements. Nitrates may reduce infarct size, improve regional myocardial function, prevent left ventricular remodeling, and provide a small relative reduction in mortality rate. In the acute setting, nitrates are often administered intravenously. Titration endpoints are control of symptoms or a decrease in mean arterial pressure by 10% (mean arterial blood pressure = $[(2 \times \text{diastolic}) + \text{systolic}] / 3$).

Antithrombotic (heparin) therapy is indicated in patients with likely or definite ACS. The combination of heparin and aspirin reduces the incidence of MI during the in-hospital period and reduces the need for revascularization procedures. Two landmark

Table 1. Differential Diagnosis of Acute Coronary Syndrome

Disease	Notes
Anxiety disorders	May be indistinguishable from angina. Often diagnosed after a negative work-up for ischemic heart disease. Often associated with palpitations, sweating, and anxiety.
Aortic dissection (see Chapter 1)	Tearing pain of abrupt onset that may radiate to the back. Blood pressure in arms may show differences >10 mm Hg. Chest X-ray may show a widened mediastinum or abnormal aortic contour in approximately 80%.
Arrhythmias (see Chapter 4)	May cause typical angina related to increased myocardial oxygen demand and/or diminished diastolic filling of the coronary arteries.
Chest wall (see Chapter 1)	Characteristically reproduced with palpation or movement. Reproduction with palpation does not exclude angina.
Cholecystitis (see Chapter 15)	Occasionally presents as chest discomfort, usually related to meals, not exertion. Diagnosis by ultrasonography.
Esophageal (see Chapter 17)	May be indistinguishable from angina. Often diagnosed after a negative work-up for ischemic heart disease.
Pancreatitis (see Chapter 16)	Occasionally chest discomfort, more commonly mid-epigastric pain with nausea and vomiting. Look for significant alcohol ingestion, gallbladder disease, abnormal amylase and lipase or liver enzymes.
Pericarditis (see Chapter 1)	Pain is often pleuritic but may resemble angina. Classically relieved by sitting up and leaning forward. May be associated with a friction rub on auscultation and diffuse ST-segment elevation on electrocardiogram or, less commonly, PR-segment depression.
Pneumothorax (see Chapter 1)	Dyspnea and chest pain. Chest x-ray confirms the diagnosis.
Pulmonary embolus (see Chapter 80)	Pain is often sharp and pleuritic, and associated with dyspnea. Syncope, hypotension, elevated neck veins, and characteristic findings on electrocardiogram are more common with large, central pulmonary emboli.
Valvular heart disease (see Chapter 7)	May cause typical angina related to left ventricular outflow obstruction and increased myocardial wall stress. Auscultation typically shows a long, late-peaking systolic murmur at the base of the heart. Aortic stenosis commonly radiates to the carotids and is associated with a weak and delayed carotid upstroke. Murmurs of subaortic hypertrophic cardiomyopathy typically increase with the Valsalva maneuver.

trials have shown low-molecular-weight heparin (LMWH) to be superior to unfractionated heparin (UFH) in this setting. LMWH has greater bioavailability and a more predictable dose-response relationship compared with UFH, but LMWH should not be used in the morbidly obese, and dosage adjustment is required in renal insufficiency.

When administered immediately upon presentation, aspirin reduces mortality in patients with unstable angina or acute infarction by diminishing platelet aggregation. The anti-inflammatory properties of aspirin may also contribute to its beneficial effects. Clopidogrel should be considered in patients with ACS who are unable to take aspirin and in high-risk patients in whom percutaneous coronary intervention is planned. Clopidogrel, a more potent antiplatelet agent than aspirin, provides additional antiplatelet activity when added to aspirin. It should be withheld if coronary bypass surgery is a possibility due to the increased risk of perioperative bleeding. Glycoprotein IIb/IIIa receptor antagonists (e.g., abciximab, tirofiban) inhibit the cross-bridging of platelets secondary to fibrinogen binding to the activated glycoprotein IIb/IIIa receptor. Glycoprotein IIb/IIIa antagonists should be considered in addition to aspirin and heparin in patients with non-STEMI and as adjunctive therapy in patients with STEMI undergoing angioplasty.

Early intravenous β-blocker therapy (i.e., atenolol, metoprolol, carvedilol) reduces infarct size, decreases the frequency of recurrent myocardial ischemia, and improves short- and long-term survival. β-blockers diminish myocardial oxygen demand by reducing heart rate, systemic arterial pressure, and myocardial contractility; in addition, prolongation of diastole augments perfusion to injured myocardium. β-blocker therapy can be used in left ventricular dysfunction if heart failure status is stable.

An angiotensin-converting enzyme (ACE) inhibitor should be administered early in the course of ACS in most patients. ACE inhibitor therapy can attenuate ventricular remodeling, resulting in a reduction in the development of heart failure and death. ACE inhibitor therapy may also reduce the risk of recurrent infarction and other vascular events. In patients who cannot tolerate an ACE inhibitor due to cough, an angiotensin-receptor blocker is a reasonable alternative.

Statin therapy appears to improve endothelial function and reduce the risk of future coronary events. A single study showed a reduction in recurrent ischemia when a high-dose statin was administered within 24-96 hours of hospital admission. The concept of plaque stabilization and improvement in endothelial function with statin therapy suggests that there is an emerging benefit to statins in ACS beyond LDL cholesterol reduction.

Eplerenone is a selective aldosterone blocker that limits collagen formation and ventricular remodeling after acute MI and also has a favorable effect on the neurohormonal profile. Eplerenone reduces mortality when started 3 to 14 days after MI in patients with left ventricular ejection fraction ≤40% and clinical heart failure or diabetes. Aldosterone antagonists should be used with great caution or not at all in patients with renal insufficiency (creatinine >2.5 mg/dL) or pre-existing hyperkalemia (>5.0 meq/L).

Percutaneous angioplasty and stent placement is the preferred therapy in specific subsets of patients with ACS (STEMI, new left bundle branch block, or true posterior infarction). In these patients, primary percutaneous coronary intervention is associated with a lower 30-day mortality rate compared with thrombolytic therapy. The incorporation of drug-eluting stents has further increased the clinical advantage of percutaneous intervention over thrombolytic therapy. A drug-eluting stent is a metallic stent with a polymer covering containing an anti-restenotic drug that is released over a period of 14-30 days. Angioplasty is also indicated in patients with a contraindication to thrombolytic therapy or in patients with cardiogenic shock. Angioplasty is most effective if completed within 12 hours of the onset of chest pain; the earlier the intervention, the better is the outcome. Prompt transfer for primary percutaneous coronary intervention may be beneficial in patients but is contingent upon transfer occurring within 2-3 hours of initial hospital arrival.

Thrombolytic agents are an alternative to primary percutaneous interventions in suitable candidates with STEMI. By lysing the clot that is limiting blood flow to the myocardium, thrombolytics restore perfusion to the ischemic area, reduce infarct size, and improve survival. Thrombolytics should be administered within 12 hours after the onset of chest pain; the earlier the administration, the better is the outcome.

The role of bypass surgery in the treatment of ACS is evolving. Bypass surgery is preferred in patients who have a large amount of myocardium at ischemic risk due to proximal left main disease, or multi-vessel disease, especially if the left ventricular ejection fraction is reduced. Bypass surgery may be preferred in patients with diabetes mellitus because of better long-term vessel patency and improved clinical outcomes. However, there is increasing evidence that drug-eluting stents may produce outcomes comparable to bypass surgery.

An intra-aortic balloon pump is indicated for ACS with cardiogenic shock unresponsive to medical therapy, acute mitral regurgitation secondary to papillary muscle dysfunction, ventricular septal rupture, or refractory angina. The intra-aortic balloon pump reduces afterload during ventricular systole and increases coronary perfusion during diastole. Patients with refractory cardiogenic shock who are treated with an intra-aortic balloon pump have a lower in-hospital mortality rate than patients who are not treated with this device.

Follow-Up

Following a MI, early cardiac catheterization during hospitalization for ACS should be considered for patients with recurrent ischemic symptoms, serious complications, or other intermediate-to high-risk features (e.g., heart failure, left ventricular dysfunction, ventricular arrhythmias). These complications or high-risk features of ACS are associated with more severe CAD and subsequent cardiac events.

Exercise testing in post-MI patients without high-risk features is performed as a prognostic assessment. By doing stress testing early post-MI, the clinician can assess functional capacity, evaluate efficacy of the patient's current medical regimen, and risk-stratify the patient according to likelihood of future cardiac events.

Patients with depressed left-ventricular systolic function are at increased risk for subsequent ventricular tachyarrhythmias. The finding of nonsustained ventricular tachycardia more than 48 hours after MI, particularly in patients with ejection fractions of <35%, usually prompts electrophysiological testing or implantation of a cardioverter-defibrillator. Studies have consistently shown that high-risk patients typically do better with an implantable cardioverter-defibrillator than with antiarrhythmic therapy.

Secondary prevention measures are an essential component of outpatient management following ACS, including management of hypertension, diabetes, lipid lowering, smoking cessation, and an exercise program. Patients should continue aspirin, β-blockers, ACE-inhibitors, statins, and nitrates.

Studies indicate that approximately 20% of patients experience depression after acute infarction and that the presence of depression is associated with increased risk for recurrent hospitalization and death. Post-infarction patients should be screened for depression.

Book Enhancement

Go to www.acponline.org/essentials/cardiovascular-section.html to access a web-based ECG tutorial and to view tables on risk stratification and management, drug therapy, and contraindications to fibrinolysis. In *MKSAP for Students 4*, assess yourself with items 12-22 in the **Cardiovascular Medicine** section.

Bibliography

Glassberg H, Desai R. Acute Coronary Syndromes. http://pier.acponline.org/physicians/diseases/d361/d361. [Date accessed: 2008 Feb 20] In: PIER [online database]. Philadelphia: American College of Physicians; 2008.

Grech ED, Ramsdale DR. Acute coronary syndrome: unstable angina and non-ST segment elevation myocardial infarction. BMJ. 2003;326:1259-61. [PMID: 12791748]

Panju AA, Hemmelgarn BR, Guyatt GH, Simel DL. Is this patient having a myocardial infarction? JAMA. 1998;280:1256-63. [PMID: 9786377]

Chapter 4

Supraventricular Arrhythmias

Charin L. Hanlon, MD

Supraventricular arrhythmias arise from impulses that originate above the ventricle and include bradyarrhythmias (sinus node dysfunction, atrioventricular nodal block) and tachyarrhythmias (atrial fibrillation and flutter, paroxysmal reentrant supraventricular tachycardia, atrial tachycardia, and preexcitation syndromes). Most supraventricular tachycardias are the product of a circulating continuous repetitive propagation of an excitatory wave traveling in a circular path, returning to its site of origin to reactivate that site (reentrant tachycardia).

Bradyarrhythmias

Sinus node dysfunction (sick sinus syndrome) is a frequent cause of pacemaker implantation. It consists of symptomatic sinus bradycardia and the tachycardia-bradycardia syndrome (alternating atrial tachyarrhythmias and bradycardia). In patients with "tachy-brady" syndrome, bradycardia usually occurs after termination of the tachycardia; atrial fibrillation is the most common tachyarrhythmia observed in this group of patients.

Atrioventricular nodal block is classified as first, second, or third degree. First-degree block is defined by prolongation of the PR interval >0.2 sec and usually is not associated with alterations in heart rate. There are two types of second-degree block, both recognized electrocardiographically by the presence of a P wave that is not followed by a ventricular complex. Mobitz type I block (Wenckebach block) manifests as progressive prolongation of the PR interval until there is a dropped beat, whereas Mobitz type II block manifests as a dropped beat without progressive PR interval prolongation. Mobitz type I block usually does not progress to complete heart block, but Mobitz type II block, which is usually associated with a bundle branch block, typically progresses to third-degree block. Second-degree block may be associated with bradycardia, depending upon the frequency of blocked atrial impulses. Third-degree block is the complete absence of conduction of atrial impulses to the ventricle and is the most common cause of marked bradycardia; ventricular rates are usually 30-50/min (Figure 1). Patients with atrioventricular block may be asymptomatic or have severe bradycardia-related symptoms (e.g., weakness, presyncope, syncope) and ventricular arrhythmias.

Therapy

The most important step in the treatment of bradycardia is the removal of all rate-affecting agents (e.g., β-blockers, calcium-channel

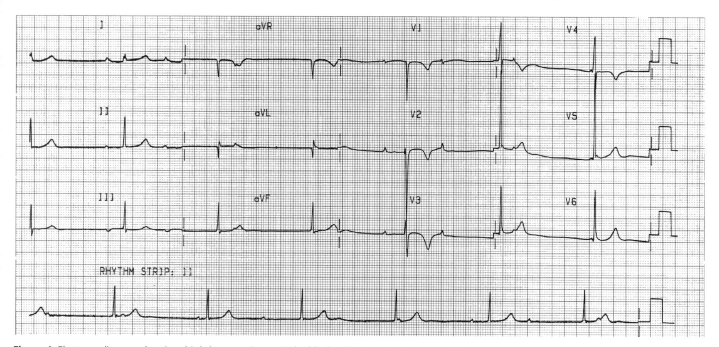

Figure 1 Electrocardiogram showing third-degree atrioventricular block with a junctional escape rhythm.

15

blockers with negative chronotropic effects, digoxin). Atropine can be used in emergency situations for symptomatic bradycardia. Pacing is indicated for symptomatic bradycardia, tachycardia-bradycardia syndrome, complete heart block, and for asymptomatic patients with asystolic pauses >3.0 seconds or a ventricular escape rate <40/min. Permanent pacing improves survival in patients with complete heart block, particularly if syncope has occurred.

Tachyarrhythmias

Atrial fibrillation is the most common sustained atrial tachyarrhythmia and is associated with loss of sinus node function, leading to uncoordinated atrial activity. The electrocardiogram is characterized by loss of P waves and irregularity of the ventricular response (Figure 2). Atrial fibrillation is classified according to its duration into acute (<48 hours), chronic (>48 hours), paroxysmal, or indeterminate; this classification determines the nature of treatment. Symptoms may include palpitations, syncope or presyncope, chest pain, dyspnea, or fatigue. Eighty percent of patients with atrial fibrillation have heart disease, including hypertension with left ventricular hypertrophy, valvular heart disease, coronary artery disease, cardiomyopathy, congenital heart disease (especially atrial septal defect), or recent open heart surgery. Heart failure and increasing age are also strongly associated with atrial fibrillation.

Chronic atrial fibrillation leads to shortening of the atrial action potential making the arrhythmia more persistent with time. This clinical observation is the basis for the aphorism "atrial fibrillation begets atrial fibrillation." Even after only 24 hours of atrial fibrillation, drug therapy becomes progressively less effective at terminating the arrhythmia.

Atrial flutter is characterized by regular atrial contractions (flutter waves or sawtooth pattern) on electrocardiography (Figure 3). Untreated, the atrial rate is 240-300/min and is usually associated with a 2:1 or 3:1 atrioventricular block, resulting in a ventricular rate of approximately 100-150/min. Sustained atrial flutter is less common than atrial fibrillation, and flutter typically converts to atrial fibrillation over time.

For atrial fibrillation and flutter, screen for noncardiac causes including substances (alcohol, caffeine, cocaine, amphetamines, inhaled β-agonists) pulmonary disease (hypoxia, chronic obstructive pulmonary disease, pulmonary embolism, pulmonary hypertension, obstructive sleep apnea), and hyperthyroidism. Obtain an electrocardiogram, complete blood count, electrolytes, glucose, serum TSH, pulse oximetry, digoxin level (if taking), baseline coagulation tests, and stool for occult blood before initiating warfarin or heparin. Obtain a transthoracic echocardiogram to evaluate for valvular heart disease and determine chamber size and function. Transesophageal echocardiography may be needed to detect or exclude the presence of intracardiac thrombi, a finding that may influence the timing of cardioversion and the initiation of anticoagulation.

The most common paroxysmal reentrant supraventricular tachycardia involves reentry within atrioventricular nodal tissue. It is a regular, narrow complex tachycardia with a ventricular rate of 160-180/min. A retrograde P wave is typically buried within the QRS complex but may occur shortly before or shortly

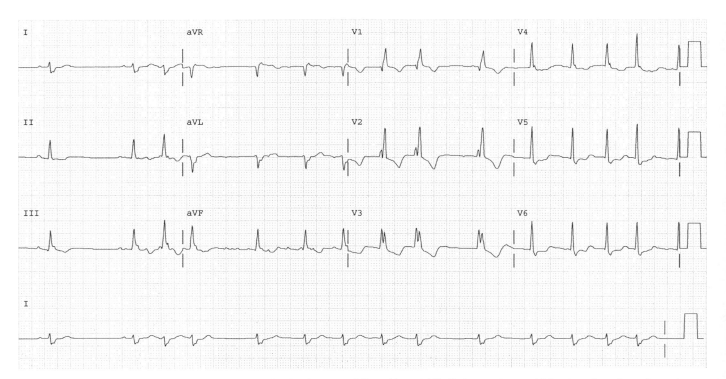

Figure 2 Electrocardiogram showing two sinus beats and a slow heart rate followed by atrial fibrillation consistent with bradycardia-tachycardia syndrome. The rhythm is irregular, and fibrillatory waves are clearly seen in lead aVF. Right bundle branch block is also present.

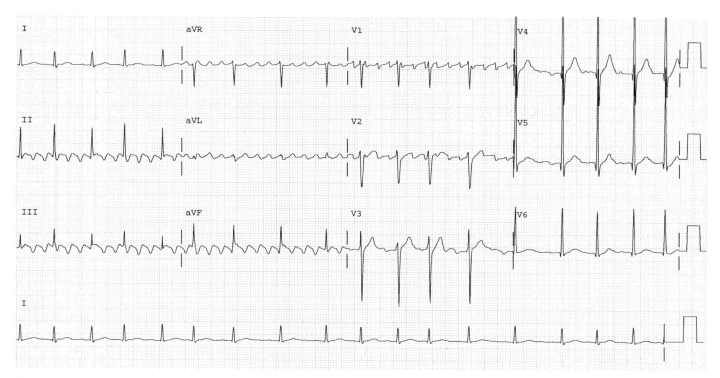

Figure 3 Electrocardiogram showing an irregular rate and a saw-tooth pattern in leads II, III, and aVF characteristic of atrial flutter.

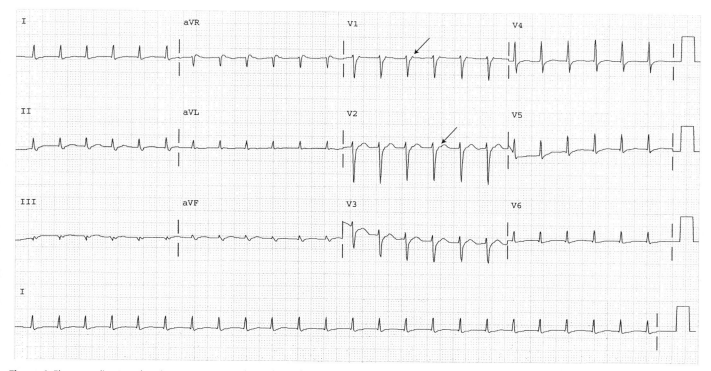

Figure 4 Electrocardiogram showing a narrow complex tachycardia with P waves buried in the T wave, most easily seen in lead V_2, characteristic of atrioventricular nodal reentrant tachycardia.

after it (Figure 4). In the absence of structural heart disease, it is a benign rhythm.

Atrial tachycardia can arise from almost any region of the right or left atrium; the most common mechanism is reentry. The P-wave morphology may be upright, biphasic, or inverted in the inferior leads, depending on the site of origin. Reentrant atrial tachycardia is frequently associated with structural heart disease; also look for possible digitalis toxicity.

Preexcitation refers to the presence of an accessory pathway that can conduct impulses from the atrium to the ventricle, bypassing the atrioventricular node. Most patients with preexcitation demonstrate a short PR interval and an initial slurring of the upstroke of the QRS complex (the delta wave), establishing the diagnosis of Wolff-Parkinson-White syndrome. Because the bypass tract may be capable of rapid antegrade conduction, patients with Wolff-Parkinson-White syndrome who develop atrial fibrillation may experience a very rapid ventricular response that can degenerate into ventricular fibrillation. The risk of sudden cardiac death in these patients is 0.15%-0.39% over 3-10 year follow-up. Table 1 summarizes a differential diagnosis of supraventricular tachycardia based on electrocardiographic features.

Therapy

Consider teaching patients with well-tolerated atrioventricular-nodal-dependent supraventricular tachycardia the Valsalva maneuver or carotid massage to help terminate episodes of arrhythmia. These maneuvers may terminate an episode of supraventricular tachycardia by increasing vagal tone, slowing atrioventricular nodal conduction, and increasing atrioventricular nodal refractoriness.

Electrical cardioversion is indicated for hemodynamically unstable patients, regardless of the tachyarrhythmia. Intravenous heparin is started immediately in patients with atrial fibrillation of unknown duration before cardioversion. Potential risks of urgent electrical cardioversion include thromboembolism (2%), tachyarrhythmias, or bradyarrhythmias. Electrical cardioversion is an alternative to pharmacologic cardioversion of atrial fibrillation of any duration; patients are anticoagulated prior to cardioversion and for up to 4 weeks after cardioversion. Cardioversion is successful in 70%-90% of patients with atrial fibrillation of less than 48 hours duration and is effective in 50% of patients with longer duration of atrial fibrillation.

Other options to control ventricular rate include atrioventricular-nodal catheter ablation techniques or surgery. Pulmonary vein catheter ablation is increasingly used to treat paroxysmal atrial fibrillation in patients with a structurally normal heart. Foci for atrial fibrillation are commonly located around the ostia of the pulmonary veins; up to 80% of patients with paroxysmal atrial fibrillation will remain arrhythmia-free after pulmonary vein catheter ablation. Catheter ablation of the accessory bypass tract is the treatment of choice for symptomatic Wolff-Parkinson-White syndrome. The "maze" surgical procedure consists of multiple atrial

incisions to reduce effective atrial size and prevent formation of atrial fibrillation wavelets; it is 99% effective with operative mortality of 1%-3%.

Consider a calcium-channel blocker (i.e., verapamil or diltiazem) to treat patients who have atrioventricular nodal re-entrant tachycardia to terminate an acute event or to prevent recurrences. Calcium-channel blocking drugs work by slowing atrioventricular conduction and increasing nodal refractoriness.

With cardiology consultation, consider using class I and class III antiarrhythmic agents (Table 2) to treat atrial tachycardia, particularly re-entrant atrial tachycardia. Amiodarone has the least proarrhythmic effect and is the preferred agent in patients with left ventricular dysfunction and structural heart disease.

The stroke rate with nonrheumatic atrial fibrillation is about 5% per year. Risk factors for stroke are history of previous transient ischemic attack or stroke, myocardial infarction, hypertension, age >65 years, diabetes, left atrial enlargement, and left ventricular dysfunction. Warfarin (target INR of 2.0-3.0) reduces the risk of stroke by an average of 64% in nonvalvular atrial fibrillation. Chronic anticoagulation is considered if there is high risk for recurrence of atrial fibrillation following successful conversion, current asymptomatic atrial fibrillation, evidence of intracardiac thrombus, or any known risk factors for thromboembolism.

The $CHADS_2$ scoring system has been well validated to estimate patient stroke risk. The $CHADS_2$ acronym is derived from the individual stroke risk factors: congestive heart failure, hypertension, age >75 years, diabetes mellitus, and prior stroke or transient ischemic attack (TIA). Patients are assigned 2 points for a previous stroke or TIA and 1 point for each of the other risk factors. In patients with a $CHADS_2$ score of 0, the risk of stroke is low and anticoagulation is not required; the risk of major bleeding in this category is greater than the benefit from anticoagulation. Those with a $CHADS_2$ score ≥ 3 and those with a prior TIA or stroke are at high risk and anticoagulation is indicated; the benefit from anticoagulation exceeds the risk of major bleeding. For patients at intermediate risk for stroke (score 1 or 2) warfarin therapy should be assessed individually, taking into account the risk of major hemorrhage and patient preference. In these patients, and those in whom full anticoagulation with warfarin is contraindicated, aspirin alone decreases stroke risk by 22%.

In patients aged >65 years, heart rate control is preferred to using antiarrhythmic drugs to maintain sinus rhythm because the

Table 1. Differential Diagnosis of Supraventricular Tachycardia Based on Electrocardiographic Features

Disease	Notes
Atrial fibrillation, atrial flutter	Atrial fibrillation is an irregular rhythm with no definitive P waves. Atrial flutter typically has saw-tooth pattern flutter waves, most noticeably in the inferior leads.
Atrial tachycardia (reentrant)	Long RP tachycardia.* Commonly associated with structural heart disease.
AV-nodal reentrant tachycardia	In the typical variety, the atria and ventricles are simultaneously activated, and either no P wave is visible or a small pseudo r-prime deflection in lead V1 and a pseudo S-wave deflection inferiorly are seen.
AV reentrant tachycardia	Short RP tachycardia.* P wave is usually located within the ST segment. Accessory AV pathways can conduct anterograde (atrium to ventricle), retrograde (ventricle to atrium), or in both directions. Only accessory pathways with anterograde conduction will show pre-excitation (Wolff-Parkinson-White pattern) on the ECG (during sinus rhythm).

* RP is the measured interval from the onset of the QRS complex to the onset of the P wave. If the RP interval is longer than the PR interval during tachycardia, the tachycardia is referred as a *long-RP tachycardia*, whereas if the RP interval is shorter than the PR interval, it is referred as a *short-RP tachycardia*.
AV = atrioventricular; ECG = electrocardiogram.

Table 2. Antiarrhythmic Agents

Class Ia

Procainamide	Prolongs conduction and slows repolarization by blocking inward sodium flux. Recommended for Wolff-Parkinson-White syndrome. Not for use in patients with severe left ventricular dysfunction; avoid in patients with renal impairment.
Quinidine gluconate	Prolongs conduction and slows repolarization. Blocks fast inward sodium channel. Adjust dose in patients with renal insufficiency.
Disopyramide	Similar electrophysiologic properties to procainamide and quinidine. Rarely used.

Class Ic

Flecainide	Blocks sodium channels (and fast sodium current). Not for use in patients with structurally abnormal hearts.
Propafenone	Blocks myocardial sodium channels. Antiarrhythmic and weak calcium channel and β-blocking properties.

Class III

Amiodarone	Blocks sodium channels (affinity for inactivated channels). Noncompetitive α- and β-receptor inhibitor. Safest agent for use in patients with structural heart disease and can be used for Wolff-Parkinson-White syndrome.
Dofetilide	Blocks rapid component of the delayed rectifier potassium current, prolonging refractoriness without slowing conduction. Must be strictly dosed according to renal function, body size, and age.
Ibutilide	Prolongs action potential duration (and atrial and ventricular refractoriness) by blocking rapid component of delayed rectifier potassium current.
Sotalol	Nonselective β-blocking properties but some positive inotropic activity. Lethal arrhythmias possible. Adjust dose in patients with renal insufficiency.

former strategy results in fewer hospitalizations and serious drug reactions. The goal of rate control is to reduce the ventricular rate to <80/min at rest and <100/min during exercise. Calcium-channel blockers (i.e., diltiazem or verapamil) or β-blocking agents (i.e., atenolol or metoprolol) are first-line therapy. Digitalis is not recommended as a single agent for rate control due to its slower onset, increased toxicity, and less efficacy of controlling the ventricular rate during exercise.

Rhythm control can be accomplished with Class Ia, Class Ic, and Class III antiarrhythmic agents (see Table 2). Oral or intravenous antiarrhythmic agents result in successful cardioversion of 60%-90% of patients with atrial fibrillation of <48 hours duration but are less effective in chronic atrial fibrillation. In patients with recurrent symptomatic atrial fibrillation, the choice of an antiarrhythmic drug depends on the presence or absence of underlying structural heart disease. Propafenone or flecainide may be initiated in the absence of structural heart disease, whereas amiodarone is typically used when underlying heart disease is present. Because these drugs can be proarrhythmic, consultation with cardiology is recommended.

Follow-Up

In patients with atrial fibrillation, assess rate control by asking about easy fatigability and exertional dyspnea and observe for heart rate >100/min while walking. If rate is >100/min, increase the atrioventricular nodal blockade with higher doses of current agent or additional drugs. In patients on warfarin, check INR as often as required to achieve a stable target INR of 2.0-3.0 in non-valvular atrial fibrillation or 2.5-3.5 in valvular atrial fibrillation.

In patients on antiarrhythmic drugs, obtain a 12-lead electrocardiogram to check QRS and QT intervals for drug toxicity.

Increases in the QRS duration or QT interval may indicate an increased risk of proarrhythmia. Monitor levels of antiarrhythmic drugs when feasible in all patients who are taking pharmacologic therapy for supraventricular tachycardia. Routinely screen patients for side effects of antiarrhythmic therapy. Obtain periodic thyroid function tests, liver chemistry tests, and pulmonary function tests (including diffusing capacity) for patients treated with amiodarone and periodic complete blood counts for patients treated with procainamide. Amiodarone has several severe side effects, including pulmonary fibrosis, hyperthyroidism, hypothyroidism, and hepatitis. Procainamide can cause agranulocytosis.

Book Enhancement

Go to www.acponline.org/essentials/cardiovascular-section.html to view the mechanism of atrioventricular nodal reentry and atrioventricular reentry tachycardias, a description of electrocardiographic recording devices, and risk estimates of atrial fibrillation related stroke and to access a tutorial on electrocardiography interpretation. In *MKSAP for Students 4*, assess yourself with items 23-29 in the **Cardiovascular Medicine** section.

Bibliography

Delacrétaz E. Clinical practice. Supraventricular tachycardia. N Engl J Med. 2006;354:1039-51. [PMID: 16525141]

Ferrari VA, Callans D, Wiegers S. Atrial Fibrillation. http://pier.acponline .org/physicians/diseases/d027. [Date accessed: 2008 Jan 23] In: PIER [online database]. Philadelphia: American College of Physicians; 2008.

Mangrum JM, DiMarco JP. The evaluation and management of bradycardia. N Engl J Med. 2000;342:703-9. [PMID: 10706901]

Chapter 5

Ventricular Arrhythmias

Steven J. Durning, MD
Mark C. Haigney, MD

Ventricular tachycardia is a potentially life threatening arrhythmia due to rapid, depolarizing impulses originating from the His-Purkinje system, the ventricular myocardium, or both. Ventricular tachycardia requires immediate evaluation and, at times, treatment as it can lead to sudden cardiac death.

The pathophysiology of ventricular tachycardia is most commonly due to abnormalities of *impulse conduction* (i.e., a reentrant pathway). Once the reentrant pathway is initiated, repetitive circulation of the impulse over the loop can produce ventricular tachycardia. Ventricular tachycardia may also arise through abnormal *impulse formation* such as enhanced automaticity or triggered activity. Enhancement of normal automaticity in latent pacemaker fibers or the development of abnormal automaticity due to partial resting membrane depolarization can serve as a nidus for ventricular tachycardia. Triggered activity does not occur spontaneously; it requires a change in cardiac electrical frequency as a "trigger" such as early depolarizations.

Ventricular tachycardia often accompanies structural heart disease, most commonly ischemic heart disease, and is associated with electrolyte disorders (e.g., hypokalemia and hypomagnesemia), drug toxicity, prolonged QT syndrome, valvular heart disease, and nonischemic cardiomyopathy.

Ventricular tachycardia is typically subdivided into *sustained ventricular tachycardia* (persists >30 seconds or requires termination due to hemodynamic collapse) and *nonsustained ventricular tachycardia* (≥3 beats and ≤30 seconds). Ventricular tachycardia is also categorized by the morphology of the QRS complexes; ventricular tachycardia is *monomorphic* if QRS complexes in the same leads do not vary in contour (Figure 1) or *polymorphic* if the QRS complexes in the same leads do vary in contour (Figure 2). Proper use of these terms and the patient context in which ventricular tachycardia occurs are essential for accurate diagnosis and therapy. It is also imperative to determine the underlying cause of ventricular tachycardia.

Prevention

Because ventricular tachycardia often occurs in the setting of ischemic heart disease, identification and reduction of risk factors for coronary artery disease is indicated.

Screening

Routine screening for ventricular tachycardia in asymptomatic persons is not recommended. Asymptomatic patients with a family history of sudden cardiac death may have long QT syndrome, arrhythmogenic right ventricular dysplasia, or Brugada syndrome (an ion channel disorder associated with incomplete right bundle branch block). A screening electrocardiogram is reasonable in these patients.

Diagnosis

Symptoms are dependent upon several factors, including the ventricular rate, the duration of tachycardia, and the presence of underlying heart disease. Patients with *nonsustained ventricular tachycardia* usually are asymptomatic but may experience palpitations. Patients with *sustained ventricular tachycardia* usually present with syncope or near syncope and can also present with sudden cardiac death.

Ventricular tachyarrhythmias consist of ventricular tachycardia, ventricular fibrillation, and torsades de pointes (a special subset of polymorphic ventricular tachycardia). Ventricular tachyarrhythmias are characterized by wide complex QRS morphology (QRS >0.12 sec) and ventricular rate >100/min. In ventricular tachycardia, the ventricular rate typically ranges from 140-250/min, ventricular fibrillation rate is typically >300/min, and torsades is characterized by a ventricular rate of 200-300/min.

Premature ventricular contractions and other ventricular arrhythmias increase in both prevalence and complexity as the population ages. Although premature ventricular contractions appear to be more frequent in patients with heart disease, they have minimal prognostic significance if left ventricular function is preserved. Among persons with a depressed ejection fraction, frequent premature ventricular contractions are associated with increased mortality, but suppression of premature ventricular contractions with antiarrhythmic drugs does not improve clinical outcome.

Supraventricular tachycardia with a wide QRS complex, usually due to coexisting bundle-branch block or pre-excitation syndrome (Wolff-Parkinson-White), can mimic ventricular tachycardia. Differentiating *ventricular tachycardia* from *supraventricular tachycardia* with aberrant conduction is important because the treatment differs markedly. Ventricular tachycardia is more common than supraventricular tachycardia with aberrancy, particularly in individuals with structural heart disease. A key point is that any wide QRS tachycardia should be considered to be ventricular tachycardia until proven otherwise (Figure 3). The most important differentiating point is the history of ischemic heart disease. In the presence of known structural heart disease, especially a prior myocardial infarction, the diagnosis of ventricular tachycardia is almost certain. Other clues include more profound hemodynamic

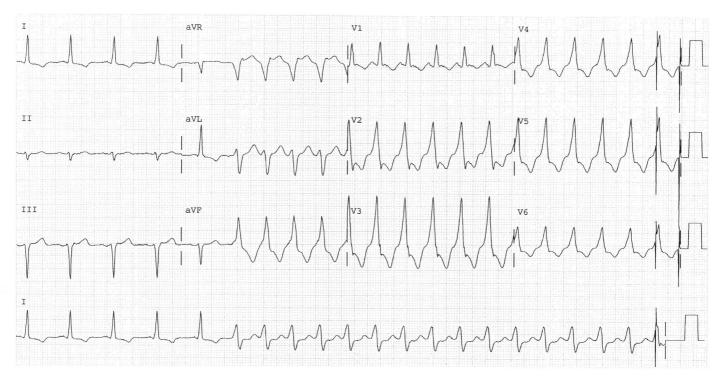

Figure 1 Approximately one quarter of the way into this ECG, monomorphic ventricular tachycardia begins; it is associated with an abrupt change in the QRS axis.

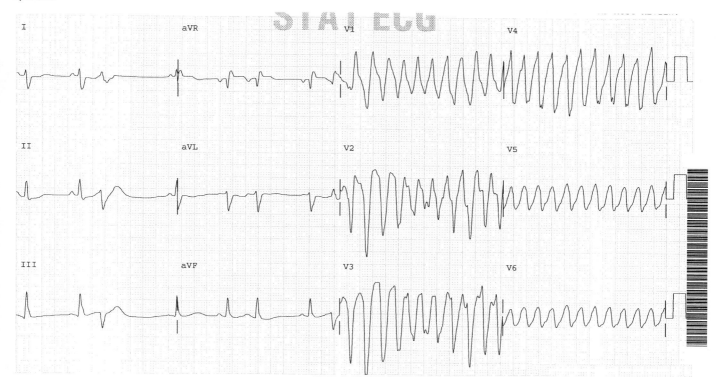

Figure 2 ECG showing degeneration of sinus rhythm into polymorphic ventricular tachycardia.

deterioration in ventricular tachycardia; however, a normal blood pressure does not rule out ventricular tachycardia. Additionally, supraventricular tachycardia and ventricular tachycardia may be distinguished at times by looking for evidence of atrioventricular dissociation on physical examination. The presence of cannon waves (large *a* waves) in the jugular venous pulsations and varying intensity of the first heart sound support atrioventricular dissociation. At times, physical examination and electrocardiography are insufficient to identify the cause of a wide-complex tachycardia; electrophysiologic testing provides definitive diagnosis and is

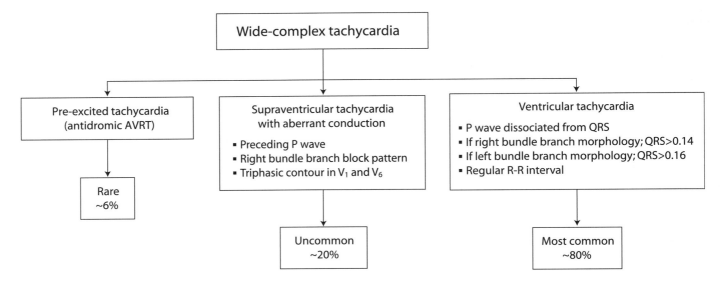

Figure 3 Differentiating ventricular tachycardia from supraventricular tachycardia with aberrancy.

indicated in these patients. In the absence of immediate expert consultation, it is always preferable to assume the patient has ventricular tachycardia and treat accordingly with immediate cardioversion.

Torsades de pointes is a specific form of polymorphic ventricular tachycardia associated with long QT syndrome which may be congenital or acquired. Risk factors for acquired long QT syndrome include female sex, hypokalemia, hypomagnesemia, structural heart disease, and a history of previous long QT or drug-induced arrhythmias. An extensive list of offending agents can be found at www.torsades.org.

Obtain an electrocardiogram immediately in suspected ventricular tachycardia. Look for clues of ischemic heart disease and review prior electrocardiograms for evidence of long QT syndrome and baseline electrocardiographic abnormalities. Search for reversible causes including electrolyte abnormalities (e.g., hypokalemia, hypomagnesemia), cardiac ischemia, heart failure, and drug toxicity. After restoring normal sinus rhythm, obtain an echocardiogram to help establish the presence of structural heart disease and to assess ventricular function.

Therapy

Ventricular tachycardia associated with hemodynamic compromise requires urgent synchronized DC cardioversion if a pulse is present and unsynchronized defibrillation if a pulse is absent. In the absence of structural heart disease, radiofrequency ablation is curative in >90% of patients and is preferred to life-long drug therapy. Primary therapy for ventricular tachycardia with structural heart disease and ejection fraction <35% is an implanted cardiac defibrillator. Several randomized clinical trials have demonstrated a reduction in mortality associated with implantation of a cardiac defibrillator in patients at risk for sudden cardiac death due to left ventricular systolic dysfunction (ejection fraction <35%) regardless of the underlying etiology.

Antiarrhythmic drugs in ventricular tachycardia are used in three primary situations: to terminate an acute episode, to prevent recurrence of ventricular tachycardia, and to prevent life-threatening ventricular fibrillation. The risk-benefit of the pharmacologic treatment of ventricular tachycardia should be considered; antiarrhythmic agents can produce or worsen ventricular tachycardia.

Most patients without heart disease who have monomorphic ventricular tachycardia have a good prognosis and a very low risk of sudden cardiac death. These patients with asymptomatic, nonsustained ventricular tachycardia need not be treated because their prognosis will not be affected.

Pharmacologic therapy for *nonsustained ventricular tachycardia* is usually avoided unless the patient has a history of structural heart disease or long QT syndrome or (rarely) intolerable symptoms. First-line therapy is a usually a β-blocker. When antiarrhythmic drug therapy is necessary due to refractory symptoms in patients with structural heart disease, amiodarone should be considered.

In patients with long QT syndrome, any medication which prolongs the QT interval should be avoided (e.g., class Ia and III antiarrhythmics and certain antihistamines). Intravenous magnesium sulfate can be used to suppress polymorphic ventricular tachycardia in patients with a prolonged QT interval.

Patients with sustained monomorphic ventricular tachycardia in the absence of structural heart disease usually require therapy with a β-blocker because the tachycardia causes symptoms. For acute treatment of sustained monomorphic ventricular tachycardia, intravenous lidocaine, procainamide, or amiodarone may be used. Patients with recurrent sustained ventricular tachycardia require chronic treatment, usually with amiodarone.

Drug therapy in most patients with ventricular tachycardia and structural heart disease is inferior to an implanted cardiac defibrillator and is used only as an adjunct except when an implanted cardiac defibrillator is contraindicated. The β-blockers and the class III agent sotalol are effective for this purpose.

Follow-Up

Appropriate treatment for heart failure, including β-blockers, angiotensin-converting enzyme inhibitors, and spironolactone has been shown to reduce the incidence of sudden death in selected patients with systolic dysfunction.

Book Enhancement

Go to www.acponline.org/essentials/cardiovascular-section.html to access a tutorial on electrocardiographic interpretation and an algorithm for the management of ventricular fibrillation, and to view tables on causes of ventricular arrhythmias and indications for an intracardiac defibrillator. In *MKSAP for Students 4*, assess yourself with items 30-32 in the **Cardiovascular Medicine** section.

Bibliography

American College of Physicians. Medical Knowledge Self-Assessment Program (MKSAP) 14. Philadelphia: American College of Physicians; 2006.

Chapter 6

Heart Failure

James L. Sebastian, MD

Heart failure is a complex clinical syndrome resulting from a structural or functional abnormality that impairs the ability of the ventricles to fill with or eject blood. Although new-onset heart failure often results from acute pump dysfunction caused by myocardial ischemia or infarction, the development and progression of chronic heart failure is typically mediated by ventricular remodeling and activation of endogenous neurohormonal pathways (e.g., renin-angiotensin-aldosterone system, sympathetic nervous system) that have long-term deleterious effects on the heart and play pivotal roles in the pathophysiology of this disorder.

In patients with chronic heart failure, the left ventricle dilates and/or hypertrophies; this causes the chamber to become more spherical in a process called ventricular remodeling. The geometric changes that affect the left ventricle increase wall stress, depress myocardial performance and activate various neurohormonal compensatory responses that result in salt and water retention despite the presence of excess intravascular volume. In addition to causing peripheral vasoconstriction, elevated levels of circulating neurohormones, such as epinephrine, aldosterone, and angiotensin II, may exert direct toxic effects on cardiac cells by promoting further hypertrophy, stimulating myocardial fibrosis and triggering programmed cell death (apoptosis).

Chronic heart failure represents a broad spectrum of disease ranging from asymptomatic persons with risk factors (Stage A) or structural cardiac abnormalities (Stage B) to patients with overt signs and symptoms of heart failure (Stage C), including those with end-stage disease (Stage D) who may require specialized treatments, palliation, and end-of-life care (Figure 1).

Heart failure, which is predominately a disease of the elderly, represents a major United States public health problem, with a prevalence of over 5 million and an incidence of over 500,000 cases each year. Approximately 80% of patients hospitalized with heart failure are over age 65, making heart failure the most common and most expensive Medicare diagnosis-related group.

Prevention

Longstanding untreated hypertension is associated with the development of both systolic and diastolic heart failure and is an independent risk factor for coronary artery disease. Even modest decreases in systolic blood pressure markedly reduce mortality and the risk of developing heart failure.

Diabetes produces morphologic and functional myocardial abnormalities independent of coronary artery disease and hypertension. Diabetes is associated with left ventricular hypertrophy and arterial wall stiffening, which may result in impaired left ventricular relaxation and distensibility. Aggressive blood pressure and lipid control appears to provide additional benefits to patients with diabetes above those seen in the general population. Angiotensin-converting enzyme (ACE) inhibitors and angiotensin-receptor blockers can prevent the development of heart failure and also provide renal protection in patients with diabetes.

Advise patients to avoid exposure to cardiotoxic substances such as alcohol, tobacco, and illicit drugs, particularly cocaine. Alcohol is a direct myocardial toxin and can cause heart failure. In some patients, abstinence from alcohol can reverse left ventricular dysfunction. Tobacco use significantly increases the risk of coronary artery disease, which in turn can lead to heart failure. Cocaine has direct, as well as indirect, effects on the myocardium that increase the risk of heart failure and sudden cardiac death.

Prolonged tachycardia may be associated with the development of a reversible form of left ventricular dysfunction. Control rapid ventricular responses in patients with atrial fibrillation and other supraventricular tachycardias in order to prevent the development of tachycardia-induced cardiomyopathy. Cardioversion to normal sinus rhythm or improved rate control can restore left ventricular function.

Screening

Because ischemic heart disease is one of the major causes of heart failure in the United States, patients at high-risk for developing coronary artery disease are screened as recommended by national guidelines. Cardiac perfusion imaging at the time of exercise stress testing may establish coronary artery disease as the underlying cause of left ventricular dysfunction. Revascularization may reduce the risk of myocardial infarction and subsequent heart failure. Coronary artery bypass graft surgery in patients with diminished left ventricular function improves ventricular performance and survival compared with medical therapy alone.

Evaluate asymptomatic patients with diastolic, holosystolic, or midsystolic heart murmurs grade ≥3 and all patients with a heart murmur accompanied by symptoms of myocardial infarction, syncope, endocarditis, or thromboembolism with an echocardiogram to detect the presence of significant valvular heart disease. Early identification of a significant valvular abnormality may prevent the development of left ventricular dysfunction if the valve can be repaired or replaced.

Look for familial patterns of heart failure by obtaining detailed family histories that focus on episodes of unexplained heart failure, sudden cardiac death, and progressive heart failure in

At Risk for Heart Failure　　　　　　　　　　　　**Heart Failure**

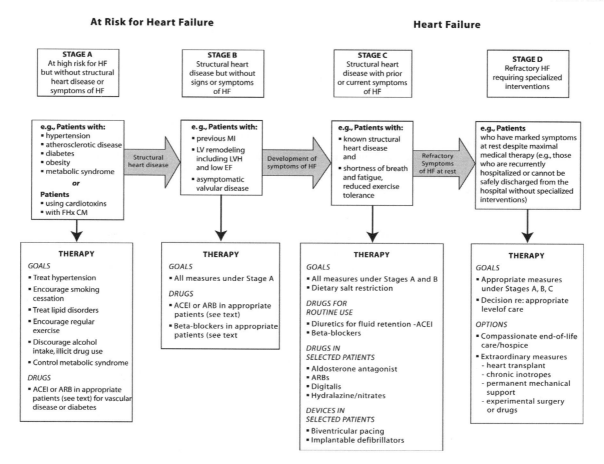

Figure 1　Stages in the development of heart failure and recommended therapy by stage. (ACEI = angiotensin-converting enzyme inhibitors; ARBs = angiotensin receptor blockers; EF = ejection fraction; FHx CM = family history of cardiomyopathy; HF = heart failure; LV = left ventricular; LVH = left ventricular hypertrophy; MI = myocardial infarction.) (From Circulation. 2005;112:154-235. Copyright © 2005 by American College of Cardiology Foundation and American Heart Association; with permission.)

young family members. Dilated cardiomyopathies may be familial in a significant percentage of cases. Identification of asymptomatic ventricular dysfunction may allow earlier intervention. A personal or family history of hemochromatosis, Wilson's disease, hypertrophic cardiomyopathy, or amyloidosis may also warrant echocardiographic screening of asymptomatic family members.

Diagnosis

In addition to establishing the diagnosis of heart failure, determine the underlying etiology, differentiate between systolic and diastolic dysfunction, and identify any specific exacerbating or precipitating factors.

The classical manifestations of heart failure include fatigue, dyspnea on exertion, orthopnea, paroxysmal nocturnal dyspnea, and fluid retention. Dyspnea at rest and fatigue may indicate a low cardiac output state. It is important to note that older patients with heart failure often present with nonspecific symptoms such as nocturia, insomnia, irritability, and anorexia that are misdiagnosed as age-related changes or ascribed to age prevalent co-morbidities.

The medical history is also used to assess functional capacity, most commonly expressed in terms of the New York Heart Association (NYHA) classification that describes the effort needed to elicit symptoms:

- *Class I:* Asymptomatic left ventricular dysfunction
- *Class II:* Dyspnea with significant exertion
- *Class III:* Dyspnea with minimal activity including usual activities of daily living
- *Class IV:* Dyspnea at rest

Although the presence of jugular venous distention, abdominal jugular reflux, pulmonary rales, ventricular gallops (S_3 or S_4), any cardiac murmur, and lower extremity edema all increase the likelihood of heart failure, these findings often do not predict the hemodynamic impairment in chronic heart failure. For example, pulmonary rales may reflect the rapidity of onset of heart failure, rather than the degree of volume overload. Elevated jugular venous pressure and an S_3 are each independently associated with adverse outcomes, including progression of heart failure.

Obtain a resting 12-lead electrocardiogram in any patient with new-onset heart failure or an exacerbation of preexisting heart failure to identify the cardiac rhythm and determine the presence of ischemia, prior infarction, left ventricular hypertrophy, and/or conduction system abnormalities.

Common radiographic findings in heart failure patients include cardiomegaly, pulmonary vascular congestion, and pleural effusions, which are often bilateral. Although a chest x-ray may be helpful in determining the cause of a patient's dyspnea, serial chest films are not sensitive to small changes in pulmonary vascular congestion and are not recommended.

Measurement of b-type natriuretic peptide (BNP), a sensitive marker of ventricular pressure and volume overload, should be considered in the evaluation of heart failure when diagnostic uncertainty exists. Higher BNP levels are suggestive of heart failure and may provide additional prognostic information. Conversely, low serum BNP levels are most useful for excluding a diagnosis of heart failure in patients with symptoms of acute dyspnea. In one recent review, a serum BNP level <100 pg/mL was determined to be the most useful test for ruling out heart failure in an emergency department setting, with a negative likelihood ratio of 0.11.

Transthoracic echocardiography is routinely used to determine the underlying etiology of heart failure and is critically important in formulating an effective, individualized treatment plan. Transthoracic echocardiography differentiates between systolic and diastolic dysfunction, and this distinction informs treatment strategies. Systolic dysfunction is usually defined as a left ventricular ejection fraction <40%. The echocardiogram typically shows evidence of ventricular remodeling with an increased left ventricular end diastolic volume and impaired indices of left ventricular contractility. Coronary artery disease, which is the underlying cause of systolic heart failure in about two-thirds of patients, may show echocardiographic evidence of regional wall motion abnormalities and/or post-myocardial infarction ventricular remodeling.

Patients with diastolic dysfunction have ejection fractions >40%. These patients typically have echocardiographic evidence of left ventricular hypertrophy, normal left ventricular end-diastolic volume, and abnormalities of left ventricular diastolic properties, including delayed active relaxation and increased passive stiffness. Because the actual measurement of diastolic function is complex and lacks sensitivity and specificity, the diagnosis of diastolic dysfunction is usually based on the typical symptoms and signs of heart failure associated with normal left ventricular ejection fraction and no valvular abnormalities on echocardiogram. Diastolic heart failure is common, especially in elderly patients, and in conditions causing significant left ventricular hypertrophy, such as hypertension, aortic stenosis, and hypertrophic cardiomyopathy.

Traditional exercise stress tests or pharmacologic stress tests may be useful in selected patients to differentiate heart failure from other conditions, confirm functional capacity, and identify myocardial ischemia. Functional class assessed by stress testing is among the most powerful predictors of survival and outcomes in heart failure.

Therapy

Limiting dietary sodium to 2 g daily and fluid to 2 quarts per day results in fewer hospitalizations for decompensated heart failure. Patients with more severe heart failure may need more rigorous limitations.

Because exercise may improve both physical and psychological well-being, encourage patients to participate in a long-term aerobic exercise program that is tailored to their functional capacity. Improvement in metabolic and hemodynamic indices occurs in patients with heart failure who undergo exercise conditioning.

All forms of sleep-disordered breathing are common in patients with cardiovascular diseases, especially heart failure and hypertension. Effective therapy of sleep-disordered breathing is associated with significant improvement in blood pressure control, exercise capacity, and quality of life, as well as decreased rates of disease progression and re-hospitalizations for heart failure.

Angiotensin-converting enzyme inhibitors, β-blockers, and, in selected patients, aldosterone antagonists improve survival in heart failure due to systolic dysfunction. Judicious use of digitalis can prevent hospitalization. In one study, the addition of a fixed dose of hydralazine and nitrates increased survival among black patients already taking standard therapy including angiotensin-converting enzyme inhibitors and β-blockers. Drug therapy for patients with systolic dysfunction is summarized in Table 1.

The management of patients with diastolic heart failure is based largely on theoretical concepts and extrapolations from trials in heart failure patients with low ejection fractions. There is general agreement that the approach to such patients includes control of heart rate and blood pressure, maintenance of normal sinus rhythm, and identification and management of myocardial ischemia.

Refer patients with NYHA class III or IV heart failure and a prolonged QRS duration (>120 msec) on electrocardiography for biventricular pacing. Cardiac resynchronization therapy in these patients improves functional capacity, quality of life, and mortality.

Implantation of a cardioverter defibrillator in patients with significant left ventricular systolic dysfunction (ejection fraction ≤30%-35%) is associated with a reduction in mortality regardless of whether the underlying cardiomyopathy was secondary to an ischemic or nonischemic etiology.

Cardiac transplantation improves survival, functional status, and quality of life in patients with NYHA class III or IV heart failure. Refer patients with severe intractable heart failure despite maximal medical therapy to a cardiac transplantation program for evaluation. Relative contraindications to cardiac transplant include age >65, end-organ damage from diabetes or vascular disease, malignancy, previous stroke, lack of psychosocial support, or active psychiatric illness.

Follow-Up

Once the diagnosis of heart failure and its underlying etiology are established, identify and correct factors responsible for any symptomatic exacerbation. Common reasons for an increase in symptoms or decline in functional status include myocardial ischemia and/or infarction, cardiac arrhythmias (i.e., atrial fibrillation), severe hypertension, worsening renal function, and noncompliance with medications or diet. In general, any condition that causes tachycardia (e.g., fever, infection, anemia, thyrotoxicosis) has the potential to exacerbate heart failure symptoms by

Table 1. Drug Treatment for Heart Failure due to Systolic Dysfunction

Drug	Notes
Angiotensin-converting enzyme inhibitors (enalapril, captopril, lisinopril)	For all classes of heart failure. Inhibits angiotensin-converting enzyme, resulting in decreased conversion of angiotensin I to angiotensin II and decreased metabolism of bradykinin. Improves exercise tolerance, hemodynamic status, and survival. May halt progression and cause regression of HF. Avoid in patients with history of ACE inhibitor-induced angioedema.
β-blockers (carvedilol, metoprolol, bisoprolol)	For all classes of heart failure. Inhibits adrenergic nervous system and improves survival. Reduces sudden death risk and may halt progression and cause regression of HF. Use with caution in patients with NYHA class IV HF. Avoid in patients with significant asthma and high-grade conduction system disease.
Aldosterone antagonists (spironolactone, eplerenone)	Improves survival in patients with NYHA III-IV HF. Improves survival after myocardial infarction with LV dysfunction. Follow potassium level, especially in patients taking ACE inhibitors.
Angiotensin-receptor antagonists (losartan, valsartan, candesartan)	Use in patients who cannot take ACE inhibitors. Inhibits renin-angiotensin system at angiotensin receptor level. Improvement in hemodynamics, symptoms.
Hydralazine and nitrates (isosorbide dinitrate, isosorbide mononitrate)	Reserved for patients intolerant to ACE inhibitors and ARB. Reduces afterload and preload. Improves survival in patients with HF but not so well as ACE inhibitors. May further reduce mortality in black patients when added to ACE inhibitors and β-blockers.
Digitalis glycoside (digoxin)	Positive inotropic agent. Slows heart rate through vagal effects, improves exercise tolerance, and reduces hospitalizations. No survival benefit. Aim for level <2.0 ng/mL. Use lower dose in elderly and in patients with renal insufficiency. Avoid hypokalemia.
Loop diuretics (furosemide, torsemide, bumetanide, ethacrynic acid)	Palliative in patients with congestive symptoms. No survival benefit.
Positive inotropic agents (dobutamine, milrinone)	Used to improve hemodynamics in patients with severe HF and to maintain patients until cardiac transplantation; can also be used continuously at home in nontransplant candidates for palliation. Arrhythmogenic; no survival benefit.

ACE = angiotensin-converting enzyme; ARB = angiotensin-receptor blocker; HF = heart failure; NYHA = New York Heart Association; LV = left ventricular.

shortening diastole and impairing left ventricular filling. Since polypharmacy is a frequent problem in older patients, be aware that concomitant use of noncardiac medications such as nonsteroidal anti-inflammatory drugs and thiazolidinediones may cause significant fluid retention and worsen heart failure.

Serial measurements of a patient's weight will determine clinical stability or the need to adjust diuretic doses. Electrolyte disturbances in heart failure are common due to the effect of medications as well as the pathophysiology of heart failure. Serum sodium ≤134 meq/L is an independent risk factor for mortality in heart failure.

Book Enhancement

Go to www.acponline.org/essentials/cardiovascular-section.html to view a chest x-ray showing pulmonary edema and to access tables on the differential diagnosis of heart failure, heart failure mimics, commonly used tests to evaluate heart failure, and a schema outlining the pathophysiology of heart failure. In *MKSAP for Students 4*, assess yourself with items 33-41 in the **Cardiovascular Medicine** section.

Bibliography

Cook DJ, Simel DL. The Rational Clinical Examination. Does this patient have abnormal central venous pressure? JAMA. 1996;275:630-4. [PMID: 8594245]

Goldberg LR, Eisen H. Heart Failure. http://pier.acponline.org/physicians/diseases/d105. [Date accessed: 2008 Jan 17] In: PIER [online database]. Philadelphia: American College of Physicians; 2008.

Wang CS, FitzGerald JM, Schulzer M, et al. Does this dyspneic patient in the emergency department have congestive heart failure? JAMA. 2005;294:1944-56. [PMID: 16234501]

Wilson JF. In the Clinic. Heart failure. Ann Intern Med. 2007;147:ITC12-1-ITC12-16. [PMID: 18056658]

Chapter 7

Valvular Heart Disease

H. Douglas Walden, MD

Introduction

Prevention

Antibiotic treatment of group A streptococcal infections and long-term prophylactic antibiotic therapy of patients with a history of rheumatic carditis may decrease the likelihood of rheumatic valvular heart disease. Endocarditis prophylaxis is indicated only for patients with prior episodes of endocarditis or with prosthetic heart valves.

Screening

Routine screening for valvular heart disease is not recommended, although a high degree of suspicion should be present whenever a patient presents with chest pain, heart failure, arrhythmias, congenital abnormalities (Marfan's), or a history of rheumatic fever.

Approach to Cardiac Murmurs

Cardiac murmurs result from increased blood flow across a normal orifice (e.g., anemia, thyrotoxicosis, pregnancy), turbulent flow through a narrowed orifice (e.g., aortic and mitral stenosis), or regurgitant flow through an incompetent valve (e.g., aortic and mitral regurgitation). Determining the timing in the cardiac cycle, chest wall location, radiation, intensity (Table 1), configuration, duration, and pitch all assist in the differential diagnosis. Not all systolic murmurs are pathologic. Asymptomatic patients with short, soft systolic murmurs (grade < 3) often do not require further investigation. The presence of any diastolic or continuous murmur, cardiac symptoms (chest pain, dyspnea, or syncope), abnormalities on examination (clicks, abnormal S_2, abnormal pulses) requires evaluation by echocardiography (Figure 1).

Various interventions may alter the intensity of murmurs (Table 2). The murmur of hypertrophic cardiomyopathy may increase with standing or Valsalva (decreased venous return decreases left ventricular chamber size and increases the degree of obstruction). The click and murmur of mitral valve prolapse may move earlier in systole and increase in intensity with standing or Valsalva (mitral prolapse increases with decreased ventricular volume and chamber size).

Aortic outflow murmurs increase in intensity the beat following a premature ventricular contraction (increased left ventricular volume). Murmurs of mitral regurgitation, ventricular septal defect, and aortic regurgitation augment with handgrip (increased cardiac output and peripheral resistance). Right-sided heart murmurs may increase during inspiration (increased venous return).

Aortic Stenosis

Aortic stenosis in adults occurs as a result of rheumatic heart disease, degeneration of a congenital bicuspid valve, or senile degeneration of a normal tri-leaflet valve. A prolonged asymptomatic period of many years is marked by progressive left ventricular hypertrophy and is followed by a shorter (1-3 years) symptomatic period characterized by angina, syncope, and heart failure. Surgical valve replacement is the definitive therapy.

Diagnosis

Exercise intolerance is an early symptom; symptoms of more advanced disease include dyspnea, angina, or exertional syncope. Physical examination reveals a crescendo-decrescendo systolic murmur loudest at the second right intercostal space with radiation to the carotids. The murmur becomes longer and peaks later in systole with more advanced disease. It may soften in the presence of left ventricular dysfunction. The second heart sound may be diminished in intensity because the valve loses mobility in patients with calcific disease. In patients with mild-to-moderate aortic stenosis due to a bicuspid valve, S_2 may be accentuated and

Grade	Description
1	Murmur heard with stethoscope but not at first
2	Faint murmur heard with stethoscope on chest wall
3	Murmur heard with stethoscope on chest wall, louder than grade 2 but without a thrill
4	Murmur associated with a thrill
5	Murmur heard with just the rim of the stethoscope held against the chest
6	Murmur heard with the stethoscope held close to but not touching the chest wall

Table 1. Grading the Intensity of Cardiac Murmurs

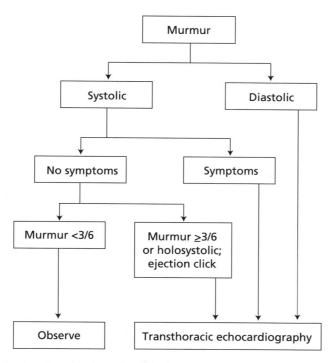

Figure 1 Decision pathway for ordering transthoracic echocardiography. (From MKSAP 14. Philadelphia: American College of Physicians; 2006.)

Table 2. Characteristics of Selected Heart Murmurs

Type	Description	Effect of Maneuvers
Systolic		
Innocent flow murmur	Mid-systolic, soft, crescendo-decrescendo; at base	None
Aortic stenosis	Systolic, harsh, crescendo-decrescendo; at right second intercostal space with radiation to carotids	↓ Handgrip or standing
Hypertrophic obstructive cardiomyopathy	Systolic, late-peaking; at base with radiation to the carotids	↓ Handgrip; ↑ Valsalva or standing
Mitral regurgitation	Pansystolic, blowing; at apex and may radiate to axilla	↑ Handgrip
Mitral valve prolapse	Mid- to late-systolic preceded by one or more clicks; at apex	Murmur and clicks move closer to S_1 with Valsalva or standing
Tricuspid regurgitation	Pansystolic, blowing; at lower left sternal border with radiation to lower right sternal border	↑ with inspiration
Pulmonic stenosis	Systolic, crescendo-decrescendo; at left second intercostal space with radiation to left sternal border	↑ with inspiration
Ventricular septal defect	Pansystolic at lower left sternal border	↑ Handgrip
Diastolic		
Aortic insufficiency	Pan-diastolic or early diastolic, decrescendo, high-pitched	Loudest with patient leaning forward
Mitral stenosis	Early diastole, decrescendo, low-pitched rumble; at apex	Loudest with patient in left lateral decubitus position
Pulmonic insufficiency	Pan-diastolic or early diastolic, decrescendo; at left second intercostal space with radiation to left sternal border	None

associated with an aortic ejection click heard best at the right upper sternal border. An S_4 gallop may accompany left ventricular hypertrophy. Pulsus parvus et tardus (dampened and delayed carotid pulsations) may be present, but carotid upstrokes can be brisk in elderly patients with noncompliant vessels.

Chest x-ray may demonstrate a boot-shaped silhouette of left ventricular hypertrophy. Electrocardiography may demonstrate left atrial or left ventricular enlargement. Echocardiograms often demonstrate thickened and calcified aortic valve leaflets with restricted motion. Doppler studies can estimate the transvalvular pressure gradient and aortic valve area. A coronary angiogram is obtained in patients aged >35 years prior to aortic valve surgery and all patients aged <35 years with left ventricular systolic dysfunction or risk factors for premature coronary disease.

Therapy

Aortic valve replacement is indicated in patients with symptomatic severe disease (<1.0 cm^2 valve area) but not for most asymptomatic patients. Left ventricular failure is associated with an increased mortality rate, but is not a contraindication to surgery. Balloon aortic valvuloplasty does not improve survival and is associated with a high rate of restenosis but can be considered as a temporizing measure in selected patients.

Cardioversion or atrioventricular nodal blocking agents (e.g., diltiazem, metoprolol) are used to manage atrial fibrillation. Careful use of angiotensin-converting enzyme inhibitors, digoxin, and diuretics may result in symptomatic improvement in heart failure but are of limited value if surgical therapy cannot be utilized. Marked changes in blood pressure may not be well tolerated because patients with aortic stenosis are dependent on adequate preload.

Follow-Up

Asymptomatic patients with mild disease typically remain stable for years. The degree of aortic valve calcification, the presence of coronary disease, and more severe valvular disease predict worse outcomes without surgery. A history, physical examination, and transthoracic echocardiogram are performed at least annually, with more frequent clinical evaluation in patients with more advanced disease.

Aortic Insufficiency

Acute severe aortic insufficiency is caused by infective endocarditis, aortic dissection, or trauma, often presents as cardiogenic shock, and usually requires emergent valve replacement. Chronic aortic insufficiency may result from rheumatic heart disease, previous endocarditis, calcific degeneration, aortic root disease, or tertiary syphilis. The clinical presentations of acute and chronic disease differ. Chronic disease improves with vasodilator therapy, although definitive surgical treatment prior to left ventricular dysfunction remains the optimal long-term choice.

Diagnosis

The diagnosis of acute aortic insufficiency is suggested in patients with rapid onset of dyspnea, exercise intolerance, or chest pain (aortic dissection). Physical findings include tachycardia, hypotension, a soft S_1 (due to premature closure of the mitral valve), an S_3 and/or S_4 gallop, an accentuated pulmonic closure sound, and pulmonary crackles. Heart size may be normal and pulse pressure may not be widened. The typical murmur of aortic insufficiency may not be prominent in acute disease as aortic and left ventricular diastolic pressures equilibrate quickly, resulting in a short and soft (sometimes inaudible) diastolic murmur.

Symptoms of chronic disease include dyspnea on exertion, orthopnea, paroxysmal nocturnal dyspnea, angina, and palpitations. Some patients remain asymptomatic for long periods as the left ventricle insidiously dilates. Physical findings include cardiomegaly, tachycardia, a widened pulse pressure, a thrill at the base of the heart, a soft S_1 and sometimes absent aortic closure sound, and an S_3 gallop. The characteristic high-pitched diastolic murmur begins immediately after S_2 and is heard at the second right or third left intercostal space, heard best with the patient seated, leaning forward, and in end-expiration. Manifestations of the widened pulse pressure may include Traube's sign (pistol shot sounds over the peripheral arteries), de Musset's sign (head bobs with each heartbeat), Duroziez's sign (systolic and diastolic murmur heard over the femoral artery), and Quincke's sign (systolic plethora and diastolic blanching in the nail bed with nail compression).

Chest x-ray may reveal cardiomegaly, valve calcification, enlargement of the aortic root, or pulmonary congestion. Electrocardiography can show left axis deviation and left ventricular hypertrophy. A serologic test (i.e., VDRL, RPR) is needed to exclude tertiary syphilis. Doppler echocardiography with color flow can confirm the presence and severity of disease and assess etiology.

Therapy

Immediate aortic valve replacement is indicated in acute disease because a normal left ventricle cannot accommodate the large regurgitant volume. Aortic valve replacement is also the treatment of choice for patients with severe chronic disease. Left ventricular systolic function is the most important determinant of survival. Valve replacement is indicated for all patients with more than mild symptoms, patients with progressive left ventricular dilatation, and for left ventricular ejection fraction of $<50\%$.

Vasodilators are the predominant drug therapy. In acute disease, sodium nitroprusside or intravenous nitroglycerin leads to augmentation of forward cardiac output, reduction of regurgitant flow, and an improved ejection fraction. Intravenous diuretics and inotropic agents (dobutamine) may also support blood pressure and improve cardiac contractility. In chronic aortic insufficiency, oral hydralazine or nifedipine improves forward stroke volume and reduces the regurgitant volume. Nifedipine may significantly reduce or delay the need for aortic valve replacement in patients with severe aortic insufficiency and normal left ventricular function. Angiotensin-converting enzyme inhibitors may also be helpful.

Follow-Up

A history, physical examination, and echocardiogram are performed every 2 to 3 years in asymptomatic patients with normal left ventricular size and function. Evaluation every six to twelve months is needed in asymptomatic patients with severe aortic insufficiency and in patients with dilated left ventricles. Echocardiography should also be obtained if there are new or changing symptoms, worsening exercise tolerance, or clinical findings suggestive of progressive disease.

Mitral Stenosis

Nearly all mitral stenosis in adults is due to rheumatic heart disease. Rare causes include malignant carcinoid, systemic lupus erythematosus, rheumatoid arthritis, and amyloidosis. Valve thickening and calcification impair flow from the left atrium to left ventricle leading to pulmonary hypertension and right heart failure. Symptoms develop after years of valvular dysfunction. Surgical valve repair is the definitive treatment of severe disease.

Diagnosis

Symptoms of mitral stenosis consist of dyspnea, fatigue, edema, orthopnea, paroxysmal nocturnal dyspnea, cough, hemoptysis, hoarseness, anginal chest pain, palpitations, and symptoms suggestive of systemic embolism. Physical findings include a prominent a-wave in the jugular pulse (decreased right ventricular compliance with pulmonary hypertension), a palpable thrill at the apex, a right ventricular heave, and signs of right-sided heart failure (e.g., jugular venous distention, hepatomegaly, ascites, and edema). Cardiac auscultation reveals accentuation of P_2 (evidence of elevated pulmonary arterial pressure), an opening snap (a high-pitched apical sound best heard with the diaphragm), and a low-pitched, rumbling diastolic murmur best heard at the apex using the bell with the patient in the left lateral decubitus position. Presystolic accentuation of the murmur may be present in both sinus rhythm and atrial fibrillation. As the severity of the stenosis worsens, the opening snap moves closer to S_2 as a result of increased left atrial pressure and the murmur increases in duration.

A chest x-ray may reveal chamber enlargement and interstitial edema. An electrocardiogram often demonstrates rhythm abnormalities (i.e., atrial fibrillation), right axis deviation, or left atrial and right ventricular enlargement. A transthoracic echocardiogram with Doppler assesses valve morphology, involvement of other valves, chamber size and function, presence of left atrial thrombus and can exclude other conditions that mimic mitral stenosis. The valve surface area, the pressure gradient across the valve, and concomitant mitral regurgitation can be determined utilizing Doppler techniques.

Therapy

Mitral valvotomy or valve replacement is the treatment of choice in symptomatic patients. Percutaneous balloon valvotomy is suitable in symptomatic patients with moderate-to-severe disease and pliable noncalcified leaflets with minimal mitral regurgitation. Valve replacement is recommended for patients with moderate or severe disease (marked limitation of physical activity or inability to perform any physical activity) who are not candidates for valvotomy or valve repair, or for patients with severe pulmonary hypertension. Open valvotomy is associated with an operative mortality of 1%-3%. Mortality associated with mitral valve replacement depends on functional status, age, left ventricular function, and

the presence of coronary artery disease, but may be as high as 10%-20% in older patients with comorbidities.

β-blockers or calcium-channel blockers with negative chronotropic properties increase diastolic filling time and are utilized for patients with symptoms associated with tachycardia. Diuretics are useful if pulmonary vascular congestion is present. Atrial fibrillation is usually treated with anticoagulants and atrioventricular nodal blockers to control heart rate but anti-arrhythmic agents or electrical cardioversion may be considered for worsening symptoms. Warfarin therapy (goal INR, 2.0-3.0) is recommended for patients with a history of previous embolic events, atrial fibrillation, sinus rhythm and an enlarged left atrium, and those with left atrial thrombi. Patients with a mitral bioprosthesis with concomitant atrial fibrillation, left ventricular dysfunction, a previous thromboembolism, or a hypercoagulable state also receive warfarin. Treat patients with a mechanical mitral prosthesis with warfarin to a target INR of 2.5-3.5 and low-dose aspirin.

Follow-Up

Asymptomatic and mildly symptomatic patients are evaluated annually by history, physical examination, electrocardiography, and chest x-ray. Patients who have undergone percutaneous or surgical mitral valvuloplasty are evaluated with a post-procedure echocardiogram and an annual evaluation thereafter. An echocardiogram is obtained if symptoms recur or if a change in physical examination is noted.

Mitral Regurgitation

Acute mitral regurgitation may result from ruptured chordae tendineae, ruptured papillary muscle, myxomatous degeneration, infective endocarditis, trauma, and acute myocardial ischemia. Mitral valve prolapse is currently the most common cause of chronic disease, followed by ischemic mitral valve disease. Mitral annular calcification is a common cause of mitral regurgitation in older individuals, whereas rheumatic heart disease is now a relatively uncommon cause.

Diagnosis

Acute, severe mitral regurgitation causes abrupt onset of dyspnea, pulmonary edema, or cardiogenic shock. Physical findings may include hypotension, an apical holosystolic murmur radiating to the axilla (the murmur may be short or absent), an S_3 or S_4 gallop, pulmonary crackles, and signs of right-heart failure (e.g., jugular venous distention, hepatomegaly and edema).

Chronic mitral regurgitation results in exercise intolerance, dyspnea, or fatigue. Physical findings include brisk carotid upstrokes, a laterally displaced apical impulse, decreased intensity of S_1, increased intensity of P_2, a widely split S_2 during inspiration and an S_3 gallop. The holosystolic murmur is best heard with the diaphragm at the apex with the patient in the left lateral decubitus position; the murmur may radiate to the left axilla and left scapular region. In advanced cases, the chest x-ray may reveal cardiomegaly and pulmonary vascular congestion. An electrocardiogram may demonstrate an abnormal rhythm (i.e., atrial fibrillation), left atrial enlargement, and left ventricular hypertrophy. An echocardiogram with Doppler allows for assessment of left atrial and left ventricular volumes, ejection fraction, and other valvular disease. The left ventricular ejection fraction may be normal or falsely elevated due to systolic ejection of a portion of left ventricular volume into the low pressure left atria.

Therapy

Repair or replacement of the mitral valve is indicated in symptomatic patients with acute disease. Intra-aortic balloon counterpulsation can improve coronary perfusion and reduce afterload in hemodynamically unstable patients. In chronic disease, survival is dependent upon left ventricular function, and surgery is most effective prior to development of heart failure, atrial fibrillation, and pulmonary hypertension. Patients who display echocardiographic features of left ventricular dilatation and/or depressed function are candidates for surgical intervention. Valve repair has advantages to replacement, including the avoidance of anticoagulants and future mechanical valve failure.

In acute mitral regurgitation, vasodilators (sodium nitroprusside and nitroglycerin) and diuretics reduce pulmonary congestion and improve forward cardiac output. An inotropic agent (dobutamine) may be used if hypotension develops; intra-aortic balloon counterpulsation may be needed. In chronic mitral regurgitation with depressed left ventricular function, diuretics, β-blockers, and angiotensin-converting enzyme inhibitors (or angiotensin II receptor blockers) are indicated. Anticoagulants and atrioventricular nodal blocking agents are used in patients with atrial fibrillation.

Follow-Up

An annual history, physical examination, and echocardiogram are appropriate for mild disease. More frequent monitoring is indicated for advanced disease. Patients with evidence of progressive left ventricular dysfunction require surgical intervention. Anticoagulation with warfarin (goal INR, 2.5-3.5) and perhaps aspirin is indicated for patients with mechanical mitral prostheses, atrial fibrillation, left ventricular dysfunction, or previous thromboembolism.

Mitral Valve Prolapse

Mitral valve prolapse results from myxomatous degeneration and is the most common congenital valvular abnormality with a prevalence of 4%-5%. Many patients are asymptomatic, others require symptomatic treatment, and occasional patients may progress to severe mitral regurgitation requiring valve surgery or repair.

Diagnosis

Patients may experience chest pain, palpitations, dizziness, syncope, dyspnea, fatigue, or symptoms of embolic phenomena.

Auscultation may reveal a high-pitched, midsystolic click sometimes followed by a late systolic murmur loudest at the apex. The click and murmur are accentuated and move earlier into systole as left ventricular volume decreases (standing or Valsalva).

Chest x-ray may reveal chamber enlargement, thoracic aneurysm formation, and skeletal abnormalities (e.g., pectus excavatum or carinatum, abnormalities of the thoracic spine). Electrocardiography may reveal a prolonged QT interval and arrhythmias. Echocardiography is used to assess severity of mitral regurgitation, mitral leaflet morphology, and left ventricular size and function. Severe regurgitation, thick and redundant leaflets, flail leaflets, and left atrial and left ventricular enlargement are associated with adverse outcomes. Ambulatory electrocardiographic monitoring may detect arrhythmias in patients with palpitations, dizziness, or syncope.

Therapy

Dietary and lifestyle modifications (restriction of alcohol, caffeine, and smoking) are the initial treatment of palpitations, chest pain, anxiety, and fatigue. Surgical intervention (mitral valve repair or replacement) is indicated for severe mitral regurgitation.

β-blockers are used for persistent palpitations, chest pain, anxiety, or fatigue. Anticoagulation with warfarin is indicated if structural cardiac disease and atrial fibrillation are present.

Follow-Up

Patients with asymptomatic prolapse and no significant mitral regurgitation are evaluated every 3-5 years. Serial echocardiography is useful for patients with thickened, redundant mitral leaflets, chest pain or syncope, or left ventricular dysfunction/mitral regurgitation. The development of significant mitral regurgitation may ultimately require mitral valve surgery.

Book Enhancement

Go to www.acponline.org/essentials/cardiovascular-section.html to view a video and listen to the murmurs of aortic stenosis, mitral stenosis, and mitral regurgitation and to access tables on the differential diagnosis of valvular heart lesions and indications for endocarditis prophylaxis. In *MKSAP for Students 4*, assess yourself with items 42-49 in the **Cardiovascular Medicine** section.

Bibliography

Choudhry NK, Etchells EE. The rational clinical examination. Does this patient have aortic regurgitation? JAMA. 1999;281:2231-8. [PMID: 10376577]

Etchells E, Bell C, Robb K. Does this patient have an abnormal systolic murmur? JAMA. 1997;277:564-71. [PMID: 9032164]

Moore M. Aortic Regurgitation. http://pier.acponline.org/physicians/diseases/d450 [Date accessed: 2008 Feb 13] In: PIER [online database]. Philadelphia: American College of Physicians; 2008.

Moore M, Rogers J. Aortic Stenosis. http://pier.acponline.org/physicians/diseases/d414 [Date accessed: 2008 Feb 13] In: PIER [online database]. Philadelphia: American College of Physicians; 2008.

Moore M, Rogers J. Mitral Stenosis. http://pier.acponline.org/physicians/ diseases/d451 [Date accessed: 2008 Feb 13] In: PIER [online database]. Philadelphia: American College of Physicians; 2008.

Rogers J. Mitral Regurgitation. http://pier.acponline.org/physicians/ diseases/d452 [Date accessed: 2008 Feb 13] In: PIER [online database]. Philadelphia: American College of Physicians; 2008.

Rogers J. Mitral Valve Prolapse. http://pier.acponline.org/physicians/ diseases/d452 [Date accessed: 2008 Feb 13] In: PIER [online database]. Philadelphia: American College of Physicians; 2008.

Section II
Endocrinology and Metabolism

Chapter 8

Diabetes Mellitus and Diabetic Ketoacidosis

Erik K. Alexander, MD

Diabetes Mellitus

Diabetes mellitus is a heterogeneous disorder with a common clinical phenotype of inappropriate glucose metabolism. Diabetes affects nearly 20 million people in the United States. This number is increasing and largely parallels the epidemic of obesity. Diabetes remains a major contributor to heart disease, blindness, renal failure, and other complications, making it a major focus for public health initiatives. Type 2 diabetes is a common disorder, often asymptomatic, and frequently not diagnosed for several years because of the lack of initial symptoms.

Two processes are central to the development of all diabetes mellitus; β-cell failure to produce insulin in a sufficient and reliable manner, or insulin resistance by peripheral tissues (i.e., muscle and liver). Type 1 diabetes mellitus is primarily a disease of complete β-cell failure and lack of circulating insulin; insulin resistance usually remains quite normal. This is evident by the fact that insulin doses required to treat type 1 diabetic patients are similar to a healthy individual's daily endogenous production (30-60 U per day). Type 1 diabetes can occur any time throughout life, but the majority of cases occur in children or young adults. Because of the acute onset of symptoms, most cases are detected soon after symptoms begin.

Type 2 diabetes is almost always associated with significant insulin resistance; in insulin-treated patients total daily doses of 100-200 U are often required, confirming the resistance of peripheral tissues to the effects of insulin. Though initial resistance results in augmented insulin secretion from the β-cells, this is unsustainable over the long term; this fact is crucial toward understanding the natural history of type 2 diabetes. Over 5 to 10 years, most patients with type 2 diabetes mellitus require increased medication (or increased insulin) to maintain glycemic control.

Screening

There is no recommendation to screen individuals for type 1 diabetes. Screening the general population for type 2 diabetes is not recommended. The U.S. Preventive Task Force (USPTF) has concluded that the current evidence is insufficient to assess the balance of benefits and harms of routine screening for type 2 diabetes in asymptomatic adults with blood pressure of 135/80 mm Hg or lower. The USPTF recommends screening for type 2 diabetes in asymptomatic adults with sustained blood pressure (treated or untreated) greater than 135/80 mm Hg, because in patients with diabetes lowering the blood pressure to less than 130/80 mm Hg reduces cardiovascular events and cardiovascular mortality.

Diagnosis

Medical history, physical examination, and appropriate laboratory testing are required for the diagnosis of diabetes. Target any patient with symptoms consistent with the disease such as unexplained weight loss, frequent infections, polyuria, or impotence, and in patients with physical findings such as acanthosis nigricans, peripheral neuropathy, or proliferative retinopathy.

A random serum glucose value of >200 mg/dL is predictive of diabetes, although it should be confirmed on repeat analysis in a fasting state. Fasting plasma glucose >126 mg/dL is highly specific (~98%) for the diagnosis (Table 1). Measurement of hemoglobin A_{1c} (HbA_{1c}) is not recommended to diagnose type 2 diabetes, although it is a useful marker of disease severity and risk of future diabetic complications. Once diabetes mellitus is diagnosed, HbA_{1c}, fasting lipid profile, serum electrolyte panel, urinalysis, and electrocardiogram are performed to screen for complications and establish baseline values.

All patients with diabetes are at risk for both microvascular and macrovascular complications. For this reason, test for evidence of urine microalbumin and refer to an ophthalmologist for a dilated examination of the retina. Interventions that reduce HbA_{1c} reduce rates of diabetes complications. The presence of microalbuminuria prompts initiation of an angiotensin-converting enzyme (ACE) inhibitor for its renal-protective effects. Blood pressure and cholesterol levels are aggressively managed (<135/80 mm Hg; LDL <100 mg/dL). Patients aged >40 years or with other cardiovascular risk factors are begun on low-dose aspirin. Most patients can be effectively treated in the ambulatory setting, although hospitalization may be required for hyperosmolar states, marked dehydration, diabetic ketoacidosis, or severe, symptomatic fasting hyperglycemia (>300 mg/dL) refractory to outpatient intervention.

Therapy

Therapy for all types of diabetes is focused on reducing elevated blood glucose concentration and preventing diabetic complications. The target HbA_{1c} level is <7% for both type 1 and type 2 diabetes. Home glucose monitoring should be instituted and patients counseled on keeping a log book of all values. Nonpharmaceutical therapies including diet and exercise programs

Table 1. Screening and Diagnostic Tests for Diabetes Mellitus

Test	Threshold Value
Fasting plasma glucose	>126 mg/dL diagnostic for type 2 diabetes. Confirm by repeat testing on another day.
Fasting plasma glucose	100-125 mg/dL suggests "impaired fasting glucose."
Random plasma glucose	>200 mg/dL plus symptoms (polyuria, polydipsia) suggests type 2 diabetes. Confirm with fasting plasma glucose or OGTT performed on another day.
OGTT (2-hour)	≥200 mg/dL diagnostic for type 2 diabetes. Confirm with second OGTT or fasting plasma glucose level on another day.
OGTT (2-hour)	140-199 mg/dL suggests impaired glucose tolerance.

OGTT = oral glucose tolerance test.

Table 2. Drug Therapies for Type 2 Diabetes

Drug	Notes
Metformin	First- or second-line therapy in patients with serum creatinine <1.6 mg/dL; use alone or in conjunction with sulfonylurea. Avoid in heart and liver failure.
Sulfonylureas (glyburide, glipizide)	First- or second-line therapy; use alone or in conjunction with metformin.
Thiazolidinedione (pioglitazone, rosiglitazone)	Possible third-line agent usually in conjunction with other oral therapies; rosiglitazone is associated with increased cardiovascular risk and should be used with caution. TZDs are contraindicated in heart failure.
Insulin (NPH, glargine, regular, lispro, aspart)	Second- or third-line agent. Can be used as solitary evening dose (NPH; glargine) in conjunction with oral medications or as part of multidose regimen.
Exenatide or DPP-IV inhibitor (sitagliptin, vidagliptin)	Second- or third-line agents; subcutaneous injection twice daily for exenatide; once- or twice-daily pill for DPP-IV inhibitors. Nausea, mild weight loss, or weight-neutral effects.

constitute cornerstones of therapy for all patients. Healthy lifestyle changes, such as regular exercise (>150 minutes weekly) and weight loss (as little as 7%), reduce the incidence of type 2 diabetes in high-risk populations. Any patient with impaired fasting glucose (110-126 mg/dL), obesity, a strong family history of diabetes, or prior gestational diabetes during pregnancy can benefit from these preventive strategies. All patients are strongly counseled to stop smoking.

For all patients with diabetes, institute foot-care strategies to prevent ulceration and amputation in patients with documented diabetic neuropathy. Educate patients regarding daily inspection of feet, wearing appropriate shoes, avoiding high-impact exercise, not going barefoot, and testing water temperature before entering.

Emphasize increased surveillance by the patient and health care team for decreased foot sensation, callus formation, deformities, and structural changes. Testing for sensory neuropathy with a 5.07/10 g monofilament has been demonstrated to predict ulcer and amputation risk (Plate 1). Monofilament testing has superior predictive value compared with test modalities such as the 128-Hz tuning fork, pin-prick, cotton wisps, or the presence or absence of neuropathic symptoms.

Prescribe orthotic footwear for patients with foot deformities and to cushion high-pressure areas. A foot ulcer, defined as any transdermal interruption of skin integrity, is predictive of amputation. For patients with foot ulcers, refer to a multidisciplinary foot clinic, if available; multidisciplinary clinics that specialize in diabetic foot care can improve outcomes in the diabetic foot.

Drug therapy is initiated in type 2 diabetes if diet and exercise do not adequately control hyperglycemia (Table 2). Metformin is frequently a first-line agent in patients with baseline creatinine

levels <1.6 mg/dL (<1.5 mg/dL in women) and without known liver disease or alcohol abuse. It is contraindicated in patients with increased risk for metabolic acidosis, although this complication is rare. Metformin must be stopped prior to receiving radiocontrast agents. Patients should be counseled about the risk of loose stools, bloating, gas, or other gastrointestinal side effects.

Sulfonylureas such as glyburide and glipizide are also first-line agents or can be given in combination with metformin. Sulfonylureas are well tolerated and have few contraindications, although they can cause hypoglycemia (unlike metformin) and are used with caution in the elderly, especially with renal failure.

Many patients fail to achieve optimal glucose control (HbA$_{1c}$ <7.0%) with metformin and/or sulfonylureas. In such patients, many strategies for further therapy are available, including:

- *Initiating exenatide or a DPP-IV inhibitor while continuing oral medications.* Exenatide is a twice-daily injectable medication that reduces HbA$_{1c}$ approximately 0.5%-1.0% and promotes a modest weight loss. It is used only in combination with metformin, a sulfonylurea, or a combination of metformin and sulfonylurea. Up to 40% of patients experience nausea, precluding continuation of this medication. DPP-IV inhibitors (sitagliptin and vidagliptin) also reduce HbA$_{1c}$ approximately 0.5%-1.0%, though without change in body weight. These oral drugs are administered once or twice daily and are often associated with mild-to-moderate nausea.

- *Initiating insulin therapy while continuing oral medications.* Because type 2 diabetes is associated with loss of β-cell function, insulin therapy is a rational option. Initially, a single dose of a long-acting insulin (NPH or glargine) can be given in the evening. Glycemic control throughout the day is improved if morning fasting glucose concentrations <100 mg/dL are achieved.

- *Initiating a third oral medication such as a thiazolidinedione.* Pioglitazone and rosiglitazone are effective at further lowering HbA$_{1c}$ approximately 0.5%-1.0%. Recent meta-analyses have suggested that rosiglitazone is associated with increased cardiovascular adverse events compared with placebo. Further investigation is pending. Nonetheless, because of this finding, the risks and benefits of using rosiglitazone (and possibly pioglitazone) must be carefully weighed. Routine monitoring of liver function tests is required during the first year, and lower extremity edema and fluid retention are common side effects. These agents are contraindicated in patients with heart failure or liver dysfunction.

If these strategies are unable to achieve the desired level of glycemic control, initiate multidose insulin therapy. In these circumstances, discontinue previous oral therapy (with the possible exception of metformin) before beginning multidose insulin regimens. There are several insulin protocols, varying in the number of daily injections and the types of insulin. With all strategies, a combination of a long-acting (such as NPH or glargine) and short-acting (such as lispro or aspart) insulin are used. Commonly, twice-daily NPH (in the morning and before bedtime) is combined with lispro (or aspart) injections given before breakfast and dinner. Alternatively, once-daily glargine (before bedtime) is combined with premeal lispro (or aspart), three times daily. Regardless, patients should be counseled that consistency in their routine (both time of insulin administration and eating patterns) is paramount to success. Many type 2 diabetics will require a total daily insulin requirement equal to 1 unit per kilogram weight, although highly insulin-resistant patients may require more.

Insulin is the mainstay of therapy for patients with type 1 diabetes and is required in all patients to avoid ketoacidosis. Without insulin, patients will become hyperglycemic (and ultimately ketotic) within 24-48 hours. Insulin therapy most frequently consists of multiple daily subcutaneous injections of long- and short-acting insulins. A common regimen is a combination of evening insulin glargine and insulin lispro (or aspart) before each meal. An alternative regimen is to administer a combination of NPH insulin twice daily and insulin lispro (or aspart) at breakfast and dinner.

Alternatively, patients can be treated with an insulin pump. With this therapy, a continuous infusion of short-acting insulin is delivered through a subcutaneous needle implanted under the skin every 72 hours. Patients are able to deliver standard basal rates of insulin throughout the day, and bolus insulin to themselves at meal times. This strategy allows for greater flexibility and precision. The goal of therapy is to reduce the HbA$_{1c}$ to <7%; however, achieving this goal commonly results in mild hypoglycemia, and patients need to be educated to avoid hypoglycemia or to recognize and treat hypoglycemia. Frequent daily monitoring of capillary blood glucose is required.

Follow-Up

Measure the degree of glycemic control with HbA$_{1c}$ every 3 to 6 months (Table 3). Obtain an annual fasting lipid profile, including low-density lipoprotein (LDL) cholesterol, triglyceride, high-density lipoprotein, and total cholesterol levels, and adjust treatment to meet goals. Screen annually for diabetic nephropathy with a spot urine for microalbuminuria. Perform a foot examination at each visit. Obtain an annual dilated funduscopic examination from a specialist, unless otherwise dictated by the specialist. Reinforce the key issues of self-care, hypoglycemia, medication, blood glucose monitoring, and lifestyle.

Diabetic Ketoacidosis

Prevention

Provide education regarding sick-day management to patients with type 1 diabetes to prevent diabetic ketoacidosis. On sick days instruct patients to increase the frequency of home blood glucose monitoring; measure urinary or fingerstick ketones; continue insulin and maintain fluids; and proceed to an emergency department if nausea and vomiting persist or if home ketone testing is positive. Ensure that patients understand the need to continue insulin therapy even when they are unable to eat.

Screening

All type 1 diabetics should be screened for ketosis when blood sugars are >350 mg/dL or there is the presence of an anion-gap acidosis, regardless of the blood sugar.

Diagnosis

Over 10% of patients with a new diagnosis of type 1 diabetes present with diabetic ketoacidosis. Diabetic ketoacidosis occurs when insufficient insulin is present and excess glucose is metabolized via the fatty acid degradation pathway, producing metabolic ketoacidosis and ketonuria. Diabetic ketoacidosis is life-threatening and

Table 3. Glycemic Targets for All Patients with Diabetes

Parameter	Target Value
Hemoglobin A$_{1c}$ (normal range 4%–6%)	<7%*
Preprandial plasma glucose	90–130 mg/dL
Postprandial plasma glucose (1–2 hr after a meal)	<180 mg/dL

*More stringent goals (i.e., <6%) can be considered in individual patients, although currently no evidence supports that this approach offers additional benefit. Adapted from American Diabetes Association, Standards of Medical Care in Diabetes. Diabetes Care. 2005;28:S10-S11; with permission.

is treated immediately in a hospital setting. The diagnosis is based upon a triad of hyperglycemia (blood glucose >250 mg/dL), arterial pH <7.30, and ketoacidosis (serum bicarbonate <15 meq/L and positive serum ketones).

Therapy

Patients are usually severely dehydrated and have hyperkalemia and hypophosphatemia. Infusion of 0.9% sodium chloride is started immediately, along with an intravenous insulin drip; several liters of intravenous fluid may ultimately be required. Once serum glucose concentrations are <250 mg/dL, 5% or 10% intravenous dextrose solution is administered to avoid hypoglycemia as insulin infusion is continued.

Insulin is delivered via intravenous infusion; an initial bolus of regular insulin (0.15 U/kg) is followed by a constant infusion of 0.1 U/kg. Blood glucose is monitored hourly to ensure reduction to normal values. During this time, insulin will cause substantial shifts in potassium from the extracellular to the intracellular space, placing the patient at risk for hypokalemia and arrhythmias. Measure serum potassium every 1-2 hours during initial treatment and replace potassium via intravenous infusion. The goal of insulin therapy is full suppression of ketosis, not control of hyperglycemia. Premature discontinuation of insulin results in relapse of ketosis.

Follow-Up

Once stabilized, patients are converted to subcutaneous insulin. Because diabetic ketoacidosis is often precipitated by coexistent illness, all patients are evaluated for signs of infection or other illness. Patient education is paramount to promote recognition of early signs of diabetes ketoacidosis in the future.

Book Enhancement

Go to www.acponline.org/essentials/endocrinology-section.html to view a foot exam tutorial; access a foot exam worksheet, self-management checklist, and screening guidelines; and view an early diabetic foot, callus, pre-ulcer, and retinopathy. In *MKSAP for Students 4*, assess yourself with items 2-17 in the **Endocrinology and Metabolism** section.

Bibliography

Campos C. Treating the whole patient for optimal management of type 2 diabetes: considerations for insulin therapy. South Med J. 2007; 100: 804-11. [PMID: 17713307]

Lochnan H. Diabetic Ketoacidosis. http://pier.acponline.org/physicians/diseases/d644. [Date accessed: 2008 Jan 10] In: PIER [online database]. Philadelphia: American College of Physicians; 2008.

Passaro MD, Ratner RE. Diabetes Mellitus, Type 1. http://pier.acponline.org/physicians/diseases/d257. [Date accessed: 2008 Jan 10] In: PIER [online database]. Philadelphia: American College of Physicians; 2008.

Vijan S. Diabetes Mellitus, Type 2. http://pier.acponline.org/physicians/diseases/d296. [Date accessed: 2008 Jan 10] In: PIER [online database]. Philadelphia: American College of Physicians; 2008.

Chapter 9

Dyslipidemia

D. Michael Elnicki, MD
Gary Tabas, MD

Lipoproteins are lipids in the blood bound to proteins. Low-density lipoprotein (LDL) makes up 60%-70% of total serum cholesterol, is the major atherogenic component, and is the main target for therapy. High-density lipoprotein (HDL) accounts for 20%-30% of total cholesterol and levels are inversely related to coronary heart disease (CHD) risk. Very-low-density lipoproteins (VLDL) are triglyceride-rich lipoproteins produced by the liver, are precursors of LDL, and contain highly atherogenic remnant particles. Intermediate-density lipoprotein (IDL) is also atherogenic and is included in the LDL measurement. Chylomicrons are formed in the intestine, are rich in triglyceride, and when partially degraded are atherogenic.

Other lipoproteins are likely involved in the formation of an atheroma. Lipoprotein a [Lp(a)] is associated with increased risk for CHD, but treatment with statins does not lower LP(a) levels or risk. Small LDL particles and HDL subfractions are related to CHD but are not superior to LDL or HDL in predicting risk. Measurement of these other lipoproteins is not routinely indicated.

Prevention

All patients should be advised about lifestyle measures that will reduce lipid levels. These include healthy diet, regular exercise, weight control, avoidance of tobacco, and moderation of alcohol intake. The components of a healthy diet include one that does not exceed caloric needs and contains less than 25%-35% of calories from all fat sources, less than 7% from saturated fat, and less than 200 mg of cholesterol/day. Increasing dietary intake of vegetables, fruits, and high-fiber foods will help lower cholesterol. In particular, low density lipoprotein (LDL) cholesterol will be lowered by eating foods with high levels of plant stanols (2 g/day) and increased amounts of soluble fiber (10-25 g/day). Aerobic exercise has beneficial effects on lipid profiles and should be done most days for at least 30 minutes per session. However, any amount of exercise is of benefit and more is better. Body weight should be brought as close as possible to the ideal body mass index. All forms of tobacco should be avoided, and alcohol intake should be moderated to ≤2 drinks per day for men and ≤1 drink for women.

Screening

Initiate screening for lipid disorders between the ages of 20 and 35 (20 to 40 for women) using fasting lipid profiles. Repeat screening of average-risk patients with normal lipids at initial screening every 5 years and more frequently in patients with other risk factors or whose diet and/or weight have changed significantly. Screening for lipid disorders should be continued into advanced ages unless patients have a short (<1-2 years) life expectancy. Lipid disorders are more common in the elderly and, due to the higher burden of disease, carry as high a CHD attributable risk as it does in middle-aged patients, even if the relative risk change is not as great. Lowering lipids also prevents stroke, an important problem in the elderly.

If a fasting lipid profile is not feasible, total and HDL cholesterol levels can be used for initial screening. If either of these is abnormal, a fasting lipid profile should be obtained. A fasting lipid profile consists of measurements of total and HDL cholesterol, triglycerides, and calculated LDL cholesterol. LDL cholesterol is calculated using the Friedewald formula:

$$LDL = \text{total cholesterol} - HDL - (\text{triglycerides}/5)$$

Triglyceride levels >400 mg/dL invalidate the Friedewald formula. In this case, LDL cholesterol can be directly measured.

Diagnosis

Perform a thorough history to identify other cardiovascular risk factors, such as cigarette smoking, hypertension, and a family history of premature heart disease. A variety of drugs can cause dyslipidemia including estrogens, corticosteroids, thiazide diuretics, beta-blockers, and androgenic steroids. History can determine coronary disease equivalent status, such as diabetes mellitus, peripheral vascular disease (aortic aneurysm, claudication), stroke, or a 10-year risk of CHD >20%. The physical examination can identify CHD risks or CHD equivalents. The exam should include measurement of blood pressure and body mass index. Patients with existing cardiovascular disease may have abnormal cardiac exams, diminished pulses, bruits, or other signs of peripheral vascular disease. Patients with very high lipids will often have cutaneous xanthomas on extensor surfaces and xanthelasmas near the eyelids. Secondary causes of dyslipidemia, important because often treatable (Table 1), include hypothyroidism, obstructive liver disease, nephrotic syndrome, alcoholism, uncontrolled diabetes, smoking, and renal failure.

Before making the diagnosis of hyperlipidemia, obtain at least two measures of LDL cholesterol at least 1 week apart. LDL levels are the primary targets of therapy. Goals for LDL cholesterol are <100 mg/dL for those with CHD or CHD equivalent disease and <130 mg/dL for patients with ≥2 risk factors. These risk factors are

Table 1. Laboratory Tests for Evaluation of Dyslipidemia

Test	Notes
Fasting lipid profile with calculated LDL cholesterol	Obtain two measurements at least 1 week apart to confirm diagnosis. Results unreliable >24 hr after myocardial infarction, major surgery, or trauma, and for 6-8 wk after event onset.
Direct LDL cholesterol measurement	Obtain if triglycerides >400 mg/dL, which makes Friedewald equation unreliable for calculating LDL cholesterol.
TSH	Identify hypothyroidism as a secondary cause.
Fasting blood glucose (FBG)	Identify uncontrolled diabetes as a secondary cause with fasting blood glucose >126 mg/dL on two fasting samples.
Direct bilirubin	Identify obstructive jaundice as a secondary cause if bilirubin >50% above normal.
Alkaline phosphatase AST/ALT	Identify liver disease as a contraindication to some lipid-lowering drugs. Verify absence of liver disease before starting a statin.
Urine for protein	Begin with a urine dipstick for overt proteinuria to identify nephrotic syndrome as a secondary cause.

ALT = alanine aminotransferase; AST = aspartate aminotransferase; HDL = high-density lipoprotein; LDL = low-density lipoprotein; TSH = thyroid-stimulating hormone.

remembered as the first five letters of the word CHOLEsterol: Cigarette use, Hypertension, Older age (45 in men, 55 in women), Low HDL, and Elders with CHD (male first-degree relatives <55 years of age and females <65 years). Further stratification of risk in patients who are above their goal of 130 mg/dL can be calculated using the Framingham risk equation (see Book Enhancement section below), which predicts 10-year risk of CHD. Patients are classified as low risk (<10% 10-year risk), moderate risk (10%-20%), and CHD risk equivalent (>20%). For the lowest-risk patients (<2 risk factors), the LDL goal is <160 mg/dL.

Triglyceride levels are a secondary target for therapy. Levels are classified as normal (<150 mg/dL), borderline (150-199 mg/dL), high (200-499 mg/dL), and very high (>500 mg/dL). Very high triglyceride levels convey a risk of pancreatitis and are treated regardless of cardiovascular risk. Low HDL cholesterol (<40 mg/dL) is a CHD risk factor and is treated in patients with CHD.

Therapy

In patients with moderate-to-low risk for CHD, dietary interventions to reduce LDL cholesterol are appropriate. Dietary and exercise habit modifications may be able to normalize lipid levels. A diet low in saturated fat can result in a 5%-15% reduction in LDL cholesterol. Switching to high-fiber foods can result in a 5% reduction in LDL. Furthermore, diets rich in fruits, vegetables, nuts, whole grains, and mono-unsaturated oils (olive oil, canola oil), and diets low in animal fat reduce cardiovascular risk even without changing lipid levels. Diets rich in n-3 fatty acids, from fish intake or supplements, improve lipid profiles and reduce risk of CHD by 20%-30%.

Patients should be encouraged to lose weight by reducing calories, particularly calories from fats and simple carbohydrates. Regular physical activity is encouraged, and both weight loss and exercise are particularly encouraged for patients with a body mass index >25. Regular aerobic exercise facilitates weight loss and improves lipid profiles. The beneficial effects are related to the amount of exercise, rather than intensity or overall fitness. Patients should begin structured exercise programs lasting at least 30 minutes on most days. Smoking cessation improves lipid ratios and reduces CHD and should be an integral part of lifestyle therapy.

Drug therapy is initiated in high-risk patients who are not responsive to lifestyle interventions, at least to the point of reaching National Cholesterol Education Program (NCEP) target cholesterol levels. Several drug classes for lipid lowering are available. These include HMG-CoA reductase inhibitors (statins), fibrates, niacin, bile acid binding resins, and intestinal cholesterol absorption blockers (Table 2). Statins, the most effective drugs for lowering LDL cholesterol, can cause hepatotoxicity and myopathy, particularly when used in combination with other lipid-lowering drugs. Patients should routinely be asked about symptoms such as nausea, abdominal pain, or myalgias. Serum transaminase levels are measured at baseline, after 3 months, and every 6-12 months when patients are on statins. If a statin-induced myopathy is suspected, confirm the diagnosis by measuring serum creatine phosphokinase. In low-risk patients, 6 months of diet and exercise are appropriate before starting drugs. Drug therapy is started earlier in patients with higher overall CHD risk and in those patients whose LDL cholesterol is more than 30 mg/dL above their goal because lowering LDL cholesterol pharmacologically has been shown to reduce CHD and stroke in primary and secondary prevention.

Follow-Up

Patients are seen at regular intervals even after lipids are normalized. Patients who are on drug therapy need to be seen regularly at 4-6 month intervals. A fasting lipid profile should be obtained at least yearly, with monitoring for drug toxicity.

Book Enhancement

Go to www.acponline.org/essentials/endocrinology-section .html to access a tool to calculate the Framingham risk score and to view tables on the classification of lipid levels, goals of

Table 2. Drugs for Treating Lipid Disorders

Agent (Examples)	Mechanism of Action and Indications
Colestipol hydrochloride Colesevelam hydrochloride	Interrupts bile acid reabsorption and reduces LDL cholesterol by 10%-15%. Often used as second-line drug with statins because it acts synergistically to induce LDL receptors. Do not use in patients with triglycerides >300 mg/dL or in those with gastrointestinal motility disorders. Can interfere with absorption of other drugs given at the same time.
Atorvastatin Lovastatin Pravastatin Simvastatin	Partially inhibits HMG-CoA reductase, inducing LDL receptor formation; lowers LDL cholesterol 20%-60%, raises HDL cholesterol 5%-10%, and lowers triglycerides 15%-25%. Drug of choice for elevated LDL cholesterol. Side effects include elevated aminotransaminase levels, myositis/myalgias. Use in combination with bile acid binding resins to synergistically lower LDL cholesterol. Use in combination with niacin and fibrates in patients with combined hyperlipidemia. Use cautiously in patients on fibrates due to increased risk of myalgia/myositis. Pravastatin is least likely to cause myalgia.
Gemfibrozil Fenofibrate	Reduces VLDL synthesis and induces lipoprotein lipase. Lowers triglycerides 50%, raises HDL 15% but does not lower LDL cholesterol reliably. Use in combination with statins cautiously due to increased incidence of myositis/myalgias. Use with caution in patients with renal insufficiency and gallbladder disease.
Niacin	Reduces hepatic production of β-containing lipoproteins and increases HDL cholesterol production. Lowers LDL cholesterol and triglycerides 10%-30%. Most effective drug at raising HDL cholesterol (25%-35%). Drug of choice for combined hyperlipidemia and in patients with low HDL cholesterol. Extended-release preparations limit flushing and aminotransaminase abnormalities. Can cause nausea, glucose intolerance, gout, and elevated uric acid levels. Over-the-counter, long-acting niacin preparations are not recommended because they increase the incidence of hepatotoxicity. Use in combination with statins or bile acid binding resins in combined hyperlipidemia. To minimize flushing, aspirin can be taken 1 hour before dose.
Ezetimibe	Selectively inhibits the intestinal absorption of cholesterol. Reduces LDL by 18%, triglycerides by 8%. When used in combination with statins, yields an additional LDL reduction of 12% (total reduction 26% to 60%), an increase in HDL of 3%, and a triglyceride reduction of 8%. Do not use in combination with resins or fibrates. Contraindicated in patients with active liver disease or elevated aminotransaminase levels.

therapy using LDL cholesterol, and nutrient composition of the Therapeutic Lifestyle Change Diet. In *MKSAP for Students 4*, assess yourself with items 15-22 in the **Endocrinology and Metabolism** section.

Bibliography

Forrester JS, Libby P. The inflammation hypothesis and its potential relevance to statin therapy. Am J Cardiol. 2007;99:732-8. [PMID: 17317382]

Kopin LA, Pearson TA. In the clinic. Dyslipidemia. Ann Intern Med. 2007;147:ITC9-1-ITC9-16. [PMID: 17785482]

Chapter 10

Thyroid Disease

Erik K. Alexander, MD

The thyroid gland releases two forms of thyroid hormone: thyroxine (T_4) and triiodothyronine (T_3). All of the T_4 in the body is made within the thyroid gland, whereas 80% of T_3 is derived from the peripheral tissues. T_3 affects the physiologic function of almost all bodily tissues through binding with a specific nuclear receptor and thereby regulates the transcription of thyroid-dependent genes. The peripheral conversion of T_4 to T_3 is decreased by various medications, including propranolol, corticosteroids, propylthiouracil, and amiodarone, and is downregulated during the course of nonthyroidal illness. The synthesis and release of thyroid hormone are controlled by the pituitary-derived thyroid-stimulating hormone (TSH) under the influence of thyrotropin-releasing hormone from the hypothalamus. TSH stimulates basic thyrocyte functions such as iodine uptake and organification and the synthesis and release of thyroid hormone. Both T_3 and T_4 are bound to protein in the circulation that serves the dual purpose of preventing excessive tissue uptake and maintaining a readily accessible reserve of hormone. Several common medications affect levels of thyroxine-binding globulin without generally affecting the free-thyroid hormone levels.

Screening

Screening for hypothyroidism and hyperthyroidism is not recommended for the general population, but it is considered for certain higher-risk populations. It is reasonable to screen women aged >50 years using a sensitive TSH test given the increased prevalence of hypothyroidism in this population. Screening other high-risk populations is also appropriate. In particular, measuring TSH is appropriate in the following patients:

- Patients with evidence of Hashimoto's disease or Graves' disease in a first-degree relative
- Patients with other autoimmune diseases such as type 1 diabetes
- Patients with a history of any prior thyroid dysfunction, even if self-limited
- Patients living in an iodine-deficient region of the world
- Patients anticipating a pregnancy or currently pregnant
- Patients with conditions (e.g., cardiac arrhythmias, weight loss, osteoporosis, anxiety) that may be explained or aggravated by hyperthyroidism

Of particular note is the population of young women with hypothyroidism receiving adequate levothyroxine replacement therapy who desire to be (or are currently) pregnant. During pregnancy, the daily thyroid hormone requirement increases by approximately 40% above baseline beginning very early in gestation. In patients with hypothyroidism, the dose of levothyroxine must be increased. Failure to do so results in maternal (and possibly fetal) hypothyroidism, which can be associated with substantial morbidity to both mother and fetus. For this reason, pre-pregnancy or pregnancy screening of women for hypothyroidism is important. Patients on thyroid replacement should be counseled to contact their physician as soon as pregnancy is confirmed so that levothyroxine dose adjustment can be made early to maintain a euthyroid state throughout gestation.

Diagnosis

Consider the diagnosis of hyperthyroidism in patients with signs or symptoms of thyrotoxicosis (Table 1) or in those with diseases known to be caused or aggravated by thyrotoxicosis (e.g., atrial fibrillation). In hyperthyroidism, the TSH is low or undetectable and a free-T_4 concentration is elevated. If the TSH is suppressed and the free-T_4 is normal, measure the serum T_3 concentration. T_3 thyrotoxicosis (suppressed TSH, normal T_4, elevated T_3) is seen with increased frequency in patients with toxic multinodular goiter and autonomously functioning thyroid nodules. Look for "apathetic thyrotoxicosis" in elderly patients characterized by a lower frequency of goiter (found in 50%), fewer hyperadrenergic symptoms, and a predominance of cardiac findings including heart failure and atrial fibrillation. Patients with a low or undetectable TSH and a normal free-T_4 have subclinical hyperthyroidism. This distinction is important because subclinical hyperthyroidism can be followed with periodic thyroid function tests in otherwise healthy patients <60 years old.

Most thyrotoxicosis is due to Graves' disease or thyroiditis. Rarely, a toxic ("hot") adenoma, toxic multinodular goiter, factitious hyperthyroidism due to thyroid hormone consumption, or a struma ovarii may be causative. Pregnant women are often found to have mildly to moderately suppressed TSH values during the first trimester due to stimulation of the thyrotropin (TSH) receptor by chorionic gonadotropin (hCG) resulting in normal or slightly increased free T_4 and T_3 concentrations. Most commonly, this does not require treatment. A radioactive iodine uptake (RAIU) is the optimal test to differentiate between thyrotoxicosis due to excess thyroid hormone production (Graves' disease or a toxic adenoma) and increased hormone release from a damaged thyroid (thyroiditis). An elevated RAIU is consistent with excess thyroid hormone production, whereas a suppressed RAIU (usually <5%) is

Table 1. Signs and Symptoms of Hyperthyroidism and Hypothyroidism

Hyperthyroidism	Hypothyroidism
Common symptoms	*Common symptoms*
Nervousness or emotional lability	Fatigue
Increased sweating	Weight gain
Heat intolerance	Alopecia
Palpitations	Cold intolerance and constipation
Fatigue	Sluggish affect or depression
Weight loss	Fluid retention
Hyper-defecation	Delayed deep tendon reflexes
Menstrual irregularity	Loss of the lateral portion of the eyebrow
Common signs	*Common signs*
Tremors	Dry, coarse skin and hair
Tachycardia or evidence of atrial fibrillation	Periorbital puffiness
Proptosis of the eyes or extraocular muscle palsy	Bradycardia
Stare, lid lag, or signs of optic neuropathy	Slow movements and speech
Goiter	Hoarseness
Pretibial myxedema	Diastolic hypertension
	Goiter

consistent with hormone release from an inflamed thyroid gland (Figure 1). An RAIU should not be performed if a patient is suspected or confirmed to be pregnant or is breast-feeding. Patients with acute nonthyroidal illness may have TSH suppression that is part of the "euthyroid sick syndrome" and not due to underlying thyrotoxicosis. The free-T_4 may be normal, elevated, or low. Additional testing is sometimes required to make the diagnosis of "euthyroid sick syndrome."

Thyroid storm is defined as a life-threatening condition manifested by an exaggeration of the clinical signs and symptoms of thyrotoxicosis accompanied by systemic decompensation. It is usually caused by rapid release of thyroid hormone (e.g., large iodine load, withdrawal of antithyroid drugs, or treatment with radioactive iodine) in the setting of other illness such as surgery, infection, or trauma. Early recognition, prompt hospitalization, and consultation with endocrinology are the keys to a successful outcome. In hyperthyroid patients, thyroid storm is a clinical diagnosis; there is no concentration of thyroid hormone elevation that is diagnostic.

The risks of hyperthyroidism are primarily related to cardiac function and arrhythmias, bone loss and osteoporosis, and a hypermetabolic state. Graves' ophthalmopathy (soft tissue inflammation, proptosis, extraocular muscle dysfunction, and optic neuropathy) is present in 10%-25% of affected patients, although subclinical enlargement of extraocular muscles may be present in up to 70% of patients without overt eye disease. Pretibial myxedema (infiltrative dermopathy characterized by nonpitting scaly thickening and induration of the skin) is a rare complication of Graves' disease. Once treated effectively, the overall risk associated with hyperthyroidism can be substantially diminished.

Hypothyroidism has a wide range of clinical symptoms and signs (see Table 1). The serum TSH is elevated (>10 μU/mL)

in primary hypothyroidism (thyroid gland failure), and is low or normal in conjunction with a low free-T_4 in rare cases of hypothyroidism due to pituitary or hypothalamic disease (secondary hypothyroidism). Patients with a mildly elevated TSH (5-10 μU/mL) and a normal free-T_4 have subclinical hypothyroidism. This distinction is important because patients with subclinical hypothyroidism may not require treatment if asymptomatic and not desiring pregnancy (or not currently pregnant).

The most common causes of hypothyroidism are chronic lymphocytic thyroiditis (Hashimoto's disease), post-thyroidectomy, and radioactive iodine administration (Table 2). Hashimoto's disease is an autoimmune disease that may present at any time but increases in prevalence with age. Onset is usually insidious and is usually associated with a goiter. The presence of thyroid peroxidase (TPO) antibody is highly correlated with the presence of Hashimoto's disease and can be useful in confirming the disease or assessing the risk of developing hypothyroidism in the future. Subacute and painful thyroiditis are other illnesses that can lead to hypothyroidism. Most patients demonstrate a triphasic thyroid hormone response once activated: mild hyperthyroidism, followed by mild hypothyroidism, followed by a return to normal thyroid function. If the final phase of thyroid normalization is not attained, TSH will remain elevated and hypothyroidism will persist.

Therapy

Early in the treatment of thyrotoxicosis, iodine avoidance (such as the contrast agent used in CT scans) and exercise restriction are recommended. Thyroidectomy is a reasonable choice in thyrotoxic patients with concomitant suspicious (malignant) nodules and in patients who cannot tolerate or refuse radioactive iodine or antithyroid drugs.

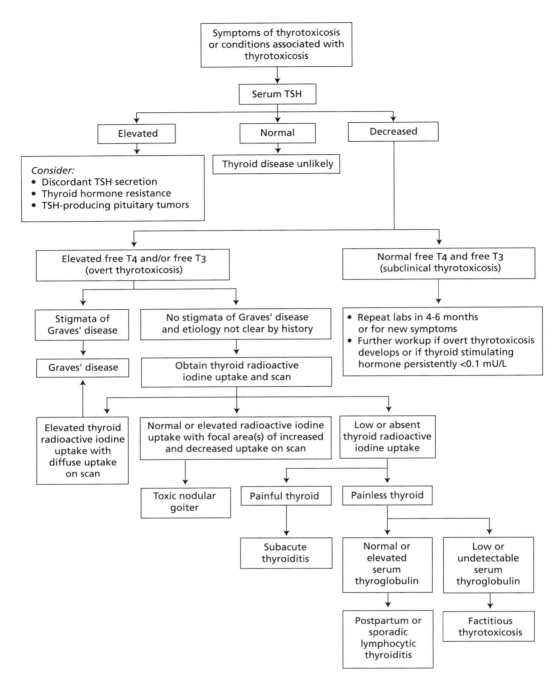

Figure 1 Diagnostic approach to thyrotoxicosis.

Thyrotoxicosis due to thyroiditis is managed conservatively because it is often self-limited. Repeated measurements of thyroid function (monthly) are indicated over a 3-4 month period.

β-blockers can be used for sympathomimetic symptoms (tachycardia, tremor, and anxiety). Nonsteroidal anti-inflammatory drugs and, rarely, corticosteroids, are administered to reduce inflammation and discomfort. For patients with Graves' disease and autonomously functioning thyroid nodules, antithyroid drugs or radioiodine can be used, although patient preference, patient age, comorbidity, severity of thyrotoxicosis, and the presence of Graves' ophthalmopathy must be taken into account.

Antithyroid drugs are used for primary therapy of thyrotoxicosis, attainment of euthyroidism in preparation for thyroidectomy, and for use in conjunction with radioiodine therapy in selected patients. Antithyroid drugs are also preferred to radioactive iodine in the presence of severe Graves' ophthalmopathy and thyroid storm. Most patients, however, ultimately select radioiodine as therapy for thyrotoxicosis caused by Graves' disease, toxic multinodular goiter, or autonomously functioning thyroid nodules. Radioiodine is also indicated in patients failing to achieve a remission after a course of antithyroid drugs. When antithyroid drugs are prescribed, methimazole is effective for most patients.

Table 2. Differential Diagnosis of Hypothyroidism

Disease	Notes
Hashimoto's disease	TSH high; positive family history for hypothyroidism; TPO antibodies present; slowly progressive
Iodine deficiency	TSH high; urine iodine low; iodine- deficient area; rare in United States
Postpartum thyroiditis	TSH triphasic (low, high, normal) over 2-4 months but often ultimately elevated; recent pregnancy
Silent thyroiditis	TSH triphasic (low, high, normal) over 2-4 months; self-limited in most cases
Subacute thyroiditis	TSH triphasic (low, high, normal) over 2-4 months; ESR elevated; painful thyroid
Drug induced	TSH high; use of amiodarone, lithium, sunitinib, interferon, iodine, or thioamides in past 1-6 months
Pituitary/hypothalamic mass	TSH low or normal; FT_4 low; headaches; most often a pituitary or sellar lesion noted on MRI/CT scan, or evidence of prior pituitary surgery
Pituitary/hypothalamic radiation therapy	TSH low or normal; FT_4 low; history of cranial radiation therapy

CT = computed tomography; ESR = erythrocyte sedimentation rate; FT_4 = free T_4; MRI = magnetic resonance imaging; TPO = thyroid peroxidase.

Alternatively, propylthiouracil is preferred in pregnant patients and in those with an allergy to methimazole. With either drug, patients should be counseled for the risk of hepatitis, vasculitis, and agranulocytosis, rare but potentially severe side effects. If immediate control of severe thyrotoxicosis is required, inorganic iodine (SSKI) can be administered orally and is highly effective. This therapy, however, is self-limited in duration (3 weeks) and precludes further use of radioactive iodine for months thereafter. The response of Grave's ophthalmopathy to the treatment of hyperthyroidism is complex and requires consultation with an ophthalmologist and endocrinologist.

Levothyroxine is the preferred treatment of hypothyroidism, and it safely, effectively, and reliably relieves symptoms and normalizes lab tests in hypothyroid patients. Levothyroxine is converted to T_3 (the active hormone) primarily in peripheral tissues at an appropriate rate for overall metabolic needs. Treatment with a combination of T_4 and T_3 is not recommended. While all patients with overt hypothyroidism (TSH >10 µU/mL) should be treated, there is limited evidence that treatment of subclinical hypothyroidism is beneficial in non-pregnant patients. At present, most patients can be safely monitored with TSH measurements every 4-6 months, evaluating for progression of disease. This recommendation excludes women seeking pregnancy or currently pregnant, who should be treated once TSH is outside the normal range because of greater maternal and fetal risk.

Follow-Up

Following treatment for thyrotoxicosis, TSH and free-T_4 are monitored every 3-6 months for the first year, and every 6-12 months thereafter. Radioactive iodine is likely to cause permanent thyroid destruction requiring life-long levothyroxine therapy.

Once initiated for the treatment of hypothyroidism, levothyroxine therapy is life-long. Serum TSH should be monitored 6-8 weeks after initiating therapy, and adjustments made to obtain a value within the normal range. A full replacement dose of levothyroxine is approximately 1.7 µg/kg, although many patients require less due to partial thyroid dysfunction. Finally, an annual evaluation of serum TSH is recommended in patients receiving levothyroxine therapy; studies have demonstrated that up to 30% of such patients may be unintentionally under- or over-replaced.

Book Enhancement

Go to www.acponline.org/essentials/endocrinology-section.html to view an example of Graves' ophthalmopathy, cervical goiter, and a nuclear scan of a hyperfunctioning nodule and to access a classification of thyrotoxicosis based upon radioactive scan results and a table of important facts on hypothyroidism. In *MKSAP for Students 4*, assess yourself with items 21-26 in the **Endocrinology and Metabolism** section.

Bibliography

Brent GA. Graves' disease. N Eng J Med. 2008;358:2594-605. [PMID: 18550875]

Burch HB. Hyperthyroidism (Thyrotoxicosis). http://pier.acponline.org/physicians/diseases/d175. [Date accessed: 2008 Feb 27] In: PIER [online database]. Philadelphia: American College of Physicians; 2008.

McDermott MT. Hypothyroidism. http://pier.acponline.org/physicians/diseases/d238. [Date accessed: 2008 Feb 27] In: PIER [online database]. Philadelphia: American College of Physicians; 2008.

Nayak B, Hodak SP. Hyperthyroidism. Endocrinol Metab Clin North Am. 2007;36:617-56. [PMID: 17673122]

Chapter 11

Adrenal Disease

Cynthia A. Burns, MD

This chapter reviews four types of adrenal disease: adrenal insufficiency, hyperadrenocorticism (Cushing's syndrome), hyperaldosteronism, and pheochromocytoma.

Adrenal Insufficiency

Adrenal insufficiency may be due to disease of the adrenal glands (primary) or disorders of the pituitary gland (secondary). Autoimmune adrenalitis is the most common cause of primary insufficiency in the United States, and exogenous corticosteroid use is the most common cause of secondary insufficiency. Primary disease results in deficiencies of cortisol, aldosterone, and adrenal androgens, whereas secondary insufficiency causes only cortisol deficiency.

Diagnosis

The presentation of adrenal insufficiency may be acute or slowly progressive. Symptoms of acute adrenal crisis are nonspecific; therefore one must be alert to the causes of adrenal insufficiency and the clinical setting in which they occur. Acute adrenal crisis most commonly follows discontinuation of long-term corticosteroid therapy, and patients are vulnerable for up to 1 year. Other settings associated with acute adrenal insufficiency include sepsis, trauma, surgery, other autoimmune disease, adrenal hemorrhage/infarction, granulomatous disease (i.e., tuberculosis and sarcoidosis), AIDS, and pituitary/hypothalamic disease. Look for unexplained weight loss, anorexia, weakness, fatigue, orthostatic hypotension, and hyperpigmentation due to elevated ACTH levels (primary adrenal insufficiency). Hyperkalemia, hyponatremia, hypoglycemia, and eosinophilia may be present.

A cosyntropin stimulation test establishes the diagnosis of adrenal insufficiency. Baseline ACTH and cortisol values are obtained, as well as 30- and 60-minute values following administration of cosyntropin. A rise of serum cortisol ≥18 µg/dL rules out adrenal insufficiency. These values may not apply to critically ill patients who have low concentrations of albumin and cortisol-binding globulin; in these patients, measure serum-free cortisol concentrations. To distinguish primary adrenal insufficiency (adrenal gland failure) from secondary adrenal insufficiency (pituitary or hypothalamic failure), measure an 8:00 A.M. plasma ACTH and cortisol level. ACTH is elevated >100 pg/mL in primary adrenal insufficiency and is low or inappropriately "normal" in secondary adrenal insufficiency. Obtain a pituitary MRI in secondary insufficiency and a CT scan of the adrenal glands in primary adrenal insufficiency. The adrenal glands appear normal in the setting of autoimmune disease.

Therapy

If acute adrenal insufficiency is suspected, immediately obtain a serum ACTH and cortisol level and give high-dose corticosteroids (dexamethasone 4 mg is preferred because it does not interfere with serum cortisol assays) and large-volume (2-3 L) intravenous saline without waiting for the laboratory results. For less critically ill patients, administer oral hydrocortisone for primary and secondary adrenal insufficiency promptly; delay is potentially life-threatening. Most patients require about 20 mg/day of hydrocortisone or an equivalent corticosteroid. Fludrocortisone is required in primary, but not in secondary, adrenal insufficiency; aldosterone production is controlled by the renin-angiotensin system and is intact in secondary adrenal insufficiency. Mild stress, such as fever or viral upper respiratory infection, requires doubling or tripling the daily corticosteroid dose, and hospitalization for severe illness requires high-dose hydrocortisone 100 mg IV every 8 hours.

Follow-Up

Patients are counseled to wear a medic-alert bracelet announcing their diagnosis and must be able to articulate how to increase corticosteroids in minor illness. Adequacy of corticosteroid replacement is evaluated by looking for signs and symptoms of adrenal insufficiency (under-replacement) or Cushing's syndrome (over-replacement). Adjust the mineralocorticoid dose based on the plasma renin activity or the patient's symptoms. Patients complaining of lightheadedness with standing or who are orthostatic on exam need more fludrocortisone, whereas patients with peripheral edema and increased blood pressure need less.

Hyperadrenocorticism (Cushing's Syndrome)

Cushing's syndrome is an array of clinical features caused by excess cortisol, most commonly secondary to corticosteroid ingestion. Most endogenous cases are caused by ACTH-secreting pituitary tumors (Cushing's disease); adrenocortical tumors and ectopic ACTH-secreting malignant tumors each account for 10% of cases (Table 1). When the syndrome is due to an ectopic ACTH-secreting tumor, symptoms of weight loss, muscle weakness, and

Table 1. Differential Diagnosis of Endogenous Cushing's Syndrome

Disease	Notes
ACTH-independent forms:	ACTH level <10 pg/mL; DHEAS levels tend to be below normal, except in adrenal carcinoma
Adrenal adenoma	Unilateral mass and small contralateral gland on CT
Adrenal carcinoma	Unilateral mass and small contralateral gland on CT; may observe elevated DHEAS levels
Bilateral macronodular adrenal disease	Large nodular glands on CT; more common after age 50
ACTH-dependent forms:	ACTH level >10 pg/mL
Cushing's disease	Bilateral adrenal hyperplasia with or without nodules; pituitary mass on MRI
Ectopic ACTH secretion	Bilateral adrenal hyperplasia; look for a lung cancer

ACTH = adrenocorticotropic hormone; CT = computed tomography; DHEAS = dehydroepiandrosterone sulfate.

profound hypokalemia may predominate. ACTH-dependent forms of Cushing's syndrome result in bilateral adrenal enlargement.

Diagnosis

Look for features of glucocorticoid excess including change in menses, weight and strength, history of recurrent or chronic infections, worsening diabetic control, or fractures. Exclude exogenous corticosteroid intake by any route; it is the most common cause of Cushing's syndrome. Look for physical features that provide evidence for a specific cause of Cushing's syndrome, such as feminization or virilization and abdominal mass (adrenal tumor) or visual field losses (pituitary tumor). Look for abnormal fat distribution, particularly in the supraclavicular and temporal areas, proximal muscle weakness, or wide purple striae. Examination of photographs over time can highlight otherwise subtle changes and provide an estimate of change over time.

Obtain a 24-hour urine free cortisol measurement or overnight 1-mg dexamethasone suppression test. A 24-hour urine free cortisol level >3 times normal supports the diagnosis of Cushing's syndrome. Inability to suppress serum cortisol following the overnight 1-mg dexamethasone suppression test also suggests the diagnosis. Obesity, alcohol abuse, renal failure, and depression can cause false-positive results (pseudo-Cushing's syndrome). An elevated 24-hour urine free cortisol measurement <3 times normal is likely due to pseudo-Cushing's syndrome.

In patients with unequivocal excess cortisol production, measure a plasma ACTH level to differentiate between ACTH-dependent (pituitary or ectopic) and ACTH-independent (adrenal) causes of Cushing's syndrome. Basal levels of ACTH <6 pg/mL are found in adrenal forms of Cushing's syndrome and above this level in ACTH-dependent disease. Undetectable ACTH levels may be spurious if the sample is not processed within two hours due to the high susceptibility of ACTH to proteolysis. Obtain an adrenal CT scan to localize lesions in patients with suppressed ACTH values. In patients with non-suppressed ACTH, obtain a pituitary MRI. Perform biochemical and imaging tests in patients with ectopic ACTH secretion to localize the source of ectopic production. The most common ACTH secreting tumors are small cell carcinoma of the lung, bronchial carcinoid, pheochromocytoma, and medullary thyroid carcinoma. Begin the evaluation with a chest MRI or CT; if negative, obtain an abdominal CT or MRI to look for pancreatic tumor and other masses.

Therapy

Surgical resection of the tumor is the optimal therapy for Cushing's syndrome (adrenal, pituitary, or ectopic). Radiation or "gamma knife" therapy can be used for patients with persistent or recurrent Cushing's disease after trans-sphenoidal surgery or for those in whom surgery is contraindicated.

Adjuvant drug therapy reduces cortisol production in patients undergoing surgery or as sole therapy for occult ectopic ACTH secretion or metastatic adrenal cancer. Ketoconazole, mitotane, metyrapone, and aminoglutethimide reduce endogenous cortisol levels and reverse most signs and symptoms of Cushing's syndrome. Steroidogenesis inhibitors may be needed as adjunctive agents to pituitary radiation therapy in patients with Cushing's disease, because radiation therapy can take 2-5 years to ablate the tumor.

Follow-Up

Following surgery, give corticosteroid replacement to patients with hypoadrenocorticism until the hypothalamic-pituitary-adrenal axis has recovered (up to a year) and recovery can be assessed with serial cosyntropin stimulation tests. Monitor patients for the development of panhypopituitarism after pituitary irradiation or extensive pituitary resection. Ensure that patients with presumed occult ectopic ACTH production undergo ongoing imaging surveillance to localize the tumor every 6 months the first year, then annually. More than half of tumors are initially occult.

Hyperaldosteronism

Once thought to be a rare cause of hypertension, hyperaldosteronism (also called aldosteronism) has been recognized in up to 14% of unselected hypertensive patients. Depending upon cause, hyperaldosteronism is amenable to medical or surgical treatment.

Diagnosis

Consider the diagnosis of hyperaldosteronism in difficult-to-control or worsening hypertension despite multiple antihypertensive agents, spontaneous hypokalemia, severe hypokalemia after institution of diuretic therapy, or hypertension at a young age. Hypokalemia results when hyperaldosteronism causes excess renal distal tubule exchange of sodium for potassium. In the presence of an elevated aldosterone and suppressed renin level, an 8:00 A.M. upright plasma aldosterone level to plasma renin activity ratio >23 suggests primary hyperaldosteronism, with a sensitivity of 97% and a specificity of 94%. Spironolactone, angiotensin-converting enzyme inhibitors, angiotensin receptor blockers, diuretics, and β-blockers should be stopped prior to testing because they alter the levels of renin and aldosterone. If positive, obtain a CT scan of the adrenal glands. Unilateral aldosteronoma (Conn's syndrome) is the most common cause of primary hyperaldosteronism, followed by bilateral adrenal hyperplasia and idiopathic hyperaldosteronism (no adrenal abnormalities visualized).

Therapy

Surgical resection of unilateral aldosterone-producing adrenal adenoma is the treatment of choice. Bilateral adrenalectomy is not indicated for bilateral adrenal hyperplasia due to the development of adrenal insufficiency. Hypokalemia usually resolves following surgery, but hypertension does not always resolve; long-standing hypertension results in permanent vascular changes, making normalization of blood pressure difficult.

Spironolactone is the treatment of choice for idiopathic hyperaldosteronism, bilateral adrenal hyperplasia, and nonsurgical candidates with unilateral disease. If additional antihypertensive medications are required to control blood pressure, low-dose thiazide therapy is usually effective in combination with spironolactone; calcium-channel blockers or angiotensin-converting enzyme inhibitors are used if additional antihypertensive therapy is indicated. A more selective mineralocorticoid receptor antagonist, eplerenone, can be used if the patient is unable to tolerate side effects from spironolactone, such as decreased libido, impotence, or gynecomastia. Salt restriction to <100 mmol/day will decrease urinary potassium wasting and potentiate the effect of antihypertensive therapy.

Follow-Up

Post-surgical patients should be monitored for hypoaldosteronism (hypotension and hyperkalemia) due to long-term suppression of the contralateral adrenal gland. Patients taking spironolactone or eplerenone require titration of medication to maximum effect on potassium concentration and blood pressure, as well as tapering of potassium supplementation.

Pheochromocytoma

Pheochromocytoma is a rare cause of secondary hypertension (<0.1%) and is classically described by the Rule of Tens: 10% extra-adrenal, 10% malignant, 10% familial, 10% bilateral, 10% pediatric, and 10% recur. Pheochromocytomas are paraganglioma tumors arising in the chromaffin cells of the adrenal medulla, and they can produce, store, and secrete catecholamines (norepinephrine, epinephrine, and/or dopamine). Most adrenal pheochromocytomas produce both norepinephrine and epinephrine.

Diagnosis

Consider pheochromocytoma in patients with moderate-to-severe hypertension (sustained or paroxysmal), coupled with episodes of severe headache, sweating, and palpitations. Table 2 describes some important disorders in the differential diagnosis of pheochromocytoma.

Obtain 24-hour urine metanephrine measurement. Plasma catecholamine measurements are avoided because of high false-positive rates, as is collecting urine for vanillylmandelic acid because of the need for a special diet prior to collection. Many medications can interfere with the assay, and this test is best performed and interpreted with the help of a specialist. When the diagnosis of pheochromocytoma is confirmed, localization with an adrenal CT is performed; intravenous contrast is not to be used because it can precipitate hypertensive crisis. If no adrenal abnormality is seen,

Table 2. Differential Diagnosis of Pheochromocytoma

Disease	Notes
Thyrotoxicosis (see Chapter 10)	Weight loss, tachycardia, tremor and suppressed serum TSH concentration, evaluated T_4 and/or T_3 levels.
Insulinoma	Whipple's triad: neuroglycopenia (sympathetic symptoms alone are not enough), glucose <50 mg/dL during the occurrence of symptoms, and prompt resolution of symptoms with administration of glucose.
Essential hypertension (see Chapter 37)	Labile blood pressure is quite common and is associated with normal levels of catecholamines and metanephrine.
Renovascular hypertension (see Chapter 37)	Paroxysmal hypertension can occur. Normal levels of catecholamines and metanephrines exclude pheochromocytoma.
Anxiety, panic attacks, and hyperventilation	Panic disorder is frequently confused with pheochromocytoma. Normal levels of catecholamines and metanephrines exclude pheochromocytoma.
Carcinoid syndrome	Typically presents with flushing, diarrhea, and cardiac-related symptoms. Symptoms are sometimes associated with eating. Elevated 24-hr urinary excretion of 5-hydroxyindole acetic acid is diagnostic.
Unexplained flushing spells	This is a diagnosis of exclusion. Signs and symptoms may be clinically indistinguishable from patients with pheochromocytoma, except that all catecholamines and metanephrine levels are normal.

TSH = thyroid-stimulating hormone.

obtain CT scan of the chest, abdomen, and pelvis and look for tumors along the sympathetic chain.

Therapy

Surgical resection is the treatment of choice. Patients must receive full alpha-adrenergic blockade (phenoxybenzamine) prior to surgery to avoid hypertensive emergency during resection. Beta-blockade follows alpha-blockade for further blood pressure and heart rate control. Beta-blockade prior to alpha-blockade is contraindicated due to the dangers of unopposed alpha-adrenergic activity.

Follow-Up

Screen patients for recurrence of preoperative symptoms and monitor blood pressure. Twenty-four hour metanephrine collection is performed after resection to ensure normalization and if recurrence is suspected. Blood pressure does not always normalize following resection due to the long-term vascular effects of hypertension.

Book Enhancement

Go to www.acponline.org/essentials/endocrinology-section.html to access a differential diagnosis of hyperaldosteronism, view a patient with hypoadrenalism and hyperadrenalism, and view CT scans of an adrenal adenoma and pheochromocytoma. In *MKSAP for Students 4*, assess yourself with items 27-30 in the **Endocrinology and Metabolism** section.

Bibliography

Nieman LK. Hypercortisolism. http://pier.acponline.org/physicians/diseases/d259. [Date accessed: 2008 Jan 15] In: PIER [online database]. Philadelphia: American College of Physicians; 2008.

Young WF Jr. Clinical practice. The incidentally discovered adrenal mass. N Engl J Med. 2007;356:601-10. [PMID: 17287480]

Chapter 12

Osteoporosis

Melissa A. McNeil, MD
Janine M. Frank, MD

Osteoporosis is a skeletal disorder characterized by decreased bone mass and an increased predisposition to fractures. Decreased bone mass can occur because peak bone mass is low (related to genetics, insufficient dietary intake of calcium and vitamin D, and physical inactivity), excessive bone resorption, or decreased bone formation during remodeling. All three mechanisms likely contribute to osteoporosis. The prevalence of low bone mineral density increases rapidly above age 50, approaching 80% in women aged >80 years. Effective screening modalities and treatments are available.

Screening

The goals of screening are to identify individuals at increased risk for developing osteoporosis and to identify patients with osteoporosis. Modifiable risk factors for osteoporosis are responsive either to lifestyle intervention or are secondary to another disease. Lifestyle risk factors include low calcium intake, inadequate physical activity, low body weight (<127 lb [57.6 kg]), cigarette smoking, and alcoholism. Secondary causes of osteoporosis include hyperthyroidism, corticosteroid use for >3 months, and sex hormone deficiency. Nonmodifiable risk factors include increasing age, female gender, race (white or Asian), and family history of fragility fracture in a first-degree relative. A fragility fracture is a spontaneous fracture or a fracture due to a fall from standing height or less. All are important in risk assessment but only the modifiable factors are relevant to a therapeutic intervention.

The screening modality of choice is a dual-energy x-ray absorptiometry (DEXA) scan. Generally, spine and hip screening provides the most reliable measurements and can be followed for change. Results of DEXA scans are provided as both T and Z scores. T scores represent the number of standard deviations from the normal gender-matched young adult mean bone density values. T scores <–2.5 are considered to be diagnostic of osteoporosis; scores between –1 and –2.5 define osteopenia. Z scores represent the number of standard deviations from the normal mean value for age and gender matched control subjects. Z scores are used in assessing osteoporosis risk in individuals aged <40 years. In individuals aged >40 years, abnormally low Z scores suggest the presence of a secondary cause of osteoporosis.

All women aged >65 years, regardless of risk factors, are screened, as well as male or female individuals with a previous fragility fracture. Postmenopausal women <65 years old with one additional risk factor are also screened. Younger women are screened if menopausal at age <40 years or have amenorrhea >1 year. Younger men and women are screened if they have a chronic disease associated with bone loss (e.g., seizure disorder on seizure medications or renal failure), have immobilization >1 year, or have received solid organ or bone marrow transplant.

Diagnosis

Look for secondary causes of osteoporosis in premenopausal women or in men aged <75 years if standard risk factors are absent. The most common secondary causes are hyperthyroidism, hyperparathyroidism, renal or liver disease, malabsorption, eating disorders, and hypogonadism in men, multiple myeloma, and Cushing's syndrome. If secondary causes have been excluded, dietary and lifestyle habits are assessed. Calcium intake (past and current), physical activity, smoking, and alcohol use are part of the assessment of every patient with osteopenia or osteoporosis.

Physical examination clues for evidence of osteoporosis or spinal fracture include kyphosis, loss of height, low body weight (<112 lb [51 kg]), inability to place the back of the head against the wall when standing upright, rib-pelvis distance greater than two finger breadths, and inability to raise from a seated position without using arms (poor proximal muscle strength). Reasonable screening tests include complete blood count, serum TSH, calcium and phosphorus, creatinine, alanine aminotransferase, aspartate aminotransferase, alkaline phosphatase, erythrocyte sedimentation rate, serum testosterone in males, serum 25-hydroxyvitamin D (if vitamin D deficiency is suspected), and tissue transglutaminase antibodies (if gluten enteropathy is suspected). In the absence of fractures, primary osteoporosis is associated with no abnormalities on laboratory testing. Look for medications besides corticosteroids that can cause bone loss including neuroleptics (e.g., phenothiazines) and anticonvulsants (e.g., phenytoin, phenobarbital, primidone, carbamazepine).

Therapy

Ensuring adequate oral calcium intake is a mainstay for both the prevention and treatment of osteoporosis. The recommended calcium intake varies by age and gender (Table 1). The daily dietary calcium intake can be estimated by multiplying each dairy product serving by 300 mg and then adding 250 mg, representing the average calcium intake from other foods. Calcium supplements (calcium carbonate or calcium citrate) are recommended for patients who do not routinely consume adequate amounts of daily calcium in their diets. Encourage smoking cessation, reduced alcohol use, and resistance exercise. For frail, elderly

Table 1. Optimal Calcium Requirements

Group	Optimal Daily Intake
Men	
25-65 years	1000 mg
>65 years	1500 mg
Women	
25-50 years	1000 mg
>50 years (postmenopausal)	1500 mg
On estrogens	1000 mg
Not on estrogens	1500 mg
>65 years	1500 mg
Pregnant and nursing	1200-1500 mg

Data from National Institutes of Health, Optimal Calcium Intake, 1994.

patients, stress the importance of the prevention of falls. This is best accomplished by home safety evaluations, minimized use of sedatives and anxiolytics, and leg-strengthening exercises.

Vitamin D is required for the absorption of calcium in the small intestine. Vitamin D deficiency is surprisingly common and often undiagnosed. The recommended vitamin D intake is 400-600 IU/day for all adults aged >50 years or 800 IU/day for those at risk of deficiency including the elderly, chronically ill, homebound, or institutionalized individuals.

The integrity of bone is determined by the balance between osteoblasts and osteoclasts. Most pharmacologic interventions decrease the resorption of bone, thus altering the balance in favor of the formation of new bone. Antiresorptive therapy is effective in patients with or at risk for osteoporosis (Table 2). Therapy is begun in patients with a DEXA T score of <–2.0 or in patients with a DEXA T score of <–1.5 if additional risk factors are present, or in any patient with a prior fragility vertebral or hip fracture.

Bisphosphonate therapy is the first line of intervention. Bisphosphonates are antiresorptive agents, which reduce risk of fracture. Treatment results in a 30%-60% decrease in fracture rates,

with the greatest efficacy shown in the prevention of new vertebral fractures. Three oral bisphosphonates are currently available: alendronate, risedronate, and ibandronate. Bisphosphonates are taken on an empty stomach with at least 8 oz of water, and patients must remain upright for at least 30 minutes (60 minutes for ibandronate) to prevent pill-induced esophageal ulceration. Bisphosphonates are contraindicated in patients with renal failure or esophageal disease. Intravenous ibandronate (every 3 months) and intravenous zoledronate (once yearly) are also FDA-approved for the treatment of osteoporosis in postmenopausal women. Intravenous bisphosphonates are contraindicated in patients with severe hypocalcemia and renal insufficiency. Bisphosphonate therapy (mainly intravenous) in patients with metastatic cancer has been associated with osteonecrosis of the jaw.

Raloxifene is a selective estrogen receptor modulator. It has an estrogen agonist effect on bone and an antagonist effect in breast and uterus and may be used in women who cannot tolerate bisphosphonate therapy. Side effects include increased risk of thromboembolism and increased vasomotor symptoms. The effect of raloxifene on bone mass is less than that of estrogen or alendronate, reducing the risk of vertebral but not hip fracture rates. While effective, estrogen therapy is no longer recommended for women with or at risk of osteoporosis due to an overall unfavorable risk/benefit profile.

Teriparatide is the first FDA-approved agent that stimulates bone formation rather than decreasing bone resorption. It is indicated for treatment of patients with severe osteoporosis who have failed or cannot take other drugs. Teriparatide reduces vertebral fractures by 65% and nonvertebral fractures by 53%, a reduction that continues even after therapy is discontinued. The drug is given as a subcutaneous injection once daily for 18 months. Side effects include lightheadedness, nausea, arthralgias, leg cramps, and, rarely, an increase in post-injection calcium level. Teriparatide is ten times more expensive than other therapies for osteoporosis

Table 2. Drug Treatment for Osteoporosis

Agent	Notes
Oral bisphosphonates (alendronate, risedronate, ibandronate)	Decreases bone resorption by attenuating osteoclast activity. First-line treatment of osteoporosis. Increases bone mass; decreases vertebral and nonvertebral fractures. May cause esophageal irritation. Must take in morning without food and with 8 oz of water and not recline for 30-60 min.
Intravenous bisphosphonates (zoledronate, ibandronate)	Decreases bone resorption by attenuating osteoclast activity. First-line treatment of osteoporosis. Increases bone mass; decreases vertebral fracture, hip fracture, and nonvertebral fractures. Flu-like symptoms after first dose. Zoledronate is given every 12 mo and ibandronate every 3 mo.
Raloxifene	Selective estrogen receptor modulator suppresses osteoclasts and decreases bone resorption; estrogen antagonist in uterus and breast. Increases bone mass; decreases vertebral fractures; decreases risk of breast cancer; increases thromboembolic risk, increases vasomotor symptoms; increases risk of fatal stroke. Not recommended for premenopausal women or women using estrogen replacement.
Teriparatide	Recombinant parathyroid hormone. Stimulates bone formation. Increases bone mass; decreases vertebral and nonvertebral fracture rates. Maximum duration of 18 months. Contraindicated if a history of bone malignancy, Paget's disease, hypercalcemia, or skeletal radiation.
Calcitonin	Decreases bone resorption by attenuating osteoclast activity. Slight increase in bone mass; decreased vertebral fracture rates. Rhinitis. Decreases pain associated with vertebral fracture. Calcitonin is *not* considered first-line treatment for osteoporosis.

and cannot be continued beyond 18 months because of concern about the risk of osteosarcoma.

Calcitonin is indicated for patients with bone pain from osteoporotic fractures or in patients with contraindications to other therapies. An anti-resorptive agent administered as a nasal spray, calcitonin is not used as a first-line agent, because other therapies are more effective.

Follow-Up

Use DEXA scan to measure bone mineral density 12 to 24 months after initiating therapy and periodically thereafter. Look for percent improvements in the bone density value to determine treatment efficacy and the T score to assess current fracture risk. Consider possible secondary causes, poor adherence, and need for additional treatment in patients with continuing bone loss after 12 to 18 months of therapy.

Book Enhancement

Go to www.acponline.org/essentials/endocrinology-section .html to access a differential diagnosis of osteoporosis and to see a clinical photograph of an elderly man with kyphosis secondary to osteoporosis, a lumbar radiograph showing osteopenia and vertebral compression fracture, and an example of a dual-energy X-ray absorptiometry report. In *MKSAP for Students 4*, assess yourself with items 31-33 in the **Endocrinology and Metabolism** section.

Bibliography

Green AD, Colon-Emeric CS, Bastian L, et al. Does this woman have osteoporosis? JAMA. 2004;292:2890-900. [PMID: 15598921]

Inzucchi S. Osteoporosis. http://pier.acponline.org/physicians/diseases/ d297. [Date accessed: 2008 Jan 24] In: PIER [online database]. Philadelphia: American College of Physicians; 2008.

Section III
Gastroenterology and Hepatology

Chapter 13

Approach to Abdominal Pain

Priya Radhakrishnan, MD

bdominal pain is a common symptom, accounting for 18%-42% of hospital admissions. Although some patients have classic symptoms pointing to a particular diagnosis, in other patients the diagnosis is obscure. Pain in the abdomen is generally of visceral or parietal origin, originates from the abdominal wall, or is referred from other sites. Visceral pain is usually caused by stretching of the organ and is not associated with signs of peritoneal inflammation. In contrast, parietal pain is secondary to inflammation or irritation of the overlying peritoneum and is associated with tenderness, guarding, or rebound. Abdominal wall pain tends to be chronic and to be precisely located by the patient. Referred pain generally follows a dermatomal distribution and is not associated with underlying tenderness or signs of peritoneal inflammation.

Evaluation

The history and physical examination help develop a differential diagnosis and direct the relevant investigations. Important clues to the underlying diagnosis can be discovered through carefully characterizing the abdominal pain with respect to onset (acute or insidious) duration, nature (intermittent or constant), relation to eating, association with bleeding, and location. Pain that is acute in onset generally points to acute inflammatory, infectious, or ischemic causes. Upper abdominal pain is usually of gastric, hepatobiliary, or pancreatic origin, whereas pain in the lower abdomen originates from the hindgut and genitourinary organs. The origin of periumbilical pain is midgut and pancreas. Hematemesis definitely points to an upper gastrointestinal etiology, but melena, maroon stools, hematochezia, or occult blood can be from either upper or lower gastrointestinal sources. General symptoms such as anorexia, nausea, or vomiting are insensitive in diagnosing abdominal pain. Associated medical problems can often suggest a diagnosis such as embolic or ischemic infarction due to cardiovascular disease, arrhythmia, or infective endocarditis. A history of multiple sexual partners, unprotected intercourse, or previous sexually transmitted disease highlights the possibility of pelvic inflammatory disease in women. The evaluation of abdominal pain is never complete until a physical examination, including pelvic and rectal examination, has been performed (Table 1).

Acute Abdominal Pain

Acute abdominal pain is defined as pain of <1 week duration; the three most common diagnoses are appendicitis, biliary disease, and non-specific abdominal pain. Patients with acute abdominal pain,

peritoneal signs, and hemodynamic instability require an urgent investigation and may need early surgical intervention. Obtain a chest x-ray and flat and upright abdominal x-rays in every patient with significant acute abdominal pain to exclude bowel obstruction or perforation (free peritoneal air localized under the diaphragm) or intrathoracic processes (e.g., pneumonia, pneumothorax, or aortic dissection) that can present as abdominal pain. In older patients, consider an electrocardiogram to exclude an atypical presentation of myocardial infarction.

Upper Abdominal Pain

Biliary pain is the commonest cause of abdominal pain among patients aged >50 years. Cholelithiasis should be suspected in patients with postprandial, right upper quadrant pain associated with ingesting fatty foods. Murphy's sign (respiratory arrest on deep inspiration while palpating right upper quadrant) suggests cholecystitis and Charcot's triad (pain, fever, and jaundice) suggests cholecystitis or ascending cholangitis. Abdominal ultrasound is the imaging modality of choice for cholelithiasis, with a sensitivity and specificity approaching 100%. Cholescintigraphy scans (e.g., HIDA scan) are an alternative to diagnose acute cholecystitis and can be used when ultrasonography is equivocal.

Peptic ulcer disease and gastritis commonly present with burning abdominal pain, but the pain may be vague or even cramping. In two-thirds of cases the pain is epigastric, but in the remainder it is in either the upper right or left upper quadrants. Pain that radiates through to the back is unusual with peptic ulcer disease or gastritis and suggests either pancreatitis or penetrating peptic ulcer disease; hematemesis or blood in the nasogastric aspirate excludes pancreatitis. Ingestion of food worsens gastric ulcer pain and improves duodenal ulcer pain, but this relationship is found in less than half of patients with confirmed peptic ulcer disease. The presence of peritoneal signs strongly suggests perforation and is supported by finding free air under the diaphragm on chest x-ray or upright abdominal x-ray.

Acute pancreatitis presents with acute epigastric pain, often radiating to the back; vomiting is found in >85% of cases. The absence of vomiting favors another diagnosis. Bending forward or lying curled up on the side may relieve the pain, but many patients report no alleviating factors. Jaundice is frequently present in gallstone pancreatitis, and a history of alcohol abuse supports alcoholic pancreatitis. Occasionally patients may have flank ecchymoses from retroperitoneal bleeding (Gray-Turner sign). Perform ultrasonography to evaluate the biliary tract for stones; obtain an abdominal CT scan, ideally with oral and intravenous contrast, when the diagnosis of acute pancreatitis is in question

Table 1. Differential Diagnosis of Acute Abdominal Pain

Type of Pain	Notes
RUQ Pain	
Acute cholangitis (see Chapter 15)	Right upper quadrant pain, fever, jaundice. Bilirubin generally >4 mg/dL; AST and ALT levels may exceed 1000 U/L.
Pneumonia (see Chapter 53)	Cough and shortness of breath, chest or upper abdominal pain.
Acute viral hepatitis (see Chapter 21)	Jaundice; AST and ALT levels generally >1000 U/L.
Acute alcoholic hepatitis	Recent alcohol intake. Fever, leukocytosis; AST level usually 2-3× greater than ALT level; bilirubin level generally >4 mg/dL.
Fitz-Hugh-Curtis syndrome (gonococcal perihepatitis)	Pelvic adnexal tenderness and leukocytosis. Cervical smear shows gonococci.
Cholecystitis (see Chapter 15)	Epigastrium and RUQ pain that radiates to the right shoulder. Mildly elevated bilirubin and aminotransferase levels. Ultrasound shows thickened gallbladder, pericholecystic fluid.
Mid-epigastric/Periumbilical Pain	
Acute pancreatitis (see Chapter 16)	Mid-epigastric pain radiating to the back, nausea, vomiting, elevated amylase and lipase. Usually secondary to gallstones or alcohol. Pain from penetrating peptic ulcer may also present similarly.
Inferior myocardial infarction (see Chapter 3)	Chest/mid-epigastric pain, diaphoresis, shortness of breath, elevated cardiac enzymes, acutely abnormal electrocardiogram.
Perforated peptic ulcer (see Chapter 18)	Sudden RUQ or mid-epigastric pain, possible hematemesis and/or melena. Normal bilirubin, aminotransferase levels. Amylase and lipase may be high; free air under the diaphragm.
Mesenteric ischemia	Postprandial abdominal pain, weight loss, and abdominal bruit. Pain out of proportion to tenderness on palpation. Anion-gap metabolic acidosis may be present. Abdominal plain films may show the classic thumbprinting sign.
Small bowel obstruction	Pain is colicky. Obstructive pattern is seen on CT or abdominal series.
Aortic dissection/rupture	Elderly patient with vascular disease and sudden onset with very severe pain that radiates to the back and lower extremity.
Diabetic ketoacidosis (see Chapter 8)	Blood glucose is always elevated, anion gap present.
RLQ Pain	
Acute appendicitis	Mid-epigastric pain radiating to RLQ. Ultrasound and CT may confirm diagnosis.
Ectopic pregnancy, ovarian cyst/torsion	May be RLQ or LLQ. Abdominal pain, nausea, fever, leukocytosis. Suspect in female with unilateral pain.
Pelvic inflammatory disease	May be RLQ or LLQ. Fever, abdominal tenderness, uterine/adnexal tenderness, cervical motion tenderness, cervical discharge.
Nephrolithiasis	Right or left flank pain that may radiate to the groin; hematuria.
Pyelonephritis (see Chapter 48)	Fever, dysuria, pain in the right or left flank that may radiate to the lower quadrant. Urinalysis shows leukocytes and leukocyte casts.
LLQ Pain	
Acute diverticulitis	Pain usually in the LLQ but can be RLQ if ascending colon is involved. CT scan can diagnose complicated diverticular disease with abscess formation.
Toxic megacolon	Dilation of the transverse and descending colon and systemic toxicity. Associated with inflammatory bowel disease and infection (e.g., *C. difficile*).

ALT = alanine aminotransferase; AST = aspartate aminotransferase; LLQ = left lower quadrant; RLQ = right lower quadrant; RUQ = right upper quadrant.

or to stage the severity or determine the presence of complications such as abscess or pseudocyst.

Central and Lower Abdominal Pain

Appendicitis is the most common cause of acute abdominal pain in patients aged <50 years. Despite the development of sophisticated diagnostic techniques and algorithms, appendicitis is missed in at least 20% of cases. The pain classically begins in the periumbilical region and migrates to the right lower quadrant and may be followed by nausea and vomiting. The diagnosis of appendicitis is doubtful if nausea and vomiting are the first signs of illness. Physical examination will reveal tenderness over McBurney's point; abdominal rigidity and a positive psoas sign (pain elicited by extending the right thigh with the patient on the left side) increase the pre-test probability of appendicitis. Leukocytosis and fever, although sensitive, are not specific for appendicitis. CT scan of the abdomen with oral and intravenous contrast is the diagnostic test of choice in non-pregnant patients (sensitivity and specificity >92%; positive likelihood ratio = 18). Ultrasound and plain abdominal x-rays have poor sensitivity and specificity in the diagnosis of appendicitis.

Small bowel obstruction presents as central or generalized abdominal pain associated with vomiting or constipation. History of prior abdominal surgery, hyperactive bowel sounds, and abdominal distension increase the probability of small bowel obstruction. Small bowel air-fluid levels are detected on abdominal x-ray. Other causes of small bowel obstruction include neoplasms, strictures, intussusception and volvulus. CT scans with contrast are superior to plain x-rays in detecting complete small bowel obstruction, but early or partial obstruction may be missed by either modality. Acute colonic distension is most likely due to mechanical obstruction, toxic megacolon (e.g., as a complication of inflammatory bowel disease or *Clostridium difficile* infection), and colonic pseudo-obstruction. Mechanical obstruction presents with crampy abdominal pain. On abdominal x-ray, dilated loops of small and large bowel and lack of gas in the distal colon or rectum suggest mechanical obstruction but can also be seen in pseudo-obstruction. Mechanical obstruction is most commonly due to tumors and sigmoid volvulus. Acute colonic pseudo-obstruction (Ogilvie's syndrome) is characterized by dilatation of the cecum and right hemicolon in the absence of mechanical obstruction; the three most common causes are trauma, infection, and cardiac disease (i.e., myocardial infarction and heart failure). Toxic megacolon presents with fever, tachycardia, and abdominal tenderness, and there is usually a history of bloody diarrhea. Abdominal films may show "thumbprinting" due to the presence of submucosal edema, or thickening of the colonic wall.

While diverticular disease is very common (50%-70% prevalence in patients aged >80 years) and often asymptomatic, acute diverticulitis presents with left lower quadrant abdominal pain and tenderness to palpation. Patients may have a history of chronic constipation and intermittent low-grade abdominal pain prior to an acute attack. Abscess formation should be suspected if guarding, rigidity, or a tender fluctuant mass is present. Abdominal and pelvic CT scan with contrast is the test of choice.

Non-specific abdominal pain is the third most common cause of acute abdominal pain presenting to the emergency department. It includes all causes of abdominal pain for which no specific surgical, medical, or gynecologic diagnosis can be made, including dyspepsia, constipation, irritable bowel syndrome, viral gastroenteritis, mesenteric adenitis, and dysmenorrhea.

Renal stones, acute urinary obstruction, and urinary tract infection including pyelonephritis are common causes of abdominal pain. Pain due to renal stone is typically acute and colicky and may radiate from the flank to the groin, particularly as the stone travels down the ureter. Renal colic may be associated with hematuria and dysuria. Helical CT scan is the most sensitive and specific imaging study available for stones and excels in making the diagnosis of nonrenal causes of flank pain as well.

Acute urinary obstruction presents with suprapubic discomfort, oliguria or anuria. It is common in older males, secondary to prostatic hypertrophy. Insertion of a catheter relieves the obstruction and pain. Testicular torsion may cause referred pain to the lower abdomen; therefore, examine the testicles for tenderness and unilateral elevation in men, particularly young men, with lower abdominal pain. Women presenting with lower abdominal or pelvic pain must have a pelvic examination and a urine pregnancy test; pelvic inflammatory disease and ectopic pregnancy are often overlooked causes of lower abdominal pain.

Generalized Abdominal Pain

Diffuse abdominal pain is seen in acute peritonitis, ischemic bowel and obstruction. The most common cause of ischemic bowel is a mesenteric arterial embolism originating from the heart (50%), followed by mesenteric arterial thrombosis (25%), and mesenteric venous thrombosis (10%). Initially, abdominal pain is poorly localized and is more severe than the findings suggested by abdominal palpation. Peritoneal signs may signify an infarction. Selective mesenteric angiography is the diagnostic study of choice.

Abdominal pain can be a presenting feature of metabolic disorders such as diabetic and alcoholic ketoacidosis, adrenal crises, sickle cell crisis, porphyria, and familial Mediterranean fever. Vasculitides (Henoch-Schönlein purpura, systemic lupus erythematosus, and polyarteritis nodosum) should also be considered in the differential diagnosis, particularly if the abdominal pain is associated with other, extra-abdominal manifestations such as rash, arthralgias, pleuritic pain, hematuria, or renal failure.

Chronic Abdominal Pain

Abdominal pain is chronic if it has persisted for >3 months. Chronic abdominal pain is a common cause of ambulatory visits; within this category irritable bowel syndrome is one of the most common causes of chronic abdominal pain. Abdominal wall pain is an often overlooked cause of chronic pain and includes entities such as hernia and rectus sheath hematomas. The pain is precisely localized by the patient with one finger.

Irritable Bowel Syndrome

The pain of irritable bowel is localized to the lower abdomen and may be associated with bloating, nausea, and diarrhea or constipation. Pain is often exacerbated by psychological stress, and the physical examination characteristically reveals only non-specific tenderness over the sigmoid colon. Irritable bowel frequently co-exists with other chronic conditions such as depression, fibromyalgia, and chronic pelvic pain syndrome. For many years, irritable bowel syndrome has been considered a diagnosis of exclusion, but this approach leads to unnecessary additional tests. Recent clinical and epidemiologic studies have led to the development of symptom-based diagnostic criteria that can accurately discriminate irritable bowel syndrome from other disorders. The Rome criteria (Table 2) for the diagnosis of irritable bowel syndrome have a sensitivity of approximately 48% and specificity of 100%. The Manning criteria are also used to diagnose irritable bowel syndrome; diagnostic accuracy of Manning criteria is better in women, younger patients, and when more criteria are positive (Table 2). Red flags that make the diagnosis of irritable bowel syndrome unlikely and that should prompt an early investigation for other causes include onset of abdominal pain in older age, anorexia, weight loss, signs of malnutrition, and recent change in bowel habits.

Table 2. Criteria for Diagnosis of Irritable Bowel Syndrome

Rome Criteria

≥3 months of continuous or recurrent symptoms of abdominal pain or discomfort that is:	Relieved with defecation and/or
	Associated with a change in frequency of stool and/or
	Associated with a change in consistency of stool
and ≥2 of these 5 symptoms on >25% of occasions or days:	Altered stool frequency (>3 bowel movements daily or <3 bowel movements weekly)
	Altered stool form (lumpy/hard or loose/watery stool)
	Altered stool passage (straining, urgency, or feeling of incomplete evacuation)
	Passage of mucus
	Bloating or feeling of abdominal distension

Manning Criteria

The presence of abdominal pain and at least 2 of the following 6 symptoms: pain relief with defecation, looser stools at pain onset, more frequent stools at pain onset, abdominal distention, mucus per rectum, feeling of incomplete evacuation

Book Enhancement

Go to www.acponline.org/essentials/gastroenterology-section
.html to view x-rays of small bowel obstruction, pneumoperi-
toneum, thumbprinting, diverticular abscess, and toxic megacolon. In *MKSAP for Students 4*, assess yourself with items 10-17
in the **Gastroenterology and Hepatology** section.

Bibliography

American College of Physicians. Medical Knowledge Self-Assessment Program 14. Philadelphia: American College of Physicians; 2006.

Jacobs DO. Clinical practice. Diverticulitis. N Engl J Med. 2007;357:2057-66. [PMID: 18003962]

Mayer EA. Clinical practice. Irritable bowel syndrome. N Engl J Med. 2008; 358:1692-9. [PMID: 18420501]

Trowbridge RL, Rutkowski NK, Shojania KG. Does this patient have acute cholecystitis? JAMA. 2003;289:80-6. [PMID: 12503981]

Chapter 14

Approach to Diarrhea

Sarang Kim, MD

Diarrhea is physiologically defined as >200 g of stool per day. In clinical practice, diarrhea is generally defined as ≥3 loose or watery stools per day, or a decrease in stool consistency and increase in frequency from a patient's baseline. Start the evaluation by differentiating acute diarrhea from chronic diarrhea.

Acute Diarrhea

Acute diarrhea is defined as diarrhea lasting <14 days and is most commonly caused by an infectious agent. Acute infectious diarrhea is transmitted predominantly through the fecal-oral route by ingestion of contaminated food and water. Most cases are self-limited and do not require extensive evaluation.

Diagnosis

The first step in evaluation of patients with acute diarrhea is to obtain a detailed history and physical examination to assess severity, quality, and duration of diarrhea and to identify epidemiologic clues for potential diagnosis. Ask patients about food, antibiotic use, recent travel, sexual activity, and sick contacts. Ingestion of preformed bacterial toxins, such as *Staphylococcus aureus*, *Bacillus cereus*, *Clostridium perfringens*, or enterotoxigenic *Escherichia coli* results in nausea and vomiting followed by diarrhea within 12 hours. Bacteria that require colonization to produce symptoms, such as nontyphoid *Salmonella*, *Campylobacter jejuni*, and enteropathic *E. coli* produce diarrhea 48 hours after ingestion. Outbreaks of diarrhea in families, nursing homes or schools, or after ingestion of undercooked shellfish are commonly associated with noroviruses. For hospitalized patients, or those with recent antibiotic use, *C. difficile* infection should be considered. Proctitis in sexually active adults is characterized by tenesmus and small volumes of stool and may be caused by herpesvirus, gonococcal, chlamydial, or syphilitic infection. Noninfectious causes of acute diarrhea include medications and ingestion of substances that can cause osmotic diarrhea, such as sorbitol, fructose, and laxatives. The temporal relationship between ingestion and acute onset of diarrhea is usually straightforward.

Diagnostic testing is generally reserved for patients with severe diarrheal illness characterized by fever, blood in stool, or signs of dehydration (e.g., weakness, thirst, decreased urine output, or orthostasis) or diarrhea lasting >7 days. For community-acquired or traveler's diarrhea, send stool cultures for *Salmonella*, *Shigella*, *Campylobacter*, *Giardia*, *Cryptosporidium*, *Cyclospora*, and *Isospora*. In the setting of blood in stool or hemolytic uremic syndrome, test for *E. coli* O157:H7 and Shiga toxin. For health care–related diarrhea, test for *C. difficile* toxin. Fecal specimens from patients with diarrhea that develop after 3 days of hospitalization have a very low yield for standard bacterial pathogens such as *Campylobacter*, *Salmonella*, and *Shigella*, and testing for these organisms is usually not indicated unless there is evidence of a specific outbreak. If the patient is immunocompromised, also test for *Mycobacterium avium* complex and *Microsporidia*.

Therapy

Empiric therapy is often appropriate for an otherwise healthy patient with acute, noninvasive diarrhea that is most likely secondary to a transient infection. Adequate hydration and avoidance of easily malabsorbed carbohydrates (e.g., lactose, sorbitol) are often sufficient. If needed for convenience or to help reduce dehydration, antidiarrheal agents such as loperamide or atropine/diphenoxylate may be used. Empiric antibiotics (i.e., a quinolone) are often appropriate for patients with acute travelers' diarrhea. Antidiarrheal agents should be avoided in patients with suspected inflammatory diarrhea (e.g., ulcerative colitis, *C. difficile*, Shiga-toxin-producing *E. coli*) because of their association with toxic-megacolon.

Chronic Diarrhea

Chronic diarrhea is diarrhea lasting >4 weeks. Differential diagnosis of chronic diarrhea is broad and can be classified as predominantly osmotic, secretory, malabsorptive, or inflammatory, but these classifications often overlap. A patient-centered approach focuses on attributes that are most apparent to the patient: duration of the diarrhea, severity of the symptoms, and characteristics of the stool is often helpful (Table 1).

Diagnosis

Ask the patient about the frequency and characteristics of stools, association with food, medications, previous surgery, or radiation treatment. Ask specifically about fecal incontinence because patients may not volunteer this symptom but instead report it as diarrhea. Diet history may reveal large quantities of indigestible carbohydrates (osmotic diarrhea) or intolerance to wheat products (celiac disease, Whipple's disease). A patient's fixation on body image and weight loss may be a clue to laxative abuse. Frequent, high-volume, watery stools suggest a disease process affecting the small intestine. High-volume diarrhea that is exacerbated with

Table 1. Causes and Evaluation of Chronic Noninfectious Diarrhea

Condition	Notes
Ulcerative colitis	Bloody diarrhea, tenesmus. Obtain colonoscopy and biopsies.
Crohn's disease	Weight loss, anemia, and hypoalbuminemia. Obtain small bowel imaging and/or ileocolonoscopy with biopsy.
Microscopic colitis (collagenous colitis, lymphocytic colitis)	Diarrhea unrelated to food intake (e.g., nocturnal diarrhea). Colonoscopy or sigmoidoscopy with biopsy.
Irritable bowel syndrome	Bloating, abdominal discomfort relieved by a bowel movement; no weight loss or alarm features.
Celiac sprue	Dermatitis herpetiformis, iron deficiency anemia. Obtain anti-tissue transglutaminase antibody and (if positive) small bowel biopsy.
Whipple's disease	Arthralgias, neurologic or ophthalmologic symptoms. Polymerase chain reaction for *T. whippleii*; small bowel biopsy.
Carbohydrate intolerance	Excess lactose—use of artificial sweeteners (sorbitol, mannitol), or fructose. Attempt dietary exclusion or breath hydrogen test.
Pancreatic insufficiency	Chronic pancreatitis, hyperglycemia, history of pancreatic resection. Obtain tests for excess fecal fat, x-ray for pancreatic calcifications, and pancreatic function tests (e.g., secretin stimulation test).
Small bowel bacterial overgrowth	Intestinal dysmotility (e.g., diabetes mellitus, systemic sclerosis), jejunal diverticula. Response to empiric antibiotics, duodenal aspirate.
Common variable immunodeficiency	Pulmonary diseases, recurrent *Giardia* infection. Obtain tests for hypogammaglobulinemia (multiple subclasses).
Medications	History. Review a drug database.
Enteral feedings	History. Classic osmotic diarrhea.
Bile acid malabsorption	History of resection of <100 cm of distal small bowel. Diagnosis of exclusion, empiric response to cholestyramine.
Bile acid deficiency	Cholestasis, history of resection of >100 cm of small bowel. Diagnosis of exclusion, test for excess fecal fat.
Dumping syndrome	Postprandial flushing, tachycardia, diaphoresis. History of previous gastrectomy or gastric bypass surgery.
Self-induced diarrhea	Somatization or other psychiatric syndromes. History of laxative use. Obtain tests for stool pH, sodium, potassium, and magnesium.

eating and relieved with fasting or a clear liquid diet suggests carbohydrate malabsorption, whereas persistent or nocturnal diarrhea suggests a secretory process. The presence of persistent, severe or aching abdominal pain suggests an invasive process associated with inflammation or destruction of the mucosa. Skin findings, when present, may provide significant diagnostic clues. For example, flushing may indicate carcinoid syndrome; dermatitis herpetiformis may occur in patients with celiac sprue; and erythema nodosum or pyoderma gangrenosum may suggest underlying inflammatory bowel disease. Bloody diarrhea typically indicates an invasive process with loss of intestinal mucosal integrity. An oily residue or evidence of undigested food in the toilet bowl is more suggestive of malabsorption.

Consider irritable bowel syndrome in patients with a long-standing history of abdominal pain and abnormal bowel habits (constipation, diarrhea, or variable bowel movements) in the absence of other defined illnesses. The presence of weight loss, blood, or nocturnal diarrhea almost always indicates that the patient does not have irritable bowel syndrome.

The number and variety of diagnostic tests available for patients with chronic diarrhea is extensive, and further testing should be guided by information obtained from history and physical. A complete blood count and chemistry panel can reveal anemia, leukocytosis, electrolyte and nutritional status. Bacterial infections rarely cause chronic diarrhea in immunocompetent patients, but common infectious causes of acute diarrhea such as *Campylobacter* or *Salmonella* can cause persistent diarrhea in immunocompromised patients. Infection should always be ruled out in patients with

chronic diarrhea before proceeding with more extensive testing (Table 2).

A fecal fat study is usually indicated for evaluating a patient with noninvasive diarrhea. However, test results are valid only if the patient ingests an adequate amount of dietary fat (>100 g/d). Any cause of diarrhea may mildly elevate fecal fat values (6-10 g/24 hr), but values in excess of 14 g/24 hr almost always indicate primary fat malabsorption.

The presence of fecal leukocytes or lactoferrin suggests an inflammatory process but rarely provides more specific clues about the cause of diarrhea. If infection is excluded in a patient with chronic inflammatory diarrhea, colonoscopy or flexible sigmoidoscopy with biopsies are usually required for diagnosis.

Measurement of stool electrolytes is valuable for only a subset of patients who remain a diagnostic challenge despite the exclusion of infectious, iatrogenic, and inflammatory causes of diarrhea. Stool electrolytes help differentiate osmotic from secretory diarrhea. If factitious diarrhea is suspected, a fresh liquid stool sample should be obtained for determination of total osmolarity, stool sodium and potassium concentrations, and the osmotic gap should be calculated.

Celiac sprue (gluten-sensitive enteropathy) occurs in approximately 1:120 to 1:300 persons in the United States and other northern European countries. Classic symptoms include steatorrhea and weight loss, but many have only mild or nonspecific symptoms that often result in erroneous diagnosis of irritable bowel syndrome. Laboratory tests that aid the diagnosis include anti-tissue transglutaminase and antiendomysial antibodies; confirmation is by endoscopic small-bowel biopsy.

Table 2. Common Tests for Chronic Noninfectious Diarrhea

Condition	Notes
Qualitative fecal fat (Sudan stain of stool)	Detects >90% of significant steatorrhea; low dietary fat leads to false-negative results.
Quantitative fecal fat (48- or 72-hour)	Gold standard. Must be on high-fat diet (>100 g/d); Values >10–24 g/24 hr indicate fat malabsorption.
Fecal leukocytes or lactoferrin	For inflammatory bowel diseases. Limited usefulness (poor sensitivity and specificity).
Stool osmolarity	Normal is 280–300 mosm/kg; <250 mosm/kg suggests factitious diarrhea.
Stool electrolytes (sodium, potassium)	Osmotic gap [290 mosm/kg – 2 (Na + K)] >125 mosm/kg suggests osmotic diarrhea; <50 mosm/kg suggests secretory diarrhea.
Stool magnesium	Spot sample >90 meq/L is abnormal; use of antacids is a common source.
Stool pH	pH <6.0 suggests carbohydrate malabsorption.
Anti–tissue transglutaminase (anti-tTG) antibody assay	Most reliable screening test for celiac sprue; diagnosis is confirmed by small bowel biopsies.
Breath hydrogen test	For carbohydrate malabsorption. Increased hydrogen excretion after carbohydrate challenge.
Small bowel biopsy	For malabsorption. Loss of villi (e.g., celiac sprue)- inflammatory infiltrates (Whipple's disease, mastocytosis).
Duodenal aspirates	For small bowel overgrowth. Quantitative bacterial culture >10^5 is positive.
Neuropeptide assays (gastrin, vasoactive intestinal peptide, glucagon, somatostatin, pancreatic peptide, neurotensin, substance P, calcitonin, motilin, urine 5-hydroxyindoleacetic acid)	For secretory diarrhea. Useful if persistent diarrhea >1 L/24 hr despite fasting and other indications of possible tumor (hypokalemia, mass, skin findings, etc.) are present.
Radiographic small bowel follow-through	For inflammatory diarrhea or bacterial overgrowth. Strictures, ulcers, fistulas suggests Crohn's disease; diverticulosis predisposes to bacterial overgrowth.
Colonoscopy with biopsies	For inflammatory or secretory diarrhea. Diagnostic for ulcerative colitis, microscopic colitis, strictures, radiation enteropathy.

From Medical Knowledge Self-Assessment Program (MKSAP) 14. Philadelphia: American College of Physicians; 2006.

Excessive bacterial colonization of the small bowel lumen may result in diarrhea and malabsorption. A clue to the presence of bacterial overgrowth is finding a low-serum vitamin B_{12} level and a high-serum folate level (from bacteria production). Common conditions that predispose patients to bacterial overgrowth include diabetes, systemic sclerosis, and surgically created blind loops (i.e., gastrojejunostomy). Although the gold standard is aspiration of duodenal luminal contents for quantitative culture at the time of upper endoscopy, many clinicians first attempt an empiric trial of antibiotics (e.g., amoxicillin–clavulanate or norfloxacin) to see if the patient's symptoms improve.

Therapy

Treatment of chronic diarrhea should be based on the underlying cause. Symptomatic therapy may be considered if a diagnosis is pending, if a diagnosis cannot be confirmed, or if the condition diagnosed does not have a specific treatment. Symptoms may be controlled with stool-modifying agents such as fiber, opiate-based medications, bile-acid binding agents, and bismuth-containing medications.

Book Enhancement

Go to www.acponline.org/essentials/gastroenterology-section.html to view a DFA stool test for Giardia, and to review the skin lesions and gastrointestinal histopathology associated with celiac disease. In *MKSAP for Students 4*, assess yourself with items 18-20 in the **Gastroenterology and Hepatology** section.

Bibliography

American College of Physicians. Medical Knowledge Self-Assessment Program 14. Philadelphia: American College of Physicians; 2006.

Fine KD, Schiller LR. AGA technical review on the evaluation and management of chronic diarrhea. Gastroenterology. 1999;116:1464-86. [PMID: 10348832]

Guerrant RL, Van Gilder T, Steiner TS, et al. Practice guidelines for the management of infectious diarrhea. Clin Infect Dis. 2001;32:331-51. [PMID: 11170940]

Chapter 15

Diseases of the Gallbladder and Bile Ducts

Nora L. Porter, MD

Gallstones are the most common cause of biliary disease in the United States. The incidence of gallstones increases with increasing age and is higher in women than in men. Ninety percent of gallstones in the United States are cholesterol stones. Gallstones form when there is excess cholesterol relative to bile salts and lecithin in bile, resulting in cholesterol crystal precipitation. Risk factors for the formation of cholesterol stones include age, estrogen (female gender, pregnancy, estrogen therapy), obesity, physical inactivity, Native American or Mexican-American ancestry, impaired gallbladder emptying (total parenteral nutrition, biliary strictures), rapid weight loss, and medications (thiazide diuretics, ceftriaxone). Risk factors for pigment stones include hemolytic disease (including sickle cell disease), biliary stasis, and biliary infection.

The majority of patients with gallstones remain asymptomatic. When gallstones obstruct the cystic duct, symptoms of biliary colic develop. Prolonged obstruction can cause inflammation of the gallbladder (cholecystitis). Gallstones may migrate to the common bile duct (choledocholithiasis) where obstruction can lead to the more serious complications of cholangitis (infection of the biliary tree) and pancreatitis.

Prevention

As obesity and a sedentary lifestyle are major modifiable risk factors for gallstones, primary prevention includes counseling patients about the importance of eating a diet high in fiber and plant-based foods, increasing physical activity, and maintaining a normal body weight. In most patients with asymptomatic gallstones, the risks of developing symptoms or complications are less than the risk of surgery, so prophylactic cholecystectomy is not indicated. Some patient populations have an increased risk of developing complicated gallbladder disease or gallbladder cancer: Pima Indian women, patients with calcified (porcelain) gallbladders, gallstones >3 cm, patients with sickle cell anemia, and organ transplant candidates. These patients may be candidates for prophylactic cholecystectomy.

Diagnosis

No single sign or symptom is sensitive or specific enough to establish or rule out the diagnosis of biliary disease. An appropriate history and physical examination, with selected laboratory and imaging studies, is required. History should focus on eliciting characteristic symptoms as well as evaluating risk factors. Classic biliary colic is constant epigastric abdominal pain that develops over 1 hour or less, radiates to the right scapula or shoulder, and subsides in several hours. Associated symptoms may include bloating, flatulence, and dyspepsia. In acute cholecystitis, the pain frequently starts in the epigastric area then localizes in the right upper quadrant. Pain lasting >6 hours, especially if accompanied by fever, chills, and diaphoresis, suggests cholecystitis. A history of jaundice, pruritis, acholic stools, and dark urine indicates biliary obstruction due to choledocholithiasis. The physical exam in biliary colic may be benign, although there may be right upper quadrant tenderness and a positive Murphy's sign (inspiratory arrest when the gallbladder fossa is palpated during deep inspiration). Patients with cholecystitis infrequently have a tender right upper quadrant mass. Jaundice supports the diagnosis of choledocholithiasis and, in the presence of fever, cholangitis. Peritoneal signs point to a perforated or inflamed viscus.

Suspect cholecystitis or cholangitis in patients with leukocytosis. Mild increases in transaminase and bilirubin concentrations may be seen. Bilirubin >4 mg/dL is not a feature of cholecystitis and should prompt an evaluation for cholangitis (Table 1).

Ultrasound is the initial imaging modality of choice in suspected biliary disease. It is the most sensitive and specific test for detecting gallstones, has no risk, is widely available, and is relatively inexpensive (Table 2). Ultrasound will demonstrate dilatation of the cystic or biliary duct if there is an obstructing stone. In cholecystitis, ultrasound will show pericholecystic fluid and a thickened gallbladder wall. A sonographic Murphy's sign further supports the diagnosis. If ultrasound is nondiagnostic, cholescintigraphy (e.g., HIDA scan) should be obtained; nonvisualization of the gallbladder suggests cholecystitis. Abdominal CT scan should be used when other studies are equivocal or when complications of cholecystitis, such as perforation, cholangitis or gangrenous cholecystitis, are suspected. If bile duct stones are suspected, magnetic resonance cholangiography is more sensitive than ultrasonography and is the preferred noninvasive imaging modality. Untreated acute cholecystitis can progress to perforation, gangrenous cholecystitis (especially in diabetic patients), and acute cholangitis. In cholangitis, bacterial infection proximal to a bile duct obstruction may result in bacteremia and rapid septic shock.

Acalculous cholecystitis may present with fever and abnormal transaminases without characteristic abdominal pain, particularly in critically ill and elderly patients. Biliary dyskinesia may have symptoms indistinguishable from biliary colic.

Table 1. Differential Diagnosis of Acute Cholecystitis

Disease	Notes
Acute cholecystitis	Epigastric and RUQ pain with Murphy's sign. Bilirubin <4 mg/dL (unless complicated by choledocholithiasis), AST, ALT may be minimally elevated.
Biliary crystals (microlithiasis, sludge)	Typical biliary pain and no gallstones on imaging studies. Diagnosis made by aspiration of gallbladder bile from the duodenum or directly from the gallbladder at ERCP and microscopic examination. May cause pain, cholecystitis, or pancreatitis. Treated with cholecystectomy.
Biliary dyskinesia	Typical biliary pain, no gallstones on imaging studies and a gallbladder ejection fraction less than 35%-40% at scintigraphy with cholecystokinin infusion. Symptoms usually relieved with cholecystectomy. This is a controversial diagnosis.
Acute cholangitis	Charcot's triad (RUQ pain, fever, jaundice) or Reynold's pentad (Charcot's triad plus shock and mental status changes). Bilirubin >4 mg/dL. AST and ALT levels may exceed 1000 U/L.
Acute pancreatitis	Mid-epigastric pain radiating to the back, nausea, vomiting, elevated amylase (>2 x normal) and lipase. Vomiting and hyperamylasemia are generally more pronounced than in acute cholecystitis.
Pyelonephritis (right)	Costovertebral angle tenderness, evidence of urinary infection. Urinalysis helps to establish the diagnosis.
Peptic ulcer disease	RUQ or mid-epigastric pain. Perforated ulcer can mimic acute cholecystitis; free air on upright x-ray.
Acute viral hepatitis	Prodromal syndrome, jaundice, AST and ALT levels generally >1000 U/L. Bilirubin level generally >4 mg/dL and usually much higher.
Acute alcoholic hepatitis	Recent significant alcohol intake. RUQ pain, fever, jaundice, coagulopathy, leukocytosis, AST level usually two to three times greater than ALT level. Bilirubin level generally >4 mg/dL.
Fitz-Hugh-Curtis syndrome (gonococcal perihepatitis)	RUQ pain, pelvic adnexal tenderness, leukocytosis. Cervical smear shows gonococci.

AST = aspartate aminotransferase; ALT = alanine aminotransferase; RUQ = right upper quadrant.

Table 2. Imaging Studies for Acute Cholecystitis

Test	Notes
Right upper quadrant US scan	81%-98% sensitive, 70%-98% specific. Sonographic Murphy's sign (showing maximal tenderness directly over the visualized gallbladder) is >90% predictive of acute cholecystitis.
HIDA scan	85%-97% sensitive, 90% specific.
CT scan	Expensive; most useful to diagnose complications such as perforation, cholangitis, and gangrenous cholecystitis.
MRI scan or MRCP scan	100% for cystic duct obstruction; 69% for gallbladder wall thickening; 93% for cystic duct obstruction; 83% for gallbladder wall thickening. Extremely expensive; not universally available.

CT = computed tomography; HIDA = hepato-iminodiacetic acid; MRCP = magnetic resonance cholangiopancreatography; MRI = magnetic resonance imaging; US = ultrasound.

Therapy

Surgery provides definitive management for most patients with symptomatic gallbladder disease. In patients with cholecystitis, early cholecystectomy (within 24 to 48 hours) is associated with fewer complications and earlier hospital discharge. Compared with open cholecystectomy, laparoscopic cholecystectomy results in shorter hospital stays, less pain, and a more rapid recovery period. When bile duct stones are suspected, intraoperative cholangiography should be performed at the time of the cholecystectomy. If this procedure is not available, postoperative endoscopic retrograde cholangiopancreatography (ERCP) with sphincterotomy is an alternative. In patients with severe cholangitis or sepsis, urgent ERCP is essential to remove obstruction and allow biliary drainage.

In most patients with gallstone disease, drug therapy is supportive until definitive surgery can be performed. Diclofenac provides pain relief in biliary colic and decreases the risk of developing acute cholecystitis. Nonsteroidal inflammatory drugs are also helpful in patients with acute cholecystitis with mild to moderate pain; patients with more severe pain may require narcotic analgesia. Treat patients with acute cholecystitis, especially those with fever, leukocytosis, or complications, with broad-spectrum antibiotics. Select antimicrobials to cover *E. coli*, *Klebsiella* sp., group D *Streptococcus* sp., and *Enterobacter* sp. In critically ill patients, including those with acute cholangitis, provide coverage for *Bacteroides* and *Pseudomonas* as well. Appropriate antibiotic regimens include ampicillin, gentamicin and metronidazole; ceftazidime and metronidazole; or monotherapy with piperacillin/tazobactam, ampicillin/sulbactam, or ticarcillin/clavulanic acid.

Ursodeoxycholic acid may be used in highly selected patients who are unable or unwilling to undergo surgery. Its use is limited to patients with cholesterol stones, patent biliary tracts, and functioning gallbladders.

Follow-Up

Most patients with asymptomatic gallstone disease should be followed for the development of symptoms. Patients who have had a cholecystectomy should follow up with their surgeons for evaluation of post-operative complications such as biliary tract injury or infection. This is particularly important for patients who undergo surgery for cholecystitis because they have a higher rate of post-operative complications.

Book Enhancement

Go to www.acponline.org/essentials/gastroenterology-section .html to view an x-ray showing pneumobilia. In *MKSAP for Students 4,* assess yourself with items 21-24 in the **Gastroenterology and Hepatology** section.

Bibliography

Cohen SM, Kim AI, Faust TW. Acute Cholecystitis. http://pier.acponline .org/physicians/diseases/d642. [Date accessed: 2008 Jan 11] In: PIER [online database]. Philadelphia: American College of Physicians; 2008.

DiSario JA. Gallstones. http://pier.acponline.org/physicians/diseases/ d183. [Date accessed: 2008 Jan 11] In: PIER [online database]. Philadelphia: American College of Physicians; 2008.

Trowbridge RL, Rutkowski NK, Shojania KG. Does this patient have acute cholecystitis? JAMA. 2003;289:80-6. [PMID: 12503981]

Chapter 16

Acute Pancreatitis

Nora L. Porter, MD

Acute pancreatitis occurs when the pancreatic enzyme trypsinogen is prematurely activated to trypsin, which in turn activates pancreatic zymogens. The resulting pancreatic autodigestion leads to an inflammatory response which causes further pancreatic damage. In severe cases, the inflammation may progress to a systemic inflammatory response, resulting in multiorgan system failure and death. The most common etiologies of acute pancreatitis in the United States are biliary obstruction and alcohol. Pancreatitis may be caused by medications such as sulfonamides, estrogens, valproic acid, thiazide diuretics, and furosemide. Other etiologies include familial pancreatitis, hypertriglyceridemia, hypercalcemia, sphincter of Oddi dysfunction, biliary ductal obstruction, vasculitis, trauma, surgery, endoscopic retrograde cholangiopancreatography (ERCP), cystic fibrosis, and penetrating peptic ulcer. As much as 20% of acute pancreatitis is idiopathic. Mild pancreatitis is usually self-limited, but more severe disease causes significant morbidity and mortality. Repeated episodes of acute pancreatitis may result in chronic pancreatitis and pancreatic endocrine and exocrine insufficiency.

Prevention

The best preventive measures for pancreatitis involve avoiding known etiologic agents and medical or surgical management of other precipitating factors. Endoscopic retrograde cholangiopancreatography is a well-established cause of acute pancreatitis. Use of safer, non-invasive imaging such as magnetic resonance cholangiopancreatography (MRCP) decreases the risk of procedure-related pancreatitis. However, MRCP cannot replace ERCP for therapeutic drainage of the biliary system.

Diagnosis

The most common symptom of acute pancreatitis is abdominal pain (Table 1). The pain may be epigastric or diffuse. It typically peaks in 30 minutes to a few hours, is moderate to severe, constant, and radiates to the back. The pain usually is not positional, although it may improve when sitting up or leaning forward. Nausea and vomiting are common; the pain of acute pancreatitis is usually not alleviated with vomiting.

Abdominal tenderness is common in pancreatitis, but peritoneal signs should prompt a search for a perforated viscus. Diminished bowel sounds may point to an associated ileus. Some physical findings may suggest a specific etiology; jaundice suggests biliary obstruction, and eruptive xanthomas suggest hypertriglyceridemia. History and physical exam should also evaluate the possibility of complications of acute pancreatitis. Nausea, vomiting, and anorexia frequently result in dehydration, hypotension, and tachycardia. High fever suggests infection. Large pseudocysts may be palpable and painful. Grey-Turner or Cullen's signs (painless ecchymosis of the flanks and periumbilicus, respectively) suggest retroperitoneal bleeding.

The diagnosis of pancreatitis relies heavily on the serum amylase and lipase, which are elevated in 75%-90% of patients. Serum lipase is more specific and stays elevated longer than amylase. Leukocytosis and electrolyte abnormalities are common.

Table 1. Differential Diagnosis of Acute Pancreatitis (AP)

Disease	Notes
Perforated viscus (see Chapter 13)	Very sudden onset; intraperitoneal air present on x-ray. In AP, the pain gradually increases over 30 minutes to 1 hour.
Acute cholecystitis and biliary colic (see Chapter 15)	Pain tends to be located in the epigastrium and right upper quadrant and radiates to the right shoulder or shoulder blade. In AP, the pain tends to radiate to the back. Ultrasound shows thickened gallbladder, pericholecystic fluid.
Intestinal obstruction (see Chapter 13)	Pain is colicky. In AP, the pain is constant. Obstructive pattern is seen on CT or abdominal series.
Mesenteric vascular occlusion (see Chapter 13)	The classic triad for mesenteric ischemia is postprandial abdominal pain, weight loss, and abdominal bruit.
Dissecting aortic aneurysm (see Chapter 1)	Sudden onset. Pain may radiate to the lower extremity. In AP, the pain gradually increases over 30 minutes to 1 hour and does not radiate to the lower extremity.
Myocardial infarction (see Chapter 3)	Myocardial infarction should be in the differential diagnosis in all patients with upper abdominal pain.
Appendicitis (see Chapter 13)	The pain may start in the epigastrium but eventually migrates to the right lower quadrant. Ultrasound and CT are very helpful in the diagnosis of appendicitis.
Diabetic ketoacidosis (see Chapter 8)	Blood glucose is always elevated, anion gap always present. Blood glucose may be elevated in severe AP but usually develops later in the clinical course. Acidosis may be present in severe AP.

CT = computed tomography.

Calcium and triglycerides should be measured to evaluate possible etiologies.

Chest and flat and upright abdominal radiographs are obtained to exclude bowel perforation or obstruction. Abdominal ultrasonography is performed to exclude gall stones. In patients with moderate or severe pancreatitis, or those who do not improve clinically within 48 to 72 hours, use contrast-enhanced, thin-section CT scan of the abdomen to confirm the diagnosis, to exclude other intra-abdominal processes, to grade the severity of pancreatitis, and to diagnose local complications such as pancreatic necrosis, pseudocyst, or abscess. MRI is used if there is a contraindication to intravenous radiocontrast.

In addition to local complications, pancreatitis may cause significant systemic complications including hypocalcemia, hyperglycemia, renal insufficiency, disseminated intravascular coagulation, and acute respiratory distress syndrome. Therefore, obtain in all patients with pancreatitis a complete blood count, electrolytes, calcium, blood glucose, BUN, creatinine, prothrombin time, and partial thromboplastin time. Pulse oximetry or, in more critically ill patients, arterial blood gases should also be obtained (Table 2).

Scoring systems such as the Ranson, Glasgow, and Acute Physiology and Chronic Health Evaluation II (APACHE II) scores are used to determine prognosis. However, these scoring systems lack sensitivity and specificity and should not supplant clinical findings such as third-space fluid loss or remote organ failure in determining risk. Organ failure, the most important indicator of severity, is defined by the presence of shock (systolic blood pressure <90 mm Hg), pulmonary insufficiency (PaO_2 <55 mm Hg), renal failure (serum creatinine >2 mg/dL), or gastrointestinal bleeding (>500 mL/24h).

Therapy

Keep patients without oral intake until there is clear clinical improvement, and treat aggressively with intravenous fluids. In more severe cases, where patients are not able to receive oral nourishment for a few weeks, nutritional support with enteral jejunal feeding, or with total parenteral nutrition if enteral feeding is contraindicated, may be required. Use of nasogastric suction is limited to patients with refractory vomiting due to ileus.

Obtain early ERCP in patients with bile duct stones, cholangitis, or biliary pancreatitis. Patients with persisting pancreatitis, persistent elevation of transaminase levels, or dilated bile ducts may have retained bile duct stones and may also benefit from ERCP. Stone extraction with biliary sphincterotomy improves the outcome, prevents further attacks of acute biliary pancreatitis, and reduces pancreatitis-related complications. Surgery is indicated for pancreatic necrosis and pancreatic abscess because the mortality rate with medical management is >50%. Pancreatic pseudocysts that fail to resolve may need surgical drainage. Cholecystectomy is indicated in patients with biliary pancreatitis to prevent recurrence.

There is no specific drug therapy for acute pancreatitis. Provide symptomatic treatment of pain, nausea, and vomiting. Treat documented infections (cholangitis, abscess, infected pseudocyst) with antibiotics. Choice of antibiotics should be based on bacterial identification and susceptibility when available. Empiric antibiotic therapy for non-infected pancreatic necrosis is controversial. If antibiotics are used, evidence-based regimens include ceftazidime, amikacin, and metronidazole; ofloxacin and metronidazole; or monotherapy with imipenem, meropenem, or cefuroxime. Patients with interstitial (non-necrotizing) pancreatitis without evidence of infection do not receive antibiotics.

Follow-Up

In general, acute pancreatitis is a self-limited condition that does not recur if the precipitating factor is removed. In patients with alcohol abuse, advise abstinence from alcohol or refer for counseling and appropriate treatment. In patients with high triglyceride levels, control with a combination of a dietary regimen and, if indicated, triglyceride-lowering medications. In patients with

Table 2. Laboratory and Other Studies for Acute Pancreatitis (AP)

Test	Notes
Serum amylase levels	Cutoff values just above normal: 90% sensitive; 70% specific. Cutoff values three times the upper limit of normal: 60% sensitive; 99% specific.
Serum lipase levels	Cutoff values three times the upper limit of normal: 90%-100% sensitive; 99% specific.
Aminotransferase levels	Elevated levels raise the suspicion for biliary pancreatitis.
Triglyceride level	Hypertriglyceridemia can be the underlying etiology of AP.
Calcium level	Hypercalcemia is a cause of AP and hypocalcemia can be a complication of AP.
BUN and creatinine levels	The incidence of renal insufficiency is 4%, 22%, and 45% in patients with interstitial, noninfected necrotic and infected necrotic AP, respectively.
Glucose level	Glucose levels can increase and are negative prognostic factor.
PT/PTT	May be elevated in AP complicated by DIC.
Abdominal and chest radiographs	Can exclude perforated viscus or obstructed bowel.
Abdominal ultrasound	Evaluate for presence of gallstones.
CT	The test of choice to determine the presence of local complications.
Test for arterial hypoxemia	Pulse oximetry in mild cases of AP and arterial blood gas in severe cases of AP.

BUN = blood urea nitrogen; CT = computed tomography; DIC = disseminated intravascular coagulation; PT = prothrombin time; PTT = partial thromboplastin time.

elevated calcium levels, begin appropriate medical or surgical management to prevent recurrence of hypercalcemia. If a specific drug precipitated the pancreatitis, discontinue its use and substitute another as needed.

Book Enhancement

Go to www.acponline.org/essentials/gastroenterology-section .html to view CT scans showing pancreatic calcifications and interstitial and necrotizing pancreatitis. In *MKSAP for Student 4,* assess yourself with items 25-29 in the **Gastroenterology and Hepatology** section.

Bibliography

Draganov P, Toskes P. Acute Pancreatitis. http://pier.acponline.org/ physicians/diseases/d268. [Date accessed: 2008 Jan 13] In: PIER [online database]. Philadelphia: American College of Physicians; 2006.

Whitcomb DC. Clinical practice. Acute pancreatitis. N Engl J Med. 2006; 354:2142-50. [PMID: 16707751]

Chapter 17

Gastroesophageal Reflux Disease

Brown J. McCallum, MD

Gastrointestinal reflux disease (GERD) is an extremely common disorder characterized by symptoms of heartburn and regurgitation. GERD is a multifactorial disorder that is associated with impaired esophageal motility and defects in the lower esophageal sphincter (LES) and the antireflux barrier located at the gastroesophageal junction. These findings result in the prolonged exposure of the esophagus to gastric contents. The most common cause of GERD is transient LES relaxations. Although the presence of acid is central to the pathogenesis of GERD, increased gastric acid secretion is not a risk factor for GERD, and few patients with this disorder actually secrete excess acid. The major complication of GERD is Barrett's esophagus, which can progress to esophageal adenocarcinoma.

Diagnosis

The diagnosis of GERD is suggested by symptoms of heartburn and regurgitation occurring after meals, aggravated by recumbency, bending, or physical exertion, and relieved by antacids. Patients with classic symptoms rarely require confirmatory testing (including testing for *H. pylori*). Atypical, extra-esophageal manifestations may occur and can include wheezing, shortness of breath, chronic cough and hoarseness, chest pain, choking, halitosis, and sore throat. Physical exam findings are less prominent, but may include wheezing, pharyngitis, and dental erosions.

Response to empiric therapy confirms the diagnosis; patients not responding may require further investigation with 24-hour ambulatory pH testing. GERD associated with dysphagia may represent a complication of long-term acid reflux, including stricture, ulceration, or adenocarcinoma, and requires evaluation with upper endoscopy. GERD presenting atypically or unresponsive to empiric therapy also warrants the consideration of an alternative diagnosis such as infectious esophagitis, pill esophagitis (alendronate and doxycycline are common causes), esophageal motility disorders, esophageal cancer, nonulcer dyspepsia, peptic ulcer disease, cardiac disease, and biliary disease (Table 1).

Therapy

Smoking cessation, elevation of the head of the bed, avoiding recumbency after eating, and sleeping in the left lateral decubitus position can be helpful. Alcohol, fatty foods, chocolate, peppermint, tomato juice, citrus juices, onions and garlic are avoided. Theophylline, nitrates, anticholinergic agents, calcium-channel blockers, alpha-adrenergic antagonists, and diazepam may all induce GERD, and their elimination (if possible) may improve symptoms. Surgical intervention is an option for patients who wish to avoid life-long medication, but it is not likely to improve symptoms that were unresponsive to proton pump inhibitors.

Treatment aims to eliminate symptoms, heal esophagitis, prevent complications, and maintain remission. Antacids are

Table 1. Differential Diagnosis of Gastroesophageal Reflux Disease (GERD)

Disease	Notes
Achalasia	Dysphagia for both liquids and solids; also may be associated with chest pain. Heartburn/chest pain in achalasia is not due to reflux but to fermentation of retained esophageal contents or esophageal muscle spasm.
Coronary artery disease (see Chapter 3)	Chest pain that may be clinically indistinguishable from chest pain associated with GERD. Coronary artery disease should be ruled out before evaluating GERD as a cause.
Diffuse esophageal spasm	Dysphagia for both liquids and solids; also may be associated with chest pain. May be coincident with GERD.
Esophageal cancer	Presents with dysphagia for solids and later liquids and weight loss, often in patients with longstanding GERD. Usually incurable by the time it presents clinically.
Infectious esophagitis	Presents with dysphagia/odynophagia. Often in immunocompromised patients with candidal, CMV, or HSV esophagitis.
Pill esophagitis	Presents with dysphagia/odynophagia. History of offending pill ingestion (e.g., potassium chloride, quinidine, tetracycline, NSAIDs, alendronate).
Peptic ulcer disease (see Chapter 18)	Pain or distress centered in the upper abdomen, relieved by food or antacids.
Biliary disease (see Chapter 15)	Epigastric or right upper quadrant pain, jaundice, acholic stools, dark urine, abnormal liver tests.

CMV = cytomegalovirus; HSV = herpes simplex virus.

appropriate over-the-counter therapy, and patients have often tried these before seeking medical treatment. A trial of a full-dose H$_2$-blocker provides relief in most patients with mild-to-moderate symptoms and is safe and relatively inexpensive. Proton pump inhibitors are the mainstay of therapy. If once-daily administration of a proton pump inhibitor does not control symptoms, twice-daily administration may be tried. Proton-pump inhibitors can heal esophagitis and control symptoms more completely than all other treatments. It is reasonable to stop therapy in patients with well-controlled mild-to-moderate symptoms, but most will require long-term therapy.

Follow-Up

Refer patients with "warning symptoms" such as dysphagia, odynophagia, bleeding, weight loss, early satiety, choking, anorexia, or frequent vomiting for endoscopy. These symptoms may be indicative of cancer, stricture, or ulceration. The diagnosis of Barrett's esophagus can only be made endoscopically; biopsy reveals specialized intestinal metaplasia. The risk of adenocarcinoma in patients with Barrett's esophagus is 30-40 times that of the general population, so experts recommend referring patients with GERD of at least 1 year duration for screening endoscopy to exclude Barrett's esophagus. Once Barrett's esophagus is diagnosed, repeat endoscopy with biopsy is recommended every 3 to 5 years to detect neoplastic transformation.

Book Enhancement

Go to www.acponline.org/essentials/gastroenterology-section.html to see an endoscopic view of Barrett's esophagus, erosive esophagitis, and Candida esophagitis. In *MKSAP for Students 4*, assess yourself with item 30 in the **Gastroenterology and Hepatology** section.

Bibliography

Fang JC. Gastroesophageal Reflux Disease. http://pier.acponline.org/physicians/diseases/d180. [Date accessed: 2008 Feb 20] In: PIER [online database]. Philadelphia: American College of Physicians; 2008.

Richter JE. The many manifestations of gastroesophageal reflux disease: presentation, evaluation, and treatment. Gastroenterol Clin North Am. 2007;36:577-99, viii-ix. [PMID: 17950439]

Chapter 18

Peptic Ulcer Disease

Brown J. McCallum, MD

Peptic ulcer disease is characterized by dyspepsia, nausea, and abdominal pain, and diagnosis is confirmed by upper endoscopy (Table 1). More than 90% of patients have *Helicobacter pylori* infection or have used nonsteroidal anti-inflammatory drugs (NSAIDs). Cigarette smoking, alcohol consumption, corticosteroid administration, and psychological stress no longer appear to be independent risk factors for the development of peptic ulcers in the absence of *H. pylori* infection or NSAID use. *H. pylori* expresses a host of factors that contribute to its ability to colonize the gastric mucosa and cause mucosal injury. NSAIDS likely cause ulcers by inhibiting the prostaglandin-mediated gastrointestinal release of the protective mucous and bicarbonate layer and through a direct toxic mucosal effect.

Prevention

Although it is assumed that lifestyle modifications such as alcohol, caffeine, and tobacco cessation will improve general health, no evidence exists that it prevents peptic ulcer disease. The use of misoprostol or proton pump inhibitors in the setting of regular NSAID use can prevent ulcers, particularly in high-risk individuals such as those with a past medical history of ulcer disease or cardiovascular disease, those taking prednisone or anticoagulants, those aged >65 years, and those with NSAID-associated dyspepsia.

Diagnosis

Patients with unexplained dyspepsia, weight loss, recurrent vomiting, dysphagia, anemia, gastrointestinal bleeding, abdominal mass, lymphadenopathy, or symptom onset after age 45 years are evaluated with esophagogastroduodenoscopy (EGD). Physical examination is usually not helpful. EGD allows for direct visualization of the ulcer and can identify active bleeding, stigmata of recent bleeding, or exposed vessels requiring active intervention. Endoscopy with biopsy is the best way to diagnose gastric cancer and to differentiate ulcers caused by NSAIDs and those caused by *H. pylori*. Nonendoscopic studies, including serum antibody tests, urea breath tests, urea blood tests, and stool examination for *H. pylori* antigens, can be used for the initial diagnosis of *H. pylori* infection. False-negative urea test results may occur in patients who recently took antibiotics, bismuth-containing compounds, or proton pump inhibitors; use of these drugs should therefore be stopped at least 2 weeks before a urea test is performed.

Therapy

Decreased dose or elimination of NSAID therapy may decrease ulcer formation. Stopping NSAIDs and use of misoprostol or a proton pump inhibitor can heal ulcers and prevent further ulcer formation and remain effective even in the presence of continued NSAID use. Four to six weeks of proton pump inhibitors is standard. Gastric or duodenal ulcer due to *H. pylori* is treated by eliminating *H. pylori* infection with antibiotics (typically, clarithromycin and either amoxicillin or metronidazole) combined with a proton pump inhibitor. Bismuth subsalicylate can be substituted for the proton pump inhibitor and tetracycline for clarithromycin. Repeat treatment is occasionally necessary (with different antibiotics) if complete eradication is not achieved, but the majority of patients do not require long-term therapy.

Table 1. Differential Diagnosis of Peptic Ulcer Disease

Disease	Notes
Irritable bowel syndrome (see Chapter 13)	Bloating, change in bowel habits, cramping in the absence of weight loss, bleeding, anemia, or relief with acid-suppressive agents.
Gastric cancer	Weight loss, early satiety, anemia, occult blood in the stool.
GERD (see Chapter 17)	Heartburn, dysphagia, supra-esophageal manifestations (chronic cough, laryngitis, asthma). Symptoms of heartburn may overlap with symptoms of dyspepsia. This differential diagnosis is best addressed by the response to acid-suppressive therapies or by EGD. The absence of endoscopic findings of esophagitis does not exclude GERD.
Nonulcer dyspepsia (see Chapter 19)	Pain, fullness, or bloating often related to eating and unaffected by bowel movements. The diagnosis of nonulcer dyspepsia requires endoscopic proof that ulcer disease is not present.
Biliary colic (see Chapter 15)	Pain, usually right upper quadrant, intermittent, may be associated with fever. Biliary sonography can be used to evaluate patients for the presence of cholelithiasis.

EGD = esophagogastroduodenoscopy; GERD = gastroesophageal reflux disease.

Follow-Up

An uncomplicated duodenal ulcer does not require repeat endoscopy for confirmation of cure unless symptoms reoccur. Patients with complicated duodenal ulcer (bleeding, obstruction, perforation) require confirmation of successful *H. pylori* eradication with a urea breath test or repeat endoscopy. Because antibody test results may remain positive for months after successful eradication of *H. pylori*, such tests are not recommended to document eradication. All gastric ulcers caused by *H. pylori* require follow-up upper endoscopy to confirm complete healing and to rule out gastric cancer.

Book Enhancement

Go to www.acponline.org/essentials/gastroenterology-section .html to review tables on peptic ulcer etiology and tests used to diagnose *H. pylori* infection, and an endoscopic view of a visible vessel at the base of a peptic ulcer. In *MKSAP for Students 4*, assess yourself with items 31-34 in the **Gastroenterology and Hepatology** section.

Bibliography

Koss M, Goldstein J. Peptic Ulcer Disease. http://pier.acponline.org/ physicians/diseases/d181. [Date accessed: 2008 Feb 19] In: PIER [online database]. Philadelphia: American College of Physicians; 2008.

Ramakrishnan K, Salinas RC. Peptic ulcer disease. Am Fam Physician. 2007;76:1005-12. [PMID: 17956071]

Chapter 19

Dyspepsia

Brown J. McCallum, MD

Dyspepsia is defined as nonspecific upper abdominal discomfort or nausea not attributable to peptic ulcer disease. The etiology and pathophysiology of dyspepsia are unclear, but this disorder may have multifactorial causes, including dysmotility, visceral hypersensitivity, *Helicobacter pylori* infection, acid-peptic disease, psychosocial factors, or an interaction among multiple processes.

Diagnosis

Diagnosis is based on the Rome III criteria and centers on satisfying one or more of the following criteria: bothersome postprandial fullness, early satiation, epigastric pain, or epigastric burning. Patients must also have no evidence of structural disease on endoscopy. Dyspeptic patients with pain or discomfort centered mainly in the midline of the upper abdomen have epigastric pain syndrome and patients with predominantly fullness, bloating and early satiety have postprandial distress syndrome. Heartburn and acid regurgitation almost always indicate gastroesophageal reflux disease, and dysphagia usually signifies esophageal pathology. The causes of dyspepsia are varied and may include delayed gastric emptying, efferent vagal dysfunction, proximal gastric contraction, and enhanced sensitivity to gastric distention (Table 1). Bleeding or anemia are never a part of functional dyspepsia and require further investigation.

It can also be helpful to classify symptoms into one of the three categories: ulcer-like dyspepsia, dysmotility-like dyspepsia, and unspecified dyspepsia. Understand that, although three symptom subgroups have been accepted in the definition of functional dyspepsia, these symptoms cannot be used to predict the cause. Ulcer-like dyspepsia is characterized by pain localized to the epigastrium; dysmotility-like dyspepsia is characterized by non-painful sensation or discomfort centered in the upper abdomen, fullness, early satiety, bloating, or nausea; and unspecified dyspepsia does not cleanly fit in either category.

Therapy

Though endoscopy is required for definitive diagnosis, in young patients lacking alarm symptoms such as dysphagia, weight loss, occult bleeding, or anemia, an empiric treatment trial prior to endoscopic evaluation is not unreasonable. Non-invasive testing for *H pylori* (i.e., urease breath test) can be helpful; if positive, eradication of *H. pylori* may relieve symptoms although randomized, controlled trials provide conflicting results as to the efficacy of *H. pylori* eradication in improving symptoms of functional dyspepsia. A typical treatment might include a proton pump inhibitor, bismuth subsalicylate, metronidazole, and tetracycline for 7-10 days. Patients aged >45 years or with alarm features are always evaluated with upper endoscopy. Ulcer-like dyspepsia may respond to proton pump inhibitors, whereas dysmotility-like dyspepsia may respond to trials of prokinetic agents (e.g., metoclopramide, certain antihistamines, phenothiazines). Amitriptyline has also been used with anecdotal success to treat functional dyspepsia, but firm evidence from clinical trials is lacking.

Follow-Up

In patients who do not respond to 4-6 weeks of therapy with one drug category, consider treatment of similar duration with alternative drugs. In patients who have had *H. pylori* treatment, confirmation of eradication with a urease breath test or stool antigen assay is warranted.

Table 1. Differential Diagnosis of Dyspepsia

Disease	Notes
Functional dyspepsia	No organic or biochemical evidence of disease after investigation. Up to 60% of epigastric pain cases.
GERD (see Chapter 17)	Heartburn or acid regurgitation. Between 2%-29% of epigastric pain cases.
Peptic ulcer disease (see Chapter 18)	Pain or distress centered in the upper abdomen, relieved by food or antacids. Between 7%-25% of epigastric pain cases.
Gastric or esophageal cancer	Warning symptoms or signs (bleeding, anemia, weight loss, dysphagia). Between 1%-3% of epigastric pain cases.
Medication side effect	Erythromycin, theophylline, digitalis, NSAIDs, and others. Between 2%-8% of epigastric pain cases.
Biliary disease (see Chapter 15)	Jaundice, acholic stools, dark urine, abnormal liver tests. <5% of epigastric pain cases.

GERD = gastroesophageal reflux disease; NSAID = nonsteroidal anti-inflammatory drug.

Book Enhancement

Go to www.acponline.org/essentials/gastroenterology-section
.html to use an algorithm to manage dyspepsia. In *MKSAP for
Students 4*, assess yourself with item 35 in the **Gastroenterology
and Hepatology** section.

Bibliography

Camilleri M. Functional dyspepsia: mechanisms of symptom generation and appropriate management of patients. Gastroenterol Clin North Am. 2007;36:649-64, xi-xx. [PMID: 17950442]

Inadomi JM, Fendrick AM. Dyspepsia. http://pier.acponline.org/physicians/diseases/d149. [Date accessed: 2008 Feb 12] In: PIER [online database]. Philadelphia: American College of Physicians; 2008.

Chapter 20

Approach to Gastrointestinal Bleeding

Warren Y. Hershman, MD

Gastrointestinal bleeding is classified as acute or chronic and as originating from either the upper (proximal to the ligament of Treitz) or the lower gastrointestinal tract. Patients with acute gastrointestinal bleeding typically present with melena (black, tarry, foul-smelling stools), hematochezia (bright red or maroon-colored stools), or hematemesis (vomiting blood or coffee-ground material). In other patients, occult bleeding may be identified by fecal occult blood testing, the presence of iron-deficiency anemia, or symptoms due to blood loss or anemia, such as fatigue, dyspnea, syncope, or angina. Management begins with an assessment and stabilization of the patient's hemodynamic status. Subsequent interventions focus on identifying and controlling the source of bleeding and preventing a recurrence.

Differential Diagnosis

The most common causes of upper gastrointestinal (UGI) bleeding requiring hospitalization are peptic ulcer, esophageal varices, Mallory-Weiss tears, gastric erosions, and erosive esophagitis. Peptic ulcer disease accounts for approximately 50% of all acute upper gastrointestinal bleeding. Patients taking aspirin or nonsteroidal anti-inflammatory drugs (NSAIDs) or who have *Helicobacter pylori* infection are at increased risk for ulcers and ulcer-related bleeding. *Helicobacter pylori* attaches to gastric epithelial cells and releases toxins which can cause mucosal injury and initiate an inflammatory response. NSAIDs block the enzyme cyclooxygenase and interfere with the production of prostaglandins that play a central role in the defense and repair of gastric epithelium. Hospitalized patients with severe comorbid conditions and patients who use anticoagulants are also at increased risk for ulcer bleeding. Bleeding from esophageal or gastric varices (5%-30% of acute UGI bleeding episodes) is often brisk, and can lead to hemodynamic instability. Bleeding due to portal hypertension resolves spontaneously less often and is associated with a higher mortality rate than UGI bleeding due to other causes. Mallory-Weiss tears are mucosal lacerations near the gastroesophageal junction. The classic history of vomiting and/or retching followed by hematemesis suggests this diagnosis but is noted in only a minority of patients. Erosive esophagitis and gastric erosions are more likely to present with small-volume bleeding or occult blood loss. Erosive esophagitis is usually associated with symptoms of gastroesophageal reflux disease, and gastric erosions tend to develop in patients who use NSAIDs, have heavy alcohol intake, or are severely ill with other medical illnesses.

The most common causes of acute, severe lower gastrointestinal bleeding are colonic diverticula, angiectasia (also known as angiodysplasia), colitis (e.g., inflammatory bowel disease, infection, ischemia, or radiation), and colonic neoplasia. Bleeding from a colonic diverticulum is typically acute and painless. Bleeding stops spontaneously in approximately 80% of patients, but 10%-40% will rebleed. Angiectasia are most common among the elderly and usually present as chronic or occult blood loss but can also cause acute painless, hemodynamically significant bleeding. Ischemic colitis typically occurs in older individuals with significant cardiac and peripheral vascular disease who present with abdominal pain. While colonic ischemia is usually transient and resolves with supportive care, acute small bowel ischemia is associated with a high mortality and requires an aggressive early approach to management, often involving angiography or laparotomy. Acute small bowel ischemia should be suspected in patients who have risk factors for embolism or thrombosis and who present with sudden-onset, severe abdominal pain that in the early stage is out of proportion to the physical exam findings. Perianal disease, such as hemorrhoids and fissures, may also present with lower gastrointestinal bleeding. Hemorrhoids are probably the most common cause of minor lower gastrointestinal bleeding. They are usually associated with straining on bowel movement and intermittent, bright red blood on the toilet paper or in the toilet bowl. Gastrointestinal bleeding should not be attributed solely to hemorrhoids until other causes have been excluded. Colon cancer must always be considered in patients who are over the age of 50 years or who have a recent change in bowel movements, constitutional symptoms, anemia, or family or personal history of cancer or polyps. Bleeding from a colonic polyp or carcinoma is usually occult or small-volume.

Immediate Assessment

The first step in the management of acute gastrointestinal bleeding is stabilization of the patient's hemodynamic status. This begins by measuring the blood pressure and heart rate and checking for postural changes in these measures. Two large caliber intravenous catheters are inserted to allow volume replacement with normal saline and, if necessary, blood products. The goals of volume resuscitation are to restore normal intravascular volume and prevent complications from red blood cell loss, including myocardial infarction, heart failure, and stroke. There is no absolute hemoglobin value that determines when transfusions are appropriate. The decision on whether to transfuse should incorporate an assessment of the patient's age and comorbidities, the amount of ongoing blood loss, stability of vital signs, and adequacy of tissue perfusion.

While the hemodynamic status is being stabilized, a focused history and physical examination can suggest specific causes for the bleeding and can provide prognostic information (Table 1). Particular attention should be paid to:

- Nature, amount, and duration of the bleeding and whether it is ongoing; character and frequency of stool output.
- Presence or absence of abdominal pain and other symptoms such as fever, diarrhea, retching prior to hematemesis, recent weight loss, or change in bowel habits.
- Complications from bleeding such as chest pain, dyspnea, or oliguria.
- Medications and ingestions such as the use of aspirin, NSAIDs, anticoagulants, and alcohol.
- Conditions predisposing to bleeding including abdominal-pelvic radiation, previous bleeding episodes, and abdominal surgery.

- Stigmata of chronic liver disease and previous episodes of variceal bleeding.
- Comorbid conditions that increase the risk of a poor outcome such as diabetes and cardiopulmonary, renal, or neurologic disease.
- Vital signs and postural changes, skin, cardiopulmonary, abdominal and digital rectal examination.

Evaluation and Management

Initial studies include a complete blood count, blood typing and cross matching, INR and partial thromboplastin time (PTT), serum electrolytes, blood urea nitrogen (BUN), creatinine, aminotransferase levels, and electrocardiogram (Table 2). While

Table 1. Common Causes of Gastrointestinal Bleeding

Cause	Notes
Upper Gastrointestinal Tract	
Gastric and duodenal ulcers	Dyspepsia, *Helicobacter pylori* infection, NSAID use, anticoagulation, severe medical illness.
Variceal bleeding	Stigmata of chronic liver disease on exam and evidence of portal hypertension or risk factor for cirrhosis (e.g., alcohol use, viral hepatitis).
Mallory-Weiss tear	History of retching prior to hematemesis.
Esophagitis	Heartburn, regurgitation, and dysphagia; usually small volume or occult bleeding.
Gastroduodenal erosions	NSAID use, heavy alcohol intake, severe medical illness; usually small volume or occult bleeding.
Esophageal or gastric cancer	Progressive dysphagia, weight loss, early satiety, or abdominal pain; usually small volume or occult bleeding.
Lower Gastrointestinal Tract	
Diverticula	Painless, self-limited hematochezia.
Angiodysplasia	Chronic blood loss or acute painless hematochezia in elderly; frequently involves upper gastrointestinal tract in addition to colon.
Colonic polyp	Usually asymptomatic; occult blood positive stool.
Colon cancer	Age >50 years and usually asymptomatic; change in bowel pattern or microcytic anemia.
Ischemic colitis	Risk factors for atherosclerosis and evidence of vascular disease in elderly; may present with abdominal pain.
Hemorrhoids	Intermittent mild rectal bleeding associated with straining on bowel movement.
Infectious colitis	Bloody diarrhea, fever, urgency, tenesmus, and exposure history.
Inflammatory bowel disease	History of condition and bloody diarrhea, tenesmus, abdominal pain, fever.
Meckel's diverticulum	Painless hematochezia in young patient and normal esophagogastroduodenoscopy and colonoscopy.

NSAID = nonsteroidal anti-inflammatory drug.

Table 2. Management Considerations for Acute Gastrointestinal Bleeding

Condition	Notes
Hemodynamic stabilization	Two large-bore IV access sites or central venous access: resuscitation with IV fluids and blood products; endotracheal intubation prior to endoscopy to prevent aspiration in patients who have ongoing UGI bleeding and altered level of consciousness.
Initial laboratories	CBC, blood type, cross-match; coagulation profile; serum electrolytes, blood urea nitrogen, serum creatinine.
Electrocardiogram	In all patients aged >50 years and all patients with underlying cardiac disease or features of ischemia.
Gastric and duodenal ulcers (see Chapter 18)	Intravenous PPI and endoscopic therapy* (for high-risk lesions) reduces the risk of recurrent bleeding. If ineffective, consult surgery or interventional radiology. After stabilization, triple therapy for *Helicobacter pylori*—for patients found to be infected.
Variceal bleeding (see Chapter 22)	Prophylactic antibiotics for all patients. First-line therapy: endoscopic band ligation or sclerotherapy and octreotide. Second-line therapy: TIPPS; balloon tamponade.
Colonic bleeding (diverticulosis, angiectasia)	First-line therapy: colonoscopy and endoscopic therapy.* Second-line therapy: arteriography (vasopressin infusion or embolization) when endoscopy is not feasible or for persistent or recurrent bleeding. Third-line therapy: exploratory laparotomy and segmental colectomy.

*Endoscopic therapy incorporates injection therapy (epinephrine, sclerosing agents), thermal techniques (probes, argon plasma coagulation), and mechanical modalities (clips). The type of lesion and the presence or absence of ongoing bleeding determine which technique is used.

CBC = complete blood count; IV = intravenous; PPI = proton pump inhibitors; TIPPS = transjugular intrahepatic portosystemic shunt; UGI = upper gastrointestinal bleeding.

an isolated elevation of the BUN or elevated BUN-to-creatinine ratio suggests an upper gastrointestinal source of blood loss, they do not reliably discriminate between upper and lower gastrointestinal bleeding. In acute, severe bleeding, the initial hematocrit often is an unreliable indicator of the volume of blood loss; it can take 24-72 hours before the hematocrit reveals the true reduction in oxygen-carrying capacity.

Clinical risk factors are used to assess the patient's risk for rebleeding and mortality including: increased age; large-volume bleeding, as indicated by hemodynamic instability; significant comorbid medical conditions (e.g., diabetes, liver failure, heart failure, renal failure); and endoscopic characteristics (see below). Obtain early consultation with a gastroenterologist and surgeon for high-risk patients.

After hemodynamic stabilization the next step is to distinguish upper from lower gastrointestinal bleeding. Although melena and hematemesis are generally associated with upper gastrointestinal bleeding and hematochezia is more often a sign of lower gastrointestinal bleeding, these distinctions are not absolute. Melena indicates that blood has been present in the gastrointestinal tract for at least 14 hours, but some patients with melena have bleeding distal to the ligament of Treitz, and 10%-15% of patients with hematochezia may have upper gastrointestinal bleeding. Most gastrointestinal bleeding is self-limited, and emergent diagnostic studies are usually required only for patients with persistent bleeding or who are hemodynamically unstable. For patients with melena or hematemesis, evaluation begins with esophagogastroduodenoscopy (endoscopy). Endoscopy identifies the bleeding source with considerable accuracy, provides important prognostic information, and allows for immediate treatment for many patients. Bleeding from varices or ulcers with specific features (i.e., adherent clot, nonbleeding visible vessel, or active bleeding) has a higher risk for recurrent bleeding, need for surgery, and mortality. Endoscopic therapy reduces morbidity and mortality in these patients. In patients with a bleeding peptic ulcer, the use of intravenous proton pump inhibitor therapy has been shown to reduce the risk of recurrent hemorrhage following endoscopic hemostasis (see Table 2). If bleeding persists despite endoscopic therapy, further options include endoscopic retreatment, angiographic embolization, and surgery. If endoscopy does not identify a bleeding source in a patient with melena, the evaluation proceeds to colonoscopy.

In patients with hematochezia and large-volume blood loss, exclude an upper gastrointestinal bleeding source with nasogastric tube aspiration of gastric contents or endoscopy. The presence of blood or coffee-ground-like material on gastric lavage indicates ongoing or recent upper gastrointestinal bleeding and the need for upper endoscopy. Negative nasogastric tube lavage is reliable only if the aspirate contains bile (a yellow or green fluid that tests positive for bile with a urine dipstick), indicating passage of the tube beyond the pylorus into the duodenum. Therefore, if nasogastric aspirate contains bile but no blood, it is appropriate to proceed to colonoscopy (see Table 2); otherwise, upper endoscopy is performed.

Ongoing rectal bleeding without an identifiable source despite upper endoscopy and colonoscopy can be evaluated with a ^{99m}Tc pertechnate-labeled red blood cell scan or angiography. The tagged red blood cell scanning is positive in 45% of patients with an active bleed, and has an overall accuracy for localizing the bleeding of 78%. It can detect ongoing bleeding occurring at a rate of 0.1-0.5 mL/min. This is often the first radiologic test performed, as it is much more sensitive than angiography in detecting a bleed, but not very specific. Visualization of the bleeding site (usually a diverticulum or vascular ectasia) by angiography necessitates a bleeding rate of at least 1 mL/min but the advantage of angiography is the ability to provide selective embolization to control bleeding. A Meckel scan (which identifies aberrant gastric mucosa) should be considered in younger patients with lower gastrointestinal bleeding to diagnose Meckel's diverticulum. Barium studies have low sensitivity and may interfere with subsequent testing and are not done in the setting of an acute gastrointestinal bleed.

Patients aged <40 years at low risk for colorectal cancer who present with small-volume, self-limited hematochezia may not require colonoscopy. If the bleeding consists of blood on toilet paper or a few drops of blood in the stool, a bleeding hemorrhoid is the most likely cause. Patients with pain on defecation may have an anal fissure. These patients can often forego colonoscopy if a digital rectal exam and anoscopy confirm a benign anorectal process and there are no other concerning features such as constitutional symptoms, anemia, blood within the stool, change in bowel movements, or a family history of colorectal polyps or cancer.

Obscure Gastrointestinal Bleeding

Gastrointestinal bleeding of obscure origin refers to recurrent or persistent bleeding in which endoscopic studies do not reveal the source of blood loss. In many instances, the bleeding site is in the upper gastrointestinal tract or colon, but is not recognized. The evaluation of gastrointestinal bleeding of obscure origin usually begins with repeat endoscopy directed at the most likely site. If repeat endoscopy is unrevealing in a patient who is not actively bleeding, examination should focus on the small intestine, utilizing such tests as enteroscopy or capsule endoscopy (Table 3).

Book Enhancement

Go to www.acponline.org/essentials/gastroenterology-section.html to view x-ray and colonoscopic images of ischemic colitis, endoscopic views of gastric antral vascular ectasia and the "visible vessel" sign, and a proctoscopic view of radiation proctitis. Access an image of cutaneous telangiectasias associated with hereditary hemorrhagic telangiectasias. In *MKSAP for Students 4*, assess yourself with items 36-38 in the **Gastroenterology and Hepatology** section.

Bibliography

American College of Physicians. Medical Knowledge Self-Assessment Program 14. Philadelphia: American College of Physicians; 2006.

Barkun A, Bardou M, Marshall JK, for the Nonvariceal Upper GI Bleeding Consensus Conference Group. Consensus recommendations for managing patients with nonvariceal upper gastrointestinal bleeding. Ann Intern Med. 2003;139:843-57. [PMID: 14623622]

Table 3. Selected Diagnostic Studies for the Evaluation of Obscure Gastrointestinal Bleeding

Examination	Notes
Repeated upper endoscopy	Angiectasias, esophagitis, Cameron's erosions (erosions at the diaphragmatic hiatus), gastric antral vascular ectasia (GAVE).
Repeated colonoscopy with ileal intubation	Angiectasias, Crohn's disease, distal ileal tumors.
Small bowel follow-through or enteroclysis	Crohn's disease, small bowel tumors. Enteroclysis is a double-contrast study performed by passing a tube into the proximal small bowel and injecting contrast and air.
CT scan of the abdomen and pelvis	Crohn's disease, malignancies, aortoenteric fistula.
Meckel's scan (in selected patients)	Meckel's diverticulum.
Capsule endoscopy (capsule enteroscopy)	Angiectasias of small bowel, Crohn's disease.
Labeled red blood cell scan*	Localization of active bleeding.
Mesenteric angiography*	Localization and possible treatment of active bleeding.
Intraoperative endoscopy	Transfusion-dependent or life-threatening bleeding.

*Especially if active bleeding is present.

Modified from Medical Knowledge Self-Assessment Program (MKSAP) 14. Philadelphia: American College of Physicians; 2006.

Bjorkman DJ, Eisen GM. Gastrointestinal Bleeding, Non-variceal Upper. http://pier.acponline.org/physicians/diseases/d184. [Date accessed: 2008 Jan 25] In: PIER [online database]. Philadelphia: American College of Physicians; 2008.

Zuccaro G Jr. Management of the adult patient with acute lower gastrointestinal bleeding. American College of Gastroenterology, Practice Parameters Committee. Am J Gastroenterol. 1998;93:1202-8. [PMID: 9707037]

Chapter 21

Viral Hepatitis

Carlos Palacio, MD

Viral hepatitis can be acute or chronic. The laboratory hallmark of acute hepatitis is elevation of serum aminotransferase levels; the clinical course ranges from asymptomatic disease to fulminant hepatic failure. Chronic hepatitis is an inflammatory process that persists >6 months and can progress to cirrhosis. Histologically, hepatitis is characterized by inflammatory cell infiltration involving the portal areas or the parenchyma, often with associated necrosis; significant fibrosis may be seen in chronic hepatitis.

Viral hepatitis is caused by infection with any of at least five distinct viruses, of which the most commonly identified in the United States are hepatitis A virus (HAV), hepatitis B virus (HBV), and hepatitis C virus (HCV). HAV is transmitted through the fecal-oral route, spreading primarily through close personal contact with an HAV-infected person. HBV is transmitted parenterally through exposure to the blood or body fluids of an infected person by injection-drug use, sexual contact with an infected person, and from an infected mother to her infant during delivery. HCV, also transmitted parenterally, is the most prevalent blood-borne infection in the United States. All three viruses can cause an acute illness characterized by nausea, malaise, abdominal pain, and jaundice. HBV and HCV also can produce a chronic infection that is associated with an increased risk for chronic liver disease and hepatocellular carcinoma.

Prevention

Administer hepatitis A vaccine to adults whose departure to endemic areas for hepatitis A virus is >2 weeks away. These areas include Africa, Central and South America, the Middle East, and Asia (see www.cdc.gov/travel/default.aspx for relevant countries); if departure is <2 weeks away, immunoglobulin should be administered singly or in combination with the vaccine. Immunoglobulin ensures passive immunity for several months. Other risk groups for hepatitis A include men who have sex with men (MSM), illegal drug users (oral and parenteral), persons with occupational risks (i.e., sewage handlers, persons working with nonhuman primates), persons with clotting factor disorders and chronic liver disease.

Administer hepatitis B vaccine to MSM and others with high-risk sexual behavior, current or recent injection-drug users, persons with chronic liver disease or endstage renal disease on hemodialysis, health care workers and public-safety workers exposed to blood or potentially infectious body fluids, household or sexual contacts of hepatitis B virus carriers, clients and staff members of institutions for persons with developmental disabilities,

international travelers to countries endemic for HBV infection, and any adult seeking protection from HBV infection.

Administer hepatitis A immunoglobulin as postexposure prophylaxis (within 2 weeks of exposure) to household, sexual, and day care contacts of persons with confirmed cases of hepatitis A, and to individuals who have consumed hepatitis A-contaminated products. Administer hepatitis B immunoglobulin as postexposure prophylaxis, along with hepatitis B vaccine, for exposure to hepatitis B-positive blood, sexual exposure to a hepatitis B-positive person, or household exposure to a person with acute hepatitis B. There is no passive or active immunization for hepatitis C virus.

Screening

Screen all persons at risk for hepatitis B and C; risk factors for hepatitis C include intravenous drug use, receipt of blood products before 1992, and needle-stick exposure to hepatitis C-positive blood. Other potential exposures that may warrant screening for hepatitis C include high-risk sexual exposures, tattoos, body piercing, and non-intravenous illicit drug use. Screen patients with unexplained acute and chronic hepatitis for hepatitis B and C infection.

Diagnosis

Hepatitis A is typically associated with abrupt onset of constitutional symptoms, such as fatigue, anorexia, malaise, nausea, and vomiting. Low-grade fever and right upper quadrant pain are often present as well. Change in color of skin, sclera, or urine are particularly helpful historical findings. Approximately 50% of patients with hepatitis A have no identifiable source for their infection, so the absence of classic risk factors cannot exclude the diagnosis. Physical examination often reveals jaundice, hepatomegaly, and abdominal tenderness. Confirm the diagnosis with serologic testing, specifically IgM antibody to hepatitis A. In most patients, IgM antibody is detectable by the time a person is symptomatic. Although rare, acute liver failure can occur; test all patients with unexplained acute liver failure for hepatitis A

Symptoms of acute hepatitis B infection are similar to those of acute hepatitis A infection. It is not uncommon for persons to have anicteric or subclinical acute infection. Approximately 30%-40% of patients with acute hepatitis B have no risk factors identified. A characteristic pattern of serologic tests is usually seen in acute hepatitis B (Table 1). During the course of acute infection, a "window period" exists wherein hepatitis B surface antigen levels have fallen but anti-hepatitis B surface antibody has not yet become

Table 1. Serologic Diagnosis of Hepatitis B Infection

	Acute Hepatitis B	Inactive Carriers	Chronic Hepatitis	Prior Exposure	Prior Vaccination
HBsAg	Positive	Positive	Positive	Negative	Negative
Anti-HBc	Positive (IgM)	Positive	Positive	Positive	Negative
Anti-HBs	Negative	Negative	Negative	Positive	Positive
HBV DNA	Positive	Negative	Positive	Negative	Negative
HBeAg	Positive	Negative	Positive or Negative	Negative	Negative
Anti-HBe	Positive or Negative	Positive	Positive or Negative	Positive or Negative	Negative

HBsAg = hepatitis B surface antigen; anti-HBc = hepatitis B core antibody; anti-HBs = hepatitis B surface antibody; HBV = hepatitis B virus; HBeAg = hepatitis B e antigen; anti-HBe = hepatitis B e antibody.

Table 2. Differential Diagnosis of Viral Hepatitis

Disease	Notes
Alcoholic liver disease	Common cause of chronic hepatitis or cirrhosis. History of excessive alcohol consumption and improvement with discontinuation; AST/ALT ratio >2.
Autoimmune hepatitis	90% female. Other autoimmune disorders may be present. 25% of cases can present with acute hepatitis. Test for ANA, smooth muscle antibody, and elevated immunoglobulins; characteristic liver biopsy.
Chronic hepatitis B	Test for HBsAg and anti-HBc.
Chronic hepatitis C	Test for anti-HCV (ELISA); if positive, test for HCV-RNA using qualitative PCR.
Drug-induced chronic hepatitis	May affect men and women of all ages, but more often in women and elderly. History of drug consumption and improvement with discontinuation.
Hemochromatosis	Most common genetic liver disease with prevalence of 1 in 400; iron overload not usually evident until midlife. Cardiac dysfunction, diabetes, and arthritis. Elevated fasting serum iron, transferrin saturation, and ferritin. Quantitative hepatic iron index on liver biopsy and HFE genotyping assist with diagnosis.
Nonalcoholic fatty liver	Most common cause of chronic hepatitis in United States; spectrum of liver disease ranges from steatosis to steatohepatitis to cirrhosis. Associated with diabetes mellitus, obesity, dyslipidemia, and insulin resistance.
Other metabolic liver disease	Wilson's disease prevalence is 1 in 30,000, and is rarely diagnosed after age 40. May present with speech or gait difficulties. Low serum ceruloplasmin, elevated urine copper, and Kayser-Fleischer ring on slit-lamp exam screening. Quantitate hepatic copper for diagnosis. Alpha-1-antitrypsin deficiency: serum level and phenotyping. Stain liver biopsy for periodic acid-Schiff (PAS)-positive inclusions.

ALT = alanine aminotransferase; ANA = antinuclear antibodies; AST = aspartate aminotransferase; ELISA = enzyme-linked immunosorbent assay; HCV = hepatitis C virus; PCR = polymerase chain reaction; RNA = ribonucleic acid.

detectable; diagnosis is based on the presence of antibody to hepatitis B core antigen (IgM). Test patients with evidence of chronic liver disease for chronic hepatitis B, in addition to patients with glomerulonephritis, polyarteritis nodosa, and cryoglobulinemia, which are extrahepatic manifestations of chronic hepatitis B infection. Serologic assays can distinguish between chronic hepatitis B infection and the inactive carrier state (Table 1). Obtain a liver biopsy to determine the grade and stage of liver injury in chronic hepatitis B, as well as to exclude additional etiologies of liver injury. Although rare, acute liver failure can occur in acute hepatitis B, and all patients with unexplained acute liver failure should have serologic testing.

Hepatitis C usually manifests as chronic liver disease because the acute infection is usually asymptomatic. Test patients with chronic liver disease for anti-hepatitis C antibody. Consider testing patients with extrahepatic complications of hepatitis C, including cryoglobulinemia, glomerulonephritis, and porphyria cutanea tarda. A positive antibody test indicates only exposure, not immunity; therefore hepatitis C virus RNA must be measured to confirm ongoing infection. Since normal aminotransferase levels occur in up to 40% of patients with chronic hepatitis C, this feature cannot exclude the diagnosis. Consider liver biopsy to evaluate the severity of disease, though this is not essential before initiating treatment. Table 2 summarizes a differential diagnosis for viral hepatitis.

Therapy

Hepatitis A infection is usually self-limiting, and treatment is supportive. Patients with acute or chronic viral hepatitis are counseled to avoid alcohol and acetaminophen and eat a balanced, nutritionally adequate diet. Fulminant hepatitis is a rare complication of acute hepatitis A and B and is heralded by symptoms and signs of liver failure, including mental status changes, ascites, and a prolonged prothrombin time. In these patients, liver transplantation may be life-saving. Criteria for hospitalization in acute viral hepatitis include inability to maintain oral hydration and symptoms or signs of liver failure.

Antiviral drug therapy is used in selected patients with chronic hepatitis B infection (Table 3); such treatment reduces the likelihood of progression to cirrhosis and hepatocellular carcinoma. Agents include high-dose interferon-α, lamivudine, adefovir, and entecavir. Criteria for treatment include elevated serum alanine aminotransferase (ALT) levels, detectable hepatitis B DNA, and

Table 3. Treatment of Chronic Hepatitis B

Chronic hepatitis B is defined as persistent HBsAg for more than 6 months.

HBeAg	HBV DNA	ALT	Treatment
Positive	Positive	<2 × normal	Observe
Positive	Positive	>2 × normal	IFNa, lamivudine, or adefovir
Negative	Positive (+ HBV = chronic active hepatitis despite negative HBeAg)	>2 × normal	IFNa, lamivudine, or adefovir; long-term treatment required
Negative	Negative	<2 × normal	No treatment
Positive or Negative	Positive	Compensated cirrhosis	IFNa (cautiously), lamivudine, or adefovir, or liver transplant
Positive or Negative	Positive	Decompensated cirrhosis	Lamivudine or adefovir, or liver transplant

ALT = alanine aminotransferase; DNA = deoxyribonucleic acid; HBeAg = hepatitis B e antigen; HBV = hepatitis B virus; IFNa = α-interferon; HBSAg = hepatitis B surface antigen.

chronic hepatitis on biopsy. All treatments can result in sustained loss of hepatitis B e antigen and hepatitis B virus DNA levels.

Interferon-α, which is administered subcutaneously, is associated with frequent side effects, including flu-like symptoms, myelotoxicity, depression, and exacerbation of autoimmune conditions. Pegylated interferon allows for less frequent administration than standard interferon and is more efficacious. Long-term monotherapy with oral lamivudine is associated with the frequent development of drug-resistant mutant strains, although this does not necessitate cessation of treatment as long as clinical and serologic benefit persists. Oral adefovir has efficacy in patients with lamivudine-resistant chronic hepatitis B, although patients on adefovir must be monitored carefully for the development of nephrotoxicity. Another problem with the oral agents is the frequent development of relapse after stopping treatment; the optimal duration of therapy with these agents, and the long-term implications of mutant strains is unclear. Endpoints to assess efficacy of treatment include normalization of serum alanine aminotransferase (ALT) level, loss of detectable hepatitis B virus DNA and hepatitis B surface antigen, and improvement in liver histology.

Antiviral therapy can induce sustained clearance of hepatitis C virus. Treatment is offered to patients with compensated liver disease (i.e., absence of ascites, encephalopathy, or variceal bleeding) in whom hepatitis C RNA is detectable and serum alanine aminotransferase (ALT) levels are elevated. An alternative strategy for patients with mild histological disease on liver biopsy is periodic liver biopsy and antiviral therapy if the disease progresses. The optimal treatment regimen is a combination of pegylated interferon-α and ribavirin. Ribavirin can be associated with hemolytic anemia. Response rates vary according to the specific hepatitis C genotype, with genotype 1 (the most common in the United States) being the most refractory to treatment. Because most patients with chronic hepatitis C never develop cirrhosis, there is controversy about the treatment of patients with persistently normal aminotransferase levels and minimal histological evidence of hepatitis.

Follow-Up

Patients on antiviral therapy must have regular laboratory and clinical monitoring to assess response to treatment and development of side effects. Patients with cirrhosis due to either hepatitis B or C are at risk for hepatocellular carcinoma, and periodic screening with ultrasonography and serum alpha-fetoprotein is recommended. The optimal time to initiate a screening program and its ideal frequency are unknown.

Book Enhancement

Go to www.acponline.org/essentials/gastroenterology-section .html to access schematic representations of the serologic course for hepatitis A, B and C, a differential diagnosis of aminotransferase elevations, see the slit lamp appearance of Kayser-Fleischer rings associated with Wilson's disease, and hepatitis C associated porphyria cutanea tarda. In *MKSAP for Students 4*, assess yourself with items 39-42 in the **Gastroenterology and Hepatology** section.

Bibliography

Dentinger CN, McMahon BJ. Hepatitis A. http://pier.acponline.org/ physicians/diseases/d471. [Date accessed: 2008 Jan 9] In: PIER [online database]. Philadelphia: American College of Physicians; 2008.

Fontana RJ, Lok ASF. Hepatitis B. http://pier.acponline.org/physicians/ diseases/d476. [Date accessed: 2008 Jan 9] In: PIER [online database]. Philadelphia: American College of Physicians; 2008.

Green RM, Flamm S. AGA technical review on the evaluation of liver chemistry tests. Gastroenterology. 2002;123:1367-84. [PMID: 12360498]

Jou JH, Muir AJ. In the clinic. Hepatitis C. Ann Intern Med. 2008;148: ITC6-1–ITC6-16. [PMID: 18519925]

Koff RS, Muir A. Hepatitis C. http://pier.acponline.org/physicians/ diseases/d163. [Date accessed: 2008 Jan 9] In: PIER [online database]. Philadelphia: American College of Physicians; 2008.

Chapter 22

Cirrhosis

Mark J. Fagan, MD

irrhosis is defined as a pathologic state of the liver characterized histologically by extensive fibrosis and regenerative nodules. Liver fibrosis begins with the activation of hepatic stellate cells, which produce excess extracellular matrix proteins, including type I collagen. Failure to degrade the increased interstitial matrix leads to progressive fibrosis. A variety of toxic, infectious, and inflammatory insults to the liver may result in cirrhosis (Table 1). Patients with cirrhosis may present with symptoms related to hepatocyte dysfunction (jaundice, coagulopathy, and edema) or symptoms due to an increase in portal venous pressure (ascites, bleeding esophageal varices, hepatic encephalopathy, and hypersplenism).

Prevention

Counsel patients who consume hazardous amounts of alcohol to reduce or stop drinking alcohol. Cessation of alcohol intake is effective in reducing the risk of cirrhosis. Treatment of hepatitis B and C infections may reduce the risk of cirrhosis in some patients. Counsel patients with chronic hepatitis B or C infection to avoid alcohol because concomitant alcohol use increases the risk for cirrhosis.

Screening

Screen patients for hazardous drinking using validated questionnaires such as the CAGE or AUDIT instruments. Test patients with risk factors for chronic hepatitis B and C infection.

Diagnosis

Patients with cirrhosis may be asymptomatic for years before developing evidence of hepatocyte dysfunction or portal hypertension. Patients may report a change in skin, sclera, or urine color due to jaundice, and they may develop pruritis related to cholestasis. The relative estrogen excess of the cirrhotic state may lead to symptoms of decreased libido, erectile dysfunction or amenorrhea. Decreased hepatic production of clotting factors may lead to abnormal bleeding. Portal hypertension may cause esophageal varices, which may lead to hematemesis or melena. Patients may report weight gain, increased abdominal girth, or ankle swelling related to ascites and edema. Family members may report changes in behavior and mental status characteristic of hepatic encephalopathy.

Search for clues to the cause of cirrhosis. Take a thorough alcohol history. Question patients about risk factors for hepatitis C infection such as intravenous drug use, blood transfusion prior to 1992, having a sexual partner who uses intravenous drugs, or incarceration. Similarly, ask patients about risk factors for hepatitis B infection, such as birth in an endemic country, having multiple sex partners, or intravenous drug use. Inquire about other diseases that may result in cirrhosis, such as right-sided heart failure, or risk factors for nonalcoholic fatty liver disease (obesity, diabetes, and hyperlipidemia). Ask about medications associated with increased risk for cirrhosis, such as methotrexate, amiodarone, or high-dose vitamin A. A family history of liver disease

Table 1. Differential Diagnosis of Cirrhosis

Disease	Characteristics
Biliary obstruction	Dilated intrahepatic ducts and common bile duct on US, CT, or MRCP; imaging may identify etiology (e.g., bile duct stone).
Chronic exposure to drugs and toxins	Exposure history, most commonly alcohol, but may be medications (methotrexate, amiodarone, high-dose vitamin A) or chemical (hydrocarbons). Long-term TPN can lead to cirrhosis.
Viral hepatitis	Etiology most commonly hepatitis A, B, and C. Diagnosis made by typical viral hepatitis serology.
Autoimmune hepatitis	Typically young women with fatigue and jaundice. Look for specific autoantibodies (ANA, ASMA).
Primary biliary cirrhosis	Typically women in their 50s. AMA typically positive (>90%).
Primary sclerosing cholangitis	Typically men in their late 30s, often with ulcerative colitis. Diagnosis usually made by endoscopic cholangiography.
Nonalcoholic fatty liver disease	Typically obese, diabetic women with hyperlipidemia. US of liver shows fatty infiltration.
Hereditary hemochromatosis	Typically men. Diagnosis suspected with elevated transferrin saturation and ferritin. Hemochromatosis gene test to confirm diagnosis.
Wilson's disease	Diagnosis is suggested by a low serum ceruloplasmin, raised serum free copper levels, and Kayser-Fleischer rings on slit-lamp examination.
α_1-Antitrypsin deficiency	Diagnosis is established by serum α_1-antitrypsin phenotyping.
Cryptogenic cirrhosis	Typical clinical features of cirrhosis but no obvious cause after extensive evaluation.

AMA = antimitochondrial antibody; ANA = antinuclear antibody; ASMA = antismooth muscle antibody; CT = computed tomography; MRCP = magnetic resonance cholangiopancreatography; MRI = magnetic resonance imaging; TPN = total parenteral nutrition; US = ultrasound.

should prompt a consideration of genetic diseases that cause cirrhosis, such as hemochromatosis, alpha-1-antitrypsin deficiency, or Wilson's disease.

Jaundice is usually first noticed in the conjunctiva, with more severe degrees apparent in other mucous membranes or the skin. Spider angiomata, thought to be the result of an increased ratio of serum estradiol to testosterone, may be found over the face, neck, shoulders, and upper thorax. Palmar erythema, gynecomastia, and testicular atrophy are thought to be related to the same hormonal effects. The breath may have a characteristic odor, fetor hepaticus, caused by the presence of dimethlysulphide due to portal-systemic shunting. The liver may be palpable or reduced in size, and the spleen may be palpable due to engorgement from portal hypertension. Bulging flanks, shifting dullness, or a fluid wave suggests ascites. The presence of leg edema in patients with cirrhosis increases the likelihood that ascites is present. Rarely, portal hypertension causes markedly dilated abdominal wall veins, "caput medusae." Impaired mental status, confusion, agitation, hyperreflexia, or asterixis (the inability to maintain a fixed posture) suggests hepatic encephalopathy. Other physical examination findings in cirrhosis include parotid enlargement, Dupuytren's contracture, clubbing, axillary hair loss, and white nails.

Laboratory tests and imaging studies, in combination with physical examination findings, can be used to estimate the likelihood of cirrhosis (Table 2). The serum albumin level, prothrombin time, total and direct bilirubin levels, and transaminase levels are useful in assessing hepatic function. Thrombocytopenia suggests hypersplenism due to portal hypertension.

In patients with newly identified ascites, perform a paracentesis and calculate the serum-ascites albumin gradient to differentiate among causes of ascites. A gradient >1.1 g/dL is compatible with cirrhosis. In patients with ascites and a change in their clinical status, perform a paracentesis and obtain an ascites granulocyte count and culture to detect spontaneous bacterial peritonitis. An ascitic fluid granulocyte count >250/µL is compatible with infection. Patients with cirrhosis should undergo upper endoscopy to search for esophageal varices (Table 2).

Therapy

The goals of therapy for cirrhosis are to slow the progression of the underlying liver disease; prevent superimposed liver insults;

Table 2. Laboratory and Other Studies for Cirrhosis

Test	Notes
Tests for the Diagnosis of Cirrhosis	
AST/ALT ≤1	Sensitivity, 44%; specificity, 94%.
Platelets <100,000	Sensitivity, 38%; specificity, 97%. Suggests presence of splenomegaly.
PT, bilirubin, albumin	Measures of liver function.
Liver ultrasound	Sensitivity, 71-100%; specificity, 88%. Compared to liver histology.
CT abdomen	Sensitivity, 84%; specificity, 100%. Based on caudate lobe/right lobe ratio exceeding 0.65.
MRI abdomen	Sensitivity, 93%; specificity, 92%. Based on enlargement of the hilar periportal space as sign of early cirrhosis.
Serum ascites albumin gradient	Sensitivity, 97%; specificity, 91%. Serum albumin minus ascites albumin: >1.1 g/dL compatible with cirrhosis.
Tests to Determine the Etiology of Cirrhosis	
Viral hepatitis studies	Hepatitis B surface antigen, hepatitis B surface antibody, hepatitis B core antibody, hepatitis C antibody helpful in diagnosing viral hepatitis.
Alkaline phosphatase	Increased in primary sclerosing cholangitis/primary biliary cirrhosis.
Antimitochondrial antibody	Positive in PBC >90%.
Antinuclear antibody	May be present in cirrhosis from autoimmune hepatitis and PBC.
Anti-smooth muscle antibody	May be present in cirrhosis from autoimmune hepatitis.
Anti-LKM antibody	May be present in cirrhosis from autoimmune hepatitis.
Total protein, globulin	Elevation seen in autoimmune hepatitis, viral hepatitis, and PBC.
Iron studies	Transferrin saturation, ferritin are increased in hemochromatosis.
GGT	May be the only abnormality in nonalcoholic steatohepatitis.
Ceruloplasmin	Decreased in Wilson's disease.
α_1-antitrypsin	Decreased in patients with α_1-antitrypsin deficiency
Tests to Detect Complications from Cirrhosis	
α-fetoprotein	Levels >500 ng/mL highly suggest HCC.
Ultrasound abdomen	Screening for HCC; gold standard for the detection ascites.
Ascites granulocytes	>250/µL suggests SBP.
Serum electrolytes	Abnormal in cirrhosis due to diuretic therapy for ascites; alcoholism.
Serum BUN, creatinine	Elevated in hepatorenal syndrome.
Hematocrit, stool occult blood	GI bleeding due to portal hypertension or other causes.
Upper endoscopy	To document and treat varices.
Serum ammonia	May be helpful in unusual presentations of hepatic encephalopathy.

ALT = alanine aminotransferase; AST = aspartate aminotransferase; BUN = blood urea nitrogen; CT = computed tomography; GGT = gamma glutamyl transpeptidase; GI = gastrointestinal; HCC = hepatocellular carcinoma; MRI = magnetic resonance imaging; PBC = primary biliary cirrhosis; SBP = spontaneous bacterial peritonitis; US = ultrasound.

prevent and treat complications such as esophageal varices, ascites, and hepatic encephalopathy; and evaluate the patient for liver transplantation. Protein-calorie malnutrition and hypermetabolism are common in patients with cirrhosis, and nutritional assessment is important. Provide alcoholic patients with folate and thiamine supplementation. Sodium restriction (<2 g/day) is important for patients with ascites. Abstinence from alcohol is critically important to reduce further liver injury. Vaccinate non-immune patients against hepatitis A and B. Administer pneumococcal and yearly influenza vaccines.

Endoscopic variceal band ligation is indicated for primary prophylaxis of variceal bleeding in patients with high-risk varices found on upper endoscopy and contraindications to or intolerance of β-blockers (see below). Endoscopic band ligation is also recommended for secondary prophylaxis in patients who have already experienced an episode of variceal bleeding. Patients who rebleed despite variceal banding may be considered for alternative treatments such as transjugular intrahepatic portosystemic stent shunt (TIPSS) or portosystemic shunt surgery. TIPSS creates a low-resistance channel between the hepatic vein and the intrahepatic portion of the portal vein using angiographic techniques. The channel is kept open by an expandable metal stent. Refractory ascites can be treated with repeated large-volume paracentesis. TIPSS is an alternative when repeated large-volume paracentesis is impractical or ineffective.

Liver transplantation is the definitive treatment for patients with end-stage liver disease and complications such as variceal bleeding, ascites, or hepatic encephalopathy. Some patients with cirrhosis and hepatocellular carcinoma can also be treated with liver transplantation. The MELD (Model for End-Stage Liver Disease) scoring system uses the patient's bilirubin, creatinine, and INR to prioritize transplant candidates. Contraindications to liver transplantation include cardiopulmonary disease that constitutes prohibitive risk for surgery, non-skin malignancy outside of the liver within 5 years of evaluation or not meeting oncologic criteria for cure, and active substance abuse.

Thirty to fifty percent of patients with portal hypertension will bleed from varices. Drug treatment with nonselective β-blockers such as propanolol or nadolol is effective for primary prophylaxis for high-risk varices and secondary prophylaxis following an episode of variceal bleeding. The dose is titrated to produce a 25% reduction in resting heart rate.

Diuretics and sodium restriction are the mainstays of treatment for ascites. Combination therapy with spironolactone plus furosemide is most effective; in one trial 90% of patients had their ascites controlled with these two drugs.

Subacute bacterial peritonitis commonly develops in hospitalized patients with ascites and an ascitic fluid protein <1.0 g/dL, variceal bleeding, or prior spontaneous bacterial peritonitis. Such patients benefit from short-term prophylactic administration of an antibiotic (i.e., trimethoprim-sulfamethoxazole, ciprofloxacin, or norfloxacin) directed at the common organisms causing spontaneous bacterial peritonitis. Long-term antibiotic prophylaxis of spontaneous bacterial peritonitis has not been shown to prolong survival.

The hepatorenal syndrome is the development of renal failure in patients with portal hypertension, ascites, and normal renal tubular function. Vigorous diuretic therapy, paracentesis without volume expansion, and gastrointestinal bleeding may precipitate hepatorenal syndrome. Other causes of renal failure should be excluded, particularly spontaneous bacterial peritonitis. Failure to improve following withdrawal of diuretics and administration of 1-1.5 L of normal saline is indicative of the hepatorenal syndrome. Dialysis is indicated for patients with significant volume overload or severe electrolyte abnormalities. Albumin and vasopressin or norepinephrine may improve renal arterial blood flow but almost all patients with the hepatorenal syndrome will require liver transplantation.

The treatment of hepatic encephalopathy begins with a search for precipitating causes such as hypovolemia, electrolyte and acid-base disturbances, gastrointestinal bleeding, infections (including spontaneous bacterial peritonitis), and medication effects. To lower serum ammonia levels and prevent or treat hepatic encephalopathy, lactulose is the mainstay of drug treatment. Titrate the lactulose dose to produce two to three soft stools per day.

Follow-Up

Follow-up issues for patients with cirrhosis include counseling about substance abuse; monitoring for complications such as bleeding, ascites, spontaneous bacterial peritonitis, hepatic encephalopathy, or hepatorenal syndrome; monitoring for medication side effects; screening for hepatocellular carcinoma; and assessing for liver transplantation. Cessation of substance abuse is critical for reducing further liver damage from toxins such as alcohol and to permit consideration for liver transplantation. Instruct patients to report any symptoms such as melena, weight gain, increased abdominal girth, edema, abdominal pain, change in mental status, or decreased urine output that suggest complications from cirrhosis. For patients taking diuretics, careful monitoring of the BUN, creatinine, and electrolytes is important to detect potential volume depletion, hyperkalemia, hypokalemia, or hyponatremia. Because patients with cirrhosis develop hepatocellular carcinoma at a rate of approximately 4% per year, many hepatologists recommend screening patients for hepatocellular carcinoma using serum α-fetoprotein and ultrasound every 6 months. The efficacy of such screening for improving survival has not yet been demonstrated.

Book Enhancement

Go to www.acponline.org/essentials/gastroenterology-section .html to view patients with massive ascites, spider angioma, gynecomastia, parotid gland enlargement, Dupuytren's contractures, palmar erythema, and white nails. Review the Cirrhosis Discriminate Score to noninvasively predict the presence of cirrhosis, and the MELD score to determine prognosis, and access alcohol screening tools and a table of drugs used to manage cirrhosis. In *MKSAP for Students 4*, assess yourself with items 43-49 in the **Gastroenterology and Hepatology** section.

Bibliography

Falck-Ytter Y, McCullough AJ. Cirrhosis. http://pier.acponline.org/ physicians/diseases/d269. [Date accessed: 2008 Jan 12] In: PIER [online database]. Philadelphia: American College of Physicians; 2008.

Garcia-Tsao G, Sanyal AJ, Grace ND, Carey W; Practice Guidelines Committee of the American Association for the Study of Liver Diseases; Practice Parameters Committee of the American College of Gastroenterology. Prevention and management of gastroesophageal varices and variceal hemorrhage in cirrhosis.Hepatology. 2007;46:922-38. [PMID: 17879356]

Runyon BA; Practice Guidelines Committee, American Association for the Study of Liver Diseases (AASLD). Management of adult patients with ascites due to cirrhosis. Hepatology. 2004;39:841-56. [PMID: 14999706]

Wong CL, Holroyd-Leduc J, Thorpe KE, Straus SE. Does this patient have bacterial peritonitis or portal hypertension? How do I perform a paracentesis and analyze the results? JAMA. 2008;299:1166-78. [PMID: 18334692]

Chapter 23

Inflammatory Bowel Disease

Brown J. McCallum, MD

Crohn's disease is an inflammatory bowel disease characterized by chronic inflammation of all layers of the bowel. It can occur anywhere within the gastrointestinal tract and frequently is non-contiguous. Biopsy will reveal full-thickness inflammation of the bowel wall and non-caseating granulomas. Peak incidence is in the third decade, but there is a second peak occurring at around age 50.

Ulcerative colitis is characterized by inflammation of the colonic mucosa. It typically causes superficial ulcerations that begin at the rectum and progress proximally through the colon. Peak incidence is similar to Crohn's disease. Unlike Crohn's disease, ulcerative colitis is a strong risk factor for colon cancer and primary sclerosing cholangitis. Table 1 summarizes differences between Crohn's disease and ulcerative colitis.

Both genetic and environmental factors play a role in the development of inflammatory bowel disease. In genetically predisposed individuals, an uncontrolled inflammatory response is stimulated by environmental triggers. The inflammatory response is the result of an imbalance in activity between pro-inflammatory mediators (e.g., interleukin-1β, tumor necrosis factor-α, thromboxane A_2) and anti-inflammatory mediators (e.g., prostaglandin E2, interleukin-10). Immunoregulatory cytokines (e.g., interleukin-2) that regulate the process of lymphocyte differentiation also appear to be imbalanced in patients with inflammatory bowel disease.

Diagnosis

Patients with Crohn's disease may have abdominal pain, diarrhea (or constipation), tenesmus, hematochezia, hematuria, weight loss, and fever. Physical examination is often normal or nonspecific. Look for perianal induration, erythema, tenderness, skin tags, and fissures. Extra-articular manifestations may include uveitis, erythema nodosum, pyoderma gangrenosum, spondyloarthritis, and aphthous ulcers. Occasionally, a tender mass may be noted in the abdomen.

Laboratory examination is characteristically nonspecific, but culture for enteric pathogens, *Clostridium difficile* toxin assay, and stool for ova and parasites are obtained to exclude other diseases. Anti-*Saccharomyces cerevisiae* antibodies (ASCA) have low sensitivity for diagnosing Crohn's disease but relatively high specificity and support a clinical diagnosis. The addition of anti-CBir1 antibody increases the specificity to 98%. Patients with Crohn's disease frequently have anemia of chronic inflammation. Abdominal x-rays are used to evaluate intestinal obstruction and toxic megacolon. An upper gastrointestinal barium study with small bowel follow-through can document the extent of involvement, areas of strictures ("string sign"), and presence of intestinal fistulae. Barium enema can be helpful for diagnosing colonic disease. The diagnosis is established with colonoscopy and biopsy. Upper endoscopy can be of value if upper gastrointestinal symptoms are present. Capsule endoscopy may play a role in the diagnosis of patients with small bowel disease that cannot be detected by endoscopy or barium contrast studies.

Patients with mild ulcerative colitis disease may have intermittent rectal bleeding (frequently after eating or while sleeping), diarrhea, or constipation, whereas patients with moderate to severe disease report bloody diarrhea, abdominal pain, and fever. Extraintestinal manifestations include uveitis, erythema nodosum, pyoderma gangrenosum, sclerosing cholangitis, spondyloarthritis, fibrotic lung disease, aortic insufficiency, venous and arterial thromboembolism, and autoimmune hemolytic anemia. Physical examination is often normal early in the course, but findings may include evidence of weight loss and abdominal tenderness.

Table 1. Essential Points Differentiating Ulcerative Colitis from Crohn's Disease

Factors	Ulcerative Colitis	Crohn's Disease
Pathology	Crypt abscesses and superficial inflammation from rectum to colon	Linear ulcerations with "skip" areas of inflammation involving entire gastrointestinal tract
Clinical presentation	Diarrhea (prominent), hematochezia, weight loss, and fever	Abdominal pain (prominent), diarrhea, inflammatory masses, fever, and weight loss
Anti-*Saccharomyces cerevisiae* antibodies and anti-CBir1 antibody	10% of cases	60% of cases
Perinuclear antineutrophil antibodies (p-ANCA)	75% of cases	10% of cases
Smoking	Alleviates symptoms	Risk factor for disease
Colon cancer risk	High risk, particularly with pancolitis	Increased risk, but lower than ulcerative colitis
Primary sclerosing cholangitis	5% incidence	Incidence increased but less than ulcerative colitis

As in Crohn's disease, laboratory evaluation is directed at excluding other infectious causes of abdominal pain, diarrhea, and fever. Perinuclear antineutrophil antibody (p-ANCA) is frequently positive in ulcerative colitis; anti-*Saccharomyces cerevisiae* and anti-CBir1 antibodies are typically negative and help differentiate it from Crohn's disease.

Diagnosis is made by endoscopic evaluation of the colon, which shows continuous mucosal involvement without "skip lesions." Biopsy confirms the diagnosis. Table 2 summarizes a differential diagnosis for inflammatory bowel disease.

Therapy

Lifestyle modification can make a dramatic difference in the treatment of Crohn's disease. All patients with Crohn's disease should be encouraged to stop smoking. There is a strong association between smoking and Crohn's disease, and the use of tobacco products both reduces the effectiveness of therapy and increases recurrence rates after surgical resection. Patients should avoid nuts, seeds, popcorn, and lettuce, particularly if they have fibrostenosing small-bowel disease. Patients with extensive ileal resection should reduce intake of fat and oxalate rich foods to avoid renal stones. Intra-luminal fatty acids bind calcium, which allows free oxalate to be absorbed in the colon, leading to hyperoxaluria and oxalate stones. Drug therapy for Crohn's disease is based on location and severity of the disease. The goal is to induce and maintain clinical remission. Mild-to-moderate colonic disease (ambulatory, eating and drinking, and no fever, weight loss, dehydration, or abdominal pain) involving the colon with or without small intestine disease is treated with sulfasalazine; budesonide is used for ileal or right colonic disease; and mesalamine or metronidazole for small or large bowel disease. Patients with moderate-to-severe disease (fever, weight loss, dehydration, or abdominal pain without obstruction) achieve remission with prednisone but require the addition of azathioprine, 6-mercaptopurine, or methotrexate for maintenance therapy. Infliximab is also useful in these individuals. Patients with severe-to-fulminate disease (resistant to oral corticosteroid therapy), require parenteral corticosteroids and perhaps infliximab; cyclosporine has also been used effectively in these patients. Patients who develop fistulae are best treated with metronidazole or ciprofloxacin. If patients show hemodynamic instability, peritoneal signs, or persistent fevers, surgical consultation should be sought. If disease is complicated by strictures, abscesses, fistulae, or is medically refractory or associated with intolerable medication side-effects, surgical resection may be indicated.

In contrast to patients with Crohn's disease, patients with ulcerative colitis who use tobacco products have decreased numbers of exacerbations and their disease may worsen with smoking cessation. Patients with mild ulcerative colitis are treated with sulfasalazine or nicotine. Moderate disease may additionally require the use of corticosteroids for remission and azathioprine or 6-mercaptopurine for maintenance. Severe disease frequently requires the use of intravenous corticosteroids. Cyclosporine, tacrolimus, and infliximab have also been used in refractory cases with some degree of success. Colectomy is curative in ulcerative colitis, and

Table 2. Differential Diagnosis of Inflammatory Bowel Disease

Disease	Notes
Ulcerative colitis and Crohn's disease	Ulcerative colitis shows continuous disease from the rectum and limited to the colon with diffusely inflamed mucosa. Crohn's disease has skip lesions and can involve entire gastrointestinal tract. Typical serology in ulcerative colitis is pANCA-positive and ASCA-negative, whereas the opposite is found in Crohn's disease.
Bacterial enteritis (see Chapter 14)	Acute onset of diarrhea with fever, chills, diarrhea, hematochezia, or pus in stool (*Campylobacter, Shigella, Salmonella, E. coli, Yersinia*). Stool cultures may be positive for enteric pathogens.
Protozoan enteritis (see Chapter 14)	Relatively acute onset of diarrhea, bloating (*Entamoeba, Giardia*). *Entamoeba* may be associated with blood in stool or RUQ pain if it is complicated by amebic liver abscess. History of travel or drinking untreated water. Giardiasis is diagnosed by stool microscopy. Both *Giardia* and *Entamoeba* have stool antigens detectable by ELISA.
Clostridium difficile infection (see Chapter 51)	Diarrhea with loose, watery stool and lower abdominal cramping. Fever and leukocytosis. History of recent antibiotic use or hospitalization. Diagnosis is by detection of *C. difficile* toxin in stool.
Irritable bowel syndrome (see Chapter 13)	Alternating diarrhea and constipation, absence of nocturnal symptoms, fever, weight loss, or hematochezia. Normal physical examination. Colonoscopy is not necessary to diagnose, but is normal if done.
Lactose intolerance (see Chapter 14)	Abdominal pain, bloating, diarrhea after lactose ingestion from a young age. A diagnostic trial of a lactose-free diet for a short period can be helpful.
Appendicitis (see Chapter 13)	Nausea, vomiting, fever, RLQ pain. Often a rapid course in a previously well patient.
Diverticulitis (see Chapter 13)	LLQ pain, fever and diarrhea, sometimes with blood, usually in an elderly patient. Abdominal CT scanning may show inflamed diverticula.
Ischemic colitis (see Chapter 13)	Abdominal pain, diarrhea, hematochezia. Pain may be out of proportion to examination findings of tenderness. in older age group with history of other vascular disease. Imaging of the mesenteric vessels is ideally required for diagnosis.
Infectious proctitis (see Chapter 49)	Pain with defecation, diarrhea, hematochezia (*Neisseria, Chlamydia, Treponema*, HSV). History of recent anal sex. Positive bacterial or viral cultures may confirm diagnosis.

ASCA = anti-*Saccharomyces cerevisiae* antibodies; CT = computed tomography; ELISA = enzyme-linked immunoassay; HSV = herpes simplex virus; LLQ = left lower quadrant; p-ANCA = perinuclear antineutrophil antibody; RLQ = right lower quadrant; RUQ = right upper quadrant.

should be considered in patients with cellular dysplasia on mucosal biopsy, confirmed cancer, refractory disease, toxic megacolon, or corticosteroid-dependent disease.

Follow-Up

Patients with inflammatory bowel disease are followed for response to therapy, exacerbations, complications of both the disease and the therapy, and emotional health. In addition, nutritional needs should be evaluated frequently. All individuals taking azathioprine or 6-mercaptopurine are monitored for pancreatitis, allergic reactions, and leukopenia.

Patients with a history of prolonged ulcerative colitis are at risk for colon cancer and should undergo periodic surveillance with colonoscopy and biopsies beginning 10 years after diagnosis.

Book Enhancement

Go to www.acponline.org/essentials/gastroenterology-section.html to review a standard evaluation for inflammatory bowel disease, view the colonoscopic appearance of ischemic colitis, *C. difficile* colitis, and an anal fissure. In *MKSAP for Students 4*, assess yourself with items 50-51 in the **Gastroenterology and Hepatology** section.

Bibliography

Bamias G, Nyce MR, De La Rue SA, Cominelli F; American College of Physicians; American Physiological Society. New concepts in the pathophysiology of inflammatory bowel disease. Ann Intern Med. 2005;143:895-904. [PMID: 16365470]

Hanauer SB, Sparrow MP. Crohn's Disease. http://pier.acponline.org/physicians/diseases/d356. [Date accessed: 2008 Feb 12] In: PIER [online database]. Philadelphia: American College of Physicians; 2008.

Section IV
General Internal Medicine

Chapter 24

Test Interpretation

D. Michael Elnicki, MD

One of the most interesting and exciting aspects of medicine is the search for diagnoses to explain patient symptoms. Clinicians start with medical histories and physical examinations and use the findings to order diagnostic tests to confirm their suspicions. To use test results in an evidence-based fashion, a clinician needs to ask a series of questions: Is there valid evidence that the test is accurate? Does the test accurately distinguish between patients with the condition in question and those without the condition? Does this test apply to my patient?

Evaluating Tests

For the evidence supporting the use of a new test to be valid, the assessment of the test should follow certain steps. First, the subjects should be recruited in a systematic fashion from a population that is appropriate for the disease being studied. All subjects should receive the reference or "gold standard" test. The gold standard test is not necessarily perfect but represents the current practice standard. The results of the new test are compared with the gold standard. The results of the two tests, the gold standard and the new test, are assessed independently. That is, the investigators are blinded to the results of one test when evaluating the other to avoid biasing their decisions. For example, knowing the result of a patient's angiogram could bias the interpretation of a nuclear medicine study.

Test Characteristics

Clinicians use quantifiable terms to describe the accuracy of tests. Sensitivity and specificity describe test results for patients with and without a condition (Figure 1). Sensitivity is the proportion of people with the disease who have a positive test. This proportion can be expressed as $a / (a + c)$. Specificity is the proportion of people without the disease who have a negative test or $d / (b + d)$. These test characteristics do not change as disease prevalence changes. Note that this assertion can be checked by multiplying the values of a and c by 10 in Figure 1.

If a test is highly sensitive, it is very useful in excluding a disease when negative. This concept is referred to as "SNout." That is, a sensitive test, when negative, rules out disease. Conversely, a very specific test, when positive, establishes the presence of disease. This concept is described as "SPin."

Positive predictive values refer to the proportion of people with positive test results who do have the disease. Negative predictive values refer to the proportion of people with negative test results

who do not have the disease. It is the same as post-test probability. They can be described as follows:

- *Positive predictive value* (PPV) = $a / (a + b)$
- *Negative predictive value* (NPV) = $d / (c + d)$

Positive and negative predictive values will change as disease prevalence changes. Again, this assertion can be checked by multiplying the values of a and c in Figure 1 by 10.

A likelihood ratio (LR) determines how much the results of a given test will increase or decrease the pretest probability. A positive likelihood ratio, used when a test is positive, is expressed as:

$$LR+ = \text{sensitivity} / (1 - \text{specificity})$$

The negative likelihood ratio, used after a negative test, is expressed as:

$$LR- = (1 - \text{sensitivity}) / \text{specificity}$$

Likelihood ratios between 0.5–1 and 1–2 do not change probability much. Some easy likelihood ratios to remember are 2, 5, and 10, which increase probability by 15%, 30%, and 45%, respectively. Likelihood ratios of 0.5, 0.2 and 0.1 decrease disease probability by 15%, 30% and 45%, respectively. Larger positive likelihood ratios and smaller negative likelihood ratios are more apt to affect clinical decisions.

Using likelihood ratios requires that the chance be expressed in terms of odds:

$$\text{Pre-test odds} \times LR = \text{Post-test odds}$$

DISEASE

		Positive	Negative
T E S T	Positive	18 a	20 b
	Negative	2 c	60 d

Sensitivity (SN) = a / (a+c)
Specificity (SP) = d / (b+d)
Positive Predictive Value (PPV) = a / (a+b)
Negative Predictive Value (NPV) = d / (c+d)

Figure 1 Test characteristics.

Therefore, probabilities need to be converted to odds. These conversions can be done using the following equation: odds = probability/ (1 – probability).

For example, if a patient's pre-test probability of disease is 0.2, the pre-test odds would then be 0.2/ (1 – 0.2) = 0.25. To convert back to probability, the following equation is used: probability = odds/(odds + 1).

In the above example, the probability is 0.25 / (0.25 + 1) = 0.2. These concepts become clearer when used in a specific case. Imagine that you are evaluating a new test to screen for hemachromatosis, a relatively common genetic disease involving iron storage. You know that hemachromatosis has a 20% prevalence in the study population (when screening, prevalence is equal to the pretest probability of disease). You appropriately select 100 patients and all undergo liver biopsy (the gold standard test). The screening test characteristics are: sensitivity = 90%; negative predictive value = 0.97; LR+ = 3.6; specificity = 75%; positive predictive value = 0.47; LR− = 0.13.

A patient from this population with a positive test will have a post-test probability of 47% of having hemachromatosis, whereas someone with a negative test will have a 3% post-test probability.

As with anything we measure, sensitivity and specificity cannot be determined absolutely, so some uncertainty remains. You will often see the precision of sensitivity and specificity expressed in terms of 95% confidence intervals (95% CI). A way to conceptualize 95% CI is that if an experiment were performed 100 times, the measured outcome value would fall 95 times within these parameters. For example, if a nuclear medicine scan has a sensitivity of 84% (95% CI; 76%-92%) for the diagnosis of a disease, you can be 95% confident that the actual sensitivity of the scan is between 76%-92%.

Many test outcomes are continuous variables, which we arbitrarily divide at some point into normal and abnormal values. Some common examples of continuous variables are troponin and prostate specific antigen (PSA) concentrations. By increasing the level at which we define abnormal (the cut point), we will decrease the number of false positive tests but at the price of increasing false negatives (less sensitive but more specific). The opposite effect (more sensitive but less specific) happens if we decrease the cut point, as shown in Figure 2. If we change our cut point for "abnormal" from 4 to 2, we will increase our specificity from 70% to 90%, but our sensitivity drops from 90% to 70%. For the test shown in Figure 2, a compromise might be to pick the value 3 as a cut point, yielding sensitivity and specificity of 80%.

A test with both good sensitivity and specificity will "crowd" the upper left margins of the ROC (receiver operator characteristics) curve. This concept is particularly valuable when comparing two tests. The test with the greatest overall accuracy will have the

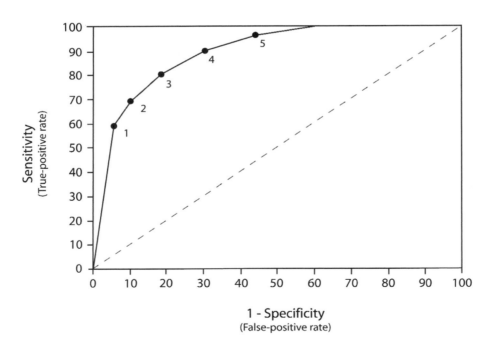

Cutpoint	Sensitivity	Specificity
1	60	95
2	70	90
3	80	80
4	90	70
5	95	60

Figure 2 Receiver operator characteristic (ROC) curve.

largest area under the ROC curve. A perfect test (100% Sn and Sp) would have an area of 1.0, so a good test might have an area of .9 while one less good would have an area of .8.

Applying Results to Patients

Before applying test results to patient care, and ideally before even ordering tests, a clinician must estimate the pre-test probability of a patient's having a condition or disease. The pretest probability of disease is based on demographic variables, history, and physical exam findings. When screening large asymptomatic populations, the prevalence of disease is often used as the pretest probability. For many symptomatic conditions, pretest probabilities in varying populations have been calculated and published. For example, a 50-year-old man with atypical angina has a pre-test probability of coronary disease that is >60%, but a 30-year-old woman with the same chest pain has <15% chance of having coronary disease (see Acute Coronary Syndrome). For less common conditions, a clinician may estimate pre-test probability from personal experience or that of colleagues. Knowing pre-test probability can dramatically affect testing strategy.

Using likelihood ratios, clinicians can assign probabilities of disease to patients based on test results. At some point, however, clinicians need to apply clinical judgment and the test results to patient care. The threshold for giving or withholding treatment will vary based on consequences of the disease and the risks of treatment. For example, a woman presented to an emergency department with pleuritic chest pain and dyspnea and her pretest probability of pulmonary embolism was estimated to be >70%, but a D-dimer test was normal and a ventilation-perfusion scan was interpreted as low probability. The physician calculated a 2%-30% post-test probability for pulmonary embolism and knew that untreated it conveyed a >20% mortality. In spite of the earlier negative tests, he obtained pulmonary angiography (the gold standard). It demonstrated multiple pulmonary emboli, for which she was successfully treated.

In some cases, the diagnosis can be made easier by sequential testing. If two tests are independent, the post-test probability after the first test can become the pre-test probability for the second. A strategy often employed for sequential testing is the initial use of a non-invasive, sensitive test. If it is positive, a more specific (and often more invasive) confirmatory test follows (e.g., exercise stress test followed by cardiac catherization).

We use sequential testing to move us toward a treatment threshold, the point at which we act upon our information. For serious diseases, like the above case, we need to be very certain. However, for less serious illnesses, we might accept more uncertainty. For patients with chest pain we might need a post test probability of <2%-5% to feel comfortable with a diagnosis. However, when treating an upper respiratory infection in a healthy person, we may feel comfortable withholding antibiotics with a 10%-20% probability of infection, since serious harm is unlikely.

As medical technology continues to advance at rapid rates, clinicians will increasingly be confronted with new diagnostic tests. A variety of factors, including cost, availability and risks, will compete in the decision-making process. However, having a solid, evidence-based foundation will enable a clinician to more easily assess new tests and appropriately apply them to patients.

Book Enhancement

Go to www.acponline.org/essentials/general-internal-medicine -section.html to view a glossary of terms commonly used in the medical literature and to see a figure that illustrates how different cutoff points alter a test's sensitivity and specificity. In *MKSAP for Students 4*, assess yourself with item 1 in the **General Internal Medicine** section.

Bibliography

Jaeschke R, Guyatt G, Sackett DL. Users' guides to the medical literature III. How to use an article about a diagnostic test. A. Are the results of the study valid? JAMA. 1994;271:389-91. [PMID: 8283589]

Jaeschke R, Guyatt GH, Sackett DL. Users' guides to the medical literature III. How to use an article about a diagnostic test. B. What are the results and will they help me in caring for my patients? JAMA. 1994;271:703-7. [PMID: 8309035]

Chapter 25

Health Promotion, Screening, and Prevention

L. James Nixon, MD

Appropriate care by internists includes not only recognition and treatment of disease but also the routine incorporation of preventive health care into clinical practice. The periodic health examination includes counseling patients in order to maintain health, screening for disease, and immunization to prevent future disease. All physicians should be familiar with the principles of preventive health care. Details of screening procedures are provided in disease-specific chapters.

One goal of the periodic health examination is to assess an individual's health risks, understand their value system, and help that individual achieve optimal health. In general, interventions that address personal health practices have a greater potential to improve health than does screening for disease. As an example, a periodic health examination with a young woman is an opportunity to discuss healthy lifestyle choices including dietary intake of fats and cholesterol, exercise and activity levels, substance use (e.g., tobacco, alcohol) and its effects, psychosocial stresses, environmental risks (e.g., seat belts, sun exposure), safe sexual practices, and contraception.

Primary prevention is the prevention of disease before its onset. Examples include immunizing patients against disease and reminding patients to wear seatbelts. Secondary prevention measures include most forms of screening during which asymptomatic individuals with risk factors for disease or preclinical disease are screened. Examples include mammography for early detection of breast cancer and colonoscopy, flexible sigmoidoscopy, or fecal occult blood testing to screen for colon cancer. Tertiary prevention includes treating a disease with the goal of restoring the patient to their previous level of health, minimizing the negative effects of disease, and preventing complications. An example is treating a patient after a myocardial infarction with cholesterol-lowering drugs to prevent a second cardiovascular event.

Principles of Screening

The goal of screening is to prevent or delay the development of disease by early detection. Early detection may result in diagnosis at a more treatable stage or before the disease has caused complications. The following criteria may be used as a guide:

- Screen for a clinically important disease, that is, a disease that is common and associated with substantial morbidity or mortality.
- Screen for a disease that has an asymptomatic period during which the disease can be detected.

- Use an effective and acceptable screening method, that is, one that is accurate, readily available, affordable, and acceptable to both patient and provider.
- There should be an acceptable and efficacious treatment for the disease.
- Early treatment is more beneficial than treatment once the patient is symptomatic.

Bias

When determining whether a particular screening test meets these criteria, be aware of certain biases that have the potential to make a screening test appear to perform better than it actually does.

Lead-time bias is the artificial increase in survival time introduced with every screening test by simply advancing the time of diagnosis without necessarily increasing overall life expectancy. For example, the lead-time associated with prostate cancer is estimated at 5-10 years.

Length-time bias occurs with every screening test because screening is less likely to detect fast-growing cancers than to detect slow-growing, more indolent cancers. It will always appear that cancer detected by screening will have better outcome than those detected by signs or symptoms. For example, lung cancers detected by spiral CT scan appear to have doubling times nearly twice as long as those detected by routine chest x-ray.

An extreme form of length-biased sampling is over-diagnosis, in which the cancer is so indolent that it probably would never have been detected during the screened person's lifetime had it not been for screening. For such a person, early detection and associated cancer treatment can only do harm, yet the person seems to benefit because he or she is "cured."

Screening Guidelines

Screening guidelines change due to availability of new evidence, and recommendations vary depending on the organization. An excellent resource for the most recent recommendations for screening is the National Guidelines Clearinghouse (www.guidelines.gov).

Cancer

Cancers for which there is good evidence that screening is beneficial include breast, colon, and cervical. Screening for HPV in conjunction with routine Pap smear has been proposed as a method to improve detection of cervical cancer based on evidence that cervical cancer is linked to HPV infection. The American College of Obstetricians and Gynecologists propose this method indicating evidence that women with negative concurrent test results have a risk of unidentified CIN 2 and CIN 3 or cervical cancer of approximately 1 in 1,000. At present the US Preventive Services Task Force (USPSTF) has indicated that the evidence is insufficient to recommend either for or against routine screening for HPV. Prostate cancer is common, but evidence regarding efficacy of screening is still lacking.

Obesity

The periodic physical exam should include periodic height and weight measurement, and those with a BMI >25 (overweight) and >30 (obese) should receive counseling regarding weight loss and lifestyle modification.

Fall Prevention

Falls are a common cause of morbidity and mortality among persons aged >70 years. A minimum assessment includes inquiring about a history of falls and assessing risk for future falls. Although little direct evidence supports the reduction of adverse outcomes in screened populations, screening in all at-risk populations is warranted given the combination of disease burden, available screening tools, and effective risk-intervention therapies. A number of screening tools are available to help with this assessment, including the "Get Up and Go" test.

Abdominal Aortic Aneurysm

One-time screening for abdominal aortic aneurysm (AAA) with ultrasound is recommended for all men aged 65 to 75 years who have ever smoked. Data from randomized clinical trials indicate that ultrasound identification and repair of AAA >5 cm diameter reduces AAA-related mortality in older men.

Dyslipidemia

Screening for adults should begin between ages 20-35 for men and ages 20-40 for women. Individuals who have other risk factors for coronary vascular disease, or who have a suspected heritable familial lipid disorder should be screened at an earlier age. Usual screening consists of a fasting lipid panel, although the combination of serum total cholesterol and HDL cholesterol can be used as a screening test in nonfasting individuals who may not return for a fasting blood draw. Repeat lipid screening every 5 years or when the patient's risk-factor profile changes.

Osteoporosis

The USPSTF recommends that women aged 65 and older be screened routinely for osteoporosis and that routine screening begin at age 60 for women at increased risk for osteoporotic fractures. This recommendation is based on good evidence that bone density measurements accurately predict the risk for fractures in the short-term, and that treating asymptomatic women with osteoporosis reduces their risk for fracture. Women at increased risk for low bone density include those with a smoking history, physical inactivity, prolonged hyperthyroidism, celiac sprue, family history of osteoporosis, and inadequate calcium intake. The evidence is not as strong for men, but screening men may be indicated with certain risk factors (e.g., long-term corticosteroid use, androgen deprivation). The most widely used and validated screening test for osteoporosis is dual-energy x-ray absorptiometry.

Type 2 Diabetes

While there is no direct evidence that screening for diabetes reduces adverse outcomes, screening for diabetes is recommended in persons with hypertension, dyslipidemia, and other coronary artery disease risk factors. Detecting diabetes in these groups may increase their risk to a level worthy of interventions that have been shown to reduce coronary artery disease events. Also consider screening adults aged ≥18 years with risk factors for type 2 diabetes (family history, obesity, gestational diabetes, polycystic ovary syndrome, high-risk ethnic group) and repeating every 3 years. The American Diabetes Association now recommends screening all adults older than age 45 for diabetes. All abnormal tests must be repeated on a subsequent day.

Chlamydia

Sexually active women <25 years should undergo screening with PCR assay from cervix or urine based on evidence that screening reduces the incidence of pelvic inflammatory disease by 50%.

HIV

The Centers for Disease Control and Prevention now recommends routine voluntary screening for HIV infection for all patients aged 13 to 64 years unless the prevalence of undiagnosed HIV infection in the screened population is documented to be <0.1%. Targeted screening should still continue in high-risk patients including all patients initiating treatment for tuberculosis and patients seeking treatment for sexually transmitted diseases.

Coronary Artery Disease

Routine screening for coronary artery disease in asymptomatic persons without cardiovascular risk factors is not recommended. Screening electrocardiograms are not recommended because abnormalities of the resting electrocardiogram are rare, not specific for coronary artery disease, and do not predict subsequent mortality from coronary disease. Exercise testing may identify persons with coronary artery disease, but two factors limit routine testing in asymptomatic adults. First, the prevalence of significant coronary artery disease is low in this population, rendering the predictive value of a positive exercise test low (i.e., false-positive results are common). Second, abnormalities of exercise testing do not accurately predict major coronary events in asymptomatic persons. There may still be a role for screening for coronary artery disease, however, in patients with diabetes prior to beginning an exercise program and in selected asymptomatic persons whose occupations may affect public safety or who engage in high-intensity physical activity. The role of coronary artery calcium (CAC) scoring by computed tomography is still evolving. In 2007 a report of the American College of Cardiology Foundation Clinical Expert Consensus Task Force concluded that it may be reasonable to consider use of CAC measurement in patients with an estimated 10%-20% 10-year risk of coronary events. This conclusion is based on the possibility that such patients might be reclassified to a higher risk status based on high CAC score, and subsequent patient management may be modified.

Hypertension

Early detection of hypertension is essential in reducing the likelihood of target-organ damage. Cure of some secondary forms of hypertension (e.g., primary aldosterone excess) is more likely if the duration of elevated blood pressure is short. Screen at every office visit, using the correct-size cuff. The average of two readings on two different occasions is used to classify the stage of hypertension.

Immunization

Most vaccines are safe and can be administered in the presence of a recent mild illness, including low-grade fever. Vaccine recommendations change frequently; for up-to-date information regarding current vaccination recommendations, two excellent Web sites are www.cdc.gov/vaccines/ and www.needletips.org/.

Influenza

Annual influenza vaccine is recommended for all persons aged ≥50 years; adults who are immunosuppressed or have chronic cardiovascular, pulmonary, metabolic (including diabetes), renal, or hematological diseases; residents of long-term care facilities; health care personnel; household members of high-risk groups; and pregnant women. The Advisory Committee on Immunization Practices (ACIP) recommends that all persons, including school-aged children, who want to reduce the risk of becoming ill with influenza or of transmitting influenza to others, should be vaccinated. Influenza vaccine is safe in pregnancy; women whose last 2 trimesters coincide with influenza season should be specifically targeted. Persons with allergies to eggs should not receive this vaccine.

Pneumococcal Vaccine

Pneumococcal vaccine is associated with substantial reductions in morbidity and mortality among the elderly and high-risk adults and is therefore recommended for all adults aged ≥65 years or with other risk factors (e.g., diabetes, cirrhosis, asplenia). Patients who receive their initial vaccine at age <65 years should receive a second dose after 5 years.

Pertussis

A new tetanus-diphtheria-acellular pertussis (Tdap) vaccine is recommended for adolescents in place of the current tetanus-diphtheria vaccine, and the Advisory Committee on Immunization Practices has recently recommended routine use of a single dose of Tdap in adults aged 19-64 years to replace the next tetanus diphtheria toxoid booster. As with other inactivated vaccines and toxoids, pregnancy is not considered a contraindication for Tdap vaccination.

Tetanus and Diphtheria

Booster tetanus diphtheria toxoid (Td) vaccinations are recommended every 10 years (as is provision of initial series of three immunizations for persons who never received this immunization series in childhood).

Measles, Mumps, and Rubella

Adults born before 1957 are generally considered immune to measles and mumps, but not necessarily to rubella. Persons born after 1956 require measles, mumps, rubella (MMR) vaccine unless there is documentation of the prior administration, physician-confirmed disease, or laboratory evidence of immunity to all three diseases. It is important to ensure that women who are considering pregnancy have positive antibody titers for rubella. MMR is not administered to pregnant women or women considering pregnancy within the next 28 days.

Human Papilloma Virus

The ACIP recommends routine vaccination of females aged 11-12 years and those <26 years who have not been previously vaccinated or who have not completed the full series (3 doses of quadrivalent HPV vaccine). Ideally, vaccine should be administered before potential exposure to HPV through sexual contact; however, females who might have already been exposed to HPV should still be vaccinated.

Hepatitis A

Hepatitis A vaccine is routine for all infants 12-23 months of age, with a second dose 6 months later. International travelers, persons relocating to areas of poor sanitation, day care staff, food handlers, military personal, illicit drug users, men who have sex with men, persons with clotting factor disorders, and persons with hepatitis B and/or hepatitis C infection are vaccinated if not already immune. The safety of hepatitis A vaccine in pregnancy has not been established.

Hepatitis B

Children are routinely vaccinated against hepatitis B. All adolescents and young adults not immunized in childhood and those at increased risk for infection (e.g., health care workers) should be immunized. Post-vaccination testing is only recommended for those who are at occupational risk or are receiving hemodialysis. To decrease the risk of perinatal viral transmission, all pregnant women are tested for hepatitis B surface antigen during an early prenatal visit. The hepatitis B vaccine is safe for pregnant women.

Varicella

Varicella vaccination is recommended for all children. Vaccination should be considered for any adult not immunized, particularly those working in high-risk environments (e.g., schools) and for women who could become pregnant. Women of childbearing age are advised to not become pregnant for 3 months after receiving the vaccine.

Varicella Zoster Virus

Varicella zoster virus (VZV) vaccine has been endorsed by the ACIP for use in immunocompetent adults aged 60 years and older to prevent or attenuate illness due to herpes zoster and can also reduce the incidence of postherpetic neuralgia. VZV vaccine is a live vaccine and is contraindicated in immunocompromised adults.

Meningococcal Vaccine

A single dose of meningococcal conjugate vaccine (MCV4) is recommended for all 11- to 12-year-olds, for adolescents at high school entry or age 15 years, and for college freshmen who will be living in a dormitory. Because freshmen living in dormitories have higher infection rates, they have been targeted for meningococcal vaccination. Others who should receive meningococcal immunization include those with deficiencies of the terminal complement components or properdin, with anatomic or functional asplenia, and those traveling to areas of the world where meningococcal infection is endemic. No data are available on the safety of MCV4 during pregnancy.

Book Enhancement

Go to www.acponline.org/essentials/general-internal-medicine -section.html to access the American College of Physicians web site on adult immunization and view a table on the current United States Preventive Services Task Force recommended interventions for the general population. In *MKSAP for Students 4*, assess yourself with items 2-15 in the **General Internal Medicine** section.

Bibliography

American College of Physicians. Medical Knowledge Self-Assessment Program 14. Philadelphia: American College of Physicians; 2006.

Hensrud DD. Clinical preventive medicine in primary care: background and practice: 2. Delivering primary preventive services. Mayo Clin Proc. 2000;75:255-64. [PMID: 10725952]

Chapter 26

Approach to Syncope

Lawrence I. Kaplan, MD

Syncope is a common symptom in adults, with a lifetime prevalence of almost 30%. Syncope accounts for 3% of emergency department visits and 6% of all hospital admissions. It is defined as a sudden, transient loss of consciousness and postural tone followed by spontaneous recovery. Presyncope is the sensation of impending syncope, without loss of consciousness. Both diagnoses are considered subgroups of dizziness, along with vertigo, the latter being the illusory sense that either the room or the patient is spinning, without loss of consciousness. The purpose of the syncope evaluation is to differentiate cardiac from other causes of syncope because the former is associated with a higher morbidity and mortality. The pathophysiology of cardiovascular syncope is a transient decrease in cerebral blood flow producing either bilateral cerebral hemisphere or brainstem hypoperfusion. Noncardiac syncope can be caused by these mechanisms, or by metabolic or electrical abnormalities.

Diagnosis

The cause of syncope is established by a combination of the history, physical examination, and simple diagnostic studies in the majority of cases. The focus of the history and physical examination is to search for precipitating causes and associated symptoms. A history of heart disease, significant cardiac risk factors, or exertional syncope suggests structural cardiac disease or arrhythmias as the cause of syncope; these conditions account for 15% of all causes. Patients with underlying cardiac disease and syncope have a 5-year mortality of approximately 50%, so it is important to identify these patients. Important structural cardiac causes include aortic stenosis and hypertrophic obstructive cardiomyopathy, and less commonly, mitral stenosis and pulmonary hypertension, the latter especially in the setting of pulmonary emboli and an acute rise in pulmonary artery pressure. Syncope associated with aortic stenosis is usually exertional, caused by an inability to increase cardiac output in response to exercise and associated decrease in systemic vascular resistance. Over 25% of patients with hypertrophic obstructive cardiomyopathy will also have syncope from dynamic outflow obstruction during exertion. Rarely, another acute structural cardiac problem such as cardiac tamponade or ascending aortic aneurysm can cause syncope. Arrhythmias cause approximately 15% of cardiac syncope, and unlike most neurocardiogenic causes, occur without warning. Tachycardias, including paroxysmal or persistent atrial fibrillation, atrial flutter, or atrial tachycardia are usually more hemodynamically unstable than bradycardias. Regardless of heart rate, arrhythmias can cause syncope by reducing cardiac output secondary to diminished stroke volume.

Approximately one third of syncope will be reflex mediated, or neurocardiogenic. Vasovagal syncope occurs as the result of sudden vasodilatation and bradycardia resulting in hypotension and cerebral hypoperfusion and is the most common cause of neurocardiogenic syncope. Vasovagal syncope precipitated by a specific trigger such as micturition, defecation, or cough is referred to as situational syncope. Carotid sinus hypersensitivity is a similar reflex provoked by carotid sinus massage or other direct manual pressure such as by a too-tight shirt collar. The etiology of neurocardiogenic syncope is either cardioinhibitory (increased parasympathetic tone with bradycardia) and/or vasodepressor (decreased sympathetic tone) secondary to baroreceptor hyperactivity. In these patients, a sudden sympathetic surge may activate mechanoreceptors in the left ventricle and stretch receptors in the great vessels via pressure or volume loading (Bezold-Jarisch reflex); such stimulation may result in inappropriately increased vagal tone producing bradycardia. The same type of blood pressure and heart rate response may be observed with the carotid sinus reflex.

Other postulated mechanisms include increased central serotonergic activity and endogenous adenosine activation. Patients with neurocardiogenic syncope are usually younger and have presyncopal symptoms such as lightheadedness, nausea, warmth, diaphoresis, or blurred vision. These presyncopal warning symptoms are highly sensitive for the diagnosis of neurocardiogenic syncope if lasting for >10 seconds.

Psychiatric illness, including anxiety attacks and pseudoseizures, are uncommon causes of syncope, as are metabolic causes such as hypoglycemia, especially in the absence of diabetes mellitus. Seizures are often mistaken for syncope, but generalized tonic-clonic movements, loss of continence, tongue biting, and postictal confusion are rare in syncope. Tonic posturing can be seen in both syncope and seizure.

Certain historical clues are strongly suggestive but not specific for particular causes of syncope. Exertional syncope occurs with aortic and mitral stenosis and hypertrophic obstructive cardiomyopathy. Chest pain and syncope suggests myocardial ischemia, pulmonary emboli, and aortic dissection. Palpitations occur in both tachycardia- and bradycardia-associated disorders, although syncope can occur without pre-syncopal palpitations. Male sex, age >54 years, and syncope lasting for only a few seconds are predictive of cardiac arrhythmia. A family history of syncope or sudden death is consistent with long QT syndrome or hypertrophic obstructive cardiomyopathy. Syncope with pain, emotional stress, cough, micturition, or defecation supports a vasovagal cause. Syncope with change in posture or prolonged standing suggests hypovolemia, disorders of the autonomic nervous system, or can be related to multiple drug effects, especially in the elderly. Drugs particularly prone to producing syncope are vasodilatory anti-hypertensive medications or preload reducing agents such as diuretics or nitrates. The association with shaving, turning one's head to the side, and tight shirt collars is consistent with carotid sinus hypersensitivity.

The physical examination is directed at signs of hypovolemia and orthostatic blood pressure changes, as well as listening for murmurs of aortic stenosis, mitral stenosis, or hypertrophic obstructive cardiomyopathy. If suggested by the history, gentle palpation of the carotid artery while the patient is on a cardiac monitor can be performed if prior auscultation of the carotid was negative for bruits. On neurological examination, look for focal findings, which may suggest a cause other than syncope for loss of consciousness such as weakness, paralysis, or dysarthria. The history and physical examination identify a cause of syncope in 45% of cases. See Table 1 for a differential diagnosis of syncope.

Diagnostic testing is guided by the history and physical examination. An electrocardiogram is done in all cases unless a clearly identified non-cardiac cause is found. The finding of an arrhythmia and conduction block may establish the diagnosis, but a normal electrocardiogram does not rule out a cardiac etiology. Rarely are diagnoses made on the basis of blood chemistries, radiographic studies, or carotid vascular studies, unless there are specific clues in either the history or physical examination. Hospital admission is appropriate when the cause of syncope is unknown or if the risk of illness or death from presumed cardiac disorders is high.

Additional diagnostic testing is based upon the pretest probability for a particular cause of the syncope (Table 2). Given the sporadic nature of neurocardiogenic syncope or cardiac arrhythmia, prolonged monitoring may be required to correlate symptoms with abrupt drops in heart rate seen in patients with vasovagal syncope or with arrhythmia. Transtelephonic electrocardiographic monitoring should be considered in patients with symptoms suggesting neurocardiogenic syncope without a precipitating event. Continuous-loop event recorders, used for up to 4 to 5 months, have correlated syncopal spells with arrhythmias in up to 20% of patients. Ambulatory monitoring should not be used for patients with suspected life-threatening arrhythmias. If structural heart disease is suspected, an echocardiogram to detect wall motion and valvular abnormalities is indicated. If there is sufficient concern for an arrhythmia, referral for an electrophysiological study may be indicated. Hospitalization and evaluation for an acute coronary syndrome is rarely indicated, unless there are additional clues suggestive of active myocardial ischemia. Stress testing is indicated for patients with exercise associated syncope, or those with significant risks for ischemic heart disease.

In suspected vasovagal syncope, a tilt-table test (patient is passively moved from supine position to head up position between 60° and 90°) can be useful, providing a diagnosis in up to 60% of cases when done with pharmacological stimulation. This test is indicated in patients with recurrent syncope, as well as those with one episode who are at high risk based upon their occupation. The poor sensitivity, specificity, and reproducibility of head-up tilt testing must be considered in the evaluation of patients with suspected neurocardiogenic syncope. Although positive results of head-up tilt testing may support a diagnosis of neurocardiogenic syncope, it is reasonable to treat selected patients empirically if the

Table 1. Differential Diagnosis of Syncope

Disease	Notes
Carotid sinus hypersensitivity	Syncope precipitated by pressure on the carotid sinus (e.g., tight collar, sudden turning of head). Can generally be diagnosed by history. Carotid massage may be confirmatory.
Situational syncope	Occurs in association with specific activities (e.g., micturition, cough, swallowing, defecation). Can generally be diagnosed by history alone.
Psychiatric disorder (e.g., anxiety, depression, conversion disorder)	More likely to experience frequent syncope and to be associated with many other symptoms. A high incidence (24%-35%) of psychiatric disorders has been reported in patients with syncope. These patients have a greater rate of recurrence.
Orthostatic hypotension	Syncope occurs on assuming the upright position. May be due to hypovolemia, drugs, or disorders of the autonomic nervous system (e.g., idiopathic hypotension, Shy-Drager syndrome).
Cerebrovascular diseases	Invariably associated with neurological signs and symptoms. Carotid Doppler not indicated, because ischemia of the anterior cerebral circulation rarely causes syncope.
Seizure disorder	Typically, history of a seizure disorder or witnessed to have seizure activity during episode. Additional findings suggesting a seizure: blue face or absence of pallor during the episode, frothing at the mouth, tongue biting, disorientation, postictal muscle aching and somnolence, age <45, and duration consciousness >5 minutes. The findings of diaphoresis or nausea before the event, postsyncopal orientation, argue against seizure.
Obstruction to left ventricular outflow (see Chapter 7)	May be exercise-related or associated with angina or heart failure. Can be diagnosed by physical exam or echocardiogram. Specific causes include aortic stenosis, hypertrophic cardiomyopathy, mitral stenosis, myxoma, pulmonic stenosis, pulmonary embolism, and pulmonary hypertension.
Bradyarrhythmias (see Chapter 4)	May be associated with near-syncopal symptoms (transient) or signs of diminished cardiac output (persistent). Can be diagnosed by ECG, ambulatory monitoring or electrophysiologic studies. Includes sinoatrial and atrioventricular node dysfunction. Either may be drug induced (β-blockers, calcium-channel blockers, antiarrhythmic drugs).
Tachyarrhythmias (see Chapters 4 and 5)	May be associated with palpitations. Ventricular arrhythmias causing syncope will typically occur in the setting of structural heart disease or with a family history of sudden cardiac death (e.g., long QT syndrome, Brugada syndrome). Ambulatory monitoring or electrophysiologic studies may be required to document arrhythmia.

Table 2. Laboratory and Other Studies for Unexplained Syncope

Test	Notes
12-lead electrocardiogram	Perform in all patients with unexplained syncope. Arrhythmias, conduction defects predisposing to complete heart block, and evidence of structural heart disease may be documented. Yields a diagnosis in approximately 5% of patients in whom the initial history and physical exam are nondiagnostic.
Routine blood tests	Rarely yield diagnostic information not suspected by the history and physical exam and not recommended. Yields a diagnosis in approximately 0.5% of patients in whom the initial history and physical exam are nondiagnostic.
Echocardiography	Should be performed in patients with syncope and clinically suspected heart disease or with exertional syncope. Can diagnose and quantify obstructive lesions and can identify abnormalities that provide a substrate for malignant arrhythmias (i.e., cardiomyopathies, valvular heart disease, and pulmonary hypertension). Yields a diagnosis in approximately 0% of patients in whom the initial history and physical exam are nondiagnostic.
Stress testing	Recommended for patients with exercise-associated syncope or in whom the clinical evaluation suggests the presence of ischemic heart disease.
Holter monitoring	Indicated in patients whose symptoms suggest arrhythmic syncope, known or suspected heart disease, and with abnormal electrocardiograms. Holter monitoring correlates symptoms with an arrhythmia in only 4% of patients. Increasing the duration of Holter monitoring (i.e., 48 or 72 hours) increases the number of arrhythmias detected but not necessarily the diagnostic yield.
Implantable loop recorders	Indicated in patients with recurrent, unexplained syncope. Long-term follow-up (median, 17 months) led to diagnosis of etiology of syncope in 41% compared to 7% assigned to conventional evaluation.
Invasive electrophysiologic studies	Performed in patients with structural heart disease and syncope that remains unexplained after appropriate evaluation. The diagnostic yield in patients without organic heart disease is 10%.
Head-up tilt-table testing	Poor sensitivity, specificity, and reproducibility; despite its limitations, head-up tilt-table testing is the only diagnostic tool available for determining susceptibility to neurocardiogenic syncope.

clinical history strongly suggests a neurocardiogenic mechanism and other cardiovascular causes of syncope have been excluded.

Therapy

Treatment of syncope is directed at the underlying cause to prevent recurrence and decrease morbidity and mortality. Structural cardiac disease and arrhythmias are covered elsewhere and will not be discussed in this section.

If hypovolemia or neurocardiogenic syncope is suspected, increased fluid and sodium intake is recommended to increase intravascular volume. For syncope refractory to volume expansion, compression stockings will decrease venous pooling. Additional treatments include elimination of drugs associated with orthostatic hypotension, including α- and β-receptor blockers and anticholinergic agents, if possible. Isometric muscle contraction to increase systemic vascular resistance and decrease venous pooling of blood at the onset of impending syncope may be useful, as is prophylactic fluid loading prior to potential situational syncope such as prolonged standing. All patients should be educated regarding the pathophysiology of syncope and strategies to avoid situational syncope. The placement of a pacemaker for neurocardiogenic syncope has been shown to reduce recurrence in up to 70% of cases.

If hypovolemia or neurocardiogenic syncope is insufficiently addressed by non-drug approaches, the addition of mineralocorticoids, to increase plasma volume by renal sodium retention, and alpha-adrenergic receptor agonists, to increase peripheral vascular tone may be successful. Alternative agents may include nonsteroidal anti-inflammatory drugs and caffeine. In elderly patients on antihypertensive medications, dose modification can be useful in resolving syncope or near-syncope symptoms.

In patients with neurocardiogenic syncope, β-blockers blunt the initial catecholamine surge and the subsequent hypercontractile activation of the left ventricular mechanoreceptors that participate in the Bezold-Jarisch reflex and reduce recurrence by up to 90%. Other therapies include midodrine, an alpha-1 receptor agonist, selective serotonin reuptake inhibitors, disopyramide, and theophylline, although none have the success rate of β -blockers.

Book Enhancement

Go to www.acponline.org/essentials/general-internal-medicine-section.html to review the important elements of the history for patients with syncope and a list of driving recommendations for patients diagnosed with various types of syncope. In *MKSAP for Students 4*, assess yourself with items 16-19 in the **General Internal Medicine** section.

Bibliography

American College of Physicians. Medical Knowledge Self-Assessment Program 14. Philadelphia: American College of Physicians; 2006.

Brignole M. Diagnosis and treatment of syncope. Heart. 2007;93:130-6. [PMID: 17170354]

Chapter 27

Depression

Hugo A. Alvarez, MD

Major depressive disorder is the most common psychiatric disorder. It affects nearly 10% of adults annually, yet less than half are diagnosed and treated. The spectrum of depressive disorders ranges from mild to severe, from brief to life-long duration, and it can present alone or coexist with other mood or psychiatric disorders, impairing social and occupational functioning. The detrimental effects of depression on quality of life and daily function match those of heart disease and exceed those of diabetes and arthritis. Socioeconomic risk factors include female gender, unemployment, poverty, low education, substance abuse, and non-married status. Medical risk factors include prior personal or family history of depression or other psychiatric disorder, postpartum state, and chronic disease such as diabetes, dementia, coronary artery disease, cancer, and stroke. The prevalence of depression in the elderly ranges from 7% to 36% in outpatients and increases to 40% in hospitalized elderly. Evidence in recent years has identified depression as an independent risk factor for increased mortality in patients with coronary artery disease, cancer, and stroke.

The biologic basis for depression involves imbalances in norepinephrine, serotonin, and/or dopamine in the prefrontal cortex, basal ganglia, hippocampus and cerebellum. Serotonergic pathways are believed to function largely in mood, while norepinephrine is likely involved with drive and energy state. Both systems function in appetite, sleep regulation, and anxiety. Depression is also strongly linked with stress, and stress systems in the brain are largely mediated by changes in norepinephrine transmission. There is also evidence of a genetic component, with elevated rates of depression in those with first-degree relatives with depression and high rates of concordance among twins. No genes that provide increased susceptibility or resistance to depression have been identified.

Prevention

Identifying and counseling asymptomatic individuals at higher risk for depression can prevent or mitigate the severity of the syndrome. In asymptomatic adults, inquire about and offer counseling to individuals with chronic disease, previous episodes of depression, recent stressful events, family history of depression, and postpartum stress. Antepartum counseling helps prevent postpartum depression in women with prior episodes of major depression, premenstrual dysphoric disorder, and psychosocial stress or inadequate social support during pregnancy.

Screening

Routine screening is recommended for all adults, including postpartum women and the elderly. Using a variety of synonyms, ask patients whether they have experienced depressed mood and anhedonia during the last month, utilizing the two-question model:

- "Over the past 2 weeks have you felt down, depressed, hopeless?"
- "Over the past 2 weeks have you felt little interest or pleasure in doing things?"

If the patient has had symptoms, ask a single follow-up question; "Is this something with which you would like help?" Begin a full diagnostic assessment for mood disorders in patients with either depressed mood or anhedonia by assessing symptoms directly using case-finding tools. The Patient Health Questionnaire (PHQ-9) is a validated screening tool that is available in English and Spanish. Repeat screening is indicated in at-risk adults, but an optimal interval is not defined.

Postpartum women should be screened 4-6 weeks after giving birth with the Edinburgh Postpartum Depression Scale, which has been well validated in this population and is available in multiple languages. In the elderly, the Geriatric Depression Screen is the best tool because it takes into account the patient's level of cognition and visual deficits that are common at this age.

Diagnosis

The diagnosis of clinical depression is based on patient history and exclusion of alternative diagnoses (Table 1); there are no additional tests that can confirm the diagnosis. Physicians trained in communication and interview skills are more likely to recognize depression. The interview must establish whether the patient meets established criteria for major depression, dysthymia, or a different psychiatric condition, and assess for substance abuse. Depressed mood and anhedonia are cardinal symptoms, and the presence of either is highly sensitive but not specific for major depression; hence, patients are evaluated with a structured instrument based on the *Diagnostic and Statistical Manual of Mental Disorders, Fourth Edition* (DSM-IV) criteria to assess symptoms of specific mood disorder syndromes. A structured approach sequences questions for maximum efficiency (average administration time from 1 to 5 minutes) and is facilitated with instruments such as the Patient Health Questionnaire (PHQ-9) to

Table 1. Differential Diagnosis of Major Depressive Disorder

Condition	Notes
Major depressive disorder	Depressed mood or loss of interest or pleasure in almost all activities. In addition, symptoms must occur nearly every day for at least 2 weeks and a total of 5 DSM-IV symptoms must be present.
Dysthymia	Characterized by depressed mood or anhedonia at least half the time for at least 2 years accompanied by two or more vegetative or psychological symptoms and functional impairment.
Subsyndromal (minor) depressions	An acute depression that is less symptomatic than major depression, and causing less impairment in social or occupational functioning.
Situational adjustment reaction with depressed mood	Subsyndromal depression with clear precipitant. Usually resolves with resolution of acute stressor without medication.
Bipolar disorder	Characterized by one or more manic or mixed episodes, usually accompanied by major depressive disorder.
Seasonal affective disorder	A subtype of major depression, occurring with seasonal change, typically fall or winter onset and seasonal remission.
Premenstrual dysphoric disorder	Characterized by depressed mood, anxiety, and irritability during the week before menses, resolving with menses.
Grief reaction	Major depression may be transiently present in normal grief; however sadness without the complete syndrome is more common. Pervasive and generalized guilt and persistent vegetative signs and symptoms should arouse concern for major depression.
Dementia	Characterized by impairment of memory, judgment, and other higher cortical functions; usually has insidious onset. Assess mini-mental status or conduct neuropsychiatric testing if diagnosis uncertain.
Hypothyroidism	Symptoms that overlap with depression include fatigue, decreased cognitive function, and depressive symptoms. Laboratory testing is confirmatory (i.e., elevated TSH).
Medication adverse effect	May have a temporal relationship to medication initiation. These include corticosteroids, interferon, propranolol, levodopa, oral contraceptives.

DSM-IV = *Diagnostic and Statistical Manual of Mental Disorders, Fourth Edition*; TSH = thyrotropin stimulating hormone.

Table 2. Criteria for Major Depressive Episode Based on DSM-IV

A) Five or more of the following symptoms have been present during the same 2-week period and represent a change from previous functioning; at least one of the symptoms is either depressed mood or loss of interest or pleasure.

1. Depressed mood most of the day, nearly every day, as self-reported or observed by others.
2. Diminished interest or pleasure in all or almost all activities most of the day, nearly every day.
3. Significant weight loss when not dieting, or weight gain; or decrease or increase in appetite nearly every day.
4. Insomnia or hypersomnia nearly every day.
5. Psychomotor agitation or retardation nearly every day.
6. Fatigue or loss of energy nearly every day.
7. Feelings of worthlessness or excessive or inappropriate guilt nearly every day.
8. Diminished ability to think or concentrate nearly every day.
9. Recurrent thoughts of death, recurrent suicidal ideation without a specific plan.

B) The symptoms do not meet criteria for a mixed episode.

C) The symptoms cause clinically significant distress or impairment in social, occupational, or other areas of functioning.

D) The symptoms are not due to the direct physiological effects of a substance (drug or medication) or a general medical condition (hypothyroidism).

E) The symptoms are not better accounted for by bereavement, i.e., after the loss of a loved one, the symptoms persist for longer than 2 months or are characterized by marked functional impairment, morbid preoccupation with worthlessness, suicidal ideation, psychotic symptoms, or psychomotor retardation.

DSM-IV = Diagnostic and Statistical Manual of Mental Disorders.
Reprinted with permission from Diagnosis and Statistical Manual of Mental Disorders, 4th ed. Washington, DC: American Psychiatric Association; 1994:148.

establish the diagnosis and the Primary Care Evaluation of Mental Disorders (PRIME-MD) or Symptom-Driven Diagnostic System for Primary Care (SDSS) to differentiate major depression from other psychiatric disorders. These tools have an additional benefit compared with other screening modalities: they assess a spectrum of psychiatric disorders in addition to the principle mood disorders. The diagnosis of depression is confirmed if patients have 2 or more weeks of anhedonia and/or depressed mood associated with 3 or 4 more symptoms for a total of at least 5 symptoms (Table 2). Up to 72% of depressed patients also present with moderate to severe anxiety.

Once the diagnosis of major depression has been established, it is critical to assess severity, functional impairment, and suicide risk. The Patient Health Questionnaire instrument uses a Likert scale for each symptom of depression and has been validated for initial severity assessment and follow-up response. Depressed patients must be asked about suicidal thoughts, intent, and plans. Such questioning does not increase the likelihood of committing suicide and is effective in detecting those at risk for carrying out a planned suicide. Patients with suicidal ideation but without a plan or intent are begun on treatment and suicidal ideation is closely monitored. Patients with a suicide plan are referred urgently to a psychiatrist or emergency referral for hospitalization and psychiatric assessment, depending upon the clinical situation. Diagnostically, the "No Harm Contract" can be used to assess the nature and severity of a patient's suicidality, uncover specific troubling issues precipitating suicidal thoughts, and evaluate the patient's competency to contract. Operationally, the "No Harm Contract" is a verbal or written agreement in which the suicidal patient is asked to agree not to harm or kill herself or himself for a particular period of time. The patient may agree with the proposal verbally or by signing a written statement, suggest modifications, refuse compliance, or choose not to answer.

The physical examination at the time of interview does not increase the diagnostic accuracy and may be normal. Symptomatic individuals may appear anxious, exhibit poor eye contact, depressed mood, decreased psychomotor activity, and tearfulness. In severe depression, affect is blunted or flat and delusions may be present. In select cases, tests to exclude conditions associated with depression such as hypothyroidism, anemia, and B_{12} deficiency should be performed.

Therapy

In patients with mild-to-moderate depression, psychotherapy and pharmacotherapy are equally effective. In patients with severe depression, combination therapy with psychotherapy and antidepressants is more effective than either alone. Of the different modalities, cognitive behavioral therapy (CBT), interpersonal, and problem-solving therapy have the greatest evidence of benefit. Cognitive behavioral therapy focuses on recognizing unhelpful patterns of thinking and reacting that lead to emotional distress, then modifying or replacing these patterns with more realistic or helpful ones. Multifaceted approaches to care that include readily accessible care, patient education, reminders, reinforcement, counseling, and additional supervision by a member of the care team are the most effective in improving adherence.

Initially, patients with major depression, dysthymic disorder, or both are started on single-agent antidepressant drug therapy. There is a wide array of drug options (Table 3); no category or agent has superior response rates. The choice of a specific agent depends on its tolerance, safety, cost, side-effect profile, and evidence of prior effectiveness with the patient or first degree relative. Rates of withdrawal from clinical trials suggest that selective serotonin reuptake inhibitors (SSRIs) are better tolerated than tricyclic antidepressants (TCAs) and have less potential overdose lethality, while monoamine oxidase inhibitors (MAOIs) have a longer list of restrictions and interactions making them the least commonly prescribed category. In mild-to-moderate depression, St. John's wort is as effective as other antidepressant agents and rarely has side effects. For patients on drug therapy with incomplete response, combination drug therapy is an option. Equal response rates have been observed when SSRIs are combined with serotonin and norepinephrine reuptake inhibitors (SNRIs) or bupropion; dose titration to achieve improvement is more important than the agents chosen. Combining MAOIs with SNRIs or TCAs is contraindicated because it may trigger the serotonin syndrome (triad of mental status changes, autonomic hyperactivity, and neuromuscular abnormalities).

The goal of treatment is to achieve complete remission within 6 to 12 weeks and continue treatment for 4 to 9 months thereafter. The duration will be longer if the precipitating event or other stressors persist, if there is a history of prior events, or if depression lasted for a long time prior to starting therapy. Up to 50% of

Table 3. Commonly Used Antidepressants*

Agent	Notes
Selective Serotonin Reuptake Inhibitors	
Citalopram	Probably helpful for anxiety disorders. Possibly fewer cytochrome P-450 interactions.
Fluoxetine	Helpful for anxiety disorders. Long half-life good for poor adherence, missed doses.
Paroxetine	FDA approved for most anxiety disorders. May have slightly greater fetal risk in 1st trimester pregnancy. Withdrawal syndrome may occur.
Sertraline	FDA approved for most anxiety disorders. Safety shown after myocardial infarction.
Serotonin and Norepinephrine Antagonist	
Mirtazapine	Few drug interactions. Less or no sexual dysfunction. Less sedation as dose increased. May stimulate appetite (and weight gain).
Norepinephrine and Dopamine-Reuptake Inhibitor	
Bupropion	Stimulating. Less or no sexual dysfunction. Less effect on weight gain. Lowers seizure threshold and may exacerbate eating disorders. Caution with impaired hepatic function.
Serotonin and Norepinephrine Reuptake Inhibitors	
Venlafaxine	Helpful for anxiety disorders. Possibly fewer cytochrome P-450 interactions. At higher doses may cause emergent hypertension, nervousness, and insomnia.
Duloxetine	Similar to venlafaxine in efficacy. May be helpful in patients with painful physical symptoms associated with depression (as may be venlafaxine and tricyclic antidepressants).
Primarily Norepinephrine Reuptake Inhibitor	
Desipramine	Like all tricyclics, anticholinergic. Caution with benign prostatic hypertrophy or in patients with cardiovascular disease.
Nortriptyline	Availability of reliable, valid blood levels. Results in lower orthostatic hypotension than with other tricyclics. Cautions same as with desipramine.

* Contraindicated with monoamine oxidase inhibitors.
Adapted from MacArthur Foundation Depression Management Tool Kit (available at www.depression-primarycare.org). FDA = Food and Drug Administration.

patients will experience recurrent symptoms and will require long-term maintenance pharmacotherapy.

Patients must be counseled about antidepressant medication to improve adherence and must receive instruction about the nature of their illness, the use of medications, strategies for coping, and the risks and benefits of treatment. Specific points of emphasis include the importance of taking the medicine daily; anticipating a 2-4 week delay before feeling better; continuation of medication even if feeling better; and potential side effects. Provide patient education materials appropriate for the patient's health literacy skills, culture, and language.

Follow-Up

Patients must be monitored at regular intervals during initiation, titration to remission, and maintenance treatment. Side effects and therapy discontinuation are common and occur in up to one-half of patients; counseling helps prevent discontinuation. Patients should be assessed 2 and 4 weeks after starting therapy for adherence, adverse drug reactions, and suicide risk and again at 6 to 8 weeks for response to therapy. At this point patients should complete a formal tool for severity assessment (e.g., PHQ-9) and are considered to have responded if a 50% or greater decrease in symptom score has occurred. After severity assessment, patients can be classified as complete, partial, and non-responders. Those with complete response should continue the same therapy modality for an additional 4-9 months. Treatment options for patients with partial response include using a higher dose of the same agent, adding a second agent, or adding psychotherapy. Patients with no response are switched to a different category of drug or to psychotherapy. Any change in therapy requires periodic follow-up as outlined above. Once patients achieve remission they are monitored regularly and receive continued counseling about medication adherence and risk of symptom recurrence.

Book Enhancement

Go to www.acponline.org/essentials/general-internal-medicine -section.html to access the Geriatric Depression Scale, the Assessment of Suicide Tool, and the Patient Health Questionnaire (PHQ) and the Patient Health Care Questionnaire-9 (mood module). In *MKSAP for Students 4,* assess yourself with items 20-25 in the **General Internal Medicine** section.

Bibliography

Depression. http://pier.acponline.org/physicians/diseases/d954. [Date accessed:2008 Jan 12] In: PIER [online database]. Philadelphia: American College of Physicians; 2008.

Fancher T, Kravitz R. In the clinic. Depression. Ann Intern Med. 2007; 146:ITC5-1-ITC5-16. [PMID: 17470829]

Williams JW Jr, Noël PH, Cordes JA, Ramirez G, Pignone M. Is this patient clinically depressed? JAMA. 2002;287:1160-70. [PMID: 11879114]

Chapter 28

Substance Abuse

Mark Allee, MD

Alcohol Abuse

Alcoholism is defined by a spectrum of problems, including a craving or compulsion to drink, a loss of control, physical dependence, and tolerance. Alcohol abuse indicates personal or legal problems with its use and dependence indicates physiologic addiction and maladaptive behavior. Dependence is best understood as a chronic disease, with peak onset by age 18 years. The differential diagnosis of alcohol abuse can be defined by a patient's drinking patterns (Table 1).

Screening

Alcoholism may be difficult to diagnose. Patients often present with complaints that may be attributable to other medical conditions or associated only with the alcohol consumption. These problems might include depression, insomnia, injuries, gastroesophageal reflux disease, uncontrolled hypertension, and important social problems. Inquire about recurrent legal or marital problems, absenteeism or loss of employment, and committing or being the victim of violence.

The US Preventive Services Task Force (USPSTF) recommends screening all adults and adolescents with either directed questioning or use of a standardized tool. The most frequently used screening tool is the CAGE questionnaire. There are four questions; a positive test is defined as "yes" answers to two or more questions:

- Have you ever felt that you should Cut down on your drinking?
- Have people Annoyed you by criticizing your drinking?
- Have you ever felt bad or Guilty about your drinking?
- Have you ever taken a drink first thing in the morning (an "Eye-opener")?

With a cutoff of two positive answers, the CAGE questions are 77%-94% sensitive and 79%-97% specific for detecting alcohol abuse or dependence in primary care settings; the test may be less accurate in women and blacks.

The World Health Organization developed the AUDIT (Alcohol Use Disorders Identification Test) screening tool that has the best operating characteristics for identifying at-risk drinking. The AUDIT uses 10 questions, including current use pattern, and takes longer to administer than the CAGE questionnaire. A modification of the AUDIT (AUDIT-C) is reduced to three questions and still performs relatively well (Table 2). With a cutoff of 4 points, sensitivity for at-risk drinking and/or alcohol abuse/dependence is 86% with a specificity of 72%. In certain groups, such as women, the elderly, and adolescents, it might be appropriate to lower the threshold for further evaluation.

In the United States, 1 in 10 women is a problem drinker; often hiding her use of alcohol. Women are more likely to develop long-term sequelae much faster than men. With women there is an increased risk of violence, sexual assault, and unplanned pregnancy. Persons older than 65 years represent the fastest growing segment of the United States population, and practitioners may

Table 1. Differential Diagnosis of Alcohol Abuse

Condition	Notes
Moderate drinking	Men, ≤2 drinks per day; Women, ≤1 drink per day; Over 65 years, ≤1 drink per day.
At-risk drinking	Men, >14 drinks per week or >4 drinks per occasion; Women, >7 drinks per week or >3 drinks per occasion; Either represent alcohol consumption above the NIAAA recommended levels.
Hazardous drinking	At risk for adverse consequences from alcohol.
Harmful drinking	Alcohol is causing physical or psychological harm.
Alcohol abuse	One or more of the following events in a year: Recurrent use resulting in failure to fulfill major role obligations; Recurrent use in hazardous situations; Recurrent alcohol-related legal problems; Continued use despite social or interpersonal problems caused or exacerbated by alcohol use.
Alcohol dependence	Three or more of the following events in a year: Tolerance; Increased amounts to achieve effect; Diminished effect from same amount; Withdrawal; Great deal of time spent obtaining alcohol, using it, or recovering from its effects; Important activities given up or reduced because of alcohol; Drinking more or longer than intended; Persistent desire or unsuccessful efforts to cut down or control alcohol use; Use continues despite knowledge of having a psychological problem caused or exacerbated by alcohol.
Substance abuse	Benzodiazepine abuse or dependence; Heroin abuse or dependence; Prescription opioid abuse or dependence; Cocaine abuse or dependence.

NIAAA = National Institute on Alcohol Abuse and Alcoholism.

Table 2. Modified Alcohol Use Disorders Identification Test (AUDIT-C)

	0 Points	1 Point	2 Points	3 Points	4 Points
How often did you have a drink containing alcohol in the past year?	Never	≤1 per month	2-4 per month	2-3 per week	≥4 per week
How many drinks did you have on a typical day when you were drinking in the past year?	0-2	3-4	5-6	7-9	≥10
How often did you have 6 or more drinks on one occasion in the past year?	Never	<1 per month	Monthly	Weekly	Daily or almost daily

From Saunders JB, Aasland OG, Babor TF, et al. Development of the Alcohol Use Disorders Identification Test (AUDIT): WHO Collaborative Project on Early Detection of Persons with Harmful Alcohol Consumption—II. Addiction. 1993;88:791–804. PMID: 8329970.

miss alcoholism in this group by thinking of it as a young person's disease. Age-related complications and illnesses (e.g., falls, cognitive decline, and depression) might present with similar symptoms. The average senior takes 2 to 7 prescriptions, so there is an increased risk of medication interaction with alcohol consumption. Fortunately, seniors are more likely to participate in and complete a treatment program when identified as having an alcohol problem.

There are no specific laboratory tests to screen for alcohol use. The main thrust of the exam and laboratory evaluation is to look for the physical and behavioral effects of alcohol such as liver disease, pancreatitis, seizure disorder, and mood disorders. Abnormal laboratory studies, including elevated aminotransaminase and pancreatic enzymes levels and macrocytic anemia, while supportive of alcohol use, do not make the diagnosis.

Therapy

Alcoholism can be treated but not cured. Non-pharmacological intervention is rooted in behavioral treatment for the patients with at-risk alcohol use. Abstinence is essential to the maintenance of a successful treatment program. A patient is encouraged to set drinking goals (I will start on this date; I will cut down by this many drinks; I will stop drinking by this date), use a diary to observe patterns of drinking, and alter environments to avoid situations that lead to alcohol use. A patient cannot do this alone and will need support from counseling.

Several studies have shown that the brief intervention counseling strategy is effective. A brief intervention is a 10- to 15-minute session where the patient receives feedback, gets advice, sets goals, and has follow-up assessments. The goal is to move the patient along the path of behavior change. Brief intervention needs to be motivational, with the practitioner offering empathetic listening and autonomy for decisions. Unfortunately, the success of brief intervention at 1 year is low and there is no demonstrable effect on morbidity and mortality.

Detoxification entails forced abstinence with treatment for withdrawal, typically with benzodiazepines. For long-term management, a multidisciplinary approach may be necessary. This approach may involve a 12-step program or a relationship with a mental health professional.

Alcoholics Anonymous has been shown to be helpful in maintaining abstinence; it provides fellowship and a support group to the alcoholic. Unfortunately Alcoholics Anonymous outpatient programs are inferior to inpatient alcohol treatment. Cognitive behavioral therapy is conducted by a mental health practitioner. With this program, patients will learn skills to cope with situations that perpetuate drinking. Spousal involvement has been shown to improve the completion of the behavioral program.

Naltrexone, an opioid receptor antagonist, is effective for short-term treatment of alcohol dependence and should be co-administered with psychosocial support. Naltrexone can be used in patients who are still actively drinking or where abstinence may be difficult. It reduces the frequency of relapse and number of drinking days by attenuating the craving and reinforcing effects of alcohol. It is contraindicated in patients with active hepatitis and opioid dependence. The most common side effects are headache and nausea.

Disulfiram, an aldehyde dehydrogenase inhibitor, leads to the accumulation of acetaldehyde if alcohol is consumed, resulting in flushing, headache, and emesis. Administration of disulfiram under supervision of another person improves abstinence and compliance with therapy. If patients use disulfiram, it is important that they avoid all alcohol-containing items, including mouthwash and cold medications. Disulfiram interferes with the metabolism of several medications such as phenytoin and should be used cautiously in patients with liver disease.

Acamprosate is a synthetic compound resembling homotaurine, a GABA analogue, and has been successful in decreasing drinking days, enhancing abstinence, and helping to prevent withdrawal symptoms. The main side effect is diarrhea, and the drug is contraindicated in patients with renal insufficiency.

Further information can be found at www.niaaa.nih.gov.

Drug Use

Although alcohol is the most commonly abused substance, illicit and legal drug use remains an important medical problem. Marijuana, cocaine, and opioids (including prescription drugs) are among the more frequently used. The USPSTF does not recommend for or against routine screening for drug abuse. Patients may be less likely to volunteer information on drug use given the legal ramifications (as opposed to alcohol). There are no formal screening tests for drug use, so a careful history is critical. Most authorities recommend that patients be considered at risk for drug abuse based on positive responses to questions about quantity and frequency of use, with the understanding that any use of illicit drugs should be considered at-risk behavior. When there is a heightened

Table 3. The US Public Health Service's Five "A's" of Behavioral Counseling

Assess	Ask about/assess health risks and factors affecting choice of behavior change.
Advise	Give clear, specific, and personalized behavior change advice.
Agree	Select appropriate treatment goals and methods based on patient interest and willingness to change.
Assist	Aid the patient in achieving agreed-upon goals with use of social/environmental support and adjunctive medical treatments when appropriate (including pharmacotherapy).
Arrange	Schedule follow-up contacts to provide ongoing support and referral as needed.

clinical suspicion, urine toxicology tests may play a confirmatory role. Some have adapted the CAGE questions to assess dependency. The US Public Health Service has advocated the use of the five "A's" construct in behavioral counseling interventions (Table 3).

Certain medical problems may arise from the use of intravenous illicit drugs. These include viral illness such as HIV, hepatitis C, and infective endocarditis. A focused history on the route of drug administration and coexistent medical problems is needed. High-risk patients should be screened with serologic testing for relevant diseases.

Detoxification has three goals: initiating abstinence, reducing withdrawal, and retaining the patient in treatment. Pharmacologic treatment of withdrawal often involves substituting a long-acting agent for the abused drug and then gradually tapering its dosage. The desirable qualities for outpatient medications include administration by mouth, low potential for abuse and overdose, and low incidence of side effects. After the substance has been identified, there may be some specific and effective treatment strategies that may be employed.

With cocaine, myocardial infarction, unstable angina, uncontrolled hypertension, and seizures are the most serious health concerns with acute intoxication. Beta-blockers are avoided in patients using cocaine because the unopposed alpha-blockade may increase the vascular tone, thus worsening the cardiovascular effects. In the acute setting benzodiazepines, vasodilators, calcium-channel blockers, and labetalol are the safest and most effective agents to treat hypertension or chest pain. Withdrawal from cocaine can produce dysphoria, sleep disturbances, anxiety, and depression. The symptoms of anxiety and depression suggest a role for antidepressants, but these agents have a delayed onset of action and may be useful only after the period of withdrawal is over. Benzodiazepines are used to terminate seizures related to acute drug toxicity; chronic anti-seizure treatment is necessary only if seizures persist following detoxification.

Opioids can depress the respiratory drive and cause sedation, requiring respiratory support with mechanical ventilation and naloxone to reverse the opioid effects. Opioid withdrawal syndrome is characterized by pupillary dilation, lacrimation, rhinorrhea, piloerection, anorexia, nausea and vomiting, and diarrhea. Beta-blockers and clonidine reduce autonomic manifestations of withdrawal. Substitution of a long-acting, orally active opioid such as methadone or buprenorphine is preferred by most patients and is associated with higher rates of retention within a treatment program and lower rates of illicit drug abuse.

Patients may benefit from referral to a formal drug treatment center that addresses motivation, teaches coping skills, provides reinforcement, improves interpersonal functioning, and fosters compliance with pharmacotherapy. One study demonstrated higher retention in the treatment program and fewer opioid positive urinalyses in patients receiving methadone and psychosocial and other services compared with patients receiving methadone alone. Patients with moderate-to-severe withdrawal symptoms, poor social support, or substantial medical or psychiatric conditions should be referred to specialized outpatient or inpatient programs.

Book Enhancement

Go to www.acponline.org/essentials/general-internal-medicine-section.html to access alcohol abuse screening tools and patterns of alcohol use. In *MKSAP for Students 4*, assess yourself with items 26-27 in the **General Internal Medicine** section.

Bibliography

Leikin JB. Substance-related disorders in adults. Dis Mon. 2007;53:313-35. [PMID: 17645897]

Saitz R. Clinical practice. Unhealthy alcohol use. N Engl J Med. 2005; 352:596-607. [PMID: 15703424]

Chapter 29

Approach to Low Back Pain

Lawrence I. Kaplan, MD

Low back pain is a common symptom in adults, with a lifetime prevalence approaching 70%. The vast majority of low back pain is musculoskeletal in etiology, and it will resolve within a 2- to 6-week period. Because most low back pain is self-limited, evaluation is focused on looking for evidence of either neurological involvement or systemic disease as the cause of the low back pain.

Prevention

Regular aerobic physical activity may decrease the likelihood of low back pain. Systematic reviews of common interventions to prevent low back pain concluded that general exercise and fitness is the only recommendation supported by evidence.

Diagnosis

The most common cause of low back pain in adults is musculoskeletal, although the precise biological rationale for the symptoms is unknown. The history and physical examination should look for the precise mechanism of injury, although often there is not an identifiable precipitant (Table 1). Musculoskeletal pain is often described as an ache or cramp, with radiation across the back in a belt-like fashion. Musculoskeletal pain will often radiate to the proximal thigh or hip, but rarely further. Radicular pain occurs in a dermatome distribution and when extending below the knee is sensitive for nerve impingement. Exacerbation of the pain with Valsalva, defecation, or cough suggests disc herniation. Pain that

occurs at rest, or progresses over time, or wakes the patient from sleep suggests a systemic illness such as infection or cancer.

There are certain "red flags" that suggest a systemic illness as the cause of back pain (Table 2) and may be an indication for early imaging. These clues are strongly sensitive, but not specific, and do not automatically warrant a more exhaustive evaluation. The evaluation depends upon the patient's description of the pain, associated symptoms, and elements in a patient's past medical history. Finding any of these may warrant a more expedited evaluation rather than conservative treatment. A previous history of cancer, unexplained weight loss, or age over 50 years with a slowly progressive or indolent history of low back pain, or pain that is unrelieved with conventional therapy increases the likelihood of cancer. A history of injection drug use, or other risk factors for bacteremia, fevers, chills, night sweats, or weight loss suggests osteomyelitis, septic discitis, or an epidural abscess as the etiology. A history of osteoporosis, or risk factors for osteoporosis, and a history of trauma are suggestive of vertebral compression fracture. Claudication alleviated by hip or lumbar flexion when walking, or by sitting, suggests spinal stenosis. In an individual with peripheral vascular disease or coronary artery disease, the description of ripping or tearing pain suggests an abdominal aortic aneurysm dissection. Bowel or bladder dysfunction or saddle anesthesia is consistent with cauda equina syndrome resulting from compression of sacral nerves from a tumor or central herniated disc.

An appropriately directed history and physical examination is the first step in the evaluation of low back pain, with focus directed at excluding both focal neurological involvement and systemic

Table 1. Differential Diagnosis of Low Back Pain

Disease	Notes
Degenerative joint disease	Common radiologic abnormality that may or may not be related to symptoms.
Degenerative disk disease with herniation	Common cause of nerve root impingement and radicular symptoms. Disk bulging is a common incidental finding on lumbar spine MRI in asymptomatic patients.
Spinal stenosis	Most common in elderly presenting with severe leg pain and pseudoclaudication aggravated by hip or lumbar flexion.
Ankylosing spondylitis	Usual onset before age 40 with chronic low back pain that worsens with rest and improves with activity. Decreased spinal range of motion.
Osteomyelitis (see Chapter 55)	Probable previous or ongoing source of infection with constitutional symptoms.
Metastatic cancer	Metastatic disease commonly from prostate, breast and lung cancer; can cause cord compression. Look for overflow incontinence, saddle anesthesia, and leg weakness.
Intraabdominal visceral disease	Gastrointestinal: peptic ulcer, pancreatitis. Genitourinary: nephrolithiasis, pyelonephritis, prostatitis, pelvic infection, or tumor. Vascular: aortic dissection. All of these illnesses can cause back pain.
Osteoporosis (see Chapter 12)	Osteoporosis with compression fracture. Accounts for ~4% of back pain complaints.
Psychosocial distress	An exacerbating factor that may delay recovery.

Table 2. "Red Flag" Indications for Early Imaging in Patients with Back Pain

"Red Flag"	Notes
Major trauma	Possible fracture
Corticosteroid use	High risk for osteoporotic fracture
Age >50 years	Increased risk for malignancy, osteoporotic fracture
History of cancer	High risk for metastatic cancer
Unexplained weight loss	Increased risk for malignancy or infection
Fever, immunosuppression, immunodeficiency, injection drug use, or active infection	High risk for spinal infection
Saddle anesthesia, bowel or bladder incontinence	Very high risk for cauda equina syndrome
Severe or progressive neurologic deficit	Increased risk for nerve root compression

disease. Attention should be paid to the quality of the patient's symptoms, as well as red flag findings. Paraspinal muscle tenderness or spasm by itself is nonspecific and can be found in all patients regardless of etiology. Spinous process tenderness on percussion is suggestive of malignancy or osteomyelitis but is not specific. A directed neurological examination should look for evidence of motor or sensory abnormalities. Ninety-five percent of all disc herniation occurs at either L_4-L_5, or L_5-S_1. Pain radiating in the anterolateral leg and great toe, associated with weakness in ankle and first toe dorsiflexion is consistent with L_5 nerve impingement from the L_4-L_5 disc. Posterior leg radiation, weakness in ankle plantar flexion, and a decreased ankle jerk reflex suggests S_1 nerve impingement from L_5-S_1 disc herniation. The presence of bilateral leg sensory deficits and saddle anesthesia is consistent with the cauda equina syndrome.

Low back pain associated with non-dermatome distribution pain and weakness that is either intermittent or persistent raises concern of psychosocial issues exacerbating the patient's symptoms. Physical examination findings suggestive of a psychosocial etiology or exacerbation of low back pain include: non-dermatome distribution pain; pain on axial load on the skull; an increase in pain with passive rotation of the spine; and a discrepancy in straight leg raising between supine and sitting positions, or with distraction.

The vast majority of patients with low back pain do not require further evaluation at the time of presentation; however, patients with history or physical examination findings suggesting potentially serious underlying systemic illness or fracture require further evaluation. Plain radiographs of the lumbar and sacral spine are most useful in the setting of trauma, or acute systemic illness, but otherwise add little to a patient's evaluation. CT and MRI are most useful for the evaluation of systemic illness, infection, and cord compression or cauda equina syndrome. In asymptomatic individuals disc bulging on MRI can be seen in 60% of studies, with true herniation in 30%, so careful correlation between imaging studies and the patient's history and physical examination findings is necessary to prevent further unnecessary diagnostic and therapeutic maneuvers. Laboratory studies, including a complete blood count, urinalysis, and erythrocyte sedimentation rate are also highly sensitive, but not specific in systemic illness, especially infections. Additional diagnostic studies including electromyography

and nerve conduction studies are rarely indicated in the initial evaluation of low back pain.

Therapy

Approximately 80% of low back pain should resolve with conservative treatment over a 4- to 6-week period. Treatment of low back pain caused by systemic illness or associated with cord compression or cauda equina syndrome requires referral and will not be discussed here.

Multiple systematic reviews have shown bed rest to be ineffective and can actually prolong low back pain. Early mobilization and continuation of normal activity is most beneficial, and back exercise should not begin until there is resolution of acute pain. There is no evidence that any specific exercise program is more beneficial, but general exercise, smoking cessation, and weight control will help prevent future episodes of low back pain. Patients with sub-acute low back pain may benefit from physical therapy, chiropractic manipulation, massage, yoga, or acupuncture, although there are conflicting data on the effectiveness of these modalities.

Initial therapy includes acetaminophen or nonsteroidal anti-inflammatory drugs (NSAIDs). Muscle relaxants and opiate analgesics are more effective than placebo, but not more effective than NSAIDs, and both may have central nervous system side effects.

Follow-Up

Schedule an office visit or telephone call at 2 to 4 weeks. The purpose of this contact is to learn whether the patient's recovery is consistent with the natural history of the condition. If recovery is delayed, consider reevaluation for more serious underlying causes of back pain. If no cause is found, reexamine for possible psychosocial factors. It may be appropriate to consider consultation with a back specialist when patients with nonspecific low back pain do not respond to standard noninvasive therapies. In general, decisions about consultation should be individualized and based on assessments of patient symptoms and response to interventions, and the availability of specialists with relevant expertise. In considering referral for possible surgery, published guidelines suggest referring patients after a minimum of 3 months to 2 years of failed nonsurgical interventions.

Book Enhancement

Go to www.acponline.org/essentials/general-internal-medicine
-section.html to view x-rays of ankylosing spondylitis and vertebral compression fracture, view an MRI of herniated disks, review
the straight leg raising sign, and laboratory tests and imaging studies for low pain. In *MKSAP for Students 4*, assess yourself with
items 28-32 in the **General Internal Medicine** section.

Bibliography

Chou R, Qaseem A, Snow V, Casey D, Cross JT Jr, Shekelle P, Owens
DK; Clinical Efficacy Assessment Subcommittee of the American
College of Physicians; American College of Physicians; American
Pain Society Low Back Pain Guidelines Panel. Diagnosis and treat-
ment of low back pain: a joint clinical practice guideline from the
American College of Physicians and the American Pain Society. Ann
Intern Med. 2007;147:478-91. [PMID: 17909209]

Shekelle PG. Low Back Pain. http://pier.acponline.org/physicians/diseases/
d304. [Date accessed: 2008 Jan 8] In: PIER [onine database]. Philadelphia:
American College of Physicians; 2008.

Wilson JF. In the clinic. Low back pain. Ann Intern Med. 2008;148:
ITC5-1–ITC5-16. [PMID: 18458275]

Chapter 30

Approach to Cough

Patrick C. Alguire, MD

Acute Cough

Acute cough is one of the most common presenting complaints in ambulatory practice and is usually self-limiting. Common causes include viral upper respiratory tract infections, bacterial sinusitis, rhinitis due to allergens or environmental irritants, acute tracheobronchitis, pneumonia (viral or bacterial), influenza, exacerbations of chronic pulmonary disease or left ventricular failure, malignancy, aspiration or foreign body, medication reactions (angiotensin-converting enzyme inhibitors), and, less commonly, pulmonary embolism.

Acute cough lasts fewer than 3 weeks, with subacute and chronic cough lasting 3 to 8 weeks and longer than 8 weeks, respectively. However, acute viral airway infection can result in protracted bronchial hyperreactivity, with secondary coughing lasting for weeks to months.

Viral upper respiratory tract infection is the most common cause of acute cough. Airway cough receptors are located in the larynx, trachea, and bronchi, and cough in the setting of rhinitis, rhinosinusitis, and pharyngitis is attributed to reflex stimulation from postnasal drainage or throat clearing. Specific viruses most frequently associated with cough are those that produce primarily lower respiratory tract disease (influenza B, influenza A, parainfluenza 3, and respiratory syncytial virus), as well as viruses that produce upper respiratory tract symptoms (corona virus, adenovirus, and rhinoviruses). Viral rhinitis or rhinosinusitis (the common cold) is characterized by rhinorrhea, sneezing, nasal congestion, and postnasal drainage with or without fever, headache, tearing, and throat discomfort. The chest examination in these patients is normal. Most viral causes of cough are treated symptomatically. Classes of cough medications include antitussives, expectorants, mucolytics, antihistamines, and nasal anticholinergics. The main indications for therapy are sleep disruption, painful cough, and debilitating cough. Elderly patients are the most vulnerable to the adverse effects of antitussive agents, including confusion, nausea, and constipation. In addition, the effect of placebo appears to be almost equal to that of antitussive agents in randomized trials. Recent systematic reviews indicate that no one antitussive agent is clearly superior in treating acute cough in adults. Among antitussives, codeine was no more effective than placebo, and evidence was mixed for dextromethorphan. Evidence suggests benefit for guaifenesin. Combination of dexbrompheniramine and pseudoephedrine was associated with significantly less severe cough than placebo but was associated with more dizziness and dry mouth (Table 1).

Viral influenza is characterized by the sudden onset of fever and malaise, followed by cough, headache, myalgia, and nasal and pulmonary symptoms. Clinical criteria for influenza include fever ≥37.7°C (≥100.0°F) and at least one of cough, sore throat, or rhinorrhea. A diagnosis of influenza can be established by analysis of viral cultures of secretions or results of several rapid diagnostic tests (immunofluorescence, polymerase chain reaction, and enzyme immunoassays). The neuroaminidase inhibitors (zanamivir and oseltamivir) are active against both influenza A and B. For any of these antiviral agents to be effective, influenza must be diagnosed and treatment initiated within 48 hours of symptom onset. Anti-influenza drugs decrease illness by about 1 day and allow return to normal activities one-half day sooner. Because of emergence of resistance, the Centers for Disease Control and Prevention no longer recommend amantadine or rimantadine for prophylaxis or treatment.

Bordetella pertussis, Mycoplasma pneumoniae, and *Chlamydia pneumoniae* are nonviral causes of uncomplicated acute bronchitis and cough in adults, accounting for 5% to 10% of total cases. Because Gram stain and culture of sputum do not reliably detect *M. pneumoniae, C. pneumoniae,* or *B. pertussis*, these tests and other diagnostic tests are not recommended. Routine antibiotic treatment of acute bronchitis does not have a consistent effect on duration or severity of illness or on potential complications and is not recommended. The one uncommon circumstance for which evidence supports antibiotic treatment is suspicion of pertussis.

Table 1. Therapies for Viral Upper Respiratory Tract Infection

Proven Effective in Randomized Trials	
Naproxen	Reduces headache, myalgias, malaise, cough
Dexbrompheniramine/pseudoephedrine	Reduces sneezing, nasal mucus/ Reduces congestion and nasal resistance
Ipratropium nasal spray	Reduces rhinorrhea, sneezing. High cost/benefit
Guaifenesin	Reduces cough
Possibly Effective (Mixed Trial Results)	
Dextromethorphan	Reduces cough
Beta-agonist inhaler	Reduces cough; may be more effective in patients with bronchial hyperresponsiveness and wheezing

Unfortunately, no clinical features allow clinicians to distinguish adults with persistent cough due to pertussis. Therefore, clinicians should limit suspicion and treatment of adult pertussis to patients with a high probability of pertussis; for example, cough lasting longer than 6 weeks or cough during documented outbreaks of *B. pertussis*. The diagnostic gold standard is recovery of bacteria in culture or by polymerase chain reaction. Antimicrobial therapy of suspected pertussis in adults is recommended primarily to decrease shedding of the pathogen and spread of disease because antibiotic treatment does not appear to improve resolution of symptoms if it is initiated beyond 7 to 10 days after the onset of illness.

Because pneumonia is the third most common cause of acute cough illness, and the most serious, the primary diagnostic objective when evaluating acute cough is to exclude the presence of pneumonia. The absence of abnormalities in vital signs (heart rate ≥ 100 /min, respiratory rate ≥ 24/min, or oral temperature $\geq 38°C$) and chest examination (rales, egophony, and fremitus) sufficiently reduces the likelihood of pneumonia to the point where further diagnostic testing is unnecessary. Cough lasting >3 weeks exceeds the case definition for "acute bronchitis." Such patients should be considered to have persistent cough or chronic cough illness (see below), and the initial diagnostic step is a chest radiograph.

Asthma is a consideration in patients presenting with an acute cough illness. However, in the setting of acute cough, the diagnosis of asthma is difficult to establish unless there is a reliable preceding history of asthma and episodes of wheezing and shortness of breath in addition to the cough. This is because transient bronchial hyper-responsiveness (and abnormal results on spirometry) is common to all causes of uncomplicated acute bronchitis. Postinfectious airflow obstruction on pulmonary function tests or methacholine challenge may be present up to 8 weeks after an acute bronchitis episode, making the distinction from asthma difficult. β-Agonists should be used in patients with cough and wheezing but are of unclear benefit in those with acute bronchitis without wheezing.

Chronic Cough

Chronic cough lasts for >8 weeks. Upper airway cough syndrome (UACS), asthma, and gastroesophageal reflux are responsible for approximately 90% of cases of chronic cough but are responsible for 99% of cases of chronic cough if the patient is a nonsmoker, has a normal chest x-ray, and is not taking an angiotensin-converting enzyme (ACE) inhibitor. Neither the patient's description of the cough, its timing (e.g., when supine), or the presence or absence of sputum production has predictive value in the evaluation of chronic cough. Chronic cough is due to more than one condition in most patients.

UACS refers to a recurrent cough triggered when mucous draining from the nose through the oropharynx triggers cough receptors. The diagnosis is confirmed when drug therapy eliminates the discharge and cough. Most patients with UACS have symptoms or evidence of one or more of the following: post-nasal drainage, frequent throat clearing, nasal discharge, cobblestone appearance of the oropharyngeal mucosa, or mucus dripping down the oropharynx. First-generation antihistamines,

in combination with a decongestant, are the most consistently effective form of therapy for patients with UACS not due to sinusitis. Additionally, the avoidance of allergens and daily use of intranasal corticosteroids or cromolyn sodium are recommended for patients with allergic rhinitis. Patients who do not respond to empiric therapy should undergo sinus imaging to diagnose "silent" chronic sinusitis.

Cough-variant asthma is suggested by the presence of airway hyper-responsiveness and confirmed when cough resolves with asthma medications. Cough-variant asthma (cough is the predominant symptom) occurs in up to 57% of patients with asthma. If the diagnosis is uncertain, inhalational challenge testing with methacholine should be considered. A normal test result is 100% sensitive in ruling out asthma but a positive test result is less helpful because it is not specific for asthma; other conditions, like chronic obstructive pulmonary disease, can be associated with a positive test. The treatment of cough-variant asthma is the same as asthma in general, but the maximum symptomatic benefit may not occur for 6 to 8 weeks in cough-variant asthma.

In patients with chronic cough who have normal chest x-ray findings, normal spirometry and a negative methacholine challenge test, the diagnosis of nonasthmatic eosinophilic bronchitis should be considered (NAEB). NAEB is confirmed as a cause of chronic cough by the presence of airway eosinophilia (obtained by sputum induction or bronchial wash during bronchoscopy) and improvement with treatment. Patients with NAEB should be evaluated for possible occupational exposure to a sensitizer. First-line treatment for NAEB is inhaled corticosteroids and avoidance of responsible allergens.

Although gastroesophageal reflux disease (GERD) can cause cough by aspiration, the most common mechanism is a vagally mediated distal esophageal-tracheobronchial reflex. There is nothing about the character and timing of chronic cough due to GERD that distinguishes it from other causes of cough. Up to 75% of patients with GERD-induced cough may have no other GERD symptoms. The most sensitive (96%) and specific (98%) test for GERD is 24-hour esophageal pH monitoring; however, a therapeutic trial with a proton pump inhibitor is recommended before invasive testing. Symptom relief may not occur until 3 months after treatment is begun.

Cough with sputum is the hallmark symptom of chronic bronchitis. Treatment is targeted at reducing sputum production and airway inflammation by removing environmental irritants, particularly cigarettes. Ipratropium bromide can decrease sputum production, and systemic corticosteroids and antibiotics may be helpful in decreasing cough during severe exacerbations. Bronchiectasis, a type of chronic bronchitis, causes a chronic or recurrent cough characterized by voluminous (>30 mL/day) sputum production with purulent exacerbations. Chest x-ray and high-resolution computed tomography scan results may be diagnostic, showing thickened bronchial walls in a tram-line pattern. Bronchiectasis should be treated with antibiotics selected on the basis of sputum cultures and with chest physiotherapy.

Although most smokers have a chronic cough, they are not the group of patients who commonly seek medical attention for cough. After smoking cessation, cough has been shown to resolve or markedly decrease in 94% to 100% of patients. In 54% of these patients, cough resolution occurred within 4 weeks.

Cough due to ACE inhibitors is a class effect, not dose related, and may occur a few hours to weeks or months after a patient takes the first dose of the ACE inhibitor. The diagnosis of ACE inhibitor-induced cough can only be established when cough disappears with elimination of the drug. The median time to resolution is 26 days. Substituting an angiotensin-receptor blocker for the ACE inhibitor can also eliminate an ACE inhibitor-induced cough.

Clinical evaluation of chronic cough includes a careful history and physical examination focusing on the common causes of chronic cough. All patients should undergo chest radiography. Smoking cessation and discontinuation of ACE inhibitors should be recommended for 4 weeks before additional workup. Cause(s) of cough may be determined by observing which therapy eliminates the symptoms associated with cough. Because cough may be caused by more than one condition, a second or third intervention should be added in the event of partial initial response. If chronic cough does not abate with empiric therapeutic trials, objective assessment should be undertaken and can include spirometry, methacholine challenge testing (if spirometry is normal), 24-hour esophageal pH monitoring, and chest computed tomography scan.

Book Enhancement

Go to www.acponline.org/essentials/general-internal-medicine -section.html to access an algorithm for the management of cough and a pneumonia prediction table. In *MKSAP for Students 4*, assess yourself with item 33 in the **General Internal Medicine** section.

Bibliography

Irwin RS, Bauman MH, Boulet LP, Braman SS, Brown KK, Change AB, et al. Diagnosis and management of cough. Executive Summary. ACCP evidence-based clinical practice guideline. Chest. 2006;129:S1-S23.

Chapter 31

Smoking Cessation

Patrick C. Alguire, MD

Nicotine is an alkaloid found primarily in tobacco and is most commonly consumed during cigarette smoking. The half-life of nicotine is about two hours and the principle metabolite is cotinine, which has a half-life of up to 20 hours. Nicotine stimulates α4-β2 neuronal nicotinic acetylcholine receptors, and like other highly addicting drugs, increases dopamine release in the nucleus accumbens and prefrontal cortex producing a pleasurable effect. The central nervous system effects of nicotine are related both to its blood level and rate of increase at nicotinic acetylcholine receptors. Cravings for nicotine are stimulated by low levels of central nervous system dopamine during periods of smoking abstinence. During this time, smokers experience the loss of the euphoric effects of nicotine and may also develop withdrawal symptoms consisting of insomnia, irritability, anxiety, shaking, hunger, and difficulty concentrating.

Smoking is the most common cause of avoidable death in the United States: 400,000 people die each year from tobacco-related diseases. Cigarettes are a known risk factor for coronary artery disease, chronic obstructive pulmonary disease and other pulmonary diseases, aerodigestive cancers, genitourinary cancers, peptic ulcer disease, and complications of pregnancy. The excess risk of death from coronary artery disease incurred by smokers drops by 50% in the first year of abstinence and continues to decline. Similarly the excess risk of lung cancer decreases steadily to 30% to 50% of

that of continued smokers after 10 years (Figure 1). Smoking cessation reduces the morbidity and mortality of other diseases such as stroke, obstructive lung disease, peripheral vascular disease, and peptic ulcer disease. Approximately 24% of adults in the United States smoke; half of them will die prematurely. The prevalence of adolescent smokers has increased dramatically in the last decade; now 33% of persons aged 18 to 24 years smoke. Up to 70% of smokers would like to quit, but only 5% to 8% can quit without therapy, usually after several attempts.

Therapy

The advice of physicians alone can improve the smoking cessation rate by 2.5%, resulting in an overall cessation rate of 10.2%. While even brief interventions can work, high-intensity counseling (more than 10 minutes) is more likely to succeed. There is no apparent advantage of group therapy over individual therapy or gradual cessation over abrupt cessation. Some patients may benefit from self-help therapy (patient pamphlets, DVDs, web sites) but the magnitude of benefit is small. The addition of self-help materials to personal counseling or drug treatment does not result in added benefit. Telephone counseling, a system of individual help that includes consistent support and reminders provided over the telephone, can be particularly helpful. Whether initiated by a

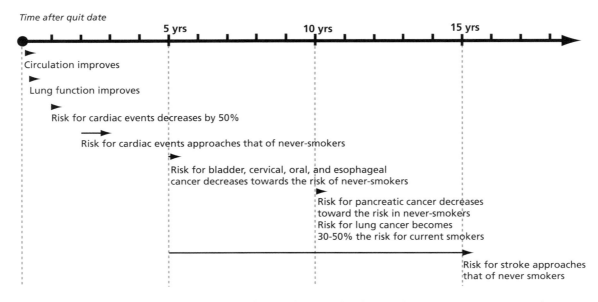

Figure 1 Time course for health benefits after smoking cessation. (From Wilson JT. In the clinic. Smoking cessation. Ann Intern Med. 2007; 146:ITC2-1– ITC2-16; with permission.)

Table 1. Five-Step Brief Intervention for Smoking Cessation

The 5 A's: For Patients Willing to Quit	The 5 R's: To Motivate Patients Unwilling to Quit
Ask about tobacco use	Encourage patient to think of Relevance of quitting smoking to their lives
Advise to quit	Assist patient in identifying the Risks of smoking
Assess willingness to make a quit attempt	Assist the patient in identifying the Rewards of smoking cessation
Assist in quit attempt	Discuss with the patient Roadblocks or barriers to attempting cessation
Arrange follow-up	Repeat the motivational intervention at all visits

physician or by the patient, telephone counseling is equally effective in helping interested smokers quit. An example of a telephone counseling system is the National Smoking Cessation hotline (1-800 QUIT NOW). There is insufficient evidence to support alternative therapies for smoking cessation such as acupuncture, aversive therapy, and hypnosis.

The U.S. Public Health Service Clinical Practice Guideline on Smoking Cessation recommends a 5-step brief intervention (Table 1). For patients unwilling to quit, the 5-R's are recommended as a motivating technique to move patients from precontemplation ("I don't want to quit") to contemplation ("I am concerned but not ready to quit now") or preparation ("I am ready to quit") stages of behavior change. Physicians should offer their patients additional therapy to improve the likelihood of successful and lasting cessation. The methods with the strongest efficacy included combinations of pharmacotherapy and behavioral counseling.

Behavioral counseling is most efficacious when combined with pharmacotherapy, including nicotine replacement products. All delivery systems of nicotine replacement therapy increase quit rates by 1.5- to 2-fold by alleviating symptoms of withdrawal. Nicotine replacement therapy is available over the counter (gum, patch, lozenge) and by prescription (inhaler, nasal spray, sublingual tablet). There is no evidence that one form of replacement is more effective or safer than another and decisions should be based upon patient preferences, side-effects, and cost. Combination forms of nicotine replacement may offer an advantage, but research results are mixed on this issue. Provision of additional behavioral support is beneficial but not necessary in order to achieve the beneficial effects of nicotine replacement therapy. In general, heavier smokers require higher doses of the nicotine replacement product to maximize efficacy. Nicotine use is contraindicated in patients with a history of recent myocardial infarction, severe angina, and life-threatening arrhythmias; replacement appears to be safe in patients with chronic stable angina. Nicotine is likely safer than smoking for pregnant women but is recommended only after failure of behavioral programs. Unlike other nicotine replacement therapies, nicotine gum has been shown to delay the weight gain associated with smoking cessation. The nicotine patch provides constant blood levels of nicotine to block withdrawal symptoms.

Bupropion was the first non-nicotine medication to be approved for smoking cessation. Bupropion inhibits serotonin, norepinephrine, and dopamine, but its mechanism of enhancing smoking abstinence is unknown. Smokers begin therapy 1 to 2 weeks before their quit date and continue for 8 to 12 weeks, but the optimal duration of therapy is unknown. A recent study showed that bupropion provided a better 1-year quit rate (30%) than nicotine replacement therapy (16%). In this study, the combination of bupropion and nicotine replacement resulted in an even higher 1-year abstinence rate of 36%. Like nicotine gum, bupropion has been shown to delay the weight gain associated with smoking cessation. Bupropion is contraindicated in patients with a current or past seizure disorder, eating disorders, or other conditions that may lower the seizure threshold. Side effects include insomnia and dry mouth. Bupropion is a category B drug for pregnancy (no evidence of risk in humans) and should be considered only if behavioral interventions are unsuccessful.

Varenicline, a novel nicotinic acetylcholine partial agonist, was approved in 2006 to treat smoking addiction. Varenicline binds to the α4β2 nicotinic receptor with greater affinity than nicotine, blocking nicotine binding and stimulating receptor mediated activity. Varenicline therapy is associated with the relaxing effect of smoking and reduces the cravings felt by smokers who quit. Varenicline has been shown to be safe and significantly more efficacious than placebo, nicotine, and bupropion for smoking cessation for up to 12 months (although never compared head-to-head with these drugs). The most common side effects are nausea, vomiting, sleep disturbance and constipation. There are no well-controlled studies in pregnant women (FDA pregnancy category C); therefore the use of varenicline is considered only when the potential benefits outweigh the potential risk to the fetus.

Book Enhancement

Go to www.acponline.org/essentials/general-internal-medicine-section.html to access a tutorial on counseling for behavior change and to access Health Tips on smoking cessation for patients and a table on pharmacologic therapy. In *MKSAP for Students 4*, assess yourself with items 34-36 in the **General Internal Medicine** section.

Bibliography

Wilson JF. In the clinic. Smoking cessation. Ann Intern Med. 2007; 146:ITC2-1-ITC2-16. [PMID: 17283345]

Chapter 32

Obesity

L. James Nixon, MD

Obesity results from an imbalance of energy intake versus expenditure and a disturbance in the factors that regulate the feedback process. The causes are multifactorial and can be considered in terms of the biopsychosocial model because there are biological (genetics, metabolic factors, comorbidities, medications), psychological (eating behaviors, activity habits, health knowledge) and social factors (socioeconomic status, neighborhoods, food policy) that all intersect to result in our current obesity epidemic. Once an individual becomes obese there are a multitude of negative effects on health including structural (e.g., obstructive sleep apnea, osteoarthritis), metabolic (e.g., diabetes, non-alcoholic steatohepatitis, hypertension) and atherosclerotic (coronary, cerebral, and peripheral vascular disease).

Obesity affects over 30% of Americans and is currently the second leading cause of preventable deaths. The best treatment for obesity is prevention. Obese individuals require education about the health risks of obesity, treatment goals, and lifestyle interventions to achieve those goals. Some patients may require the addition of counseling about drug therapy or surgery to achieve weight goals.

Prevention

One primary goal for internists is to identify and counsel people at risk for obesity. This approach, if successful, is ideal because it avoids the pitfalls associated with trying to treat obesity once it occurs. Inquire about a family history of obesity because obesity is influenced by both genetic and environmental factors. Also ask about exercise and television viewing habits because persons with a more sedentary lifestyle are at greater risk for obesity. Counsel patients who plan to stop smoking that they are at increased risk for weight gain. Other life events associated with increased risk for weight gain include pregnancy and short-term disability after surgery or injury. Other risk factors for obesity include lower socioeconomic status and certain minority groups such as Latinos, African Americans, and Polynesians. A number of medications are associated with weight gain (certain antipsychotics, antidepressants, anticonvulsants, antidiabetic drugs, and corticosteroids), so a medication history can provide useful information. Finally, ask about any recent weight gain because a weight gain of more than 1-2 pounds per year is a red flag for future weight gain.

At-risk patients are counseled to exercise regularly; 30 minutes or more, five times per week is ideal, although there is benefit from even less regular exercise (taking stairs instead of elevator). Beneficial dietary changes include controlling caloric intake by using small portion sizes. Patients should also be counseled to lower fat intake, increase dietary fiber, drink fewer carbonated, sugar-sweetened beverages, and eat breakfast in order to lower the risk of becoming overweight. Also educate patients about the adverse health effects of weight gain.

The rate of childhood obesity is increasing, and over half of overweight children will become overweight adults. Internists have a role in preventing childhood obesity because the children of overweight adults are more likely to become overweight themselves. Internists can also help by advising pregnant women about the risk that excessive weight gain poses to their health and the health of their unborn child, as intrauterine imprinting can affect long-term control of body weight. Higher maternal weight increases the risk for childhood weight above the 95th percentile and for the metabolic syndrome.

Screening

Measure height, weight, and waist circumference at each visit and calculate the body mass index:

A BMI of 18.5 to 24.9 is normal for most people; overweight is 25 to 29.9; and obesity is ≥30. Morbid obesity is defined as a BMI > 40. BMI has a good correlation with risks associated with obesity and body fat, such as diabetes, heart disease, osteoarthritis, gallbladder disease, gastroesophageal reflux, and certain types of cancer (e.g., breast, endometrium, prostate, colon, kidney, and gallbladder).

Abnormal waist circumference (>102 cm [40 inch] for males or >88 cm [35 inch] for females) is a measure for central obesity, a surrogate estimate for visceral fat. Visceral fat is a more metabolically active fat that releases free fatty acids into the portal system, which contributes to hyperlipidemia, hyperinsulinemia, and atherogenesis. Waist circumference measurement alone is as good as the waist circumference divided by the hip circumference. The co-occurrence of metabolic risk factors for both type 2 diabetes and coronary heart disease (abdominal obesity, hyperglycemia, dyslipidemia, and hypertension) defines the "metabolic syndrome" (Table 1).

Diagnosis

Patients identified as overweight, obese, or having an abnormal waist circumference are assessed for obesity-associated conditions such as hypertension, metabolic syndrome, endocrinopathies (i.e., hypothyroidism, diabetes, and Cushing's syndrome), and reproductive disorders such as polycystic ovary disease (Table 2). In all patients with a BMI of >25, obtain a blood glucose, serum

Table 1. Clinical Features of the Metabolic Syndrome

Risk Factor	Defining Level
Abdominal obesity (waist circumference)	
Men	>102 cm (>40 in)
Women	>88 cm (>35 in)
HDL cholesterol	
Men	<40 mg/dL
Women	<50 mg/dL
Triglycerides	≥150 mg/dL
Fasting glucose	≥110 mg/dL
Blood pressure	≥130/≥85 mm Hg

HDL = high-density lipoprotein.

Table 2. Differential Diagnosis of Obesity

Disease	Notes
Hypothalamic injury	Headache; endocrine dysfunction; hypothalamic symptoms. Order MRI or CT of skull.
Cushing's disease (see Chapter 11)	Central obesity; hypertension; plethora; striae. Measure urinary cortisol and adrenal suppression.
Polycystic ovary syndrome (see Chapter 34)	Oligomenorrhea; hirsutism; increases LH/FSH ratio; high testosterone levels; low SHBG; insulin resistance.
Drug-induced obesity	Antipsychotics; antidepressants; antiepileptics; steroids; serotonin antagonists; antidiabetic drugs.
Hypothyroidism (see Chapter 10)	High TSH; low thyroxine; lethargy; cold intolerance; bradycardia. Weight gain is often due to fluid retention.

CT = computed tomography; FSH = follicle-stimulating hormone; LH = luteinizing hormone; MRI = magnetic resonance imaging; SHBG = sex hormone-binding globulin; TSH = thyrotropin stimulating hormone.

creatinine, and fasting lipid profile (HDL cholesterol, triglycerides, and LDL cholesterol) to assess for comorbidities. A sleep study may be indicated to confirm sleep apnea in patients with somnolence, hypertension, plethora, or history of snoring.

Therapy

Help patients with a high BMI and/or increased central adiposity to develop a plan to prevent further weight gain and ultimately reduce body weight. Initial steps include addressing modifiable risk factors for obesity and setting goals for gradual, sustainable weight loss. A reasonable goal is to lose 10% of body weight because this is associated with significant risk reduction. Rates for weight loss vary, but 0.5-1 pound per week is a reasonable goal.

Weight loss can be achieved through alterations in both diet and exercise. Reducing energy intake is essential for weight loss. For example, in one study, participation in Weight Watchers was associated with a 5.3% weight loss at 1 year and 3.2% at 2 years. At reduced energy intake under controlled conditions, diet composition is unimportant. For some people, short-term, very-low-carbohydrate diets produce more weight loss than other diets, but sustainability is difficult. Low-fat diets produce weight loss but not more than other diets. Increased intake of high-fiber foods may enhance satiety, as may higher protein diets. The other side of the energy balance is increasing physical activity to increase energy expenditure. Recommend exercise for 30 to 60 minutes 5 or more days a week by increasing walking or other comparable activities. Exercise is particularly helpful in maintaining a lower weight once achieved. Sustained weight loss requires lifestyle changes, so consider referring obese patients to behavioral specialists such as clinical psychologists or trained dietitians.

Consider surgical treatment for patients with BMI ≥35 and obesity-related medical comorbidities (e.g., hypertension, diabetes, dyslipidemia, coronary artery disease, or sleep apnea) or BMI ≥40 without comorbidities in whom attempts at weight loss, including drug therapy, were unsuccessful. Surgery produces long-term weight loss that can be >25% of body weight in one year, and lost weight is regained slowly, if at all. Surgery may also be recommended to individuals with progressive obesity, such as continuing weight increases of more than 5 kg/year before age 30. The most common procedures are Roux-en-Y gastric bypass, stapled gastroplasty, and adjustable gastric banding. After bariatric surgery, many patients have significant improvement or resolution of obesity-related diseases including diabetes, hypertension, sleep apnea, and hyperlipidemia, and recent studies suggest decreased overall mortality. Referral for bariatric surgery should not be done lightly, however. The operative mortality in most studies ranges from 0.1% to 1%. Complications after bariatric surgery can include nutritional deficiencies (e.g., vitamin B_{12}, folate, and iron), venous thromboembolism, gallstones, infections, vomiting, and "dumping syndrome," in which the consumption of refined sugar causes abdominal cramping and diarrhea.

When lifestyle treatments are ineffective, or the patient is unable to lose excess weight, the addition of drug therapy may be helpful. Drug therapy is generally considered for patients with a BMI ≥30, or ≥27 with comorbidities. Drug therapy is generally tried before surgical intervention. Sibutramine (a non-amphetamine appetite suppressant that blocks the update of norepinephrine, serotonin and dopamine) and orlistat (blocks lipase and fat absorption in the intestine) are two drugs that produce dose-related weight loss. Criteria for success with drug therapy include >2 kg (4 lb) weight loss at 4 weeks, >5% weight loss at 6 months, and maintaining >5% weight loss at 1 year. Both of these drugs are associated with significant side effects. Orlistat can cause abdominal discomfort and increased frequency of defecation; sibutramine may cause hypertension, insomnia, and headaches. The American College of Physicians clinical guidelines for management of obesity include fluoxetine and bupropion as alternate drugs for the treatment of obesity. The data supporting the use of these drugs for the treatment of obesity is equivocal and they are not FDA approved for this indication. Among diabetic patients exenatide, an injection that improves glycemic control by mimicking the action of the hormone incretin, is associated with weight loss among users. The weight loss may be related to delayed gastric emptying causing patients to feel "full" faster and longer. Exenatide is not approved for use in non-diabetics. Drugs awaiting approval or in development include the cannabinoid receptor antagonist rimonabant. Advise patients that there is limited efficacy and safety information about the use of over-the-counter herbal preparations for weight loss. Ephedra-containing compounds have been removed from the market because of safety concerns.

Follow-Up

Schedule follow-up visits to monitor weight loss and comorbid conditions in all obese patients. Use ongoing office visits or ongoing behavioral therapy to reinforce or boost weight loss programs as the recidivism rate is high for obesity. Generally, the more support the patient receives, the more successful the weight loss.

Book Enhancement

Go to www.acponline.org/essentials/general-internal-medicine -section.html to review how to write an exercise prescription, to use a tool to classify obesity and to calculate the BMI, and to view diagrams of surgical procedures for obesity. In *MKSAP for Students 4*, assess yourself with items 37-39 in the **General Internal Medicine** section.

Bibliography

Bray GA. Obesity. http://pier.acponline.org/physicians/diseases/d161. [Date accessed: 2008 Jan 10] In: PIER [online database]. Philadelphia: American College of Physicians; 2008.

Eckel RH. Clinical practice. Nonsurgical management of obesity in adults. N Engl J Med. 2008;358:1941-50. [PMID: 18450605]

Snow V, Barry P, Fitterman N, Qaseem A, Weiss K; Clinical Efficacy Assessment Subcommittee of the American College of Physicians. Pharmacologic and surgical management of obesity in primary care: a clinical practice guideline from the American College of Physicians. Ann Intern Med. 2005;142:525-31. [PMID: 15809464]

Chapter 33

Approach to Involuntary Weight Loss

Bruce Leff, MD

Involuntary weight loss is defined as the loss of >5% of total body weight over a 6-month period or >10% over a 1-year period; it may also be identified by patient self-report if accompanied by a noticeable change in clothing size. Involuntary weight loss is common and may be associated with significant illness, malnutrition, and decline in physical function, reduced quality of life, and a two-fold increase in mortality.

Terminology used to describe weight loss is confusing and betrays an incomplete understanding of the underlying pathophysiology of involuntary weight loss. Classic definitions of involuntary weight loss are derived from syndromes first described in starving children, Kwashiorkor and marasmus, both of which are reversible with feeding. However, many adults with involuntary weight loss fail to respond to feeding and thus involuntary weight loss may result from several types of conditions which may overlap. *Wasting*, or *starvation*, is weight loss without an underlying inflammatory condition and may respond to increased caloric intake. *Sarcopenia* is age-related muscle loss without other precipitating causes. *Cachexia* is weight loss with an underlying inflammatory condition characterized by increased cytokine production and possible muscle wasting, and is associated with a number of chronic diseases such as cancer, AIDS, chronic obstructive pulmonary disease, and others. *Protein energy malnutrition* is characterized by weight loss, reduced mid-upper arm circumference, and laboratory evidence of reduced dietary intake of protein and calories. *Failure to thrive* is weight loss and decline in physical and/or cognitive functioning with signs of hopelessness and helplessness.

Differential Diagnosis

There have been remarkably few well-conducted studies on the causes of weight loss in adults. However, these studies have been relatively consistent in the proportion of patients with various causes; approximately 50%-70% of patients have a physical cause, 10%-20% have a psychiatric cause, and 15%-25% have no specific cause determined after a thorough evaluation and long-term follow-up (Table 1). Of note, the studies on which these etiologic proportions are based were mostly referred inpatient populations, and some were performed at a time when body imaging techniques were less robust than today. Thus, it is reasonable to expect that among outpatient populations, the etiologic profile of involuntary weight loss may be different.

The most common physical cause of involuntary weight loss is malignancy. Weight loss may be the presenting feature of cancer before other symptoms emerge. The second most common physical cause is nonmalignant gastrointestinal disease such as peptic ulcer disease, inflammatory bowel disease, malabsorption, oral disorders, dysphagia, and gallbladder disease. A broad spectrum of conditions accounts for the remainder of physical causes, including endocrine disorders (especially thyroid disorders and diabetes mellitus), late-stage heart failure or chronic obstructive pulmonary disease, and infections such as tuberculosis and HIV. Medications commonly cause weight loss, especially among the elderly by suppressing appetite. Such drugs include digoxin, theophylline, angiotensin-converting enzyme inhibitors, nonsteroidal anti-inflammatory drugs, selective serotonin reuptake inhibitors,

Table 1. Differential Diagnosis of Involuntary Weight Loss (IWL)

Disease	Notes
Cancer	Percent of patients with cancer and a physical cause of IWL, 30%-55%; percent of all patients with IWL, 16%-38%.
Gastrointestinal disorders	Percent of patients with a gastrointestinal disorder and a physical cause of IWL, 22%-25%; percent of all patients with IWL, 10%-18%.
Endocrine disorders	Percent of patients with an endocrine disorder and a physical cause of IWL, 6%-9%; percent of all patients with IWL, ~5%.
Infections	Percent of patients with an infection and a physical cause of IWL, 6%-9%; percent of all patients with IWL, ~5%.
Pulmonary disorders	Percent of patients with a pulmonary disorder and a physical cause of IWL, 8%; percent of all patients with IWL, 6%.
Medications	Percent of patients with physical cause of IWL due to medication, 3%-18%; percent of all patients with IWL, 2%-9%.
Cardiovascular diseases	Percent of patients with cardiovascular disease and a physical cause of IWL, 13%; percent of all patients with IWL, ~9%.
Renal disease	Percent of patients with renal disease and a physical cause of IWL, 6%; percent of all patients with IWL, 4%.
Neurologic disease	Percent of patients with neurological disease and a physical cause of IWL, 2%-13%; percent of all patients with IWL, 2%-7%.
Depression	Percent of all patients with IWL, 9%-18%.
No diagnosis	Percent of all patients with IWL, 5%-26%.

anticholinergic agents, and dopaminergic agents such as L-dopa and metoclopramide.

Weight loss is commonly associated with psychiatric disorders, especially depression. Dementia may cause weight loss that precedes the diagnosis of the underlying cognitive disorder. Eating disorders such as anorexia and substance abuse disorders such as alcoholism cause weight loss. Socioeconomic and functional problems may cause or exacerbate weight loss. Examples include difficulty in obtaining food because of functional disabilities, lack of financial resources, and social isolation and loneliness.

Evaluation

Because a substantial proportion of patients who report weight loss may not have experienced it, use documented weight measurements or objective evidence of weight loss, such as change in fit of clothes or corroboration by a trusted observer, before pursuing an evaluation. Then, confirm that changes in total body water are not the cause of weight loss. Dramatic weight changes can occur with gain or loss of total body water, which occur more quickly and erratically than changes in lean body mass.

Although the differential diagnosis of weight loss is wide ranging, it is clear from the literature that a carefully performed history and physical examination, followed by targeted use of diagnostic studies, is most likely to discover the etiology. An often overlooked clinical pearl is that the chief complaint frequently points to a specific etiology. Look for information that suggests chronic diseases such as malignancy, gastrointestinal disorders, endocrinologic disorders, infections, or severe cardiopulmonary conditions. Take a careful medication history with particular emphasis on medications known to affect appetite or whose use is temporally related to weight loss. Be certain to assess the patient's affective and cognitive state. Standard tools based on DSM IV criteria to assess for depression or the Mini-Mental State Examination to assess cognition can be very helpful in this regard.

Obtain a history of dietary practices, dietary intake, and supplement use. Inquire about the living environment, functional status, dependency, caregiver status, alcohol or substance abuse, social support, and resources. It is important to question relatives and caregivers.

Initial diagnostic testing is limited to basic studies unless the history and physical examination suggest a specific cause (Table 2). The following studies should be obtained in most patients: complete blood count, erythrocyte sedimentation rate or C-reactive protein, serum chemistry tests including calcium and liver tests, thyroid stimulating hormone level, urinalysis, chest radiograph, and stool occult blood. In patients with gastrointestinal symptoms or abnormalities in blood counts or liver tests, obtain an upper gastrointestinal series, abdominal ultrasonography, abdominal CT scan, or esophagogastroduodenoscopy, as appropriate. Indiscriminate imaging of the thorax and abdomen with CT or MRI in the absence of supporting history, physical examination, or laboratory findings is not helpful. Truly occult malignancy is not common.

It may be difficult to establish a definitive diagnosis for weight loss, and perhaps a quarter or more of patients will not have a diagnosis after an appropriate initial evaluation. For such patients, careful reevaluation over time is an appropriate course; if serious disease is present, the cause is likely to become evident within 3 to 6 months. If an etiology cannot be established over time, the prognosis is favorable.

Treatment

Once a specific diagnosis is made, treatment should, in most patients, alleviate weight loss. If weight loss continues, the putative diagnosis may not be correct or completely responsible. Consider medication and lifestyle changes for some patients. Change or eliminate medications that may be associated with anorexia and/or temporally related to weight loss. Address issues

Table 2. Laboratory and Other Studies for Involuntary Weight Loss

Test	Notes
CBC	Anemia is present in 14% with a physical cause of weight loss.
Electrolytes, blood urea nitrogen, creatinine, glucose, liver tests	The combination of decreased albumin and elevated alkaline phosphatase is 17% sensitive and 87% specific for cancer. Adrenal insufficiency is associated with electrolyte disturbances in 92% of patients.
ESR	Increased in patients with neoplasia (mean ESR 49 mm/h) compared with those with psychiatric (mean ESR 19 mm/h) and unknown cause (mean ESR 26 mm/h) of IWL.
Thyroid-stimulating hormone	To look for "apathetic" hyperthyroidism.
Chest radiography	A useful test overall in individuals with a physical cause of IWL.
HIV	If risk factors are present.
Upper GI x-ray series, EGD, abdominal ultrasonography, or abdominal CT scan	Upper GI has the highest yield in disclosing a pertinent abnormality beyond basic screening tests among persons with physical cause of weight loss if GI symptoms are present. Among patients diagnosed with cancer, the following were the most useful follow-up tests to make a diagnosis: for patients who had only an isolated abnormality in the CBC, abdominal CT scan, abdominal ultrasonography, and endoscopy; for patients who had only an isolated abnormality in liver tests, abdominal ultrasonography and abdominal CT scan; and for patients who had normal liver tests and CBC, upper endoscopy and abdominal CT scan.

CBC = complete blood count; CT = computed tomography; EGD = esophagogastroduodenoscopy; ESR = erythrocyte sedimentation rate; GI = gastrointestinal; HIV = human immunodeficiency virus; IWL = involuntary weight loss.

of social isolation and poor eating environments, if applicable. Ensure that oral health is adequate and that the patient has access to food and is able to eat it. Address personal and ethnic food preferences in the promotion of oral dietary intake. Assist those who need help with eating by seeking to improve their functional status or making certain they obtain help to eat. Eliminate restrictive diets, where appropriate.

The proven benefit of oral nutritional supplementation for weight loss is limited. In fact, the amount of regular food intake is sometimes decreased by oral nutritional supplement use. However, nutritional supplementation may be useful when access to calories is an issue due to functional impairments. Appetite stimulants are often recommended but are of limited benefit in patients not responding to treatment of the primary cause or if the cause of weight loss is unknown. Appetite-stimulant therapy has been studied mainly in patients with AIDS or cancer cachexia. In these patients, certain agents (e.g., megestrol acetate, human growth hormone) have been shown to promote weight gain. However, a survival benefit has never been demonstrated, and in some trials patients who received such agents have experienced an increase in mortality.

Book Enhancement

Go to www.acponline.org/essentials/general-internal-medicine-section.html to access tables on drug treatment, important history and physical examination elements for involuntary weight loss, nutritional syndromes, and a patient administered nutrition checklist for older adults. In *MKSAP for Students 4*, assess yourself with items 40-41 in the **General Internal Medicine** section.

Bibliography

Leff B. Weight Loss. http://pier.acponline.org/physicians/diseases/d244. [Date accessed: 2008 Jan 22] In: PIER [online database]. Philadelphia: American College of Physicians; 2008.

Vanderschueren S, Geens E, Knockaert D, Bobbaers H. The diagnostic spectrum of unintentional weight loss. Eur J Intern Med. 2005;16:160-164. [PMID: 15967329]

Chapter 34

Disorders of Menstruation and Menopause

Sara B. Fazio, MD

Disorders of menstruation are common, ranging from the complete absence of menstrual blood flow (amenorrhea) to irregular or heavy bleeding (abnormal uterine bleeding), and later in the life cycle culminate in the menopause. The normal menstrual cycle depends on a tightly regulated system that includes the central nervous system, hypothalamus, pituitary, ovaries, uterus, and vaginal outflow tract. Disruption of the axis at any level can cause a variety of menstrual disorders (Table 1).

The menstrual cycle is regulated by the pituitary-hypothalamic axis. The hypothalamus releases gonadotropin-releasing hormone (GnRH) in a pulsatile fashion, stimulating release of follicle-stimulating hormone (FSH) and leuteinizing hormone (LH) from the pituitary. FSH causes the development of multiple ovarian follicles, which in turn release estradiol. Estradiol inhibits FSH release, allowing only one or two dominant follicles to survive, and stimulates LH secretion. LH promotes progesterone

Table 1. Differential Diagnosis of Amenorrhea

Disease	Present in Primary Amenorrhea?	Present in Secondary Amenorrhea?	LH	FSH	E_2	Notes
Hypothalamus						
Hypothalamic amenorrhea	Yes	Yes	↓ or normal	↓ or normal	↓	Exercise, weight loss, stress, chronic illness
Hypogonadotropic hypogonadism	Yes	Yes	↓ or normal	↓ or normal	↓	Anosmia may be present
Hypothalamic tumors	Yes	Yes	↓ or normal	↓ or normal	↓	Brain imaging necessary
Pituitary						
Hypogonadotropic hypogonadism	Yes	Yes	↓ or normal	↓ or normal	↓	
Pituitary tumors (e.g., prolactinoma)	Yes	Yes	↓ or normal	↓ or normal	↓	Brain imaging; prolactin may ↑
Pituitary infection or infiltration	Yes	Yes	↓ or normal	↓ or normal	↓	
Sheehan's syndrome	No	Yes	↓ or normal	↓ or normal	↓	After delivery; can be acute or insidious
Ovary						
Gonadal dysgenesis	Yes	Yes	↑	↑	↓	45,XO = Turner's syndrome
Pure gonadal dysgenesis	Yes	Yes	↑	↑	↓	Karyotype either 46,XX or 46,XY
Premature ovarian failure	No	Yes	↑	↑	↓	Autoimmune syndromes
Polycystic ovary syndrome	Yes	Yes	↑ or normal	Normal	Normal	Hyperandrogenism; oligomenorrhea since menarche
Ovarian tumors	No	Yes	↓	↓	↑ or normal	Look for acute virilization
17α-hydroxylase deficiency	Yes	No	↑	↑	↓	Sexual infantilism
Uterus						
Müllerian agenesis	Yes	No	Normal	Normal	Normal	May have cyclical pelvic pain
Asherman's syndrome (uterine synechiae)	No	Yes	Normal	Normal	Normal	History dilation and curettage
Other						
Adrenal tumors	No	Yes	↓	↓	↑ or Normal	Hyperandrogenism
Thyroid disease	Yes	Yes	Normal	Normal	Normal	
Testicular feminization	Yes	No	↑	↑ or normal	↑	XY karyotype

DHEAS = dehydroepiandrosterone sulfate; E_2 = estradiol; FSH = follicle-stimulating hormone; LH = luteinizing hormone; T_3 = triiodothyronine; T_4 = thyroxine.

production, which then causes a surge of LH secretion 34-36 hours before follicle rupture and ovulation. Once this occurs, progesterone is produced by ovarian granulose cells (the corpus luteum) for approximately 14 days, which then involutes unless pregnancy is established. Estrogen functions physiologically to increase the thickness and vascularity of the endometrial lining whereas progesterone increases its glandular secretion and vessel tortuosity. The cyclical withdrawal of estrogen and progesterone results in endometrial sloughing and menstrual bleeding.

Amenorrhea

Primary amenorrhea is the failure of menstruation in girls 16 years of age or older, while secondary amenorrhea is the absence of menstruation for 3 cycle intervals or 6 consecutive months in women with prior menstrual flow. Table 2 lists common tests used in the evaluation of primary and secondary amenorrhea. Approximately 50% of primary amenorrhea is caused by chromosomal disorders, which cause gonadal dysgenesis and depletion of ovarian follicles. Turner's syndrome is the most common in this category and is classically associated with a 45 XO genotype. It is characterized by a lack of secondary sexual characteristics, growth retardation, webbed neck, and frequent skeletal abnormalities. Hypothalamic hypoandrogenism accounts for approximately 20% of causes and includes both functional and structural hypothalamic disorders, such as developmental defects of cranial midline structures, tumors, or infiltrative disorders.

Less common etiologies of primary amenorrhea include developmental disorders, such as mullerian agenesis, imperforate hymen, and defects of the cervix or vagina. Such patients have normal secondary sexual characteristics. Patients with androgen-resistance syndromes (XY karyotype) have some female secondary sexual characteristics, but absence of or minimal pubic and axillary hair, a shallow vagina, and often a labial mass (testes). Endocrine abnormalities such as prolactin excess, thyroid disease, or polycystic ovary syndrome (PCOS), while more commonly associated with secondary amenorrhea, also cause primary amenorrhea. Patients with primary amenorrhea should be examined for the presence of an intact uterus and vaginal outflow tract, secondary sexual characteristics, and signs of hyperandrogenism. If evidence of characteristic developmental disorders is present, karyotype testing should be considered. Primary ovarian failure of any etiology can be diagnosed by an elevated follicle-stimulating hormone (FSH). If the FSH is low or normal, testing of prolactin and thyroid-stimulating hormone (TSH) is warranted as well as head imaging to exclude structural disease.

Secondary amenorrhea is much more common. All previously menstruating women who present with amenorrhea should be tested for pregnancy, the most common etiology. Premature ovarian failure may occur as a result of surgical oophorectomy, chemotherapy, radiation, or autoimmune destruction of ovarian tissue. Diagnosis of secondary ovarian failure is also made by an elevated FSH. In such patients, vaginal bleeding will not occur with a progesterone challenge because estrogen levels are low, but will occur after estrogen priming followed by a progesterone challenge, demonstrating the integrity of the uterine lining and outflow tract.

Polycystic ovary syndrome (PCOS) affects 6% of women of child-bearing age and typically presents with oligomenorrhea and signs of androgen excess (hirsutism, acne, and occasionally alopecia). The cause is not fully understood, but there is abnormal gonadotropin regulation, with subsequent overactivity of the ovarian androgen pathway. Insulin resistance is an important feature of the disorder, as is overweight/obesity, though only 50%

Table 2. Laboratory and Other Studies for Amenorrhea

Test	Notes
β-HCG	Use to confirm or exclude pregnancy.
FSH	Hypergonadotropism (ovarian failure, menopause) is present when levels are >20 IU/mL. Use to rule out ovarian failure. Perform karyotyping in all patients <30 years with elevated FSH levels.
Prolactin	Because prolactin levels can be elevated by stress, breast exam, and food intake, repeat analysis on a fasting morning sample before performing cranial imaging. Hypothyroidism can also cause elevations in serum prolactin level. Phenothiazine, tricyclic antidepressants, metoclopramide, reserpine and methyldopa, can cause hyperprolactinemia. Values >100 ng/mL suggest pituitary tumor.
TSH	Hypothyroidism and, less commonly, hyperthyroidism are associated with menstrual cycle abnormalities and infertility.
Testosterone, DHEAS	Serum androgens may be helpful in the setting of hirsutism and acne; total testosterone >200 μg/dL and DHEAS >3× upper limit of normal may suggest tumor (although no tumor will be found on most occasions).
17-hydroxyprogesterone	Beneficial in screening for congenital adrenal hyperplasia.
Estradiol	Decreased in hypothalamic and pituitary amenorrhea, and in ovarian failure; should always be assessed with FSH. Very limited use in clinical practice unless evaluating primary amenorrhea.
Luteinizing hormone	Normal levels are 5-20 IU/mL, with midcycle peak three times the base level. In hypogonadotropic states (hypothalamic or pituitary dysfunction), the level is <5 IU/mL. In hypergonadotropic states (postmenopausal or ovarian failure), the level is >20-40 IU/mL. Not needed to diagnose PCOS.
Bone density test (DEXA)	May be required in a patient with amenorrhea who is estrogen deficient.
Brain MRI	Necessary to rule out a hypothalamic or pituitary mass, infection, or infiltration; critical to consider in the setting of primary amenorrhea with hypogonadotropic hypogonadism.

β-HCG = β human chorionic gonadotropin; DEXA = dual-energy X-ray absorptiometry; DHEAS = dehydroepiandrosterone sulfate; FSH = follicle-stimulating hormone; IU = international units; LH = luteinizing hormone; MRI = magnetic resonance imaging; PCOS = polycystic ovary syndrome; TSH = thyroid-stimulating hormone.

of affected women are obese. Other forms of androgen excess (androgen-producing tumor, congenital adrenal hyperplasia, Cushing's syndrome) should be excluded. Typically there is a mild elevation in testosterone and DHEA-S (dehydroepiandrosterone sulfate) levels and a luteinizing hormone (LH)/FSH ratio greater than 2:1. Diagnosis requires two out of three of the following: ovulatory dysfunction, laboratory or clinical evidence of hyperandrogenism, and ultrasonographic evidence of polycystic ovaries.

Hyperprolactinemia is a frequent cause of secondary amenorrhea and is commonly related to medications. Drugs that reduce central catecholamine and dopamine production or release can cause hyperprolactinemia. Among the most common are tricyclic antidepressants, phenothiazines, and metoclopramide. Primary hypothyroidism reduces negative feedback on the production of hypothalamic thyrotropin-releasing hormone, which stimulates prolactin production. Tumors that secrete prolactin or compress the pituitary stalk will lead to hyperprolactinemia. If the prolactin level is elevated and medication and hypothyroidism are excluded, imaging of the head is warranted.

Hypothalamic amenorrhea involves disordered gonadotropin release. It may be a result of a tumor or infiltrative lesion (e.g. lymphoma, sarcoidosis) but more commonly is functional. The usual etiologic factors are stress, excessive loss of body weight or fat, excessive exercise, or some combination thereof. Diagnosis is one of exclusion.

When amenorrhea with low or inappropriately normal FSH level is present, secondary causes (PCOS, androgen or prolactin excess, hypothyroidism) must be ruled out. If a functional etiology is suspected, reduction in exercise, improvement in nutrition, and attention to emotional needs are helpful adjuncts. Because lack of adequate estrogen predisposes to osteoporosis, it is very important to initiate adequate estrogen and progesterone replacement until etiologic factors are resolved and menstruation can return to normal.

Abnormal Uterine Bleeding

Abnormal uterine bleeding is any bleeding that is excessive or scanty or occurs outside the normal menstrual cycle. Similar to amenorrhea, the diagnosis is best approached in anatomic terms. Pregnancy must always be considered. Implantation, ectopic pregnancy, threatened or missed abortion, as well as gestational trophoblastic disease can cause abnormal bleeding. Consider anatomic lesions of the uterus in all patients with abnormal bleeding, including endometrial polyps, uterine fibroids (leiomyomata), and, particularly in the peri- or post-menopausal population, endometrial hyperplasia or carcinoma. Cervical polyps or cervical neoplasia commonly present with abnormal bleeding, though typically with intermenstrual bleeding. All patients should have a speculum examination to assess for visible lesions, a Pap smear, and a bimanual exam to assess for structural abnormality. Ultrasound imaging may be necessary to detect endometrial polyps or sub-mucosal fibroids and can assess the endometrial thickness. The latter is particularly important in a peri-menopausal or post-menopausal woman with abnormal bleeding because an endometrial biopsy may be warranted if the endometrium is >4-5 mm in thickness or is heterogeneous. Risk factors for endometrial carcinoma include chronic unopposed estrogen (as seen in chronic anovulatory states), obesity, age >45, nulliparity, and tamoxifen use.

Anovulation is the most common cause of abnormal vaginal bleeding. Estrogen is produced by FSH stimulation of the ovary, but because ovulation does not occur progesterone is never produced and the uterine lining builds up. This eventually leads to discoordinate menstrual bleeding, often presenting as bleeding at intervals shorter than the typical cycle length (metrorrhagia) or extended periods of heavy blood loss (menorrhagia). It is common for patients at extremes of the menstrual cycle to be anovulatory (adolescence and the peri-menopause). The most common cause of anovulatory bleeding in reproductive-aged women is PCOS. Anovulatory bleeding may precede amenorrhea in functional hypothalamic disorders. Endocrine etiologies must also be considered in patients with abnormal uterine bleeding. Prolactin excess will initially cause anovulation. Menorrhagia may be reported in women with hypothyroidism. Cushing's syndrome commonly causes menstrual irregularities, likely secondary to cortisol suppression of gonadotropin-releasing hormone. Ovulatory status may be determined by basal body temperature or progesterone level on day 21 of the cycle, but neither is precise.

Systemic illness, coagulopathy, or medication should also be considered in the etiology of abnormal uterine bleeding. Cirrhosis reduces the ability of the liver to metabolize estrogen and decreases clotting factor production. Renal failure interferes with estrogen clearance and is associated with abnormalities in platelet function. In adolescents with menorrhagia, up to 20% have an inherited bleeding disorder, most commonly von Willebrand's disease.

Hormonal therapy can regularize anovulatory bleeding. Options include combination oral contraceptives, cyclic progestins or a progestin containing intra-uterine device. In most cases, regularity of menstrual flow can be re-established and control of heavy blood loss can be achieved. In patients who are at risk for endometrial hyperplasia or carcinoma, a biopsy should be first obtained before hormonal manipulation. Nonsteroidal anti-inflammatory medications inhibit endometrial prostaglandins and decrease blood flow.

Menopause

Menopause refers to cessation of ovarian function. Because one-third of the lifespan of most women encompasses the postmenopausal period, physicians who care for these women must recognize the effects of estrogen deficiency. Elements that should be addressed in the history include timing of change in menstrual cycle, presence of hot flashes or night sweats, and fluctuations in mood. Patients should be questioned regarding evidence of urinary incontinence, vaginal dryness, and changes in sexual function or desire. Examination should include evaluation for height loss and kyphosis (signs of osteoporosis), breast examination (given increased incidence of breast cancer with advancing age), and evidence of vulvar or vaginal atrophy. Because the diagnosis of menopause can be made by history and physical without laboratory confirmation, obtain an FSH level only if the diagnosis is unclear or if the patient requires confirmation for reassurance.

Osteoporosis is a direct effect of estrogen loss at any age. Premenopausal women have less heart disease than men (in the absence of other risk factors), but this relative protection is lost at menopause. The role of hormone replacement therapy has become increasingly controversial. While clearly controlling many of the symptoms of menopause (e.g., vasomotor instability and vaginal dryness) and reducing the risk of osteoporotic fractures, recent research has suggested a higher frequency of cardiac events in the first 5 years of hormone replacement therapy. In addition, studies have demonstrated a small but statistically significant increase in breast cancer in women taking estrogen. Thus, the approach to management has become more individualized, where estrogen is used at the lowest dose and for the shortest duration possible to treat menopausal symptoms, typically no more than two years. Contraindications to hormone replacement therapy include unexplained vaginal bleeding, a history of clotting disorder, liver disease, coronary artery disease, stroke, breast or endometrial cancer.

Serotonin norepinephrine reuptake inhibitors, most notably venlafaxine, serotonin reuptake inhibitors, clonidine, and black cohosh may all be helpful in controlling vasomotor symptoms in selected patients. Soy preparations have minimal efficacy. Vaginal atrophy can be treated with lubricants or localized vaginal estrogen preparations that have little systemic absorption. Patients should be instructed on risk reduction for coronary artery disease. Bone density testing should be offered to all women aged >65 years or any woman at increased risk for osteoporosis.

Patients at the peri-menopause frequently experience irregular bleeding secondary to anovulation, but shortened intermenstrual cycles, longer duration of bleeding, or episodes of heavy bleeding warrant endometrial biopsy. Similarly, post-menopausal bleeding requires endometrial evaluation. While the most common etiology is endometrial atrophy, the possibility of endometrial carcinoma must be excluded.

Book Enhancement

Go to www.acponline.org/essentials/general-internal-medicine-section.html to review an extensive differential diagnosis and common laboratory studies for amenorrhea, and a table of causes of abnormal uterine bleeding organized by patient age. In *MKSAP for Students 4*, assess yourself with items 42-43 in the **General Internal Medicine** section.

Bibliography

American College of Physicians. Medical Knowledge Self-Assessment Program 14. Philadelphia: American College of Physicians; 2006.

Col N, Cyr M, Miller M, Wheeler C. Menopause and Hormone Therapy. http://pier.acponline.org/physicians/diseases/d293. [Date accessed: 2008 Jan 14] In: PIER [online database]. Philadelphia: American College of Physicians; 2008.

Fazio SB, Ship AN. Abnormal uterine bleeding. South Med J. 2007; 100:376-82. [PMID: 17458397]

Gifford SD. Dysfunctional Uterine Bleeding. http://pier.acponline.org/physicians/diseases/d295. [Date accessed: 2008 Jan 14] In: PIER [online database]. Philadelphia: American College of Physicians; 2008.

Chapter 35

Common Dermatologic Disorders

Hanah Polotsky, MD

In the United States, up to 60% of dermatologic disorders are treated by primary care physicians. Skin complaints account for approximately 5% of internal medicine visits. Rash and pruritis are particularly common complaints and frequently occur together. The presence or absence of pruritis with a primary skin lesion can dramatically change the differential diagnosis. Generalized pruritis can present as the only dermatological complaint signifying an underlying systemic disorder.

Evaluation

Obtain a detailed and targeted history including location of lesions, time of onset and evolution (acute or chronic), and any systemic symptoms such as fever, malaise, gastrointestinal, or upper respiratory symptoms. Rash accompanied by fever is common with disseminated infections (viral or bacterial), drug reactions, collagen vascular diseases, and vasculitis. Investigate external factors, such as new medications, foods, soaps, occupational, environmental, and sun exposures. Patients may self-treat skin eruptions or pruritis with over-the-counter remedies. Eliciting a detailed history of previous treatments may clarify altered natural progression of skin disorders.

It is imperative to perform an inspection of the entire skin and mucosal surfaces. Patients should be entirely undressed, wearing only a hospital gown. Natural light exposure is preferable. Skin palpation can help appreciate texture of the lesions, depth, and tenderness. Learning how to describe skin lesions is critical to correctly communicate relevant findings. Several attributes of skin lesions are paramount, including location, color, border, type, and arrangement (Table 1).

Dermatitis (Eczematous Rashes)

Eczema denotes epidermal eruptions characterized histologically by intracellular edema. Atopic, contact, seborrheic, and stasis dermatitis are common types of eczema, whereas nonspecific dermatitis is a diagnosis of exclusion when no etiology is identified. Topical corticosteroids and oral antihistamines are usually the treatment of choice for any type of eczema.

Atopic dermatitis is an allergic disorder with genetic and immunologic components characterized by intense itching leading to excoriation, lichenification (epidermal thickening), hyperpigmentation, and papulosquamous eruption (Plate 2). Typical locations are the flexural areas, head, neck, trunk, and hands. Acute eruptions are often accompanied by erythema, vesiculation, and oozing. In addition to the standard treatment of dermatitis, skin moisturizers can be used to decrease dryness and pruritis.

Contact dermatitis is precipitated by local absorption of allergen or irritant through the stratum corneum. Common allergens include metals (e.g., nickel), topical anesthetics, neomycin, poison oak, poison ivy (Plate 3), and strong soaps or personal care products. The location of eruptions may help to identify causative agents (e.g., neck rash caused by a necklace). The mainstay of treatment is avoidance of the allergens and irritants.

Table 1. Dermatologic Lexicon

Description	Definition	Examples
Macule	Flat skin lesion <1 cm in diameter	Freckle
Patch	Flat skin lesion >1 cm in diameter	Tinea versicolor
Papule	Raised skin lesion <0.5 cm in diameter	Acne
Plaque	"Plateau-like" elevated lesion >0.5 cm in diameter	Psoriasis
Nodule	Raised sphere-like lesion >0.5 cm in diameter and depth; called a *cyst* when filled with liquid or keratin	Erythema nodosum
Vesicle	Blister filled with clear fluid <.5 cm in diameter	Varicella
Bulla	Blister filled with clear fluid >0.5 cm in diameter	Poison ivy
Pustule	Vesicle filled with pus	Folliculitis
Crust (scab)	Dried pus, blood and serum from breakage of vesicles, bullae, or pustules	Herpes zoster (shingles)
Scale	Dry, whitish, and flaky stratum corneum	Seborrheic dermatitis

Other common terms include *induration* (dermal thickening), *lichenification* (epidermal thickening), *atrophy* (loss of epidermal or dermal tissue), *wheal* (dermal edema), *comedones* (lesions of acne), *ulcer* (loss of epidermal tissue and some dermis), *erosion* (superficial loss of epidermis), and *fissure* (linear opening in epidermis).

Seborrheic dermatitis (Plate 4) is characterized by erythematous plaques with a dry or oily scale occurring in hair-bearing parts of the body including scalp (dandruff), eyelashes, eyebrows, beard, chest, the external ear canal and behind the ear, the forehead, and nasolabial folds. The precise etiology is unknown but appears to be related to colonization with the yeast *Malassezia furfur*. Scalp dermatitis is treated with selenium sulfide, coal tar, or ketoconazole shampoos. The face can be cleansed and treated with topical 1% hydrocortisone and 2% ketoconazole cream.

Bacterial Skin Infections

The most common skin infections observed in the outpatient setting include cellulitis, folliculitis, and impetigo. Increasingly these infections are caused by community-acquired methicillin-resistant *Staphylococcus aureus* (MRSA), especially in patients who have had close recent contact with persons having a history of a similar infection, including household and athletic team members, prison inmates, and military personnel.

Cellulitis is a deep skin (dermis) infection most frequently caused by *Staphylococcus aureus* or Group A streptococci. A well-demarcated area of warmth, swelling, tenderness and erythema is found on physical exam (Plate 5). Cellulitis can be differentiated from contact dermatitis by absence of vesicles or pruritis. Patients with cellulitis are treated with oral antibiotics and analgesics; intravenous antibiotics may be necessary for failed outpatient treatment (Table 2).

Folliculitis and furunculosis are pustular skin infections arising from hair follicles and caused by *Staphylococcus aureus* and, less frequently, Group A *Streptococcus* (Plate 6). Topical antibiotics (e.g., mupirocin) and hot compresses may be sufficient for treatment. Furuncles (boils) are pus-filled nodules requiring incision, drainage and systemic antibiotics. Elimination of *S. aureus* nasal carriage using topical or intranasal antibiotics may decrease relapses.

Impetigo is a superficial (epidermis) skin infection that typically presents as a group of crusted pustules caused by beta-hemolytic streptococci and *Staphylococcus aureus* (Plate 7). Cephalexin, erythromycin, or dicloxacillin eradicates the lesion in 90% of cases; so does topical mupirocin ointment. Herpes simplex can be confused with facial impetigo; a history of recurrent vesicles occurring in the same location is consistent with herpes simplex.

Fungal Infections

Dermatophyte organisms are fungi infecting the stratum corneum. Tinea pedis is the most common dermatophyte infection and often presents as chronic maceration, fissuring, and scaling between the toes. Some patients have a chronic moccasin-type, or hyperkeratotic form of infection; the soles are involved with fine silvery scale extending from sole to heel and sides of the feet (Plate 8). Tinea pedis can be associated with recurrent cellulitis. Treatment consists of antifungal creams (e.g., clotrimazole, terbinafine); oral therapy is sometimes necessary with moccasin-type tinea pedis or more extensive disease.

Tinea versicolor is caused by the lipophilic yeast *Malassezia furfur*. The typical clinical features include nonpruritic, light brown or reddish brown macules or hypopigmented macules in darker persons (Plate 9). The characteristic distribution of tinea versicolor is on the chest, back, lower neck, and proximal upper

Table 2. Antibiotic Therapy for Cellulitis

Disease	Notes
Mild, uncomplicated cellulitis at low risk for MRSA (oral treatment)	• Dicloxacillin or cloxacillin • First-generation cephalosporin (cephalexin or cefadroxil) • Clindamycin or macrolide (erythromycin, azithromycin, clarithromycin) if allergic to penicillin • An advanced fluoroquinolone (moxifloxacin, levofloxacin) if intolerant to the above drugs
Mild, uncomplicated cellulitis at risk for MRSA infection (oral treatment). In outpatients, consider recent close contact with persons having similar infection including household members, athletic team members, prisoners, and military personnel.	• Trimethoprim-sulfamethoxazole* • Clindamycin (if sensitive) • Minocycline or doxycycline
Moderate-to-severe cellulitis with systemic manifestations of infection at low risk for MRSA (parenteral treatment)	• Semisynthetic penicillin (nafcillin, oxacillin) • Cephalosporin (cefazolin or cephalothin) • If penicillin-allergic: clindamycin; fluoroquinolone (moxifloxacin, levofloxacin); advanced macrolide (clarithromycin, azithromycin); oxazolidinone (linezolid); vancomycin; daptomycin; tigecycline
Moderate-to-severe cellulitis with systemic manifestations of infection at risk for MRSA (parenteral treatment). Risk categories include recent antibiotic use, recent hospitalization, hemodialysis, illicit IV drug use, diabetes, and previous MRSA infection or colonization.	• Clindamycin (if sensitive) • Vancomycin • Linezolid • Daptomycin • Tigecycline

*For non-purulent cellulitis, trimethoprim-sulfamethoxazole is not recommended because the likely cause, Group A streptococci, is in most cases resistant to this antimicrobial agent.
MRSA = methicillin-resistant *Staphylococcus aureus*.

extremities. Diagnosis is confirmed by microscopic evaluation of a potassium hydroxide preparation made from scrapings of lesions showing the classic appearance of both spores and hyphae in a "spaghetti and meatball" pattern. Therapy with topical 2.5% selenium sulfide solution or oral, single-dose ketoconazole are equally effective. Infection recurs in 60% to 80% requiring retreatment.

Onychomycosis is a fungal infection of the nail caused by dermatophytes, yeasts, or molds (Plate 10). It is common, increasing in prevalence with age. Up to half of all patients with thickened toenails have a nonfungal cause for the nail thickening such as psoriasis, subungual warts, lichen planus, and bacterial infections. Fungal infection of the nail should be confirmed with culture of nail debris or clippings before starting therapy. Treatment of onychomycosis is recommended in patients with peripheral vascular disease or diabetes mellitus to prevent development of cellulitis. Oral therapy with itraconazole or terbinafine is effective and preferred; topical therapy is ineffective. Treatment is usually for 2-3 months with close monitoring for adverse reactions (heart failure with itraconazole and hepatotoxicity with terbinafine).

Candidiasis is an inflammatory reaction to *Candida albicans* infection. It usually occurs in moist areas such as skin folds, under the breasts, perianally, and in axillae causing itching and burning (Plate 11). On physical exam, infected areas appear erythematous with scattered satellite papules and pustules. Candidiasis can often be confused with intertrigo, which is an irritant skin fold dermatitis from moisture and rubbing, especially prominent in obese patients. Intertrigo usually lacks the same degree of redness and satellite lesions found in candidiasis and a microscopic examination of a potassium hydroxide preparation will not demonstrate hyphae and pseudohyphae that is diagnostic of candidiasis. Candidiasis is treated with topical nystatin or imidazole creams and attention to hygiene, especially dryness of affected areas.

Acne

Acne vulgaris usually begins at puberty and results from hyperkeratinization of follicles, increased sebum production, proliferation of *Propionibacterium acnes*, and resulting inflammation (Plate 12). Acne is classified by severity and type as comedonal-only acne, mild-to-moderate inflammatory acne, moderate-to-severe inflammatory acne, and severe papulonodular inflammatory acne. Acne is exacerbated by creams and lotions, mechanical trauma (rubbing from clothing, picking, and repetitive scrubbing), medications (e.g., prednisone and progesterone), and sweating. Polycystic ovary syndrome should be considered in women with acne, hirsutism, and acanthosis nigricans (hyperpigmentation of flexural folds). Patients should be advised to use noncomedogenic oil-free make-up and sunscreen; dietary changes do not affect acne. Comedonal acne is treated with topical benzoyl peroxide and a topical antibiotic. Papular and pustular acne are treated with combination topical benzoyl peroxide/topical antibiotic and topical isotretinoin, adapalene, salicylic acid, or azelaic acid. If topical therapy is ineffective, systemic antibiotic therapy is indicated, followed by treatment with 0.05% isotretinoin if necessary. Oral contraceptives and spironolactone are effective for hormonal acne. Metformin may decrease acne in polycystic ovary syndrome. Tretinoin (Accutane) is the only therapy that alters the natural history but is teratogenic and is given only under the supervision of a dermatologist.

Acne rosacea is a chronic inflammatory skin disorder of unknown etiology affecting the face, typically the cheeks and nose, usually occurring after the age of 30 years (Plate 13). On physical examination there is erythema with telangiectasias, pustules, and papules without comedones. Rosacea can be differentiated from seborrheic dermatitis by the presence of pustules. In early stages, rosacea can present with only facial erythema and resemble the butterfly rash of systemic lupus erythematosus; however, the rash of systemic lupus erythematosus typically spares the nasal labial folds and areas under the nose and lower lip (Plate 14). Rhinophyma (big irregular hyperplastic nose) can develop in some rosacea patients (Plate 15). Treatment consists of metronidazole gel, low-dose oral tetracycline, or erythromycin.

Viral Skin Infections

Herpes zoster (shingles) is caused by reactivation of varicella zoster virus in older or immunosuppressed patients. Patients may report localized sensations ranging from mild itching or tingling to severe pain that precedes the development of the skin lesions by 1-5 days. Skin changes begin with an erythematous maculopapular rash followed by the appearance of clear vesicles in a dermatomal distribution; the vesicles become pustular and eventually crust with healing (Plate 16). Bacterial superinfection of cutaneous lesions occasionally occurs. Patients are treated with an oral antiviral (i.e., acyclovir, valacyclovir, or famciclovir); treatment is most effective if begun within 48-72 hours of the onset of rash. The addition of corticosteroids to antiviral therapy reduces the duration of acute neuritis but not the incidence of postherpetic neuralgia. Postherpetic neuralgia is a painful sequela of shingles treated with amitriptyline, gabapentin, or long-acting opioids. There is a 10% to 20% lifetime incidence of herpes zoster in those who have had chickenpox, and the incidence increases with age. Immunization with VZV (varicella zoster virus) live vaccine of immunocompetent adults older than age 60 years is currently recommended in order to reduce the incidence and severity of zoster and postherpetic neuralgia.

Herpes labialis is caused by reactivation of herpes simplex virus type I (HSV-1). Primary infection with HSV-1 is asymptomatic in up to 90% patients but may present as acute, painful gingivostomatitis (Plate 17). Recurrent infections are characterized by grouped vesicles on an erythematous base located on the lips ("cold sores") and usually recur in the same location, lasting 5-10 days. Treatment with oral or topical antiviral drugs does not shorten the duration. In patients with clearly identifiable prodromal symptoms of localized itching or burning, early treatment before the outbreak of vesicles reduces the duration of the rash by 1-2 days but does not prevent recurrences.

Benign Growths

Seborrheic keratosis is a painless, non-malignant growth appearing as a waxy, brownish patch or plaque (Plate 18). These lesions are more common in elderly patients and do not require treatment except for cosmetic reasons.

Warts (verruca vulgaris) are caused by infection of the epithelial tissues with human papillomavirus (HPV) (Plate 19). Diagnosis is based on the typical verrucous appearance of a papule or plaque on hands or feet. Nongenital warts in immunocompetent patients are harmless and two-thirds resolve spontaneously by 2 years. Topical salicylic or lactic acid is available over-the-counter and hastens the resolution of 60% to 80% of warts. Cryotherapy combined with topical therapy is used for warts that do not respond to initial topical management.

Miscellaneous Skin Conditions

Psoriasis is a chronic, relapsing skin disorder characterized by discrete and well-demarcated raised plaques or papules covered by a silvery white scale on the scalp, extensor surface of the extremities, low back, and intergluteal cleft, and behind the ears (Plate 20). Symptoms are primarily cosmetic, although itching and pain occur. Nail pitting, onycholysis, subungual hyperkeratosis, or discoloration of the nail surface occurs in up to 50% of patients. Limited chronic plaque psoriasis can be managed with sunlight, topical corticosteroids, and tar shampoo or lotion if the scalp is involved. Topical corticosteroids should be discontinued slowly to avoid rebound of psoriasis. Chronic plaque psoriasis involving more than 10% of the body surface, and more severe forms of psoriasis should be referred to a dermatologist. Infection, particularly streptococcal infections of the upper respiratory tract; injury to the skin; and medication (e.g., lithium and β-blockers) can exacerbate psoriasis. An inflammatory, seronegative spondyloarthropathy, psoriatic arthritis, can occur in up to 25% of patients with psoriatic skin lesions (Plate 21). Inflammatory bowel disease—including ulcerative colitis and Crohn's disease—occurs more commonly in patients with psoriasis.

Urticaria (hives) are raised, intensely pruritic red lesions with sharp borders, typically 2-4 mm in diameter (Plate 22). In acute urticaria, individual lesions may last 30 minutes to 2 hours, and an episode usually resolves within a few days or weeks. In chronic urticaria, individual lesions may last 4 to 36 hours. An attack usually continues for several days or weeks, but may persist beyond 6 weeks in one third of the patients. Common causes of urticaria are medications, foods, viral or bacterial infection, latex or other physical contacts, and stinging insects. Indiscriminate laboratory testing is rarely helpful. Urticaria, in rare cases, can precede anaphylaxis or angioedema in complement-induced allergic reactions. The standard therapy for urticaria is antihistamines. If histamine-1 blockade is not sufficient, histamine-2 receptor or leukotriene antagonists can be added. Corticosteroids are reserved for severe symptoms unresponsive to maximal doses of antihistamines.

Alopecia consists of generalized or patchy hair loss, usually from the scalp, but occurring in other sites as well. Alopecia areata is a self limiting condition associated with atopy and other autoimmune processes. Patients with alopecia areata have a well-demarcated, completely bald area with no signs of inflammation, desquamation, or scarring (Plate 23). Intralesional corticosteroids can help stimulate growth but are not routinely used. Androgen-dependent hair loss or male-pattern baldness is common, and its incidence increases with age. There is usually a genetic predisposition to the age of onset and severity of the baldness in these patients. A small proportion of postmenopausal women may also have this type of baldness. Conventional medical treatments for male-pattern baldness include oral finasteride or topical preparations of 2% or 5% minoxidil. Other causes of alopecia include drug-induced alopecia, lichen planus, trichotillomania (neurotic hair pulling) or traction alopecia (e.g., tight braiding of hair), fungal or bacterial folliculitis, and discoid lupus erythematosus.

Scabies is caused by *Sarcoptes scabiei* var. *hominis*, an obligate human parasite preferentially affecting impoverished, immobilized or immunosuppressed persons. Spread is direct, personal contact, especially during sex. Acquisition from bedding or clothes is rare. Scabies infestation causes intense itching and a papular or vesicular rash (Plate 24). Burrows are visible as short, wavy lines. Location in the interdigital webs, flexure surface of the wrists, penis, axillae, nipples, umbilicus, scrotum, and buttocks is diagnostic.

Pediculosis (head lice) and scabies are closely related conditions caused by arthropods. Pruritis is the primary symptom of this disorder; excoriations and pyoderma may also occur. The diagnosis of head lice is established by identifying crawling lice in the scalp or hair. Lice egg cases are called *nits* and are found sticking to the hair shaft in patients with lice. Nits are generally easier to see than lice because they are often found in the occipital or retroauricular portions of the scalp. Permethrin is the treatment of choice for both scabies and head lice.

Dermatologic Signs of Systemic Disease

Erythema multiforme presenting as circular erythematous plaques with a raised, darker central circle ("target lesions") is pathognomonic for this disorder (Plate 25). Palms and soles are frequently involved. Wide-spread blisters and mucosal lesions with systemic symptoms are seen in Stevens-Johnson syndrome, a severe form of erythema multiforme. Immunologic reaction to drugs or infections involving immune complexes in the skin is a possible etiology of the disease. No specific therapy is indicated for minor forms of erythema multiforme other than treating the underlying condition. Systemic corticosteroids and supportive measures are used to treat the Stevens-Johnson syndrome.

Erythema nodosum is characterized by tender, deep, erythematous nodules frequently limited to lower legs and often accompanied by fever and joint pain (Plate 26). Erythema nodosum is the result of a hypersensitivity immune reaction to infection or inflammation (e.g., streptococcal pharyngitis, sarcoidosis, inflammatory bowel disease) involving subcutaneous fat. The mainstay of management is treatment of underlying disease. Lesions usually resolve in several weeks with symptomatic relief from nonsteroidal anti-inflammatory medications. Corticosteroids can be used if infectious etiology is ruled out.

Generalized pruritis without rash usually has local or systemic causes. In elderly patients, the most common cause of pruritis is xerosis (dry skin) (Plate 27). Frequent bathing, poor chronic hydration, and dry winter weather exacerbate dry skin and the accompanying itch. The treatment of xerosis should include advice about using a humidifier in dry weather conditions, avoiding excess bathing and scrubbing of skin, use of moisturizing soaps, and routine use of moisturizers and occlusives. Pruritus may be caused by fleas or mites from pets, or by using new soap (contact dermatitis) or medication (allergic dermatitis). When more than one household member has pruritus, empiric treatment for scabies may be appropriate. Persistent pruritus in patients with no skin lesions warrants further evaluation for systemic causes, including hyperthyroidism, cholestasis (e.g., primary biliary cirrhosis), chronic renal failure, infection (e.g., HIV, hepatitis C), hematologic disease (e.g., polycythemia vera, lymphoma), and malignancy. Doxepin, a sedating antidepressant and antihistamine, may alleviate nocturnal pruritus. Nonsedating antihistamines are rarely beneficial for isolated pruritis.

Book Enhancement

Go to www.acponline.org/essentials/general-internal-medicine -section.html to view additional clinical images of common dermatologic conditions and review tables on the differential diagnosis for psoriasis and herpes zoster, drug treatment for acne and herpes zoster, and the evaluation of pruritis. In *MKSAP for Students 4*, assess yourself with items 44-57 in the **General Internal Medicine** section.

Bibliography

American College of Physicians. Medical Knowledge Self-Assessment Program 14. Philadelphia: American College of Physicians; 2006.

Chapter 36

Comprehensive Geriatric Assessment

Ivonne Z. Jiménez-Velázquez, MD

The evaluation of a geriatric patient differs from the usual medical evaluation by being comprehensive, interdisciplinary, and having an emphasis in functional ability, independence, and quality of life. The comprehensive geriatric assessment addresses functional ability, physical health, sensory capacity, cognitive and mental health, and socio-environmental limitations that can affect the lives of elderly patients and their caregivers. Possible benefits of the geriatric assessment include greater diagnostic accuracy, improved functional and mental status, reduced mortality, decreased use of nursing homes and acute care hospitals, and greater satisfaction with care.

Assessment of Functional Ability

Review the patient's ability to function by evaluating activities of daily living (ADL) and the capacity for living independently by assessing instrumental activities of daily living (IADL). Activities of daily living are self-care activities that a person must perform every day (Table 1). Patients unable to perform these activities and obtain adequate nutrition usually require caregiver support. Instrumental activities of daily living are activities that enable a person to live independently (Table 2). Patients with deficits in activities of daily living and instrumental activities of daily living are further evaluated regarding their home environment and caregiver availability.

History

To overcome communication problems due to the patient's hearing or vision loss, move close to the patient, face the patient directly, and speak clearly and slowly to allow lip-reading. Shouting to hard-of-hearing patients does not help because age-related stiffening of the tympanic membrane and ear ossicles distorts high-volume sound.

Some patients prefer to have a relative present; however, unless mental status is impaired, interview the patient alone to encourage the discussion of personal matters. Do not invite a relative to be present without asking the patient's permission because doing so implies that the patient is incapable of providing a competent history. Asking the patient to wait outside while a relative or friend is interviewed can damage the physician-patient relationship.

Determine which drugs are used, at what dose, how often, who prescribed them, and for what reason. Over-the-counter drugs and all herbal and nutritional supplements must be identified because their potential to cause drug interactions and their overuse or misuse can have serious health consequences. The precise nature of drug allergies should also be determined. The patient should be asked to bring to the office all their medications. Frequently, identical medications with different names have been prescribed by different physicians. Incorrect dosing may also occur by misunderstanding instructions.

Table 1. Katz Activities of Daily Living Scale*

Activity	Item
Eating	Eats without assistance, or needs assistance only in cutting meat or buttering bread (1 point).
	Needs assistance in eating or is fed intravenously (0 points).
Dressing	Gets clothes and dresses without assistance or needs assistance only in tying shoes (1 point).
	Needs assistance in getting clothes or in getting dressed or stays partly or completely undressed (0 points).
Bathing	Bathes without assistance or needs assistance only in bathing one part of the body (e.g., back) (1 point).
(sponge bath, tub bath, or shower)	Needs assistance in bathing more than one part of the body or does not bathe (0 points).
Transferring	Moves in and out of bed and chair without assistance (may use cane or walker) (1 point).
	Needs assistance in moving in and out of bed or chair or does not get out of bed (0 points).
Toileting	Goes to the bathroom, uses toilet, cleans self, arranges clothes, and returns without assistance (may use cane or walker for support and may use bedpan or urinal at night) (1 point).
	Needs assistance in going to the bathroom, using toilet, cleaning self, arranging clothes, or returning, or does not go to the bathroom to relieve bladder or bowel (0 points).
Continence	Controls bladder and bowel completely (without occasional accidents) (1 point).
	Occasionally loses control of bladder and bowel (0 points).
	Needs supervision to control bladder or bowel, requires use of a catheter, or is incontinent (0 points).

*The maximum score is 6. Declining scores over time reveal deterioration.

Table 2. Lawton Instrumental Activities of Daily Living Scale

Activity	Item	Score*
Can you prepare your own meals?	Without help;	2
	With some help; or	1
	Are you completely unable to prepare any meals?	0
Can you do your own housework or handyman work?	Without help;	2
	With some help; or	1
	Are you completely unable to do any housework?	0
Can you do your own laundry?	Without help;	2
	With some help; or	1
	Are you completely unable to do any laundry?	0
Do you or can you take prescribed drugs?	Without help (i.e., correct doses at the correct time);	2
	With some help (i.e., someone prepares the drug and/or reminds you to take it); or	1
	Are you completely unable to take prescribed drugs without help?	0
Can you get to places beyond walking distance?	Without help;	2
	With some help; or	1
	Are you completely unable to travel unless special arrangements are made?	0
Can you go shopping for groceries?	Without help;	2
	With some help; or	1
	Are you completely unable to do any shopping?	0
Can you manage your own money?	Without help;	2
	With some help; or	1
	Are you completely unable to manage money?	0
Can you use the telephone?	Without help;	2
	With some help; or	1
	Are you completely unable to use the telephone?	0

* The maximum score is 16. Declining scores over time reveal deterioration.

Inquire about alcohol, drugs, and tobacco use. The risk of falling asleep while smoking in bed is increased in the elderly, who should be warned against this practice. The CAGE screening questionnaire identifies patients at risk for alcohol dependence. Exercise type and amount are important and are determined in the interview.

The type, quantity, and frequency of food eaten, including the number of hot meals per week, are determined. Any special diets are noted. The intake of alcohol, dietary fiber, daily intake of water, and all vitamins and minerals are also determined. The patient's ability to eat (e.g., chewing, swallowing) is assessed. Reduced vision and decreased taste or smell may cause anorexia.

Family history is guided toward discovering disorders that may affect the patient in late life (e.g., diabetes, cancer, Alzheimer's disease). Ask about frequency of social contacts, family visits, community support groups, availability of caregivers, and family support. Have the patient describe a typical day, including activities such as reading, television watching, work, exercise, hobbies, and interactions with others.

There is a strong relationship between spirituality and health observed in the elderly. Religious involvement has been related to lower rates of hypertension, stroke, coronary artery disease, survival after open heart surgery, and even longevity. Determine the frequency of church attendance (of any religious group) which may influence coping abilities and recovery from illness.

The patient's wishes regarding measures for prolonging life, such as intubation, use of mechanical devices, and cardiac resuscitation are discussed and documented. The possession of a living will or the desire to create one is determined.

A sexual history should encompass sexual interest, activity, and function. If sexual dysfunction is present, ascertain the symptoms and onset, duration, and severity. Determine whether the problem is associated with medical illnesses, habits, medications or substance abuse, or is psychological. Rapid onset of sexual dysfunction suggests psychogenic causes or medication effects, whereas a more gradual onset suggests the presence of medical illnesses. Decreased libido suggests hormonal deficiencies, psychogenic causes, or medication effects.

Physical Examination

Normal aging changes should be considered while evaluating an elderly patient. For example, respiratory rate may be as high as 16-25/min; respiration rate >25/min may signal a lower respiratory tract infection, heart failure, or another disorder before other symptoms become obvious. Unexplained bruises may signal elderly abuse. An important part of the evaluation of an elderly patient is to offer preventive care, appropriate for the patient's age and sex.

Assessment of Cognitive Function and Mood

The most frequently used and most extensively studied screening test is the Mini-Mental State Examination. Scores <24 points (out of a possible 30) are highly correlated with cognitive loss (www .hospitalmedicine.org/geriresource/toolbox/howto.htm). Many other screening instruments can be used to identify elderly with early cognitive impairment. The most sensitive tool for assessing impairment of short-term memory is the three-word recall. The clock drawing test is useful to evaluate cognitive deterioration over time.

Early identification of patients with dementia, particularly Alzheimer's disease, is increasingly important as more treatment and palliative interventions become available. The diagnosis of dementia may be accompanied by psychiatric symptoms, such as visual and auditory hallucinations, delusions, and behavioral changes and their occurrence are explored.

Evaluation of depression is extremely important in the elderly patient because it is a well-known risk for many other diseases, including dementia. It is a treatable disorder, and successful management can have a positive impact on the quality of life for both the patient and the caregiver. The Geriatric Depression Scale (the Yesavage scale) and the Hamilton scale are the most commonly used screening tests. Most late-onset depressions emerge in the context of a chronic medical illness, particularly neurologic illness.

Assessment of Gait

A major goal of functional assessment is to promote and maintain an elderly person's independence. Gait, including mobility and balance, is assessed. The Tinetti balance and Gait evaluation is a very useful instrument for this assessment.

The "Get Up and Go" test is appropriate for screening because it is a quantitative evaluation of general functional mobility. Persons are timed in their ability to rise from a chair, walk 10 feet, turn, and then return to the chair. Most adults can complete this task in 10 seconds, and most frail elderly persons, in 11 to 20 seconds. Those requiring >20 seconds are referred to physical medicine and rehabilitation for comprehensive evaluation. A strong association exists between performance on this test and a person's functional independence in activities of daily living.

The Performance-Oriented Mobility Assessment (POMA) scale evaluates mobility and balance. This test requires 15 to 20 minutes. Patients are asked to perform a series of gait, mobility, and balance tasks while raters assign either dichotomous or quality-graded scores. Lower scores are predictive of increased risk for falls.

Assessment of Incontinence

Ask the patient and/or caregiver about incontinence. If not asked directly, most patients will not volunteer this information. Normal bladder filling and emptying require accommodation of increased bladder volumes at a low intravesicular pressure, a bladder outlet that is closed at rest and remains closed during increased abdominal pressure, and the absence of involuntary bladder contractions. Age-related physiologic changes leading to incontinence are associated with decline in bladder capacity, decrease in urethral closing pressure, uninhibited detrusor contractions, loss of elasticity of the bladder tissue, increased prostate size with outlet obstruction in men, and pelvic muscle laxity in women. The basic clinical evaluation of patients with such symptoms includes a history and physical examination, urinalysis, and serum creatinine and plasma glucose measurement. Having patients with urinary incontinence record in a diary the frequency, timing, and amount of voiding for 24 to 72 hours helps categorize incontinence as urge, stress, or overflow (Table 3). Total incontinence refers to continuous loss of urine with minimal activity. Functional incontinence refers to that caused by mental or physical activities that impede normal voiding or the ability to get to the toilet. A rectal examination is useful in identifying fecal impaction, rectal masses, and sphincter tone. In men, evaluating the prostate gland for hyperplasia or a mass is appropriate, as is evaluation of the urethra. In women, a pelvic examination may identify signs of atrophic vaginitis, pelvic prolapse, cystocele, or rectocele. Reversible conditions associated with incontinence are summarized by the mnemonic DIAPPERS (*d*elirium, *i*nfection of the urinary tract, *a*trophic urethritis/ vaginitis, *p*harmaceuticals, *p*sychologic disorders [especially depression], *e*xcessive urine output [associated

Table 3. Types of Urinary Incontinence

Type	Notes*
Urge incontinence, overactive bladder dysfunction	Characteristics: daytime frequency; nocturia; bothersome urgency. Pathophysiology: involuntary contraction of the bladder; decreased control of the detrusor muscle; decreased competence of the urethral sphincter in men. Therapy: biofeedback; bladder training; anticholinergics; oxybutynin; tolterodine.
Stress incontinence	Characteristics: involuntary release of urine secondary to effort or exertion (e.g., sneezing, coughing, physical exertion). Pathophysiology: pelvic muscle laxity; nerve injury, or urologic surgery; poor intrinsic sphincter function. Therapy: Pelvic floor muscle training for women (Kegel); biofeedback; electrical stimulation; open retropubic colposuspension; suburethral sling procedure.
Overflow	Characteristics: associated with overdistension of the bladder. Pathophysiology: underactive detrusor muscle or outlet obstruction. Therapy: pelvic floor muscle training with biofeedback in early postprostatectomy period; external penile clamp.

* Tricyclic antidepressants are an off-label treatment for urge incontinence. α-Adrenergic agonist midodrine is an off-label treatment for stress incontinence.
Modified from Medical Knowledge Self-Assessment Program (MKSAP) 14. Philadelphia: American College of Physicians; 2006.

with heart failure or hyperglycemia], restricted mobility, and stool impaction).

Socio-Environmental Situation

An adequate evaluation includes information about the caregiver and the patient's ability to finance adequate nutrition and medical treatment. The availability of social support groups, environmental safety, and special requirements due to specific disabilities are explored. A reliable informant is required for many geriatric patients. Common types of abuse in the elderly include physical, psychological, and financial abuse, and neglect. Any sign of elderly abuse should be explored, documented, and reported to adult protective services.

Assessment of the Elderly Driver

Although older drivers do not have high overall rates of motor vehicle crashes, they are involved in more fatalities and crashes per mile driven than any other age group except those aged 16 to 24 years. Any report of an accident or moving violation involving an elderly patient should trigger an assessment of the person's driving capacity. In addition, patients with known cognitive losses, limitations in movement of the neck or extremities, cardiac arrhythmias, or a history of falls should be considered as high risk and require closer evaluation. All patients who drive should be routinely asked about recent accidents or moving violations. The ability of a mildly demented person to drive satisfactorily can be markedly increased with an appropriate "co-pilot," thus preserving the mobility and self-esteem of the patient as well as the public safety.

Book Enhancement

Go to www.acponline.org/essentials/general-internal-medicine-section.html to access the Confusion Assessment Method tool, Geriatric Depression Scale, Nutrition Checklist for Older Adults, and review a table of nutritional syndromes and cause of memory loss. In *MKSAP for Students 4*, assess yourself with item 58 in the **General Internal Medicine** section.

Bibliography

American College of Physicians. Medical Knowledge Self-Assessment Program 14. Philadelphia: American College of Physicians; 2006.

Fleming KC, Evans JM, Weber DC, Chutka DS. Practical functional assessment of elderly persons: a primary-care approach. Mayo Clin Proc. 1995;70:890-910. [PMID: 7643645]

Holroyd-Leduc JM, Tannenbaum C, Thorpe KE, Straus SE. What type of urinary incontinence does this woman have? JAMA. 2008;299:1446-56. [PMID: 18364487]

Chapter 37

Hypertension

Thomas M. DeFer, MD

Hypertension is extremely common, often asymptomatic for many years, and may result in serious and sometimes mortal complications. Less than one-third of patients with hypertension in the U.S. are adequately controlled. More than 90% of cases are essential (idiopathic), due to diverse multiple factors, such as environmental influences, salt sensitivity, renin, cell membrane defects, insulin resistance, and genetic effects. Hypertension is secondary when there is an identifiable specific structural, biochemical, or genetic defect causing the increased blood pressure (Table 1).

Prevention

Therapeutic lifestyle changes should be instituted in all patients at risk for hypertension or with prehypertension (Table 2). Therapeutic lifestyle changes include weight loss to <20% above ideal body weight, sodium reduction to ≤2400 mg/day, exercise, and alcohol intake ≤2 ounces/day. Dietary recommendations include fresh fruits and vegetables, low/non-fat dairy products, low saturated/total fat, cholesterol, and sodium.

Screening

Early detection of hypertension is essential in reducing stroke, coronary artery disease, peripheral vascular disease, chronic kidney disease, and retinopathy. Screen all patients at every office visit by performing office sphygmomanometry using an appropriate-sized cuff and proper technique.

Diagnosis

The diagnosis is established by documenting office systolic blood pressure ≥140 mm Hg and/or diastolic blood pressure ≥90 mm Hg, based on the average of two or more readings obtained on each of two or more office visits. Hypertension can be diagnosed on the basis of elevated systolic blood pressure even if the diastolic blood pressure is normal (i.e., isolated systolic hypertension).

Perform ambulatory blood pressure monitoring when white coat hypertension (elevated blood pressure only in the office) is suspected or if the diagnosis is uncertain. Self-recorded measurements are not sufficiently valid for making treatment decisions.

Table 1. Causes of Secondary Hypertension

Condition	Notes
Drug induced	Nonsteroidal anti-inflammatory drugs; amphetamines/cocaine; sympathomimetics (e.g., decongestants, dietary supplements); oral contraceptives; corticosteroids.
Chronic kidney disease (see Chapter 57)	Elevated BUN, creatinine, and potassium; low calcium; elevated phosphate; anemia. These are late manifestations of renal failure; most patients present at an earlier stage, with minimal signs and symptoms.
Renovascular disease (atherosclerotic and fibromuscular)	Onset of hypertension at young age, especially in women (fibromuscular). Atherosclerotic disease is often associated with cigarette smoking; flash pulmonary edema; coronary artery disease; flank bruits; advanced retinopathy; increased creatinine (usually with bilateral renovascular disease), increase in creatinine after treatment with angiotensin-converting enzyme inhibitor or angiotensin receptor blocker.
Aortic coarctation	Headache, cold feet, leg pain; reduced or absent femoral pulse, delay in femoral compared with radial pulse, murmur heard between scapulae. "3-sign" on chest radiography.
Hypercalcemia (see Chapter 59)	Primary hyperparathyroidism is the most common cause in outpatients. Hypercalcemia and elevated parathyroid hormone; 20% have (inappropriately) normal parathyroid hormone levels.
Thyroid disease (see Chapter 10)	Hyperthyroid: sweating, tachycardia, weight loss, tremor, hyperreflexia. Hypothyroid: cold intolerance, weight gain, goiter; slowed reflexes.
Primary hyperaldosteronism (see Chapter 11)	Muscle cramping, nocturia, thirst. Physical examination normal; hypokalemia.
Cushing syndrome (see Chapter 11)	Weight gain, menstrual irregularity, hirsutism; truncal obesity, abdominal striae; hypokalemia, metabolic alkalosis, increased cortisol (urine or blood).
Pheochromocytoma (see Chapter 11)	Sweating, heart racing, pounding headache; pallor; tachycardia; hypertension may be worsened during secretion, or episodic with intervals of normal blood pressure; increased urine or plasma catecholamines or metanephrine.

BUN = blood urea nitrogen; PTH = parathyroid hormone.

Table 2. Classification of Blood Pressure in Adults

Classification	SBP (mm Hg)		DBP (mm Hg)
Normal	<120	*and*	<80
Prehypertension	120-139	*or*	80-90
Stage 1 hypertension	140-159	*or*	90-99
Stage 2 hypertension	≥160	*or*	≥100

SBP = systolic blood pressure; DBP = diastolic blood pressure.

Cardiovascular risk correlates directly with blood pressure stage, beginning at 115/75 mm Hg and doubles with each 20/10 mm Hg increment. In persons >50 years old, systolic blood pressure ≥140 mm Hg is a much more important cardiovascular risk factor than diastolic blood pressure. Determine the presence of additional cardiovascular risks including smoking, obesity, inactivity, dyslipidemia, diabetes mellitus, microalbuminuria or estimated glomerular filtration rate <60 mL/min, increased age, and family history of premature cardiovascular disease. Risk factors increase the risk for a cardiovascular event additively.

The history and physical exam can help determine the likelihood of secondary hypertension and target organ damage and whether other cardiovascular risk factors are present. A history of myocardial infarction, angina, heart failure, stroke, transient ischemic attack, renal disease, and claudication are evidence of target organ damage. Physical findings include retinopathy, cardiac findings consistent with ischemia/infarction/failure, bruits, neurologic signs consistent with stroke, and diminished or absent peripheral pulses.

Obtain the following studies in all patients: hematocrit, glucose, creatinine, electrolytes, urinalysis, fasting lipid profile, and electrocardiogram. Urinalysis showing blood and/or protein may indicate renal damage or the presence of secondary hypertension. The urinary albumin/creatinine ratio can also be used to guide treatment. An electrocardiogram showing left ventricular hypertrophy and/or signs of previous infarction is evidence of cardiovascular damage. While echocardiography is more sensitive at diagnosing ventricular hypertrophy, it is not recommended in all patients. Specific lab testing is usually needed to confirm the presence of secondary hypertension suspected from the history or physical exam.

Some patients present with severe elevations of blood pressure (>210/120 mm Hg). The clinical criteria for hypertensive emergency are markedly elevated blood pressure with symptoms/signs of acute target organ damage. Hypertensive urgency consists of critically elevated blood pressure without acute end organ damage.

Therapy

Therapeutic lifestyle changes should be instituted in all patients with hypertension and prehypertension. Use therapeutic lifestyle changes for 6 to 12 months as the sole therapy for stage 1 hypertension without target organ damage or evidence of cardiovascular disease. Therapeutic lifestyle change is continued even if drug therapy becomes necessary. Modifiable risk factors should be treated. Although relieving stress may lower blood pressure, no controlled trials have shown persistent effects.

Initial drug therapy is dictated by the degree of hypertension, risk level, specific patient factors, and compelling indications. Drug therapy is appropriate for stage 1 hypertension when therapeutic lifestyle changes have failed and is initiated immediately in conjunction with lifestyle changes for stage 2 hypertension. The general treatment goals are <140/90 mm Hg for most patients and <130/80 mm Hg for patients with diabetes or renal disease. Hypertension (including isolated systolic hypertension) in the elderly is treated according to the usual guidelines. Older patients experience greater stroke benefit from antihypertensive drug therapy.

Thiazide diuretics, angiotensin-converting enzyme (ACE) inhibitors, angiotensin-receptor blockers (ARBs), and calcium-channel blockers may all be considered for initial treatment of hypertension, and all reduce the complications of hypertension. Thiazide diuretics are the initial choice in most patients. This is particularly true in African Americans and the elderly who have a greater tendency to be sodium sensitive. Calcium-channel blockers are also relatively more effective in these groups. Diuretics equalize the response of African Americans to ACE inhibitors and ARBs. For patients with chronic kidney disease and a creatinine >1.5 mg/dL or glomerular filtration rate <30-50 mL/min, loop diuretics are preferred. Short-acting loop diuretics, such as furosemide, must be given more than once a day. ACE inhibitors and ARBs are similarly efficacious but the latter cause less cough.

Without compelling indications, β-blockers are generally no longer considered first-line treatment due to the lack of data supporting an independent effect on morbidity and mortality. The vasodilating β-blockers (e.g., labetalol and carvedilol) may be preferable to more conventional β-blockers (e.g., propranolol and atenolol). The latter have been associated with an increased rate of stroke and risk of developing diabetes. α-Blockers are not as effective as diuretic therapy and should not be used as monotherapy for hypertension. Direct renin inhibitors (e.g., aliskiren) are new agents that effectively lower blood pressure but lack outcome data.

Achievement of goal blood pressure often requires two or three antihypertensives. The typical decrease in blood pressure to a single agent is 12-15 mm Hg systolic and 8-10 mm Hg diastolic. Therefore, initiate therapy with a combination of antihypertensive medications in untreated stage 2 hypertension.

Compelling indications (Table 3) for certain antihypertensive agents include coronary artery disease or heart failure, stroke, diabetes, and chronic kidney disease, particularly with proteinuria. In these instances, the preferred agents are used first and continued regardless of whether additional agents are needed to control the blood pressure. In patients with hypertension and coronary artery

Table 3. Compelling Indications, Contraindications, and Side Effects for Antihypertensive Drugs

Class of Drug	Compelling Indications	Contraindications	Side Effects
Diuretics	Heart failure; advanced age; systolic hypertension	Gout	Hypokalemia; hyperuricemia; glucose intolerance; hypercalcemia; hyperlipidemia; hyponatremia; impotence
β-Blockers	Angina; heart failure; postmyocardial infarction; tachyarrhythmias; migraine	Asthma and COPD; heart block	Bronchospasm; bradycardia; heart failure; impaired peripheral circulation; insomnia; fatigue, decreased exercise tolerance; hypertriglyceridemia
ACE inhibitors	Heart failure; left ventricular dysfunction; postmyocardial infarction; diabetic nephropathy; proteinuria	Pregnancy; bilateral renal artery stenosis; hyperkalemia	Cough; angioedema; hyperkalemia; rash; loss of taste; leukopenia
ARB	ACE inhibitor cough; diabetic nephropathy; heart failure	Pregnancy; bilateral renal artery stenosis; hyperkalemia	Angioedema (rare); hyperkalemia
Calcium antagonists	Advanced age; systolic hypertension; cyclosporine-induced hypertension; angina, coronary heart disease	Heart block (verapamil, diltiazem)	Headache; flushing; gingival hyperplasia; edema; constipation
α-Blockers	Prostatic hypertrophy	Orthostatic hypotension	Headache; drowsiness; fatigue; weakness; postural hypotension

ACE = angiotensin-converting enzyme; ARB = angiotensinogen receptor blocker; COPD = chronic obstructive pulmonary disease.
Modified from Medical Knowledge Self-Assessment Program (MKSAP) 14. Philadelphia: American College of Physicians; 2006.

disease, β-blockers are the drugs of choice because they decrease cardiovascular mortality. Vasodilating β-blockers improve survival in patients with heart failure. The presence of asthma or chronic bronchitis may limit the use of β-blockers. ACE inhibitors are preferred for asymptomatic ventricular dysfunction and symptomatic heart failure because they decrease cardiovascular mortality. ARBs may be specifically beneficial in patients with left ventricular hypertrophy, compared to β-blockers. Combination ACE inhibitors and thiazide diuretic treatment reduces recurrent stroke rates. ACE inhibitors and ARBs reduce albuminuria and the progression of chronic kidney disease, including diabetic nephropathy. ACE inhibitors produce greater reductions in cardiac morbidity and mortality compared with calcium-channel blockers. An increase in serum creatinine by up to 33% is acceptable and not a reason to discontinue therapy; however, hyperkalemia may limit their use.

Hypertensive emergencies are treated in the hospital setting with parenteral medications (e.g., intravenous nitroprusside) and intensive care unit monitoring. Unless symptoms or progressive target organ damage are present, parenteral drugs are avoided in hypertensive urgencies. Administer one or more rapid-onset oral antihypertensive drugs (e.g., oral clonidine or long-acting calcium-channel blockers); once blood pressure is <180/110 mm Hg, administer a longer-acting formulation and recheck the blood pressure within 48 hours. Avoid short-acting calcium-channel blockers in patients with ischemic heart disease because reflex adrenergic stimulation and tachycardia may lead to myocardial ischemia.

Follow-Up

Follow-up of antihypertensive therapy should be individualized. Uncontrolled hypertension requires more vigilant follow-up, at least monthly until control is achieved. Consider regular home blood pressure measurements in selected patients. Patients should be questioned about medication side effects. If at follow-up there has been a partial response to a submaximal dose of the initial agent, the dosage should be maximized. A second drug from a different class may be added if there is a partial response to otherwise well-tolerated monotherapy. If a thiazide diuretic was not the first choice, use it as the second agent because it provides augmentation to almost any other agent used as monotherapy. If a diuretic was the first choice, add an ACE inhibitor, an ARB, or a calcium-channel blocker. A third or fourth agent can be added if the target blood pressure has not been reached. β-Blockers are reasonable to add as a third or fourth agent when maximal doses of more preferred drugs are insufficient.

Resistant hypertension is blood pressure above goal despite maximal doses of three antihypertensives, one being a diuretic. Important causes include nonadherence, inadequate therapy, excess alcohol consumption, and other drugs (e.g., nonsteroidal anti-inflammatory drugs and sympathomimetics). White coat hypertension may also contribute to the apparent occurrence of refractory hypertension, and ambulatory blood pressure monitoring is useful if suspected. Treatment strategies include addressing potential reasons for resistance. If a typical β-blocker is being used, changing to a vasodilating β-blocker may be helpful. For some patients, combining an ACE inhibitor and an ARB may provide additional blood pressure lowing. The aldosterone antagonists, spironolactone and eplerenone are potentially effective additions for resistant hypertension even in the absence of hyperaldosteronism. The addition of hydralazine or clonidine may be necessary in a few patients. Evaluation for secondary hypertension should be done when the clinical situation is suggestive or if the patient is adherent to a four-drug regimen without adequate control.

Only half of patients who start therapy continue it after 1 year. Using once-a-day therapy, maintaining close contact with patients, encouraging home blood pressure monitoring, and using drugs with fewer adverse effects and lower cost may improve patient adherence. A simple question to assess adherence in a nonthreatening and nonjudgmental manner is, "Most people have trouble remembering to take their medicine. Do you have trouble remembering to take yours?"

Book Enhancement

Go to www.acponline.org/essentials/general-internal-medicine -section.html to access the Framingham Risk Scoring System and a hypertension history checklist, to review the correct steps in blood pressure measurement, to learn ways to increase medication compliance, and to view examples of retinal changes, renal artery stenosis, and electrocardiographic signs of left ventricular hypertrophy. In *MKSAP for Students 4,* assess yourself with items 59-77 in the **General Internal Medicine** section.

Bibliography

Chobanian AV. Clinical practice. Isolated systolic hypertension in the elderly. N Engl J Med. 2007;357:789-96. [PMID: 17715411]

Moser M, Setaro JF. Clinical practice. Resistant or difficult-to-control hypertension. N Engl J Med. 2006;355:385-92. [PMID: 16870917]

Reeves RA. The rational clinical examination. Does this patient have hypertension? How to measure blood pressure. JAMA. 1995;273:1211-8. [PMID: 7707630]

Section V
Hematology

Chapter 38

Anemia

Reed E. Drews, MD

Anemia is commonly encountered in daily clinical practice. Often identified incidentally in asymptomatic patients, anemia can be "benign" or related to serious underlying disease. It has a wide differential diagnosis, including congenital and acquired disorders. Distinguishing the many causes of anemia and determining management are guided by a structured approach, which considers red cell morphology alongside other clinical and laboratory findings.

Because the life span of normal red blood cells approaches 120 days, nearly 1% of circulating red cells must be replenished daily to maintain a normal hematocrit. Normal hematopoiesis, as well as heightened production during bleeding or hemolysis, requires a healthy bone marrow microenvironment, healthy hematopoietic stem cells, endogenous growth factors (e.g., erythropoietin, thyroid hormone, and testosterone in the case of males), and ample and usable body stores of iron and vitamins (folate and cobalamin).

Defining Anemia

Anemia is defined as a reduction below normal in the number of red blood cells in the circulation. Men have higher mean hematocrit and hemoglobin values than women, largely due to testosterone production in men and borderline iron stores in menstruating women. Hematocrit and hemoglobin levels have wide normal ranges, and changes in plasma volume can influence these measurements considerably, either by hemodilution or hemoconcentration. For example, in pregnant women, red blood cell mass rises; however, plasma volume increases to a greater extent. Pregnant women therefore develop lower hematocrit and hemoglobin levels (physiologic anemia). The World Health Organization defines anemia as hemoglobin <13 g/dL in men and <12 g/dL in women.

Measuring Anemia

Multi-channel automated analyzers assess directly the red blood cell count, mean cell volume (MCV), red cell distribution width (RDW; the degree of variation in red cell size), and hemoglobin level (the concentration of hemoglobin in whole blood after lysing red cells) while calculating hematocrit, mean cell hemoglobin (MCH), and mean cell hemoglobin concentration (MCHC) from these measurements. Automated analyzers may yield spurious values in certain clinical circumstances (e.g., high leukocyte counts, lipemia, precipitating monoclonal proteins, cold agglutinins, hyperglycemia), and this should be suspected when measured hemoglobin levels do not approximate one-third the calculated hematocrit.

Clinicians should evaluate red blood cell measurements alongside leukocyte counts, platelet counts, and leukocyte differentials. Abnormalities in these other bloodlines may suggest a disorder of trilineage hematopoiesis. Reticulocyte counts suggest whether or not the bone marrow responses to anemia are adequate. Appropriately increased reticulocyte counts (>100,000/μL) almost always reflect either red blood cell loss (e.g., bleeding or hemolysis) or response to appropriate therapy (e.g., iron, folate, or cobalamin). A lower-than-expected reticulocyte count indicates underproduction anemia, including deficient erythropoietin, nutritional deficiencies (e.g., iron, folate, cobalamin), inflammatory block, or a primary hematopoietic disorder (e.g., red cell aplasia or myelodysplasia). Examination of the peripheral blood smear for morphologic features of red blood cells, leukocytes, and platelets may provide important clues to the etiology of the anemia (Table 1). Results of various blood chemistries (Table 2) help to refine or confirm diagnostic considerations suggested by the CBC, reticulocyte count, and peripheral blood smear.

Diagnosis

Anemias due to red blood cell underproduction generally develop and progress slowly over weeks to months. In contrast, anemias due to bleeding or hemolysis generally occur rapidly over days to weeks. Because anemia may be hereditary rather than acquired, knowledge of family history of anemia is useful when considering congenital and acquired causes, as well as acquired contributors to worsened congenital anemia (e.g., thalassemia).

While symptoms and signs can offer important clues to the etiology of anemia, physical examination is often normal or nonspecific. Consideration of anemia categorized by red blood cell size and other morphologic abnormalities can supplement the history and physical examination. These categories include the microcytic (MCV <80 fL), normocytic (MCV 80-100 fL), and macrocytic (MCV >100 fL) anemias.

Microcytic Anemia

Factors to consider in the differential diagnosis of microcytic anemia include reduced iron availability, globin chain production, and/or heme synthesis (Table 3). Deficiency in one or more of these will result in hypochromic, often microcytic, anemia. Severe iron deficiency and inflammation reduce iron availability. Reduced globin production characterizes the thalassemias

Table 1. Peripheral Blood Smear Findings and Associated Conditions

Finding	Association
Cigar-shaped and pencil–thin-shaped red cells	Iron deficiency anemia
Small target cells, teardrop cells, and basophilic stippling	Thalassemia
Coarse basophilic stippling	Sideroblastic anemia
Rouleau formation	Monoclonal protein, cold agglutinin, or increased fibrinogen (as in acute phase reaction)
Spherocytes	Membrane loss as in hereditary spherocytosis and immune hemolytic anemia
Schistocytes	Fragmentation hemolysis, as in micro- or macro-angiopathic hemolytic anemias (e.g., disseminated intravascular coagulation, thrombotic thrombocytopenia purpura, malfunctioning native or mechanical heart valves)
Bite cells	Oxidative hemolysis, which may be due to unstable hemoglobins or potent oxidants (with or without glucose-6-phosphate dehydrogenase or pyruvate kinase deficiencies)
Parasites (e.g., malaria, *Babesia*)	Inside red cells a cause of hemolysis
Teardrop cells, nucleated red cells, and immature myeloid forms	Myelophthisic anemia, also known as leukoerythroblastic anemia

Table 2. Laboratory Tests in Anemia Evaluation

Laboratory Test(s)	Roles in Anemia Evaluation
Absolute reticulocyte count ([RBC count × reticulocyte count]/100)	Values >100,000/μL signify increased erythropoiesis and shifts in reticulocyte pools from bone marrow to peripheral blood compatible with bleeding, hemolysis, or response to treatment.
Folate and cobalamin (vitamin B_{12}) levels	Low levels characterize vitamin B_{12} or folate deficiency anemia.
Serum iron, TIBC, and ferritin	Low serum iron and high TIBC (iron/TIBC <10%-15%) characterize iron deficiency without inflammation (low ferritin). Low serum iron and low TIBC characterize anemia of inflammation (normal to high ferritin). Caveat: 20% of patients with "anemia of inflammation" have iron/TIBC <10%.
Serum transferrin receptor concentration	Elevated in the setting of increased erythropoiesis or iron deficiency. If hemolysis or ineffective erythropoiesis is excluded, an elevated serum transferrin receptor concentration suggests iron deficiency.
ESR, fibrinogen, haptoglobin, and CRP	Increased levels indicate acute-phase reaction due to inflammatory cytokines, which decrease EPO production, decrease responsiveness to EPO, and block iron transport.
Serum creatinine	High levels signify underproduction of EPO, which is manufactured primarily by the kidneys.
EPO	Should rise logarithmically above normal levels in relation to decreasing hematocrit. Levels >500 U/mL predict poor response to recombinant EPO administration.
TSH	Assess possible hypothyroidism, which may cause anemia.
Testosterone	Assess possible hypotestosteronism in men, which may cause anemia.
LDH, bilirubin, and haptoglobin	Haptoglobin levels <20 ng/mL indicate hemolysis, supported by elevated LDH and total bilirubin levels.
Urinary hemosiderin and hemoglobin	Presence support intravascular hemolysis.
SPEP, UPEP, quantitative immunoglobulins	Hypogammaglobulinemia, positive serum monoclonal proteins, and urinary free kappa or lambda light chains suggest possible plasma cell myeloma or lymphoma.

RBC = red blood cell; TIBC = total iron binding capacity; ESR = erythrocyte sedimentation rate; CRP = C-reactive protein; EPO = erythropoietin; TSH = thyroid stimulating hormone; LDH = lactate dehydrogenase; SPEP = serum protein electrophoresis; UPEP = urine protein electrophoresis.

and other hemoglobinopathies. Certain toxins (e.g., alcohol, lead) and drugs (e.g., chloramphenicol, isoniazid) reduce heme synthesis, which is also a characteristic of the congenital and acquired idiopathic sideroblastic anemias.

Iron Deficiency

The most common cause of microcytic anemia is iron deficiency, usually related to menstrual or gastrointestinal blood loss or malabsorption syndromes. Hypochromia (decreased MCHC) is the first morphologic sign of iron deficiency, followed by microcytosis (decreased MCV). As hemoglobin levels decline, red cells become heterogeneous in shape (anisocytosis) (Plate 28). Pica, a craving for ice or other unusual substances (e.g.,

clay or cornstarch), is symptomatic of iron deficiency and quickly disappears with iron replacement. In men and postmenopausal women with iron deficiency, evaluation of the gastrointestinal tract for a source of blood loss is mandatory. In premenopausal women, evaluation also includes gynecologic examination. Chronic intravascular hemolysis with loss of iron in the urine is an uncommon cause of iron deficiency. Partial or total gastrectomy leads to decreased production of hydrochloric acid and diminished iron absorption.

Serum ferritin levels are the most useful test in the diagnosis of iron deficiency. However, because ferritin is an acute-phase reactant, it has less diagnostic value in patients with infection or inflammatory disorders. Virtually all patients with serum ferritin levels <10-15 ng/mL are iron deficient. However, 25% of menstruating

Table 3. Differential Diagnosis of Microcytic Anemia

Disease	Notes
Iron deficiency anemia	Anemia with hypochromia, microcytosis, and increased RDW. Usually due to menstrual or GI blood loss; less commonly, celiac disease or chronic intravascular hemolysis. Serum ferritin concentration and transferrin saturation usually low; serum transferrin receptor concentration usually increased. Search for a source of chronic blood loss.
α-thalassemia trait	Mild anemia with normal RDW due to homozygous single α-globin gene deletion or heterozygous double α-globin gene deletion. Seen in individuals of African, Mediterranean, Middle Eastern and Southeast Asian ancestry. Normal serum ferritin concentration and transferrin saturation. On electrophoresis, normal percentage of hemoglobin A_2 and hemoglobin F. Usually a diagnosis of exclusion.
β-thalassemia trait	Mild anemia with normal RDW due to reduced expression of β-globin gene. Seen in individuals of African, Mediterranean, Middle Eastern and Southeast Asian ancestry. Normal serum ferritin concentration and transferrin saturation. On electrophoresis, increased percentage of hemoglobin A_2 (3.6%-8%) and normal to slightly increased percentage of hemoglobin F (1%-3%).
β-thalassemia intermedia	Hemoglobin 7-10 g/dL due to reduced but not absent expression of both β-globin genes. Typically, there is evidence of ineffective erythropoiesis with a low serum haptoglobin and increased levels of indirect bilirubin and LDH in the setting of normal reticulocyte count and increased iron stores. Increased serum ferritin concentration and transferrin saturation. On electrophoresis, increased percentage of hemoglobin A_2 (5.4%-10%) and hemoglobin F (20%-80%).
Sickle-β+ thalassemia	Seen in persons of African, Middle Eastern, Mediterranean, or Indian ancestry. Serum ferritin and transferrin saturation usually normal. Hemoglobin electrophoresis shows predominantly hemoglobin S but also variable amounts of hemoglobin A (5-30%); hemoglobin A_2 increased (>3.5%); hemoglobin F normal to variably increased (2-10%).

GI = gastrointestinal; LDH = lactate dehydrogenase; RDW = red cell distribution width.

women with absent stainable bone marrow iron have ferritin levels >15 ng/mL. Assuming absence of inflammation, higher ferritin cutoff limits of 30-41 ng/mL improve diagnostic efficiency. Soluble transferrin receptor (STR), a truncated fragment of the membrane receptor that is increased in iron deficiency when availability of iron for erythropoiesis is low, is not significantly different from normal in inflammation. Therefore ratios of STR to log ferritin may be used to distinguish anemia of inflammation (where the ratio of STR to log ferritin is < 1) from iron deficiency anemia, either alone or in combination with anemia of inflammation (where ratios of STR to log ferritin are >2).

The treatment of choice for iron deficiency is almost always an oral iron preparation. Iron salts, such as ferrous sulfate, are preferred over iron polysaccharide complexes. Ascorbic acid enhances absorption of iron, while certain dietary substances, calcium, and inhibitors of gastric acid secretion decrease iron absorption. Treatment should be continued for 6 months to 1 year until hemoglobin levels and iron stores return to normal.

Anemia of Inflammation

Inflammatory cytokines block iron utilization, yielding low serum iron and total iron binding capacity levels, and high ferritin levels. Cytokines increase serum ferritin levels by as much as 3-fold. Hence, serum ferritin levels <100 ng/mL may reflect iron deficiency in patients with inflammatory states. Reticulocyte counts are inappropriately low for the degree of anemia. Bone marrow biopsies are generally not indicated unless competing causes of anemia are suspected (e.g., pure red cell aplasia, sideroblastic anemia or other myelodysplastic syndromes).

The management of anemia of inflammation is treatment of the underlying inflammatory condition. When symptomatic anemia persists despite treatment of the chronic condition (e.g.,

rheumatoid arthritis), administration of recombinant human erythropoietin can improve anemia with diminished need for red blood cell transfusion.

Thalassemia

Thalassemias are congenital disorders of imbalanced globin chain production or synthesis of abnormal globin chains. Microcytic, hypochromic red blood cells in thalassemic states are accompanied by target and teardrop cells, and basophilic stippling (Plate 29). Although patients with thalassemia trait can develop iron deficiency, this is less likely among patients with severe thalassemia where iron overload is a concern, particularly in patients who have had frequent blood transfusions. Folic acid supplementation is a supportive therapy in all patients with thalassemia. However, other treatments vary according to the severity of the thalassemia. Patients with thalassemia trait do not require specific therapy. Patients with more severe thalassemia often require blood transfusions to maintain growth, manage symptomatic anemia, and to prevent complications of extramedullary hematopoiesis. Iron chelation therapy prevents and manages iron overload. Hydroxyurea may benefit patients with beta-thalassemia intermedia. Hematopoietic stem cell transplantation is an established treatment for severe beta-thalassemia.

Macrocytic Anemia

First assess the reticulocyte count and rule out stress erythropoiesis, as in bleeding or hemolysis. Reticulocytes are larger than senescent red cells; consequently, increased reticulocyte numbers elevate the MCV but generally not above 110 -115 fL. Macrocytic anemias may be non-megaloblastic or megaloblastic (Table 4).

Table 4. Differential Diagnosis of Megaloblastic Anemia (Macrocytosis, Hypersegmented Neutrophils, Macroovalocytes)

Disease	Notes
Folate deficiency	Morphologically indistinguishable from vitamin B_{12} deficiency and drug-induced megaloblastosis. Inquire about excessive alcohol use, quality of diet, history of small bowel disease. Do serum antibody test for celiac disease (anti–tissue transglutaminase).
Vitamin B_{12} deficiency	Morphologically indistinguishable from folate deficiency. Loss of vibration or position sense favors vitamin B_{12} deficiency. However, neurologic disease due to vitamin B_{12} deficiency may occur without anemia or macrocytosis.
Drug-induced changes in erythrocytes	Numerous drugs prescribed for cancer, HIV infection, psoriasis, lupus, rheumatoid arthritis, and immunosuppression in transplant patients cause macrocytic and sometimes megaloblastic changes in erythrocytes. History should be revealing. See Web enhancement for list of drugs that commonly cause macrocytosis (www.acponline.org/essentials/hematology-section.html).
Erythroleukemia	Erythroleukemia is a morphologic diagnosis based on marrow study. Characterized by normal or high serum vitamin B_{12}. Cytogenetic abnormalities are present in about half of cases.

Table 5. Differential Diagnosis of Hemolytic Anemia*

Disease	Notes
Membrane defect (e.g., hereditary spherocytosis, hereditary elliptocytosis)	Suspected due to family history, splenomegaly, and spherocytes or elliptocytes on smear. Confirmed by osmotic fragility (and negative) direct Coombs' test.
Enzymopathies (G6PD and pyruvate kinase deficiency)	Common forms of G6PD deficiency usually have only episodic moderate hemolysis, precipitated by oxidant drugs or infection. Variable blood smear findings include bite cells, spherocytes, rarely fragments, and often little erythrocyte abnormality other than polychromasia (from reticulocytosis). Pyruvate kinase deficiency is rare with moderately severe anemia, with acanthocytes.
Hemoglobinopathies (hemoglobins S and C, thalassemias, and hereditary unstable hemoglobins; see Chapter 40)	Chronic or episodic hemolysis. Hemoglobin A_2 levels are increased with β-thalassemias (hemoglobin F may be). No structural hemoglobin abnormality is detectable with α-thalassemias; these are diagnosed based on hematocrit, MCV, smear, and family study. Abnormal hemoglobins such as E and D are uncommon in the United States. Blood smear changes suggest certain hemoglobinopathies; hemoglobin electrophoresis reveals the abnormal hemoglobin.
Autoimmune hemolytic anemias (AIHA) (warm and cold)	Spherocytes on the blood smear; erythrocyte agglutination is seen with cold agglutinin disease. Confirmed by direct and indirect Coombs' tests, and cold agglutinin titer. Most cases of warm AIHA are associated with an underlying disorder (i.e., systemic lupus and lymphoproliferative disorders, or drug-induced). Cold AIHA is direct Coombs' positive for C3 and is also frequently associated with underlying disorders including transient postinfectious (i.e., *Mycoplasma pneumoniae*) and systemic lupus.
Erythrocyte fragmentation syndromes (TTP, HUS, DIC; see Chapter 41)	TTP usually presents with neurologic symptoms and severe fragmentation anemia and thrombocytopenia. With HUS (children), renal abnormalities predominate and anemia and thrombocytopenia are milder. In other causes of microangiopathic anemia, the anemia and thrombocytopenia are usually mild to moderate; these disorders include DIC, malignant hypertension, and scleroderma renal crisis and are diagnosed by peripheral blood smear in the proper clinical context.
Infections (malaria, babesiosis)	Symptoms of infection, particularly fevers, usually dominate. Splenomegaly is the rule with malaria; babesiosis produces a usually milder malaria-like illness unless patients are asplenic. Finding intraerythrocyte parasites on blood smear is diagnostic.
Hypersplenism (see Chapter 22)	Splenomegaly of any etiology can cause hemolysis; hypersplenism may also lower leukocytes, platelets, or any combination of cell lines. Hypersplenism produces no erythrocyte morphologic changes, but the smear may show changes related to the underlying etiology (e.g., target cells with liver disease).

*Go to www.acponline.org/essentials/hematology-section.html to see examples of peripheral blood smears illustrating findings associated with these conditions.
AIHA = autoimmune hemolytic anemia; DIC = diffuse intravascular coagulation; G6PD = glucose-6-phosphate dehydrogenase; HS = hereditary spherocytosis; HUS = hemolytic uremic syndrome; TTP = thrombotic thrombocytopenic purpura.

Hemolysis

When laboratory assessments suggest hemolysis (see Table 2), consider cause by type (spherocytic or non-spherocytic), site (intramedullary or extramedullary; intravascular or extravascular), and mechanism (immune-mediated or non-immune-mediated; intrinsic versus extrinsic to the red cell). For example, spherocytic hemolytic anemia implicates a membrane defect, either acquired as in warm autoimmune hemolytic anemia or congenital as in hereditary spherocytosis. Non-spherocytic hemolytic anemias include bite cell hemolysis (as in oxidant stress) and fragmentation hemolysis (as in thrombotic microangiopathies). Intramedullary hemolysis is seen in a variety of disorders associated with ineffective erythropoiesis, including thalassemia. Extramedullary hemolysis may be extravascular (as in hemolysis mediated by the spleen) or intravascular (as in hemolysis associated with cold agglutinin disease or thrombotic microangiopathies). Immune-mediated hemolysis is distinguished by the Coombs' test. Hemolytic disorders "intrinsic" to the red cell include membrane defects, enzymopathies, and hemoglobinopathies. Table 5 summarizes various causes of hemolytic anemia. In all cases, examining the peripheral blood smear is central to identifying red cell morphologies that implicate certain hemolysis mechanisms (see Table 1).

In oxidant hemolysis, a by-product is methemoglobin (containing ferric ions), which has altered spectrophotometric properties from hemoglobin (containing ferrous ions). As a consequence, patients with methemoglobinemia have PaO_2 values (reflecting the total concentration of oxygen in blood) that appear higher than expected in relation to the percent oxygen saturation (which specifically reflects the percent of oxygen bound to hemoglobin containing ferrous ions).

Megaloblastic Macrocytosis

Macroovalocytes suggest megaloblastic maturation of red cells; hypersegmented neutrophils may also be present (Plate 30). Etiologies (see Table 4) include folate and/or cobalamin deficiencies, drugs affecting folate metabolism and/or DNA synthesis, and acquired idiopathic causes of megaloblastic maturation such as the myelodysplastic syndromes. MCVs >115 fL are almost always due to megaloblastic causes. Because megaloblastic causes of anemia impact trilineage hematopoiesis, leukopenia and thrombocytopenia may accompany anemia.

Patients with macrocytic anemia or specific neurologic symptoms should be screened for vitamin B_{12} deficiency. However, the MCV should not be used as the only indication to exclude vitamin B_{12} deficiency. Elevated serum levels of methylmalonic acid and homocysteine support B_{12} deficiency in patients with slightly low or borderline serum B_{12} levels (100-300 pg/mL). Daily oral vitamin B_{12} can be used to treat most cobalamin-deficient patients. "Time-release" formulations are avoided because they may not reliably release their vitamin B_{12} content.

Non-Megaloblastic Macrocytosis

Large target cells (MCV 105-110 fL) and echinocytes (spur cells with multiple undulating spiny red cell membrane projections) signify membrane changes associated with liver disease. Diminished splenic function (hyposplenism or asplenia) yields large target cells, acanthocytes (red cells with only several rather than multiple spiny membrane projections), Howell-Jolly bodies, and variable numbers of nucleated red blood cell.

Normochromic Normocytic Anemia

When MCV is normal (80-100 fL), assessing whether it is declining or rising over time may provide clues to evolving microcytic or macrocytic pathologies. Other etiologies of normocytic anemia (Table 6) include underproduction of erythropoietin, as in

Table 6. Differential Diagnosis of Normocytic Anemia

Disease	Notes
Acute blood loss	Anemia with variation in erythrocyte size (increased RDW) if iron deficient; increased reticulocyte count; the leukocyte count and platelet count may be slightly increased depending on the rapidity of bleeding.
Chronic renal failure (see Chapter 57)	Anemia with a low reticulocyte count due to impaired erythropoietin production. Renal endocrine function does not correlate with renal exocrine function.
Pure red cell aplasia	Anemia with severe reticulocytopenia. Diagnosis made by examination of a bone marrow aspirate in which erythroblasts will be absent or severely diminished. Red cell aplasia can be idiopathic or secondary to a thymoma, a solid tumor, a hematologic malignancy, a collagen-vascular disease, viral infections and, in particular, parvovirus B19 infection, which is common in immunosuppressed patients such as those with AIDS or those taking immunosuppressive drugs, and in patients with a hemolytic anemia from any cause. Drugs such as phenytoin, azathioprine, isoniazid, chloramphenicol, and mycophenolate mofetil have caused red cell aplasia.
Malignancy (solid tumors, lymphomas, myelofibrosis)	Anemia with a low reticulocyte count. With bone marrow involvement by tumor, leukoerythroblastosis and extramedullary hematopoiesis occur, and nucleated erythrocytes and myelocytes are seen in the peripheral blood. If there is a plasma cell dyscrasia, rouleaux formation may be present on the peripheral blood smear. If there is splenomegaly, teardrop-shaped erythrocytes will be present.
Alcoholic liver disease	Anemia with a low reticulocyte count. Target cells and acanthocytes may also be present. If there is portal hypertension with splenomegaly, the leukocyte and platelet counts will be reduced, although thrombocytopenia in liver disease is chiefly due to underproduction of thrombopoietin by the liver.
Anemia of inflammation (chronic disease)	A normocytic, but sometimes microcytic, anemia that occurs in association with another disease, usually infectious, inflammatory, and neoplastic disorders that are characterized by distinct abnormalities of iron metabolism: low serum iron and transferrin with reduced transferrin saturation and a normal or elevated serum ferritin and normal or increased bone marrow iron stores.
Hemolytic anemia	Anemia with an elevated reticulocyte count and spherocytes, sickled cells, blister cells, or fragmented erythrocytes. There may be hemoglobinuria. If reticulocyte count is sufficiently elevated, the MCV may be high. The serum haptoglobin level will be low whether the hemolysis is intravascular or extravascular, and if the hemolysis is antibody-mediated, the direct Coombs' test result will be positive. The essential laboratory test is the peripheral blood smear, which can distinguish between the different types of erythrocyte hemolysis: spherocytic hemolytic anemias, erythrocyte enzyme defects, erythrocyte fragmentation syndromes, cold agglutinin disease, hemoglobinopathies, heavy metal intoxication, and paroxysmal nocturnal hemoglobinuria. Urine hemoglobin and urine hemosiderin measurements are useful for detecting intravascular hemolysis.

AIDS = acquired immunodeficiency syndrome; ESR = erythrocyte sedimentation rate; HIV = human immunodeficiency virus; MCV = mean corpuscular volume; RDW = red cell distribution width.

renal failure; inflammation; other deficient growth factors (e.g., thyroid hormone and testosterone); or marrow infiltrative myelopathies, which yield tear drop, nucleated red cells and immature leukocytes. Except for acute blood loss, the most common cause is the anemia of inflammation. Aplastic anemia, a rare cause of normocytic normochromic anemia, is usually accompanied by severe granulocytopenia and thrombocytopenia due to deficient hematopoietic stem cells.

Book Enhancement

Go to www.acponline.org/essentials/hematology-section.html to see peripheral blood smears depicting iron deficiency, schistocytes, spherocytosis, megaloblasts, target cell, bite cells, sickle cells, acanthocytes, a list of drugs that can cause macrocytosis, and algorithms to help you assess macrocytic and microcytic anemia. In *MKSAP for Students 4*, assess yourself with items 2-13 in the **Hematology** section.

Bibliography

Bain BJ. Diagnosis from the blood smear. N Engl J Med. 2005;353:498-507. [PMID: 16079373]

Gordeuk VR. Microcytic Anemia. http://pier.acponline.org/physicians/diseases/d897. [Date accessed: 2008 Jan 8] In: PIER [online database]. Philadelphia: American College of Physicians; 2008.

Schilling RF. Macrocytic Anemia. http://pier.acponline.org/physicians/diseases/d896. [Date accessed: 2008 Jan 8] In: PIER [online database]. Philadelphia: American College of Physicians; 2008.

Spivak JL. Normocytic Anemia. http://pier.acponline.org/physicians/diseases/d895. [Date accessed: 2008 Jan 8] In: PIER [online database]. Philadelphia: American College of Physicians; 2008.

Chapter 39

Bleeding Disorders

Diane C. Sliwka, MD

Bleeding disorders are characterized by defects in primary and secondary hemostasis. Primary hemostasis involves the formation of a platelet plug at the site of vascular disruption, a process that begins with adhesion of platelets to exposed subendothelial matrix. Adhesion is mediated through interactions of specific platelet receptors, such as the collagen receptor and the platelet glycoprotein Ib-IX-V complex, which binds von Willebrand's factor with the subepithelial matrix. Adhesion induces platelet activation, with attendant platelet shape change, secretion of platelet alpha and dense granules, and exposure of fibrinogen receptors that mediate platelet aggregation through binding of the dimeric fibrinogen molecule to adjacent platelets. Platelet activation also leads to rearrangement of membrane phospholipid, with increased expression of anionic phospholipid on the platelet surface and the release of platelet microparticles. Anionic phospholipid provides a surface that supports secondary hemostasis. Secondary hemostasis is initiated by the exposure of tissue factor at the site of vascular damage; tissue factor binds activated factor VII and activates factor X and factor IX. Activated factor IX, in turn, activates additional factor X leading to the generation of thrombin and cleavage of fibrinogen to form fibrin (Figure 1).

Approach to the Patient

Detailed bleeding history includes duration, frequency, timing, and sites of bleeding. Blood transfusion history, family history, medications (e.g., aspirin, clopidogrel, nonsteroidal anti-inflammatory drugs [NSAIDs], warfarin), and medical history (e.g., liver disease, uremia, poor nutrition, antibiotic use) provide clues to etiology and bleeding risk.

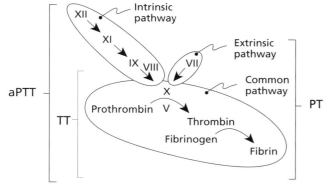

Figure 1 Coagulation cascade.

A mucocutaneous bleeding pattern is the hallmark of primary hemostasis. Epistaxis, gingival bleeding, easy bruising, and menorrhagia are characteristic. Persistent oozing after an injury is common because the initial platelet plug is not formed. Secondary hemostasis is characterized by bleeding into muscles and joints. Delayed bleeding is common because the platelet plug gradually succumbs to the pressures of blood flow without reinforcement from a strong fibrin mesh. Excessive bleeding after childbirth, surgery, or trauma can occur in either category.

The prothrombin time (PT) and the activated partial thromboplastin time (aPTT) are screening assays designed to detect clotting factor deficiencies as well as inhibitors that interfere with effective fibrin clot formation (Table 1). Factor levels <35% are needed to prolong the PT and aPTT, and reliance on these tests alone underestimates bleeding risk. A mixing study differentiates factor deficiency from factor inhibitor by mixing patient plasma with normal plasma (factor deficiencies correct with mixing). Bleeding time identifies disorders of platelets and vessel wall integrity. Thrombin time tests the conversion of fibrinogen to fibrin. Fibrinogen, fibrinogen degradation products, and D-dimer are used to identify excessive fibrinolysis.

Disorders of Primary Hemostasis

Disorders of primary hemostasis include abnormalities of platelets or the vascular endothelium. Thrombocytopenia affects bleeding time when platelet count is <100,000/µL, but spontaneous bleeding does not occur until platelet count is <10,000-20,000/µL. Dysfunction of platelet adhesion occurs in von Willebrand's disease and Bernard-Soulier syndrome. Platelet activation can be limited due to drugs such as aspirin, clopidogrel, and NSAIDs, or in uremia due to kidney disease. Ehlers-Danlos syndrome, Marfan's syndrome, and hereditary hemorrhagic telangiectasia are associated with blood vessel abnormalities affecting hemostasis.

Von Willebrand's Disease

The most common inherited bleeding disorder is von Willebrand's disease (vWD), an autosomal dominant disorder that occurs in an estimated 1:100 to 1:400 people. Clinically, patients have mild-to-moderate bleeding evidenced by nosebleeds, heavy menstrual flow, gingival bleeding, easy bruising, and bleeding associated with surgery or trauma.

Von Willebrand's factor (vWF) functions to adhere platelets to injured vessels and as a carrier for factor VIII. Secondary hemostatic dysfunction can occur due to low factor VIII levels in vWD; this distinction is important for treatment purposes. Diagnostic

Table 1. Causes of Prolonged Prothrombin Time, Partial Thromboplastin Time, Thrombin Time, and Bleeding Time

Prolonged Laboratory Test	Causes
Prothrombin time	Warfarin, factor VII deficiency or inhibitor, vitamin K deficiency (nutritional or antibiotic related), and liver disease
Partial thromboplastin time	Heparin, lupus anticoagulant (predisposes to thrombosis), von Willebrand disease, factor VIII, IX, XI, XII deficiency or inhibitor
Combined prothrombin and partial thromboplastin time	Supratherapeutic doses of heparin or warfarin; DIC (PT prolonged first); liver disease; factor V, X, prothrombin, or fibrinogen deficiency or inhibitor; warfarin and direct thrombin inhibitors
Thrombin time	Heparin, direct thrombin inhibitors, fibrin degradation products, low or high fibrinogen levels
Bleeding Time	Thrombocytopenia (<100,000/µL), platelet dysfunction, von Willebrand disease

DIC = disseminated intravascular coagulation; PT = prothrombin time.

Table 2. Laboratory Abnormalities in Hemophilia, von Willebrand's Disease, and Platelet Function Defects

Test	Hemophilia	vWD	Platelet Function Defect
vWF antigen	Normal	Decreased	Normal
Factor VIII	Decreased	Decreased or normal	Normal
vWF activity (ristocetin cofactor)	Normal	Decreased or normal	Normal
Bleeding time, PFA-100 analysis, platelet aggregation	Normal	Increased	Increased

vWD = von Willebrand's disease; vWF = von Willebrand factor; PFA = platelet function analyzer.
From Medical Knowledge Self-Assessment Program (MKSAP) 14. Philadelphia: American College of Physicians; 2006.

testing includes bleeding time, vWF antigen level, vWF activity assay, factor VIII level, and a multimer study used to diagnose subtypes of vWD (Table 2). Desmopressin releases stored vWF from endothelium and is the first line of therapy for vWD. Intermediate-purity factor VIII concentrates, which contain vWF, can also be given. Cryoprecipitate is rich in vWF but carries transfusion infection risk.

Disorders of Secondary Hemostasis

Disorders of secondary hemostasis are characterized by deficiencies of coagulation factors. These include inherited hemophilias, liver disease, vitamin K deficiency, antibodies, and consumptive processes such as disseminated intravascular coagulation. Medications such as warfarin, heparin, low-molecular-weight heparin, and direct thrombin inhibitors (e.g., argatroban, lepirudin) also interfere with secondary hemostasis (Table 3).

The Hemophilias

Factor VIII (hemophilia A) and factor IX (hemophilia B) deficiency are X-linked disorders with clinical manifestations seen almost exclusively in males. The frequency of hemophilia A is about 1:10,000 and less for hemophilia B. All daughters of patients with hemophilia are obligate carriers, whereas all sons are normal. Sons of carrier mothers have a 50% chance of having hemophilia, and daughters have a 50% chance of being carriers. The spontaneous mutation rate is 3%. Fibrinogen and factor II, V, VII, X, and XI deficiencies are usually autosomal recessive disorders and are rare in comparison.

Hemophilia A and B are classified as mild, moderate, or severe according to the baseline level of clotting factor. Patients present in childhood with muscle hematomas, hemarthroses, and persistent delayed bleeding after trauma or surgery. Mild hemophilia can be missed until adulthood. Assessing factor VIII and IX levels is indicated in any male who presents with a prolonged aPTT that corrects with a mixing study (see Table 1).

Factor VIII and IX deficiency are treated with factor replacement (recombinant or purified). Fresh frozen plasma is a diluted source of clotting factors with limited efficacy for high-level replacement.

Liver Disease

Hepatic dysfunction causes bleeding because the liver synthesizes almost all the hemostatic proteins (exceptions are vWF and tissue plasminogen activator). PT is a sensitive indicator of hepatic synthetic function due to the short half life of factor VII (6 hours), which the failing liver cannot maintain. Both PT and aPTT prolong with more severe hepatic synthetic dysfunction. Fresh frozen plasma transiently replaces all coagulation factors but is short-lived. Desmopressin may help by improving platelet function, and vitamin K administration excludes concurrent vitamin K deficiency.

Vitamin K Deficiency

Clotting factors II, VII, IX, and X as well as protein C and protein S require vitamin K–dependent gamma-carboxylation for full activity. Dietary vitamin K is obtained primarily from the intake of dark green vegetables and is modified by gut flora to the active

Table 3. Differential Diagnosis of Prolonged Screening Coagulation Tests Not Caused by Disseminated Intravascular Coagulation

Disease	Notes
Liver failure	Most coagulation factors are produced in the liver. Liver failure will cause a global coagulation factor deficiency and prolongation of PT and aPTT. Platelet count is normal unless cirrhosis (with hypersplenism) is present.
Vitamin K deficiency	May be due to dietary deficiency, impaired intestinal absorption, or derangement of intestinal vitamin K-producing bacterial flora. Leads to decreased levels of vitamin K-dependent coagulation factors. Mild deficiency produces prolongation of only PT; severe deficiency affects both PT and aPTT.
Massive blood loss	Insufficiently compensated loss of coagulation factors may be seen in massive bleeding with transfusion of red cells without concomitant transfusion of plasma, and the laboratory picture may be difficult to differentiate from that of DIC. FDP or D-dimer levels may be normal in the early phase of trauma.
Use of unfractionated heparin or vitamin K antagonists	Heparin prolongs the aPTT (and only slightly the PT), whereas vitamin K-antagonists (e.g., warfarin) prolong both PT and aPTT. Note that LMWH has no effect on aPTT. Platelet count is normal.
Inhibiting antibody, phospholipid antibody, or both	Autoimmune disorder causing antibody-mediated destruction of a coagulation factor. Diagnosed by mixing test in which there is lack of normalization of coagulation times after mixing patient plasma with normal plasma (1:1).

aPTT = activated partial thromboplastin time; DIC = disseminated intravascular coagulation; FDP = fibrinogen degradation product; LMWH = low-molecular-weight heparin; PT = prothrombin time.

form. Interruption of bile flow prevents absorption of vitamin K. Antibiotic-related elimination of enteric bacteria limits intestinal sources of vitamin K, whereas warfarin directly antagonizes vitamin K activity.

PT is first to prolong, but the aPTT will also lengthen with further factor deficiencies. In adults with normal hepatic function, oral or subcutaneous vitamin K usually corrects the clotting times within 24 hours; intravenous vitamin K has an increased risk of anaphylaxis. Fresh frozen plasma is used when urgent correction is required.

Antibodies to Blood Clotting Factors

Antibodies directed against clotting factors are rare but potentially lethal acquired bleeding disorders. Most such antibodies are considered idiopathic, but they may develop due to drugs or as part of an underlying illness such as malignancy or autoimmune disorders (e.g., systemic lupus erythematosus, rheumatoid arthritis). Diagnosis is made by a protracted clotting time that does not correct with a mixing study. Quantifying the inhibitor by obtaining an inhibitor titer helps determine treatment options. Causes include use of fibrin sealants during procedures, antiphospholipid antibodies, and antibiotics. General principles of therapy for such disorders include nonspecific immunosuppression with corticosteroids, targeted immune suppression such as rituximab (anti-CD 20 monoclonal antibody), immune globulin administration, and removal of inhibitors through plasma exchange.

Disseminated Intravascular Coagulation

The syndrome of disseminated intravascular coagulation (DIC) involves a complex series of events initiated by a systemic illness (e.g., sepsis, trauma, malignancy) manifesting with thrombosis and hemorrhage. Thrombosis is initiated by tissue factor stimulated thrombin activation. As antithrombin III is consumed, thrombin is left unopposed, leading to extensive intravascular fibrin formation and organ thrombosis.

As platelets and coagulation factors are consumed, the balance shifts toward a bleeding diathesis. This includes hemorrhage into damaged tissues and ineffective thrombus formation at new sites of injury. DIC manifests clinically with hematuria, hemoptysis, oozing at mucosal surfaces, and bleeding at puncture sites.

The usual screening tests for DIC include a platelet count, PT, aPTT, fibrinogen, and D-dimer. Treatment of the instigating disease process remains the only successful therapy; other measures are supportive. Platelet transfusions are indicated for platelet count <10,000-20,000/μL and cryoprecipitate transfusions for fibrinogen levels <100 mg/dL. Heparin is used in certain clinical situations, particularly when DIC is associated with acute promyelocytic leukemia, but effectiveness has not been shown in clinical trials.

Book Enhancement

Go to www.acponline.org/essentials/hematology-section.html to use a table to guide the evaluation of hemophilia A and B; to distinguish between von Willebrand's disease, hemophilia, and platelet disorders; and to view the mucocutaneous manifestations of hereditary hemorrhagic telangiectasias. In *MKSAP for Students 4*, assess yourself with items 14-15 in the **Hematology** section.

Bibliography

Drews RE. Critical issues in hematology: anemia, thrombocytopenia, coagulopathy, and blood product transfusions in critically ill patients. Clin Chest Med. 2003;24:607-22. [PMID: 14710693]

Chapter 40

Sickle Cell Anemia

Reed E. Drews, MD

The sickle mutation is a single base change (GAT → GTT) in the sixth codon of exon 1 of the β-globin gene, resulting in replacement of the normal glutamic acid with valine at position 6 of the β-globin polypeptide. As a consequence of this single amino acid substitution, deoxygenated hemoglobin S heterotetramers polymerize to form fibrils, causing red blood cells to sickle and hemolyze (Plate 31). Sickle cells, forming in the relatively hypoxic regions of tissues, impede blood flow in the microvasculature and promote vaso-occlusion, resulting in profound, often disabling complications, including acute pain (crises), chronic pain, and organ dysfunction or failure (Table 1). The prevalence of sickle cell trait varies widely worldwide and may be as high as 50% in certain regions, affecting individuals of African, African-American, Hispanic, Mediterranean, Asian, and Asian-Indian descent. Among persons of African ancestry, sickle cell anemia is one of the most common genetic diseases; about 10% are carriers of the sickle gene and 1:600 newborn black infants have sickle cell anemia.

Screening

The goal of newborn screening is to identify infants with sickle cell anemia early and to treat them for 5 years with prophylactic penicillin (or a macrolide if there is sensitivity to penicillin), which has been shown to reduce both mortality and morbidity from pneumococcal infections in infants with sickle cell anemia and sickle-β-thalassemia. Abnormal hemoglobin may be identified in white people; most reports indicate that universal screening is more cost effective than targeted screening. For possible future primary prevention, counseling the family of the affected infant should initiate screening of other family members, especially the parents.

Diagnosis

Sickle cell anemia is inherited in an autosomal manner. If both parents carry sickle hemoglobin or other abnormal hemoglobin, there is a 25% risk that the fetus of each pregnancy will have sickle cell anemia or another sickle cell syndrome. Prenatal diagnosis with therapeutic abortion is an option for preventing sickle cell anemia or other sickle cell syndromes. However, clinicians must offer family and genetic counseling to ensure that the parents fully understand the prenatal diagnosis, its complications, and possible outcome, including abortion.

Most patients with sickle cell anemia experience manifestations of the disease in childhood, even as early as 6 months of age. Aspects of the medical history that support the possibility of sickle cell anemia or a related hemoglobinopathy include recurring episodes of acute pain, chronic pain, and symptoms and signs of anemia and its sequelae with organ dysfunction or failure (see Table 1). The average hemoglobin level of patients with sickle cell anemia is 7-8 g/dL; the anemia is normocytic normochromic with high reticulocyte counts from stress erythropoiesis and chronic hemolysis. Microcytic hypochromic indices suggest sickle-β-thalassemia or co-inherited α-thalassemia. High platelet and leukocyte counts relate to asplenia due to auto-infarction.

Hemoglobin electrophoresis both at alkaline pH (cellulose acetate) and acidic pH (citrate agar) distinguishes most different structural variants of hemoglobin. High hemoglobin F levels are associated with less severe disease. Elevated hemoglobin A_2 levels signify the presence of β-thalassemia. Knowledge of the molecular lesion of a patient with sickle cell anemia may predict disease severity, assist family counseling and planning, and guide use of aggressive therapeutic modalities (e.g., allogeneic bone marrow transplantation).

Additional laboratory testing documents organ dysfunction caused by sickle cell anemia. Urinalysis and creatinine levels identify patients with proteinuria and renal failure. In patients who have received multiple transfusions, indirect antibody testing detects alloantibodies relevant to future transfusions, while liver enzymes, viral hepatitis serologies, and serum iron chemistries identify patients who have contracted viral hepatitis and/or developed iron overload. Pulmonary hypertension, correlating with older age and prior history of the acute chest syndrome, is the most common abnormality on echocardiogram with electrocardiography demonstrating signs of right ventricular hypertrophy or strain (marked right axis deviation, tall R wave in V_1, delayed precordial transition zone with prominent S waves in leads V_5 and V_6, inverted T waves and ST depression in V_1 to V_3, and peaked P waves in lead II due to right atrial enlargement). Physical examination findings associated with sickle cell disease are summarized in Table 2.

Therapy

Relaxation and biofeedback methods, cognitive coping strategies, and self-hypnosis are techniques that reduce emergency department visits, hospital admissions, hospital days, and analgesic use. Goals of these interventions are to improve quality of life by increasing activity and enhancing normal function and to decrease dependence on opioid analgesics.

Supplemental oxygen should be used only in the presence of demonstrated hypoxia (pulse oximetry <92% or PaO_2 ≤70 mm Hg). For severe symptomatic anemia or acute organ failure,

Table 1. Major Complications of Sickle Cell Anemia

Complication	Notes
Acute chest syndrome (ACS) vs. pneumonia, fat embolism, VTE (venous thromboembolism)	• ACS correlates with risk of pulmonary hypertension and is the most frequent cause of death. Associated with chlamydia, mycoplasma, respiratory syncytial virus, coagulase-positive *S. aureus, S. pneumoniae, Mycoplasma hominis*, parvovirus, and rhinovirus infections (in decreasing order of frequency). • Pneumonia is usually a localized infiltration, whereas ACS is usually characterized by diffuse pulmonary infiltrates. Cultures of bronchial washings or deep sputum are usually positive in pneumonia. • Fat embolism presents with chest pain, fever, dyspnea, hypoxia, thrombocytopenia, and multiorgan failure. Fat embolism is a component of ACS and is usually associated with acute painful episodes. It is best differentiated by the presence of fat bodies in bronchial washings or in deep sputum and by multiorgan involvement (e.g., stroke, renal failure). • Presence of lower extremity thrombophlebitis may differentiate VTE from ACS, but in some cases pulmonary arteriography may be needed. Newer contrast agents may be safer than hypertonic contrast agents, which precipitate intravascular sickling.
Avascular necrosis	Involves hips and shoulders; may require surgery. More common in sickle cell-α-thalassemia than in other sickle cell syndromes.
Cerebrovascular accidents	Occurs in 8%-17% of patients. Infarction is most common in children; hemorrhage is most common in adults. Brain imaging and lumbar puncture establish the diagnosis.
Cholecystitis vs. hepatic crisis	Chronic hemolysis may result in gallstones and acute cholecystitis. Fever, right upper quadrant pain, and elevated aminotransferase levels may also be due to sickle cell related ischemic hepatic crisis; abdominal ultrasonography can help differentiate.
Dactylitis vs. osteomyelitis	Painful, usually symmetrical, swelling of hands or feet, erythema, and low-grade fever. More common in children before age 5. Osteomyelitis usually involves one bone.
Heart failure	Related to pulmonary and systemic hypertension and ischemia.
Infection	Related to functional asplenia.
Leg ulcers	Most common in HbS disease.
Liver disease	Viral hepatitis and/or iron overload from transfusions and ischemic-induced hepatic crisis.
Pain syndrome vs. myocardial infarction (MI), appendicitis	• Sickle cell pain crisis involving the chest may suggest acute MI. The quality of pain of myocardial infarction (central pressure) is different from that of sickle cell pain (sharp, pleuritic). Serial determination of cardiac enzymes will differentiate the two. • Abdominal pain, fever, and leukocytosis may suggest appendicitis. A high level of lactate dehydrogenase and normal bowel sounds support sickle cell pain syndrome.
Priapism	Prolonged or repeated episodes may cause impotence.
Proteinuria and renal failure	Prevalence of proteinuria and renal failure is approximately 25% and 5%, respectively.
Pulmonary hypertension	Risk of development correlates with increasing age and prior history of acute chest syndrome.
Retinopathy	More common in patients with compound heterozygosity for HbSC.
Sickle anemia vs. aplastic crisis, hyperhemolysis	Anemia that decreases by ≥2 g/dL during a painful crisis could be due to aplastic crisis or hyperhemolysis. Aplastic crisis could be due to coexistent infection (e.g., parvovirus B19), cytotoxic drugs, or idiopathic. Hyperhemolysis could be due to infection (i.e., mycoplasma), transfusion reaction, or coexistent glucose-6-phosphate dehydrogenase deficiency. Reticulocyte count is decreased with aplastic crisis and increased with hyperhemolysis. Bilirubin, lactic dehydrogenase, and aminotransferase levels are elevated in hyperhemolysis.
Splenomegaly and splenic sequestration	Common in children aged <5 years who afterwards manifest asplenia from splenic infarction. Patients with HbSC often have splenomegaly persisting into adulthood.

HbS = hemoglobin S; HbSC = hemoglobin SC.

blood/exchange transfusions improve blood oxygen carrying capacity and microvascular perfusion by diluting circulating sick-led erythrocytes. Exchange transfusions, a pheresis technique that removes the patient's blood while transfusing normal, cross-matched donor blood, should be considered to decrease hemoglobin S levels <30% in managing cerebral infarcts, fat embolism, acute chest syndrome, unresponsive acute priapism, and non-healing leg ulcers. Similarly, an on-going program of exchange transfusions prevents first-time and recurrent strokes in children who are considered at high risk for developing stroke based on trans-cranial Doppler findings or have had a stroke already. To avoid increased blood viscosity, transfusions should not yield hemoglobin levels >10 g/dL. Incidence of iron overload, which

increases morbidity and mortality, is less in patients on blood exchange compared with those on simple blood transfusion. Allogeneic bone marrow transplantation (in patients <16 years of age with severe complications) may cure sickle cell anemia; its success depends on the availability of donors and the severity of the disease of the patient in question (75% -85% event-free survival, 15% graft rejection, and 10% mortality in recipients of HLA-matched donor marrow). Periodic retinal examinations are recommended for monitoring and managing (photocoagulation) progressive proliferative sickle retinopathy.

Effective pain relief is best achieved with combined use of acetaminophen, nonsteroidal anti-inflammatory drugs (NSAIDs), opioids, and adjuvants (antihistamines, antidepressants, and

Table 2. Physical Examination Findings Associated with Sickle Cell Disease

Complication	Notes
Fever	Acute painful episodes are often associated with low-grade fever. If temperature >38.3°C (>101°F), rule out infection.
Pulse	Anemia, infection, and pain are often associated with tachycardia.
Respiratory rate	Respiratory rate is usually 16-20/min in the steady-state. Rate <10/min suggests opioid overdose.
Blood Pressure	Usually low normal. Hypertension increases risk of morbidity and mortality.
Cardiac exam	A systolic murmur due to anemia is common. The absence of a murmur is associated with mild anemia and no cardiomegaly. Increased intensity of the pulmonic component of S2, right-sided murmurs and gallops (increased intensity with inspiration), and prominent A wave in the jugular venous pulse are findings of pulmonary hypertension and right ventricular hypertrophy or strain.
Pulmonary exam	Lungs are usually clear in the steady state. Rhonchi may be heard in patients with history of recurrent ACS. Decreased breath sounds and/or rales in a febrile patient suggest pneumonia or ACS.
Abdominal exam	With age and repeated episodes of sickling, the spleen becomes small, fibrosed, and devoid of any function (autosplenectomy). However, splenomegaly may persist into young adulthood, especially in HbSC, sickle cell-β-thalassemia, or sickle cell-α-thalassemia. Hepatomegaly could be a sign of iron overload or heart failure. Tender hepatomegaly suggests hepatic crisis.
Skin exam	5%-10% of patients develop leg ulcers. Most leg ulcers are located either on the medial or lateral aspect of the ankles.
Neurologic exam	Focal findings suggestive of stroke. Not all patients with history of stroke have residual weakness.

ACS = acute chest syndrome; HbSC = hemoglobin SC.

anticonvulsants). Meperidine is not recommended as opioid therapy, because it is less effective than morphine or hydromorphone and is associated with more side effects (e.g., seizures). NSAIDs should be avoided in patients with renal failure. Patients are hospitalized when severe acute painful episodes do not resolve at home with oral analgesics after 1-2 days or do not resolve or improve significantly after a minimum of 4-6 hours of treatment with parenteral opioids.

Hydroxyurea augments levels of hemoglobin F, which inhibits intracellular polymerization of hemoglobin S; it decreases the incidence of acute painful episodes by approximately 50% in responders, the incidence of acute chest syndrome, and the need for blood transfusion. Follow-up of patients taking hydroxyurea for 9 years showed that hydroxyurea was associated with a 40% reduction in mortality. Despite its myelosuppressive effects, hydroxyurea may improve hemoglobin levels by prolonging red cell survival.

Angiotensin-converting enzyme (ACE) inhibitors prevent progressive renal disease by lowering intraglomerular pressures. Additionally, ACE inhibitors can lower protein excretion and should be used in patients with albuminuria, even in the absence of hypertension. Recombinant erythropoietin stimulates erythropoiesis to achieve hemoglobin levels similar to steady state values (7-9 g/dL) in patients who have renal failure or to limit blood transfusions in patients who are alloimmunized and for whom crossmatch compatible blood is difficult to find. Polyvalent (23-valent) pneumococcal polysaccharide vaccine, *H. influenzae* type b conjugate vaccine, and influenza vaccine prevent infections. Supplemental folic acid prevents folate deficiency (arising from chronic hemolysis) and subsequent elevation of homocystine levels, which may be a risk factor for stroke.

Book Enhancement

Go to www.acponline.org/essentials/hematology-section.html to view a peripheral blood smear of sickled cells, a figure showing dactylitis, and tables of indications for blood transfusion, hemoglobinopathy electrophoresis patterns, and commonly used tests to evaluate patients with sickle cell disease. In *MKSAP for Students 4*, assess yourself with items 16 and 17 in the **Hematology** section.

Bibliography

Ballas SK. Sickle Cell Anemia. http://pier.acponline.org/physicians/diseases/d905. [Date accessed: 2008 Jan 8] In: PIER [online database]. Philadelphia: American College of Physicians; 2008.

Frenette PS, Atweh GF. Sickle cell disease: old discoveries, new concepts, and future promise. J Clin Invest. 2007;117:850-8. [PMID: 17404610]

Chapter 41

Thrombocytopenia

Richard S. Eisenstaedt, MD

Thrombocytopenia occurs through one of two mechanisms: decreased platelet production or accelerated destruction (Table 1). Most disorders that produce thrombocytopenia through inadequate bone marrow production also affect other marrow cell lines and cause additional cytopenias, which include bone marrow injury mediated by toxins (e.g., alcohol), idiosyncratic drug reaction, metastatic cancer, miliary tuberculosis or other infections, deficiency of vitamin B_{12} or folic acid, and bone marrow diseases such as acute leukemia, dysmyelopoietic syndrome, or aplastic anemia. Accelerated peripheral platelet destruction occurs in patients with splenomegaly and hypersplenism or disseminated intravascular coagulation. This chapter focuses on three other causes of accelerated platelet destruction: idiopathic thrombocytopenic purpura (ITP), heparin-induced thrombocytopenia (HIT), and thrombotic thrombocytopenic purpura–hemolytic uremic syndrome (TTP-HUS).

Idiopathic Thrombocytopenic Purpura

Thrombocytopenia in ITP occurs when antibodies targeting platelet antigens mediate accelerated destruction. Antibodies arise in three distinct clinical settings: drug induced, disease associated, and idiopathic.

Almost any drug can trigger platelet-targeted antibody production, but the syndrome is most often linked to quinine or quinidine. Although these drugs are infrequently used, quinine-related

Table 1. Differential Diagnosis of Thrombocytopenia

Condition	Comments
Pseudothrombocytopenia	In vitro clumping of platelets caused by EDTA-dependent agglutinins leads to falsely decreased platelet counts. Excluded by examination of peripheral blood smear.
Decreased Platelet Production	
Vitamin B_{12} and folate deficiency (see Chapter 38)	Associated with pancytopenia, macrocytosis, macro-ovalocytes, hypersegmented neutrophils, and possibly neurological signs.
Bone marrow disorders (e.g., acute leukemia, aplastic anemia, dysmyelopoietic syndrome)	Associated with pancytopenia, abnormal blood smear (e.g., nucleated erythrocytes, tear drop cells, immature neutrophils), and abnormal bone marrow examination.
Toxins/drugs	History of exposure to alcohol, environmental, occupational exposures, or drug. Mechanism may also include accelerated destruction. Often associated with anemia or pancytopenia.
Infection	Thrombocytopenia is seen in HIV, hepatitis B and C, EBV, rubella, disseminated tuberculosis, and other infections. Mechanism may also include accelerated destruction.
Accelerated Destruction	
Immune thrombocytopenia purpura (ITP)	Isolated thrombocytopenia in absence of systemic disease, lymphadenopathy and splenomegaly. Large platelets on peripheral smear and increased megakaryocytes on bone marrow (bone marrow not usually required for diagnosis).
Heparin immune thrombocytopenia	Exposure history. May be associated with modest thrombocytopenia and devastating arterial and venous thrombosis.
Chronic liver disease (see Chapter 22)	Portal hypertension can lead to splenic sequestration of platelets and thrombocytopenia. Liver disease may be associated with target cells. Liver disease may be occult.
Thrombotic thrombocytopenic purpura/ hemolytic-uremic syndrome (TTP/HUS)	TTP is characterized by thrombocytopenia, fever, microangiopathic hemolytic anemia, neurologic symptoms, and renal disease. HUS is characterized by thrombocytopenia, microangiopathic hemolytic anemia, and renal disease. Elevated serum LDH concentration and schistocytes on peripheral blood smear.
Disseminated intravascular coagulation (see Chapter 39)	Typically in setting of sepsis, metastatic cancer, or obstetrical catastrophe. Coagulopathy characterized by an elevated prothrombin time and activated partial thromboplastin time, low fibrinogen, and thrombocytopenia.
HELLP syndrome (hemolysis, elevated liver enzymes, low platelets)	Thrombocytopenia associated with microangiopathic hemolytic anemia, elevated liver enzymes, and hypertension in late pregnancy.
Chronic lymphocytic leukemia (see Chapter 43)	ITP as an autoimmune complication of chronic lymphocytic leukemia.

EBV = Epstein-Barr virus; EDTA = ethylene diamine tetra-acetic acid; HIV = human immunodeficiency virus; ITP = idiopathic thrombocytopenic purpura; LDH = lactate dehydrogenase.

compounds are found in diverse naturopathic or herbal products. A careful drug history, including a review of all prescriptions, over-the-counter drugs, herbs, and supplements, is important to identify the offending agents. Stopping the drug hastens recovery from ITP.

ITP may be part of a broader disease affecting immune regulation, such as HIV infection, systemic lupus erythematosus, and, especially in older patients, lymphoproliferative malignancy. HIV-infected patients may develop ITP before immunosuppression, and opportunistic infections suggest the presence of HIV infection. Therefore screening is warranted in all patients with ITP who have behavioral risks for HIV infection. Recent reports link ITP to *Helicobacter pylori* infection, although platelet count response to antibiotic therapy is unpredictable.

ITP commonly presents as easy bruising or petechial rash. At times, asymptomatic thrombocytopenia is noted on routine blood tests. ITP is a disease of exclusion; the diagnosis is most probable in patients with isolated thrombocytopenia. The leukocyte count should be normal, and the hemoglobin concentration is normal or reduced as a result of blood loss secondary to thrombocytopenia (Table 2). Measurement of platelet-associated antibody is not helpful, because the test lacks both sensitivity and specificity. The physical exam is normal, except for signs of bleeding, most often petechiae, which are punctuate red macular lesions that do not blanch with pressure, on the skin or mucous membranes. Patients may have ecchymoses on the skin or more overt bleeding, especially in the gastrointestinal tract. The presence of fever or hepatosplenomegaly suggests another diagnosis. The blood smear will show decreased platelets and occasional large platelets, or mega-thrombocytes. Bone marrow aspirate, if necessary to exclude other diagnoses, will show increased numbers of megakaryocytes and normal erythroid and myeloid precursors. Hematology consultation is advised in patients with severe thrombocytopenia or uncertain diagnosis.

Patients with ITP require treatment when their thrombocytopenia is severe enough to cause clinical bleeding. Such bleeding is expected when the platelet count is less than 10,000/μL. Both corticosteroids and intravenous gamma globulin (IVIG) are effective therapy, but thrombocytopenia often relapses when treatment is discontinued. In patients with chronic ITP, the risks of prolonged therapy with corticosteroids or IVIG must be balanced against the benefits. Some patients with tolerable bleeding are best managed without immunosuppressive therapy. Rarely, patients with significant bleeding unresponsive to immunosuppressive medication require splenectomy. While platelet counts will improve, perioperative and long-term asplenia complications must be anticipated (i.e., infection with encapsulated bacteria); pneumococcal, meningococcal, and *Haemophilus influenzae* vaccines are administered before splenectomy.

Heparin-Induced Thrombocytopenia

HIT is a unique drug-triggered platelet disorder: 1%-2% of patients receiving unfractionated heparin will develop HIT. The incidence is lower in patients receiving low-molecular-weight heparin. Thrombocytopenia in HIT is modest; mean platelet counts are approximately 60,000/μL, and patients typically do not bleed excessively. To the contrary, patients with HIT have a dramatic risk of thromboembolic complications, including deep venous thrombosis and pulmonary embolism, as well as unusual clotting problems such as portal vein thrombosis or acute arterial occlusion.

The early stages of HIT are asymptomatic; all patients receiving heparin should have periodic screening platelet counts. In patients on heparin who develop thrombocytopenia, laboratory tests will reveal antibodies that cause heparin-induced serotonin release or platelet aggregation, although the clinical circumstances may suggest the diagnosis before confirmatory laboratory data are available.

Heparin must be discontinued and an alternative rapidly acting anticoagulant used instead. Warfarin is not a suitable alternative. Direct thrombin inhibitors, such as lepirudin or argatroban, should be administered, often under a hematologist's guidance.

Thrombotic Thrombocytopenic Purpura–Hemolytic Uremic Syndrome

Patients with TTP-HUS develop consumptive thrombocytopenia and microangiopathic hemolysis from platelet thrombi that form throughout the microvasculature. The multi-system nature

Table 2. Laboratory Tests to Support the Diagnosis of Idiopathic Thrombocytopenic Purpura (ITP)

Test	Notes
CBC	Low platelet count with normal hemoglobin/hematocrit and leukocyte count is evidence for the diagnosis of ITP.
Peripheral blood smear	Exclude platelet clumping (pseudothrombocytopenia). Myeloid and erythroid morphology should be normal. Platelets should appear normal or large in size. Abnormal or immature leukocytes should be absent. The presence of schistocytes is associated with TTP and is evidence against ITP. The presence of polychromatophilia, poikilocytosis, and spherocytes suggests hemolytic anemia. Nucleated erythrocytes should be absent.
Bone marrow aspiration	Consider bone marrow aspiration and biopsy to establish the diagnosis in patients with atypical or nondiagnostic findings or with additional abnormalities on the peripheral blood smear; ITP will show normal or increased numbers of megakaryocytes, normal myeloid and erythroid morphology, and no malignant cells.
HIV antibodies	Indicated in patients with risk factors for HIV.
PT/PTT	Coagulation testing is not recommended for routine diagnosis; however, an abnormal PT or PTT is evidence against ITP.
ANA and other serologic tests	ANA not recommended for routine diagnosis; however, consider ANA and other serologic tests such as rheumatoid factor, complement levels, and anti-DNA in patients with rash, synovitis, arthralgias, or other signs of rheumatologic disease.

ANA = antinuclear antibody; CBC = complete blood count; DNA = deoxyribonucleic acid; HIV = human immunodeficiency virus; PT = prothrombin time; PTT = partial thromboplastin time.

of this syndrome is unpredictable. Fever, renal disease, and fluctuating neurological abnormalities are parts of the syndrome but are seldom all present during earlier phases of the illness. TTP-HUS is a syndrome with diverse triggers and pathophysiology, including abnormal von Willebrand's factor metabolism and very high-molecular-weight polymers that predispose to platelet microthrombi. Some patients with TTP have an autoantibody that inhibits a metalloproteinase (ADAMTS13) that normally cleaves unusually large von Willebrand's factor multimers into smaller fragments. Pregnant women, HIV-infected patients, and patients receiving cancer chemotherapy or immunosuppression following organ transplantation are at increased risk.

Children develop the hemolytic uremic syndrome with prominent gastrointestinal symptoms from Shiga-toxin–producing enteric bacteria such as *E. coli* 0157-H7.

Laboratory findings of a microangiopathic hemolysis, including prominent schistocytes on peripheral blood smear (Plate 32), decreased haptoglobin, and elevated serum lactate dehydrogenase along with thrombocytopenia suggest TTP-HUS syndrome. Assays for ADAMTS13 activity may help to confirm the diagnosis, but the test is neither uniformly standardized nor easily available, and therapy should not be withheld while awaiting test results. Malignant hypertension, disseminated intravascular coagulation, and prosthetic heart valves can be associated with microangiopathic hemolysis, although the additional presence of thrombocytopenia, fever, renal, and neurological findings strongly supports the diagnosis of TTP-HUS.

Treatment consists of plasma exchange and corticosteroids. Platelet transfusions in patients with untreated TTP-HUS are associated with acute renal failure, stroke, and sudden death and are contraindicated.

Book Enhancement

Go to www.acponline.org/essentials/hematology-section.html to view images of petechiae and peripheral blood smears showing platelet clumping and schistocytes, and to access a systematic review on drug causes of thrombocytopenia. In *MKSAP for Students 4*, assess yourself with items 18-22 in the **Hematology** section.

Bibliography

Sekhon SS, Roy V. Thrombocytopenia in adults: A practical approach to evaluation and management. South Med J. 2006;99:491-8; [PMID: 16711312]

Simantov R. Idiopathic Thrombocytopenic Purpura. http://pier.acponline .org/physicians/diseases/d340. [Date accessed: 2008 Jan 11] In: PIER [online database]. Philadelphia: American College of Physicians; 2008.

Chapter 42

Thrombophilia

Patrick C. Alguire, MD

Thrombosis can represent a normal response to injury or an unwanted response to an inciting factor. Factors limiting thrombosis include rapid blood flow and dilution of activated factors, a non-thrombogenic endothelium, inhibitors to coagulation factors, and a fibrinolytic system that degrades fibrin clots. Venous stasis limits blood flow and allows activated factors to accumulate, vascular injury disrupts the endothelium and exposes platelet and coagulation active surfaces, and a defect or deficiency of inhibitors or lytic factors allows coagulation activation to go unchecked. Thrombophilia refers to patients with an increased risk of thrombosis. Thrombophilia risk factors can be congenital or acquired, permanent or transient. They act by disrupting the blood flow, the blood vessel, or the procoagulant/anticoagulant regulatory pathways. In the normally functioning anticoagulant pathway, thrombin bound to thrombomodulin on the endothelial cell surface activates protein C which binds to cofactor protein S on the platelet surface resulting in the degradation of factors V and VII. Antithrombin is another major regulatory protein of the coagulation cascade. It irreversibly binds and neutralizes activated factors II, IX, and X. Genetic amino acid defects or vitamin B_{12} and B_6 deficiency may result in an elevated homocystine concentration, which in turn may result in thrombotic and atherosclerotic reactions. Thrombophilia may also be due to abnormally elevated levels of prothrombin, deficiencies of antithrombin, protein C, the cofactor protein S, thrombomodulin, or an abnormal factor V that cannot be degraded by activated protein C. The evaluation of thrombophilia begins by establishing which risk factors are present (Table 1). A family history is a particularly strong indicator of risk and prompts consideration of congenital disorders.

Until 1993, a genetic cause of thrombophilia was detected in only 5%-15% of patients and was limited to deficiencies of antithrombin, protein C, and protein S. The discovery of two prothrombotic mutations, the factor V-Arg506Gln (factor V Leiden) mutation and the prothrombin G20210A mutation, has greatly increased the percentage of patients in whom a hereditary risk factor is identifiable. The total incidence of an inherited thrombophilia in patients with deep venous thrombosis is approximately 30% compared with about 10% in patients without deep venous thrombosis. The pathogenesis of venous thromboembolism, however, is multifactorial, and more than 90% of persons with the factor V Leiden or the prothrombin G20210A mutations never have a venous thromboembolism (VTE).

Screening

A family history of thrombosis in a first-degree relative has a positive predictive value of only 14% for factor V Leiden, the most

Table 1. Risk Factors For Venous Thromboembolism (VTE)

Disease	Notes
Immobility	Prolonged immobilization (>72 hours) increases the risk for VTE. High risk includes recent stroke with paresis, MI, HF, and pulmonary disease.
Inherited thrombophilia	Family history of thrombosis or thrombophilia; personal history of VTE under age 45, recurrent thrombosis, or thrombosis at an unusual site; personal history of arterial thrombosis under age 50 (MI, stroke); personal history of pregnancy complications (fetal demise, abruption).
Malignancy	Includes solid and hematologic cancers, especially myeloproliferative disorders. Ongoing treatment, palliation, or a diagnosis within the prior 6 months all increase risk. Screen all patients with VTE for malignancy with age- and sex-appropriate screening (e.g., mammograms for women over age 50 and Pap smears for women over age 18); CBC and liver tests; chest x-ray for all smokers. The utility of screening for malignancies, with regard to morbidity and survival, is not known.
Previous thrombosis	Even in the absence of a recognized thrombophilic condition, the risk for VTE increases in any patient with a history of thrombosis.
Surgery	All but minor procedures in the last month represent an increased risk for VTE. Hip, knee, and pelvic surgeries are highest risk.
Trauma	Trauma (especially of the lower limb, with or without plaster immobilization) within the last month increases risk for VTE, especially spinal injuries.
Erythropoiesis stimulating agents	When administered to patients with cancer to treat chemotherapy-associated anemia, erythropoietin and darbepoietin are associated with increased risks of VTE and mortality.

CBC = complete blood count; HF = heart failure; MI = myocardial infarction.

common of the thrombophilias; therefore the clinical utility of thrombophilia screening has been questioned. Nevertheless, some experts believe that the benefits of screening family members of patients with documented hereditary defect can be clinically important to the individual patient, particularly if they are exposed to high-risk situations such as use of birth control pills or initiating hormone replacement therapy.

Diagnosis

Strongly consider the diagnosis of an inherited thrombophilia in:

- VTE in the absence of obvious risk factors (e.g., cancer, prolonged immobility, recent trauma, surgery)
- VTE at age <50 years or in patients who have a positive family history for thrombophilia
- Women with VTE while receiving oral contraceptive pills or hormone replacement therapy, or during pregnancy
- Women who develop myocardial infarction at age <45 years, particularly if cigarette smokers (look specifically for factor V Leiden mutation)
- Women with unexplained complications of pregnancy (e.g., unexplained recurrent miscarriages, stillbirth, intrauterine growth retardation, abruptio placenta, severe preeclampsia)
- Patients at age <50 years with unexplained cerebrovascular accident, ischemic heart disease, or peripheral vascular disease (look specifically for anticardiolipin antibodies, lupus anticoagulant, and hyperhomocystinemia)

Factor V Leiden, prothrombin gene mutations, and hyperhomocystinemia are by far the most common defects; factor V Leiden and prothrombin gene mutations are found almost exclusively in persons of European heritage. The presence of a lupus anticoagulant is suggested by the paradoxical finding of thrombosis associated with a prolonged partial thromboplastin time test.

Avoid testing during an acute episode of thrombosis, because protein levels may be transiently low as a result of consumption. Avoid testing while a patient is taking anticoagulants. In particular, heparin may decrease antithrombin levels or mimic a lupus anticoagulant, and warfarin will decrease protein C and protein S levels. Finally, confirm all test results before assigning a specific diagnosis; laboratory abnormalities can be transient and a single positive test may be unreliable (Table 2).

Therapy

Certain thrombophilias (hyperhomocystinemia, lupus anticoagulant, anticardiolipin antibodies) are associated with increased arterial vascular disease. The combination of smoking and these conditions may increase vascular risk. Dehydration and prolonged immobility are additional risk factors for VTE. Advise all patients to stop smoking and patients at risk to avoid dehydration and prolonged immobility.

Patients with VTE and certain thrombophilias are at especially high risk for recurrent VTE. The benefit of long-term anticoagulation in these high-risk patients may outweigh the risk of bleeding complications. Recommend lifelong therapeutic anticoagulation in patients with VTE and any of the following thrombophilias: lupus anticoagulant, anticardiolipin antibodies, homozygosity for the factor V Leiden mutation, homozygosity for prothrombin gene defect, combined heterozygosity for factor V Leiden mutation and prothrombin gene defect, and antithrombin III deficiency. Provide only temporary prophylactic anticoagulation in all other patients with documented thrombophilias during high-risk situations such as surgery, prolonged immobilization, and pregnancy.

Consider the use of folic acid supplementation, vitamin B_6 supplementation, and oral vitamin B_{12} supplementation in patients with VTE or arterial thrombosis who also have high

Table 2. Laboratory and Other Studies for Thrombophilia

Condition	Test
Activated protein C resistance	95% of activated protein C resistance is due to the factor V Leiden gene mutation; thus, the activated protein C resistance assay is a good screen. False-positive results in pregnancy and oral contraceptive pill use. Confirmed positive test result with testing for the factor V Leiden gene mutation.
Factor V Leiden gene mutation	A direct PCR gene test. Test of choice for activated protein C resistance in patients who are pregnant or receiving estrogen or oral contraceptive pills.
Prothrombin gene mutation	A direct PCR gene test.
Protein C deficiency	Select both antigenic and functional assay. Active thrombosis and use of warfarin may cause false-positive results.
Protein S deficiency	Select both antigenic and functional assay. Active thrombosis, use of warfarin, and pregnancy may cause false-positive results.
Antithrombin III deficiency	Select both antigenic and functional assay. Active thrombosis and use of heparin may cause false-positive results.
Fasting plasma homocysteine level	The risk for thrombosis increases as levels exceed 10 µmol/L. Renal failure and vitamin deficiencies can cause false-positive results. Pregnancy may artificially lower levels.
Lupus anticoagulant	Test with partial thromboplastin time. If prolonged, perform mixing study; mixing with normal plasma will not correct study if lupus anticoagulant is present.
Anticardiolipin antibodies (immunoglobulin G, immunoglobulin M)	ELISA testing. Levels fluctuate; thus, positive tests should be repeated several weeks apart.

PCR = polymerase chain reaction; ELISA = enzyme-linked immunosorbent assay.

plasma homocysteine levels. Hyperhomocystinemia has been implicated in the development of VTE and arterial thrombosis, which may be associated with defects in pathways using these factors or low levels of these vitamins.

Follow-Up

Follow patients with thrombophilias closely for the development of thrombotic events. Do not obtain regular laboratory studies once the diagnosis of a thrombophilia has been established, except in patients who require monitoring of anticoagulant therapy. Do not repeat thrombophilia testing or regular routine blood work in patients in whom a diagnosis of a thrombophilia has already been established. Periodically check platelet levels in patients with anticardiolipin antibodies or lupus anticoagulant, because these individuals may have thrombocytopenia as part of their clinical picture.

Book Enhancement

Go to www.acponline.org/essentials/hematology-section.html to review common sites of thrombosis and recommendations for the duration of anticoagulation therapy for inherited thrombophilias. In *MKSAP for Students 4*, assess yourself with items 23-24 in the **Hematology** section.

Bibliography

Bick RL. Hereditary and acquired thrombophilic disorders. Clin Appl Thromb Hemost. 2006;12:125-35. [PMID: 16708115]

Karovitch A, Rodger M. Thrombophilia. http://pier.acponline.org/physicians/diseases/d647. [Date accessed: 2008 Jan 18] In: PIER [online database]. Philadelphia: American College of Physicians; 2008.

Chapter 43

Common Leukemias

Mark M. Udden, MD

Leukemias are clonal malignant proliferations of hematopoietic cells. They are classified according to their cell of origin as myeloid or lymphoid and by the tempo of their progress as chronic or acute. Chronic lymphoid leukemia and chronic myeloid leukemia are indolent clonal proliferations of lymphoid or myeloid cells accompanied by maturation. Acute myeloid or lymphoid leukemias are aggressive clonal proliferations of myeloid or lymphoid cells without appropriate maturation. Acute lymphoid leukemia, which is more frequent in childhood, will not be discussed here.

Chronic Lymphoid Leukemia

Diagnosis

Chronic lymphoid leukemia (CLL) is the most common leukemia encountered in adults. Patients may be asymptomatic or have non-specific complaints of fever, night sweats, weight loss, fatigue or malaise. Patients with splenomegaly may have early satiety or left upper quadrant pain. Lymphadenopathy, often painless, may be present.

Look for signs of anemia, such as pallor and tachycardia, lymphadenopathy, and hepatosplenomegaly. The key to diagnosis is the recognition of an increased blood leukocyte count due to increased numbers of mature lymphocytes and "smudge" cells (lymphocytes which appear flattened or distorted) on peripheral smear (Plate 33). Bone marrow aspirates and biopsy may be performed to evaluate thrombocytopenia or anemia.

The diagnosis of CLL is confirmed by an absolute increase in mature lymphocytes (>5000/μL). Immunophenotyping by flow cytometry is necessary and will show a mature B cell lymphocyte phenotype with expression of CD19 and CD20 along with expression of a T lymphocyte antigen, CD5.

Staging of CLL requires clinical assessment for lymphadenopathy and enlargement of the liver and spleen. This is complemented by CT scans of chest and abdomen to confirm the extent of lymphadenopathy. Because of the association between warm autoimmune hemolytic anemia and CLL, a direct Coombs' test is obtained in anemic patients and when spherocytes are observed on the peripheral blood smear. Two staging schemes are currently in use: Rai and Binet. Early-stage patients (stage 0, 1, and 2 by the Rai system) require observation only. Later-stage disease (Rai 3 and 4), often associated with symptoms as well as anemia or thrombocytopenia, is usually treated. Specialized testing, such as cytogenetic studies and determination of the mutation status of the V gene for immunoglobulin, is becoming increasingly important in establishing risk for progression.

Therapy

CLL patients are at greater risk for infections than other older adults; pneumococcal vaccination is recommended. Radiation therapy is sometimes used to control painful or bulky lymph nodes. If transfusions are required, provide irradiated blood products to avoid development of transfusion-related graft-versus-host disease. Patients treated with fludarabine are at an increased risk for this complication.

Most symptomatic patients are treated with the purine analog, fludarabine. Patients with very advanced disease are sometimes given a combination of fludarabine, cyclophosphamide, and humanized antibody against CD20 (rituximab). Very young patients are considered for bone marrow transplantation. About 10% of patients will develop autoimmune hemolytic anemia; these patients may respond to chemotherapy for CLL, prednisone, or anti-CD20 treatment.

Follow-Up

Most patients with CLL are elderly, and many never require treatment for their leukemia. Follow the complete blood count periodically to look for a rapid increase in lymphocyte count, anemia, or thrombocytopenia. Patients who have received fludarabine-based treatment are profoundly immunosuppressed and may develop atypical infections such as pneumocystis pneumonia. About 10% of patients experience a transformation of their chronic leukemia to a very aggressive and difficult-to-treat diffuse large-B-cell lymphoma; this is known as *Richter's transformation*.

Chronic Myeloid Leukemia

Diagnosis

Chronic myeloid leukemia (CML) is a clonal proliferation of mature granulocytes associated with a (9;22)(q34;q11) translocation which results in a truncated chromosome 22, the Philadelphia chromosome. Patients usually present in chronic phase and may do well for years. CML may transform into acute leukemia (myeloid in two-thirds of patients, lymphoid in one-third). The transformation may be recognized as an accelerated phase or as blast crisis.

Patients present with fatigue, lethargy, low-grade fever, and weight loss. Splenomegaly may be associated with early satiety, abdominal swelling, or left upper quadrant pain. Physical examination may reveal pallor and splenomegaly, but lymphadenopathy is not common in the chronic phase. Occasional patients will present with leukostasis syndrome: hypoxia, altered mental status, and bleeding associated with very high leukocyte counts.

CML is recognized by an elevated blood leukocyte count and increased number of granulocytic cells in all phases of development on the peripheral blood smear (Plate 34). Very immature cells or blasts represent 1%-5% of the granulocytes, with increasing numbers of promyelocytes, myelocytes, and metamyelocytes. A myelocyte-metamyelocyte "bulge" in the differential count typifies CML. Similar to other myeloproliferative disorders, the basophils and eosinophils are increased. When blasts represent more than 10% of the leukocytes, accelerated or blast phase should be considered.

The diagnosis is confirmed by cytogenetic study of the bone marrow aspirate showing a t(9;22) chromosomal abnormality or the presence of the novel BCR-ABL gene produced by the translocation. The BCR-ABL gene is detected and quantitated by polymerase chain reaction. Patients with abdominal pain or discomfort should undergo abdominal ultrasound or CT scanning to identify splenomegaly or splenic infarct.

Therapy

Occasional patients will require transfusion to treat anemia and rarely for thrombocytopenia. Massive splenomegaly with splenic infarction may require splenectomy for patient comfort. Occasional patients have extramedullary disease that will respond to localized low-dose radiation treatment.

The treatment of CML was revolutionized by the development of therapy targeting the novel tyrosine kinase produced by the BCR-ABL gene. Inhibition of this kinase by imatinib reduces the leukocyte count, shrinks the spleen, and clears the bone marrow of Philadelphia chromosome positive cells. Imatinib treatment often achieves molecular remissions in which no BCR-ABL transcripts can be identified in blood or bone marrow. Imatinib must be given indefinitely; BCR-ABL positive cells will appear 3-4 months after discontinuation of therapy.

Transformation (which is usually lethal) of CML into the accelerated or blast phase is delayed by imatinib therapy. One to two percent of patients per year develop resistance and may require alternative drugs to overcome BCR-ABL mutations that produce kinases not inhibited by imatinib. Patients who are refractory to imatinib or who develop resistance should be considered for allogeneic bone marrow transplantation. Two new tyrosine kinase inhibitors, dasatinib and nilotinib, are effective in treatment of patients who develop resistance to imatinib.

Follow-Up

Patients are typically seen every 1-2 weeks during the initiation of treatment with imatinib. Once stable counts are achieved, patients are followed every month to monitor the blood counts. Peripheral blood or bone marrow samples are obtained periodically to asses the efficacy of treatment; the best results are associated with a four-fold reduction of BCR-ABL transcripts determined by quantitative polymerase chain reaction. Increasing leukocytes, basophilia,

fever, and enlarging spleen are signs of accelerated phase and blast crisis.

Acute Myeloid Leukemia

Diagnosis

Acute myeloid leukemia (AML) is a malignant clonal proliferation of myeloid cells that do not fully mature. AML can appear de novo or arise after exposure to radiation, benzene, or chemotherapy, or occur as a result of transformation of a myeloproliferative disorder, such as CML or polycythemia vera. Myelodysplastic syndromes also have a propensity for transformation into AML. Patients typically become symptomatic over a few weeks or months.

AML presents with nonspecific symptoms of fatigue, pallor, and easy bleeding. Of all the leukemias, patients with AML are most likely to have significant thrombocytopenia, with bleeding, bruising, and petechiae, and ineffective leukocyte function, leading to infection. Patients have a variable degree of lymphadenopathy and hepatosplenomegaly. When the leukocyte count is very high, patients may present with leukostasis syndrome.

The diagnosis is suggested by an elevated leukocyte count, anemia, thrombocytopenia, and blasts on the peripheral blood smear (Plate 35). The diagnosis is confirmed by bone marrow aspiration and biopsy showing >20% blasts. Typical myeloblasts demonstrate antigens found on immature cells such as CD34 (stem cell marker), and HLA-DR, as well as antigens more specific for granulocytic maturation such as CD33 and CD13. Cytogenetic studies are crucial because three typical abnormalities carry a good prognosis: t(8;21), t(15;17), and in(16). Loss or deletion of chromosome 7 and more complex cytogenetic abnormalities are associated with antecedent radiation, treatment with alkylating agents, or myelodysplasia and have a poor prognosis. The morphology of the bone marrow cells combined with immunophenotype and cytogenetic studies are used to further classify AML in accordance with the WHO or FAB classification systems.

Acute promyelocytic leukemia is a special case marked by the t(15;17) translocation, which disturbs a retinoic acid receptor. Patients with acute promyelocytic leukemia have significant bleeding due to fibrinolysis and disseminated intravascular coagulation.

Therapy

Patients require immediate hospitalization for initiation of therapy, irradiated and filtered blood and platelet transfusion support, and antibiotics for infection.

The standard induction regimen is 3 days of an anthracycline, such as idarubicin, and 7 days of a continuous infusion of cytosine arabinoside. After induction therapy patients remain pancytopenic for many days. Younger patients and patients with good prognosis cytogenetics do well, with remission rates of 60%-70% defined by normalization of the blood count, fewer than 5% bone marrow blasts, and normalization of the karyotype. Older patients, and those with high-risk cytogenetics, have much lower remission rates. Once remission is achieved, consolidation chemotherapy is given and patients with high-risk disease are referred for allogenic bone marrow transplantation.

Treatment for acute promyelocytic leukemia is initiated with all-*trans*-retinoic acid, which induces maturation of the promyelocyte and ameliorates disseminated intravascular coagulation.

Follow-Up

Most patients with AML relapse within 18-24 months of achieving complete remission. Patients are seen monthly during the first 2 years after remission to perform an interim history and physical examination and blood count; bone marrow aspiration is performed only if there are abnormalities in the complete blood count. Patients who have undergone stem cell transplantation are immunosuppressed; quickly investigate and treat even relatively minor complaints.

Book Enhancement

Go to www.acponline.org/essentials/hematology-section.html to view notes to help you differentiate the peripheral blood smear findings of the common leukemias and to view peripheral blood smears, staging systems, differential diagnosis and suggested laboratory evaluations. In *MKSAP for Students 4*, assess yourself with items 25-27 in the **Hematology** section.

Bibliography

Garewal H, Mahadevan D. Chronic Lymphocytic Leukemia. http://pier.acponline.org/physicians/diseases/d481. [Date accessed: 2008 Jan 14] In: PIER [online database]. Philadelphia: American College of Physicians; 2008.

Jabbour EJ, Estey E, Kantarjian HM. Adult acute myeloid leukemia. Mayo Clin Proc. 2006;81:247-60. Erratum in: Mayo Clin Proc. 2006; 81:569. [PMID: 16471082]

Maslak P. Acute Myelogenous Leukemia. http://pier.acponline.org/physicians/diseases/d482. [Date accessed: 2008 Jan 14] In: PIER [online database]. Philadelphia: American College of Physicians; 2008.

Tsimberidou AM, Giles FJ. Chronic Myeloid Leukemia. http://pier.acponline.org/physicians/diseases/d480. [Date accessed: 2008 Jan 14] In: PIER [online database]. Philadelphia: American College of Physicians; 2008.

Chapter 44

Multiple Myeloma

Mark M. Udden, MD

Multiple myeloma (MM) is a malignant clonal proliferation of plasma cells. MM arises when mutations occur in B cells committed to plasma cell differentiation. Myeloma usually evolves from a pre-malignant condition, monoclonal gammopathy of uncertain significance (MGUS). Malignant transformation is associated with immunoglobulin gene rearrangements in IgH (heavy chain) genes leading to secretion of an intact monoclonal IgG, IgA, or IgM protein that can be detected by serum protein electrophoresis (SPEP). Changes occur in λ or K genes that result in excretion of a monoclonal light chain which can be detected on urine electrophoresis (UPEP). Cytogenetic abnormalities such as 13q- and mutations in the oncogenes ras and p53 also occur in MM. Proliferation of plasma cells, elaboration of M-protein, and light chains along with activation of osteoclasts account for the protean manifestations of MM.

Diagnosis

Suspect MM in patients with anemia, bone pain, osteopenia or osteoporosis, pathologic fracture, lytic bone lesions, hypercalcemia, recurrent infections (particularly pneumococcal), or renal failure. Hyperviscosity is associated with large amounts of circulating IgG or smaller concentrations of IgA (a dimeric protein) or IgM (a tetrameric protein) and may be associated with bleeding, decreased visual acuity, retinopathy, neurological symptoms, heart failure, and dyspnea. Amyloidosis is also associated with MM or may occur as a primary disorder associated with a monoclonal protein.

Monoclonal immunoglobulins are frequently observed in older patients as a benign asymptomatic condition called *monoclonal gammopathy of uncertain significance* (MGUS). There is a 2% annual transformation of MGUS to MM. The differentiation of MM from MGUS is summarized in Table 1. Smoldering myeloma is an intermediate disorder that resembles MM in that the bone marrow shows >10% plasma cells or the serum IgG is >3.0 g/dL, but there is mild or no anemia. In smoldering myeloma, lytic bone lesions, renal disease, and hypercalcemia are absent and there is typically slow progression to MM.

Evaluation of MM (Table 2) begins with a serum protein electrophoresis and urine protein electrophoresis on a 24-hour urine sample. The specific type of monoclonal protein is determined by immunoelectrophoresis. Up to 20% of patients with myeloma do not secrete an intact immunoglobulin but secrete in the urine a λ or K light chain. Light chains are not detected in a routine urinalysis, emphasizing the need for urine immunoelectrophoresis. Additional studies include complete blood count, radiographic bone survey (Figure 1), serum creatinine, blood urea nitrogen, and calcium. Bone scans are not obtained, because the myeloma lesions are usually lytic and do not image well with nuclear scans that detect primarily osteoblastic activity.

A bone marrow aspirate and biopsy is done to document the presence of increased plasma cells. In some patients a biopsy of a mass will show the presence of a plasmacytoma. Quantitative immunoglobulin measurement will show depressed amounts of the non-myeloma immunoglobulins, predisposing the patient to recurrent infection. Serum lactic dehydrogenase concentration and β₂-microglobulin determination are used to determine tumor burden associated with MM. Table 3 describes some important disorders to consider in the differential diagnosis of MM.

Table 1. Diagnosis of Multiple Myeloma* and Monoclonal Gammopathy of Undetermined Significance (MUGA)

Multiple myeloma major criteria	I. Plasmacytoma on tissue biopsy
	II. Bone marrow clonal plasma cells >30%
	III. High M-protein (IgG >3.5 g/dL, IgA >2.0 g/dL) or Bence Jones proteinuria >1.0 g/24h
Multiple myeloma minor criteria	A. Bone marrow clonal plasma cells 10%-30%
	B. M-protein IgG <3.5 g/dL, IgA <2.0 g/dL
	C. Lytic bone lesions
	D. Diminished levels of nonmonoclonal immunoglobulins (IgM <50 mg/dL, IgA <100 mg/dL, or IgG <600 mg/dL)
MUGA	• M-protein (IgG <3.5 g/dL, IgA <2.0 g/dL)
	• Bence Jones proteinuria <1.0 g/24h
	• Bone marrow clonal plasma cells <10%
	• No end-organ damage (no symptoms, no bone lesions, no anemia, normal renal function)

*Diagnosis of multiple myeloma is made by at least 1 major and 1 minor diagnostic criteria or at least three minor criteria that include A and B.

Table 2. Laboratory and Other Studies for Diagnosis of Multiple Myeloma (MM)

Test	Notes
Complete blood count	Anemia is present in about 60% of patients at diagnosis and eventually develops in all patients. Possible thrombocytopenia and leukopenia.
Peripheral blood smear	Rouleaux formation due to increased serum proteins.
Serum calcium (see Chapter 60)	Hypercalcemia found initially in 15%-20% of patients due to cytokine-mediated destruction of bone.
Serum creatinine	20% of patients have creatinine level >2 mg/dL at diagnosis. Causes: hypercalcemia, "myeloma kidney," dehydration, and hyperuricemia.
Serum protein electrophoresis	Characteristic "M-protein" in approximately 80% of patients; presence or absence does not guarantee or exclude the diagnosis. Note whether there is a "spike" or a diffuse increase in levels. A spike in γ-globulin is more consistent with a monoclonal protein and a diffuse increase with a polyclonal increase. A polyclonal gammopathy almost never relates to MM.
Immunofixation of serum	At diagnosis 93% of patients with MM have a monoclonal protein in the serum by immunofixation.
Quantitative immunoglobulins (IgA, IgG, IgM)	Confirms monoclonal gammopathy; >90% of patients also have suppression of at least one of their uninvolved immunoglobulins at diagnosis.
β_2-microglobulin	Important for prognosis by measuring tumor burden.
24-hour urine protein electrophoresis with immunofixation	75% of patients have M-protein in their urine by immunofixation. Because approximately 20% of patients with MM have light chain only, the free monoclonal light chain may be missed in the serum in these patients; this test is essential, especially in this subgroup of patients.
Radiographic bone survey	75% of patients have punched-out lytic lesions, osteoporosis, or fractures on conventional radiography. Because myelomatous bone lesions are lytic, conventional radiography is superior to technetium-99m bone scanning.
Bone marrow aspirate and biopsy	Essential, but not sufficient, for the diagnosis. Plasma cells account for ≥10% of the bone marrow cells.
Bone marrow plasma cell labeling index	Specifically measures plasma cell proliferation. Prognostic for survival.
Cytogenetics and FISH studies	Obtained at diagnosis. Certain chromosomal abnormalities (e.g., deletions of the long arm of chromosome 13 [13q-]) are associated with shorter disease-free survival and overall survival.

FISH = fluorescence in situ hybridization; IgA = immunoglobulin A; IgG = immunoglobulin G; IgM = immunoglobulin M.

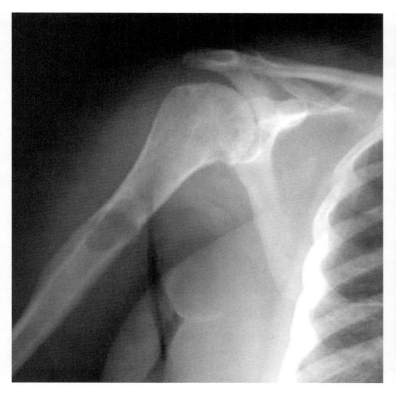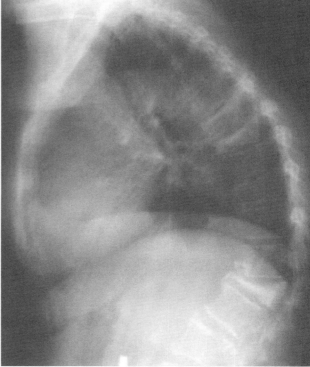

Figure 1 Lytic lesion right humerus (*left*) and osteoporosis and compression fracture of the thoracic spine (*right*) in a patient with multiple myeloma.

Table 3. Differential Diagnosis of Multiple Myeloma (MM)

Disease	Notes
Monoclonal gammopathy of undetermined significance (MGUS)	M-protein <3 g/dL; bone marrow plasma cells <10%; normal hemoglobin, serum calcium, serum creatinine, and bone survey. May be precancerous, but no therapy reduces the likelihood of malignant transformation.
Polyclonal hypergammaglobulinemia	A nonclonal increase in serum immunoglobulins. No increased risk of evolving into MM. Associated with liver disease, connective tissue disease, chronic infections (e.g., HIV), lymphoproliferative disorders, and nonhematologic malignancies.
Plasma cell leukemia	2000/μL circulating plasma cells. Worse prognosis than typical MM.
POEMS syndrome	Rare variant of MM consisting of peripheral neuropathy, organomegaly, endocrinopathy, monoclonal plasma proliferative disorder, skin changes, sclerotic bone lesion(s), papilledema, finger nail clubbing, edema, effusions, and possibly associated Castleman disease.* Not all features required; minimum of peripheral neuropathy, plasma cell dyscrasia, and either sclerotic bone lesion or Castleman disease. Better overall prognosis than MM.
Primary systemic amyloidosis (AL amyloid)	A clonal plasma cell proliferative disorder in which fibrils of monoclonal light chains are deposited in the kidney and other tissues (e.g., liver, heart, peripheral nervous system) causing nephrotic syndrome, cardiomyopathy, orthostatic hypotension, cholestatic liver disease, peripheral neuropathy, pinch purpura, fatigue, weight loss, peripheral edema, macroglossia, xerostomia, arthropathy, carpal tunnel syndrome. Most patients have small serum M-proteins and approximately 5% bone marrow plasma cells. 6%-15% of patients with AL amyloid have coexisting MM.
Waldenström macroglobulinemia	An IgM monoclonal gammopathy characterized by anemia, hyperviscosity, lymphadenopathy, and bone marrow plasmacyte infiltration. More responsive to agents like purine nucleoside analogs and anti-CD20 immunotherapy.
Plasmacytoma	A localized collection of plasmacytes that may occur as a single lytic lesion in bone or extra-medullary (upper respiratory tract, especially sinuses, nasopharynx, or larynx). May or may not have M-protein in the serum or urine. No increase in bone marrow plasma cells; no anemia, hypercalcemia, or renal insufficiency. Treated with local therapy (e.g., excision, radiation). Patients have increased risk for developing MM.

* A lymphoproliferative disorder association with HIV and human herpesvirus 8.
HIV = human immunodeficiency virus; IgM = immunoglobulin M.

Therapy

Maintain hydration and avoid nephrotoxic drugs and contrast dyes in patients with MM to prevent renal failure. Mild hypercalcemia may resolve with hydration alone, and early renal failure may improve with hydration and treatment of hypercalcemia. Patients with severe renal compromise may require dialysis. Paralysis or incontinence may occur when a vertebral plasmacytoma compresses the spinal cord. Begin corticosteroids and obtain emergent radiation oncology or neurosurgery consultation for symptomatic spinal cord compression. Consider radiation therapy or surgery to treat impending long-bone fracture unresponsive to chemotherapy. Initiate plasmapheresis for symptomatic hyperviscosity. Give all patients pneumococcal vaccination and annual influenza vaccinations. Patients aged <70 years with good performance status are candidates for autologous bone marrow transplantation.

Initiate bisphosphonates (i.e., pamidronate or zoledronate) for hypercalcemia and bone disease. Prior to their initiation pay careful attention to dentition and have any necessary dental work completed before treatment, if possible. Monitor patients carefully for side effects including renal insufficiency and osteonecrosis of the jaw, which may be more likely to occur if dental work is done after long-term bisphosphonate treatment.

Identify bone marrow transplant candidates as early as possible, and in these patients avoid melphalan-containing chemotherapy. Such patients are treated with high-dose dexamethasone alone or in combination with thalidomide. Thalidomide is a potent teratogen and must be used cautiously in women of child-bearing age. Patients receiving thalidomide and dexamethasone combination therapy have a very high risk for venous thromboembolism and require anticoagulation with low-molecular-weight heparin or warfarin. Two new agents that show efficacy in relapsed or refractory myeloma are the proteosome inhibitor bortezomide and the thalidomide analog revlimide. The response to treatment is determined by following the serum protein electrophoresis and/or urine protein electrophoresis; the amount of immunoglobulin should decrease significantly after 3-4 months of treatment. If a response is achieved, the patient is referred for autologous bone marrow transplantation.

Follow-Up

Patients with MGUS have a transformation rate to MM that is proportional to the size of their monoclonal protein peak in their serum or urine. For example, patients with IgG <1.5 g/dL have low risk of transformation over the next year compared with patients with ≥2.5 g/dL. Thus, patients with MGUS and low paraprotein concentrations are checked once a year, and those with larger concentrations are checked more often. Patients with MM are followed on a monthly basis to determine their response to therapy and to assess their renal function, complete blood count, and calcium levels.

Book Enhancement

Go to www.acponline.org/essentials/hematology-section.html to view a bone marrow aspirate, peripheral blood smear with rouleaux, bone x-ray, and a serum protein electrophoresis comparing MM, polyclonal gammopathy, and normal findings. In *MKSAP for Students 4*, assess yourself with items 28-29 in the **Hematology** section.

Bibliography

Dispenzieri A. Multiple Myeloma. http://pier.acponline.org/physicians/diseases/d189. [Date accessed: 2008 Jan 14] In: PIER [online database]. Philadelphia: American College of Physicians; 2008.

Rajkumar SV, Kyle RA. Multiple myeloma: diagnosis and treatment. Mayo Clin Proc. 2005;80:1371-82. [PMID: 16212152]

Section VI
Infectious Disease Medicine

Chapter 45

Approach to Fever

Joseph T. Wayne, MD

Fever can be the presenting symptom and/or sign in a multitude of infectious and non-infectious conditions. It is an adaptive, complex biologic response to alter the body's temperature set-point.

Central control of body temperature resides in the hypothalamus and follows a defined pathway through the limbic system to the lower brainstem and reticular formation to the spinal cord and finally the sympathetic ganglia. Normal body temperature ranges from 96°F (35.6°C) to 100.8°F (38.2°C) with a mean of 98.2°F (36.8°C). There is a diurnal variation with a nadir near 6 A.M. and a peak near 4 P.M. Fever is defined as a temperature of ≥99°F (37.2°C) in the morning and ≥100°F (37.7°C) in the afternoon. If the temperature is ≥106°F (41.1°C), hyperthermia or hyperpyrexia may be present. *Hyperthermia* occurs when thermoregulatory control is overwhelmed by the combination of exogenous heat exposure and excess heat production without a change in the hypothalamic set-point. *Hyperpyrexia* is a high fever (and change in hypothalamic set-point) observed in patients with severe infections but that most commonly occurs in patients with central nervous system hemorrhage.

Fever related to bacterial infection results from exposure to endotoxin or bacterial lipopolysaccharide and resultant production of cytokines including interleukins 1 and 6, tumor necrosis factor, the interferons, and prostaglandin E2. Cytokines stimulate the organum vasculosum laminae terminalis (OVLT) in the pre-optic region. The neurons of the OVLT cross the blood brain barrier and enter the hypothalamus. The primary neurotransmitter in the hypothalamus is prostaglandin E2 (PGE-2). There are also endogenous cryogens in the hypothalamus (arg-vasopressin and α-melanocyte stimulating hormone) that prevent the set-point from rising out of control.

Cytokines also mediate the febrile response in noninfectious, inflammatory conditions (e.g., autoimmune disorders). In response, metabolic and immunologic changes occur favorable to host survival and less favorable for bacterial proliferation. To determine the cause of fever, thorough attention must be addressed to performing a comprehensive history and physical examination appropriate to the clinical setting.

Approach to the Patient

Patient subjective reports of fever are accurate only about 50%-75% of the time. Temperature can be taken with digital thermometers, infrared tympanic thermometers, and liquid crystal thermometers, which measure surface temperature of the skin. Digital thermometers are the most accurate, with rectal temperature the most reproducible. Infrared tympanic thermometers and liquid crystal thermometers can vary as much as 0.5-1.5°C. Confirm a fever measured by infrared tympanic thermometers and liquid crystal thermometers with a digital thermometer. It is best to record the temperature from the same site every time (e.g., all oral).

Next, determine if temperature elevation is due to fever or hyperthermia. In fever, there is shivering and peripheral vasoconstriction; when there is defervescence, vasodilatation and sweating will occur. In hyperthermia, these responses are not present and there will be a history of environmental or drug exposure and/or excessive exertion immediately preceding the development of elevated body temperature. Medication history is also important. Drug reactions can cause confounding and recurrent fever, some with shaking chills. Only by eliminating the suspected drug and observing the result can it be ascertained as the cause of fever.

Outpatient Fever

Most outpatient fevers are due to viral illness and will resolve in less than 2 weeks. A seriously ill patient (e.g., pale, dyspneic, altered mental state, cool, clammy, hypotensive, tachycardic, cyanotic) makes bacterial infection more likely. Look for localizing clues (e.g., cough, dyspnea, dysuria, diarrhea, localized pain, presence of wound, vaginal or ear discharge) and focus the physical exam based upon these findings.

If there are no localizing complaints, a detailed history and physical examination, including pelvic examination in a female, is necessary. In stable outpatients, this can be done over several visits. Address recent medication use, surgery with implanted devices, transfusions, exposures to known illnesses, animals, travel history, drug use, sexual habits, dietary habits (e.g., raw seafood or undercooked meat), and family history of connective tissue disease. This process is repeated to assess any new complaints and monitor for changes.

If fever has been of short duration and no potential source for the fever is suggested at the first visit, obtain a complete blood count with differential, peripheral blood smear, and urinalysis. Immature band forms, toxic granulations, or Dohle bodies may indicate a bacterial cause of fever. Leukopenia most often is due to viral illness, but may also be seen with autoimmune or marrow infiltrative disorders. Lymphocytosis with atypical lymphocytes is associated with Epstein-Barr, cytomegalovirus, and HIV infections; monocytosis can be seen with typhoidal disease and tuberculosis.

If fever is persistent for more than one to two weeks, a more thorough evaluation is initiated (Table 1). Some experts also include an erythrocyte sedimentation rate (ESR) and C-reactive protein (CRP) as part of the evaluation. Although ESR and CRP are non-specific, significant elevations of one or both (ESR >50 mm/hr; CRP >15 mg/L) suggests the possibility of serious underlying disease. In stable patients, there is no need to initiate antibiotic therapy until a diagnosis is established. If fever persists for >3 weeks despite three or more visits and appropriate investigation, it is designated a fever of unknown origin.

Inpatient Fever

In addition to looking for localizing signs and symptoms, there are several features of inpatient fever that warrant special attention. These include identifying intravascular catheters (bacteremia), urinary catheters (urinary tract infection), nasogastric tubes (sinusitis), recent foreign body insertions (e.g., infected joint replacements, vascular grafts, and pacemakers) and blood transfusions (febrile transfusion reaction) as a potential source of infection or fever. Problems due to prolonged immobility should also be considered (e.g., deep venous thromboses, decubitus ulcers, atelectasis).

Assess any localized findings, check all invasive sites for signs of infection, inspect dependent parts of the body for skin breakdown (redness, warmth, tenderness, swelling, and discharge), examine the legs for swelling, and look for medications associated with hyperthermia or fever. Examinations should be repeated daily when in-hospital until a source is found or the fever resolves. In addition to the standard laboratory evaluation and chest x-ray, additional tests are directed by the physical findings. If fever persists for >3 days in the immunocompromised inpatient and >1 week in the immunocompetent inpatient without a diagnosis, it is designated a fever of unknown origin.

Table 1. Minimal Diagnostic Evaluation for Persistent Fever

- Comprehensive history
- Physical examination
- Complete blood cell count and differential
- Blood film reviewed by hematopathologist
- Routine blood chemistry (including lactic dehydrogenase, bilirubin, and liver enzymes)
- Urinalysis and microscopy
- Blood (x3) and urine cultures
- Anti-nuclear antibodies (ANA), rheumatoid factor
- Human immunodeficiency virus antibody
- Cytomegalovirus IgM antibodies; heterophil antibody test (if consistent with mononucleosis-like syndrome)
- Q-fever serology (if exposure risk factors exist)
- Chest radiography
- Hepatitis serology (if abnormal liver enzyme test result)

From Mourad O, Palda V, Detsky AS. A comprehensive evidence-based approach to fever of unknown origin. Arch Intern Med. 2003;163:545-51; with permission.

Fever of Unknown Origin

The most common categories of illness associated with fever of unknown origin are infectious diseases, noninfectious inflammatory diseases, malignancies, and miscellaneous causes (Figure 1). The most common infectious cause is tuberculosis. In patients with HIV infection, approximately 80% will have an additional infection causing the fever. No cause for fever of unknown origin is found in approximately 25% of patients.

If no infectious cause is identified, further evaluation is directed toward autoimmune diseases, connective tissue diseases, and granulomatous disorders (i.e., sarcoidosis). In the miscellaneous category, thyroiditis, pulmonary embolism, drug fever, and factitious fever need to be considered.

For fever of unknown origin, additional investigation beyond that for persistent fever is necessary (see Table 1). Some experts recommend a fever diary to monitor and record the fever pattern. HIV antibody (and viral load if fever is of recent onset), erythrocyte sedimentation rate, and CT of the chest and abdomen are often added. If this fails to identify a source, repeated questioning and examinations are warranted.

Treatment

Seizures, birth defects, brain damage, and death have been attributed to fever, as well as jeopardizing myocardial and pulmonary function in patients with underlying disease. However, evidence for such direct harm is lacking, whereas consistent evidence of the beneficial effects of fever exists. When antipyretics are administered, studies have shown prolonged time to crusting in varicella infection, and viral shedding is increased and neutralizing antibody production is suppressed in herpes zoster and rhinoviral infections. Cooling blankets have been shown to increase oxygen consumption (by induced shivering) and cause coronary artery vasospasm. Antipyretics are not without adverse effects: aspirin has gastrointestinal and renal effects and acetaminophen has liver and renal effects. Despite the lack of evidence that fever is harmful, and evidence demonstrating potential deleterious effects of treating fever, antipyretic therapy may be considered for patient comfort and is considered safe when appropriate dosing guidelines are followed. If the decision is made to treat a patient's fever, dosing should be around the clock to avoid discomfort from cyclical sweats during PGE-2 inhibition and chills as the set-point returns upward. Empiric antibiotic therapy is guided by the most likely source. In stable patients without localizing signs, empiric antibiotic therapy is typically withheld. In unstable patients without localizing signs, empiric broad spectrum antibiotics may be initiated (see Chapter 46).

Book Enhancement

Go to www.acponline.org/essentials/infectious-disease-section .html to review a table of infection mimics that can present with fever. In *MKSAP for Students 4*, assess yourself with item 4 in the **Infectious Disease Medicine** section.

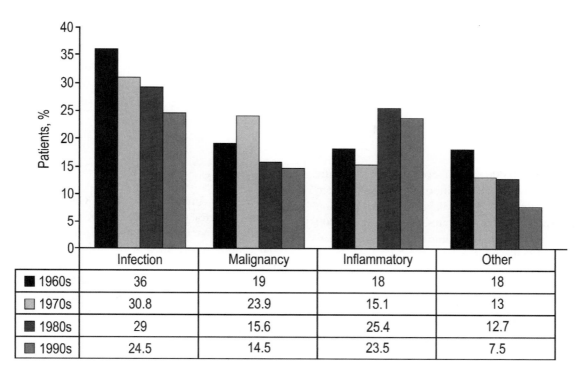

	Infection	Malignancy	Inflammatory	Other
■ 1960s	36	19	18	18
▫ 1970s	30.8	23.9	15.1	13
■ 1980s	29	15.6	25.4	12.7
■ 1990s	24.5	14.5	23.5	7.5

Figure 1 Cause of fever of unknown origin over past 40 years. (From Mourad O, Palda V, Detsky AS. A comprehensive evidence-based approach to fever of unknown origin. Arch Intern Med. 2003;163:545-51; with permission.)

Bibliography

Bleeker-Rovers CP, Vos FJ, de Kleijn EM, et al. A prospective multicenter study on fever of unknown origin: the yield of a structured diagnostic protocol. Medicine (Baltimore). 2007;86:26-38. [PMID: 17220753]

Mourad O, Palda V, Detsky AS. A comprehensive evidence-based approach to fever of unknown origin. Arch Intern Med. 2003;163:545-51. [PMID: 12622601]

Chapter 46

Sepsis Syndrome

Charin L. Hanlon, MD

Approximately 750,000 cases of severe sepsis occur in the United States each year. The mortality rate ranges from 20% to 50%. By 2020, there will be more than 1 million cases of sepsis per year in the United States, resulting in 215,000 deaths. Early diagnosis of sepsis syndrome and early goal-directed therapy reduces mortality.

Sepsis is a complex dysregulation of both inflammation and coagulation. Primary cellular injury may result directly from infection or when a toxic microbial stimulus (e.g., endotoxin) initiates a deleterious host inflammatory response. A network of inflammatory mediators is generated, including TNF-α, IL-1, and other cytokines and chemokines that activate leukocytes, promote leukocyte-vascular endothelium adhesion, and induce endothelial damage. Endothelial damage, a key component of sepsis pathophysiology, leads to tissue factor expression and activation of the tissue factor-dependent clotting cascade with subsequent formation of thrombin such that microaggregates of fibrin, platelets, neutrophils, and erythrocytes impair capillary blood flow, decreasing oxygen and nutrient delivery to tissues. In addition, cytokines stimulate nitric oxide release, smooth muscle relaxation, and systemic vasodilation, leading to impaired oxygen delivery and anaerobic metabolism on a cellular level. The most severe manifestations of this process include disseminated intravascular coagulation and metabolic (lactic) acidosis.

Higher levels of circulating and intracellular TNF-α, IL-1, IL-6, and soluble adhesion molecules, which are markers for activated or damaged endothelium, have been more common in older compared with younger patients with sepsis. Increasing age is also associated with rising circulating levels of IL-6 and D-dimer, activated factor VII, and other coagulation factors, indicating activation of inflammatory and coagulation pathways.

Diagnosis

In 1992, the American College of Chest Physicians and the Society of Critical Care Medicine issued standardized definitions for various severe infections that constitute the sepsis syndrome. Four entities were defined: systemic inflammatory response syndrome (SIRS), sepsis, severe sepsis, and septic shock (Table 1). The definitions provide a simple and practical framework for identifying these disorders. They are a continuum, with a stepwise increase in mortality from SIRS to septic shock. SIRS criteria are relatively nonspecific and can be present in many shock states (Table 2). The presence of the SIRS criteria should place sepsis on the differential and lead to an investigation for infection.

The initial evaluation of the septic patient includes a rapid yet thorough history and physical examination, with emphasis on identifying a possible source of infection. The vital signs are crucial to determining the stability of the patient and require continuous monitoring, including blood pressure, pulse, respiratory rate, and oxygen saturation.

Laboratory evaluation is focused on finding evidence for end-organ dysfunction related to the sepsis (e.g., renal failure, liver dysfunction, disseminated intravascular coagulation, mental status changes). It includes a complete blood count with differential, electrolytes, creatinine, urinalysis, liver chemistry tests, coagulation parameters, and a random serum cortisol level to inform decision making on need for adjunctive corticosteroid therapy. Serum lactate level should be measured because it has been correlated with the degree of global tissue hypoxia and the severity of sepsis. Lactate level >4 mmol/L implies significant tissue hypoxia. Obtain cultures of blood, urine, sputum, and any other sites of potential infection as soon as the diagnosis of sepsis is suspected. Obtain x-rays and other imaging studies as directed by patient symptoms.

Table 1. Definitions of Systemic Inflammatory Response Syndrome, Sepsis, Severe Sepsis, and Septic Shock

Systemic inflammatory response syndrome (SIRS)	Two or more of the following:
	  Temperature >38.0°C (100.4°F) or <36°C (96.8°F).
	  Heart rate >90/min.
	  Respiration rate >20/min or arterial blood PaCO$_2$ <32 mm Hg.
	  Leukocyte count >12,000/μL or <4000/μL with 10% bands
	    (in absence of other known cause of these conditions).

Sepsis	Systemic inflammatory response syndrome in response to confirmed infectious process.
Severe sepsis	Sepsis associated with organ dysfunction, hypoperfusion, or hypotension. Hypoperfusion and hypotension abnormalities may include, but are not limited to, lactic acidosis, oliguria, or an acute alteration in mental status.
Septic shock	Sepsis-induced hypotension and perfusion abnormalities despite adequate fluid resuscitation.

Table 2. Differential Diagnosis of Shock

Disease	Notes
Septic shock	Characterized by high cardiac output (early) that can become depressed (late), low systemic vascular resistance, and low filling pressures. Fever, leukocytosis, and source of infection are characteristically present.
Cardiogenic shock	Typically occurs in acute coronary syndromes, in valve dysfunction, or from cardiac tamponade. Characteristics include cardiogenic pulmonary edema, high filling pressures, low cardiac index, and high systemic vascular resistance. ECG is useful in evaluating patients with suspected sepsis to exclude acute coronary syndrome. Echocardiogram is also useful in this regard.
Hypovolemic shock	Characterized by low cardiac output, high systemic vascular resistance, and low cardiac filling pressures. Patients may have a history of hemorrhage, but other causes of volume depletion may be causal, such as with severe diarrhea.
Anaphylactic shock	Clinical presentation includes urticaria, angioedema, or both; shortness of breath and wheezing; stridor due to laryngeal edema; pulmonary edema; and hypotension. As may be seen in severe sepsis, the systemic vascular resistance is typically low, and the cardiac output elevated. Diagnosis is made when the typical signs and symptoms occur shortly after exposure to a suspected antigen. Treatment with epinephrine should be part of the initial management. Corticosteroids and antihistamines are also indicated.
Neurogenic shock/spinal shock	Occurs in spinal cord injury or other severe CNS injury. Thought to be caused by failure of the autonomic nervous system; as a result, it is associated with a low systemic vascular resistance and typically bradycardia. Bradycardia and hypotension in a patient with spinal cord injury should raise suspicion for this syndrome.
Adrenal crisis	Adrenal crisis may be difficult to distinguish from septic shock on clinical grounds. Patients with adrenal crisis often have shock and abdominal symptoms (tenderness, nausea, vomiting) and may have fever. In addition, weakness, fatigue, lethargy, and confusion are common. Patients may have hyponatremia and hyperkalemia suggesting adrenal insufficiency. If adrenal insufficiency is suspected, testing of adrenal function should be initiated without delay.
Obstructive shock	Characterized by hypotension, tachycardia, and low cardiac output and may mimic septic shock. Causes of obstructive shock include cardiac tamponade, pulmonary embolism, and tension pneumothorax. All of these diagnoses are life-threatening and should be excluded without delay.

CNS = central nervous system; ECG = electrocardiography.

Therapy

Almost universally, patients are admitted to the hospital if they meet SIRS criteria. If patients have sepsis, severe sepsis, or septic shock, they are managed in the intensive care unit setting. Early goal-directed therapy refers to the concept of early restoration of hemodynamic stability during the first 6 hours of hospitalization (Table 3). This therapy serves to balance oxygen delivery with oxygen demand to prevent tissue hypoxia. The goals of treatment are a central venous pressure (CVP) of 8-12 mm Hg, mean arterial pressure (MAP) >65 mm Hg ([(2× diastolic) + systolic] / 3), urine output >0.5 mL/kg/hr, and central venous oxygen saturation (SvcO$_2$) >70%. To achieve the CVP goal of 8-12 mm Hg requires placement of a central venous catheter attached to a pressure transducer, measuring the pressure in the superior vena cava or right atrium. Either crystalloid or colloid is given aggressively until the CVP goal is obtained. There is no evidence-based benefit for one fluid replacement over another. Initially, a 500-1000 mL bolus of fluid is given and the CVP monitored to direct subsequent fluid replacement. If the fluid challenge fails to achieve a mean arterial pressure >65 mm Hg, vasopressors are added. Source control is crucial initially. This includes removal of sources of infection, such as indwelling catheters, drainage of abscesses, and surgical debridement of wounds, done promptly upon the diagnosis of sepsis.

During the initial stabilization, peripheral oxygen consumption is estimated by measuring central venous oxygen saturation from blood obtained from the superior vena cava. If the superior vena cava oxygen saturation is <70%, oxygen carrying capacity needs to be increased. This is done by transfusion if the hematocrit is <30% or with inotropic agents to increase cardiac output.

Currently accepted therapy consists of treating the underlying illness and administering antibiotics directed against the causative pathogen. The septic patient requires early, empiric broad-spectrum antibiotics, which are narrowed when culture results are available and antimicrobial drug sensitivities are known. In selecting empiric antibiotics, recognize that gram-positive infections now cause most cases of sepsis but gram-negative infections are still prevalent, and fungal infections must be considered in the high risk patients (e.g., neutropenic and transplant patients receiving immunosuppression therapy). Antibiotics should be initiated within 1 hour of the sepsis diagnosis.

Vasopressors are included as part of early goal-directed therapy if the mean arterial pressure is <65 mm Hg after the initial fluid resuscitation. The most commonly used vasopressor for septic shock is norepinephrine. It is a potent peripheral vasoconstrictor reversing the endotoxin-induced vasodilation that is the hallmark of septic shock. Dopamine is also acceptable but is associated with more tachycardia and arrhythmia because it acts as an alpha- and beta-agonist. Vasopressin has been investigated in severe shock resistant to other vasopressor agents and may be associated with some benefit. Vasopressin is avoided in patients with cardiac dysfunction because it commonly depresses cardiac output.

Recombinant human activated protein C (aPC or drotrecogin alfa) significantly reduces mortality rates in patients with severe sepsis. Patients who benefited most from receiving aPC had a high

Table 3. Treatment for Sepsis

Agent	Notes
Crystalloids	Restores intravascular volume, which is depleted in patients with severe sepsis. Improves cardiac output, organ perfusion, and mortality in severe sepsis. Commonly given as repeated rapid bolus infusions as long as the patient remains in shock or on vasopressors and continues to show a beneficial response without major adverse effects. May require 4-6 L during initial stabilization.
Antibiotic therapy (fourth-generation cephalosporin, extended-spectrum antipseudomonal penicillin, carbapenem)	Early appropriate antibiotic therapy is associated with improved outcomes. Appropriate empiric therapy should be initiated rapidly, even if the source of infection is unknown. A more appropriate, source-directed antibiotic selection should be initiated if the source is known or becomes known. For example, add vancomycin if MRSA is suspected; add double coverage with an IV fluoroquinolone or aminoglycoside if a highly resistant gram-negative pathogen is suspected; add clindamycin if toxic shock syndrome is suspected; consider additional agents such as fluoroquinolones, macrolides, tetracyclines, antifungal agents, and antiviral agents depending on the clinical presentation.
Norepinephrine	Improves blood pressure and cardiac output. Associated with less tachycardia than other vasopressors with β-effects. More effective than dopamine in refractory septic shock. Currently considered by many to be the first choice of vasopressors for patients with septic shock.
Dobutamine	Improves cardiac output. May be used in combination with a vasopressor to increase cardiac output if it is inappropriately low.
Vasopressin	Improves blood pressure in patients with septic shock. Because vasopressin works on receptors other than adrenergic receptors, it may be useful in refractory septic shock treated with high-dose adrenergic vasopressors. No randomized controlled trials exist to show a mortality benefit in this setting.
Drotrecogin alfa	Replaces activated protein C, which is depleted in severe sepsis. Activated protein C has antithrombotic, profibrinolytic, anti-inflammatory, and antiapoptosis properties. Improves survival in patients with severe sepsis at high risk of death. Mild increase in the incidence of serious bleeding.

IV = intravenous; MRSA = methicillin-resistant *Staphylococcus aureus*; SVR = systemic vascular resistance.

risk of death as determined by a severity-of-illness scoring system such as APACHE II >25 (Acute Physiology and Chronic Health Evaluation II), or with the greatest degree of organ failure. Bleeding complications were significantly increased in patients taking aPC, with 3.5% of participants who received aPC developing severe bleeding compared with 2% of participants who received placebo.

Historically, the use of corticosteroids has had mixed results in the treatment of septic shock. Initial studies of high-dose corticosteroids found an increase in morbidity and mortality. Recently, moderate doses have been used with success. Evidence now supports the use of corticosteroids (hydrocortisone 300 mg/d or equivalent) in septic shock for those patients who have relative adrenal insufficiency. This term is used to describe patients who have inadequate cortisol response to their septic condition and is defined as a random cortisol level of <15 µg/dL or a failure to increase by >9 µg/dL after administration of 250 µg of cosyntropin (ACTH stimulation test). Dexamethasone will not interfere with the cortisol assay and can be given until the stimulation test is completed. Corticosteroids are usually continued until the shock state is resolved and are then tapered over approximately a week. Higher doses of corticosteroids are avoided. In the absence of shock, corticosteroids are not be used in the treatment of sepsis. No benefit of corticosteroid therapy is seen in patients with a random cortisol >34 µg/dL.

Hyperglycemia and insulin resistance are common in the critically ill. Following initial stabilization, blood glucose is maintained <150 mg/dL by continuous insulin infusion if glucose is otherwise difficult to control. Tight glucose control has been proven to benefit patients with other forms of critical illness, including diabetics

with acute myocardial infarctions or stroke, and post-surgical patients requiring mechanical ventilation, but its benefit to medical patients with severe sepsis has not been proven.

Deep vein thrombosis prophylaxis is given with either low-dose unfractionated heparin or low-molecular-weight heparin. Mechanical compression devices are an alternative if there is a contraindication to anticoagulation. Stress ulcer prophylaxis is given with proton pump inhibitors or histamine-2 receptor blockers.

Book Enhancement

Go to www.acponline.org/essentials/infectious-disease-section .html to access a table of the key elements in the history and physical examination of a patient with sepsis, an algorithm on the resuscitation of a patient with sepsis, and to view an example of livedo reticularis and meningococcemia. In *MKSAP for Students 4*, assess yourself with items 5-6 in the **Infectious Disease Medicine** section.

Bibliography

American College of Physicians. Medical Knowledge Self-Assessment Program (MKSAP) 14. Philadelphia: American College of Physicians; 2006.

Dellinger RP, Carlet JM, Masur H, et al. Surviving Sepsis. Campaign guidelines for management of severe sepsis and septic shock. Crit Care Med. 2004;32:858-73. [Erratum in: Crit Care Med. 2004;32:1448. Correction of dosage error in text. Crit Care Med. 2004;32:2169-70. [PMID: 15090974]

O'Brien JM Jr, Ali NA, Aberegg SK, Abraham E. Sepsis. Am J Med. 2007;120:1012-22. [PMID: 18060918]

Chapter 47

Common Upper Respiratory Problems

Robert W. Neilson Jr., MD

This chapter discusses four common upper respiratory problems: upper respiratory infection, pharyngitis, sinusitis and otitis media.

Upper Respiratory Infection

Upper respiratory infection (URI) is an undifferentiated, usually viral syndrome that lacks a prominent feature characteristic of other acute respiratory infections. This infection is benign and self-limited, lasting 3 to 7 days. Viruses (rhinovirus, coronavirus, respiratory syncytial virus) cause infection by gaining entrance to epithelial cells of the upper respiratory tract, leading to vasodilation and increased vascular permeability, cholinergic stimulation, and host inflammatory responses.

Prevention

Contact with secretions is probably the principal mode of respiratory virus transmission and is prevented with frequent hand washing. Prevention with vitamins C or E or *Echinacea* is not supported by strong evidence.

Diagnosis

Viral URIs have an incubation period of 24-72 hours causing a combination of sore throat, cough, rhinorrhea, fever (<102°F, lasting <72 hours), and/or laryngitis. Physical examination may reveal a red nose, glassy-appearing nasal mucosa, nasal discharge, and mild oropharyngeal erythema. Laboratory testing and imaging studies are unnecessary for diagnosis. A small percentage of patients will develop acute bacterial sinusitis. Lower respiratory tract infections with upper respiratory viruses can occur in patients with underlying cardiopulmonary disease or immunosuppression. Viral URIs can cause heightened symptoms of asthma and chronic obstructive pulmonary disease.

Therapy

Heated vapor inhalation, such as from a hot shower, may be used to decrease nasal symptoms. Other symptomatic measures include extra fluid intake, saltwater gargle, throat lozenges, saline nasal spray, and adequate rest. Although there is no good evidence that these individual methods work, they are inexpensive and safe.

For relief of nasal congestion, oral (pseudoephedrine) or topical (phenylephrine) nasal decongestants are beneficial. In patients with rhinorrhea and sneezing, consider a short course of a first-generation antihistamine or intranasal ipratropium. In patients with a productive cough and wheezing, an inhaled β-agonist will reduce cough duration. Naproxen or ibuprofen and acetaminophen may be used for headache, myalgias, and malaise. Intranasal or oral zinc-containing preparations can potentially reduce the duration of URI. Codeine and over-the-counter antitussives have not been found to be effective for acute cough in URIs. Antibiotics are not indicated for uncomplicated URIs, even when purulent cough or nasal discharge is present. However, antibiotics may be indicated in URIs of prolonged duration (>7 days) if sinusitis is suspected and in patients with chronic obstructive pulmonary disease with evidence of exacerbation. Patients should be instructed to follow up if they develop persistent cough, shortness of breath, hemoptysis, chest pain, wheezing, dysphagia, trismus, severe headache, persistent nasal discharge, or ear pain (Table 1).

Pharyngitis

Pharyngitis is defined as direct infection of pharyngeal tissue. Viral infections, such as rhinovirus, are the most common cause of pharyngitis. Much less common causes include Epstein-Barr virus and acute retroviral syndrome. Group A β-hemolytic streptococcus (GABHS), *Chlamydia pneumoniae*, and *Mycoplasma pneumoniae* are the most common bacterial causes of pharyngitis. GABHS causes 5%-15% of acute pharyngitis in adults. With the exception of rare pharyngeal infections caused by other bacterial pathogens, GABHS is the only bacterium for which antimicrobial therapy is of proven benefit. Complications from GABHS pharyngitis include toxic shock syndrome, suppurative complications (peritonsillar abscess, pneumonia, sepsis), and nonsuppurative postinfectious sequelae (rheumatic fever, glomerulonephritis, reactive arthritis).

Prevention

GABHS pharyngitis is a very common and usually self-limited infection that is treated easily in both index cases and contact cases that become symptomatic. Do not use antibiotics to protect asymptomatic normal individuals.

Diagnosis

Consider the prevalence and severity of GABHS pharyngitis in the community. The following relevant epidemiologic factors should also be kept in mind: age (most commonly ages 5-15), season of

Table 1. Differential Diagnosis of Upper Respiratory Infection

Disease	Characteristics
Streptococcal pharyngitis	Criteria suggesting group A streptococcal pharyngitis: history of fever, tonsillar exudates, tender anterior cervical adenopathy, and no cough. Trismus, unilateral tonsillar swelling, and uvula deviation suggest peritonsillar abscess.
Sinusitis	Purulent nasal discharge, unilateral sinus pain or tenderness, maxillary toothache, poor response to decongestants, and worsening illness after initial improvement suggests sinusitis. Recurrent sinusitis is an indication for ENT consultation.
Acute cough illness (bronchitis, pneumonia)	Chest pain, wheezing, dyspnea, fever. Obtain chest x-ray to exclude pneumonia if pulse >100/min, respiratory rate >24/min, or temperature >38°C (100.4°F).
Epiglottitis	Severe sore throat with benign appearing oropharynx. Adults may have dyspnea, drooling, and stridor. Obtain urgent ENT consultation and do not attempt to examine the throat. Lateral neck film may show enlarged epiglottis (the "thumb sign").
Mononucleosis (Epstein-Barr virus)	1-2 week prodrome of fatigue, malaise, and myalgia. Adenopathy (predilection for posterior cervical nodes), sore throat, fever, splenomegaly and hepatomegaly, and lymphocytosis with atypical lymphocytes.
Allergic rhinitis	Seasonal nasal symptoms; clear rhinorrhea, watery, itchy eyes, and possible history of asthma.
Asthma	Wheezing, dyspnea, persistent dry cough; symptoms may worsen at night, triggered by cold air, exercise, or strong smells.
Influenza	Coryza, fever to 41°C (105.8°F); myalgias, headache, and sore throat. Severity of symptoms associated with high fever and myalgias suggest influenza.
Otitis media	Ear pain, fever, decreased hearing acuity; tympanic membrane red, opaque, bulging, or retracted. More common in children than adults.
Meningococcal disease	Patients with meningococcal disease may have sore throat, rhinorrhea, cough, headache and conjunctivitis before invasive disease.

ENT = ear, nose, and throat.

the year (most commonly winter and early spring in temperate climates), crowded living conditions, and recent close contact with a person with pharyngitis. Characteristic symptoms include sudden onset of sore throat, pain on swallowing, headache, fever, and malaise. Coryza, cough, and hoarseness are not usual symptoms. Look for tonsillopharyngeal erythema with or without exudates. Examine for tender and enlarged anterior cervical lymph nodes. Two laboratory methods are available to detect GABHS in the pharynx: culture of a throat swab (the gold standard) and rapid antigen testing. Rapid antigen testing is popular because of the speed with which results are obtained (a few hours or less). Because the incidence of streptococcal pharyngitis and risk of acute rheumatic fever are low in adults, throat culture is not indicated unless rapid antigen testing is unavailable, the sensitivity of the method of rapid antigen testing is <80% (however, most commercially available tests have reported sensitivities of 80%-90%), or gonococcal pharyngitis is suspected.

Therapy

Antimicrobial therapy should be used only when GABHS pharyngitis is highly likely. Clinical criteria for streptococcal infection include history of fever, tonsillar exudates, tender anterior cervical lymphadenopathy, and absence of cough or other URI symptoms. Patients with all clinical criteria should be treated with antibiotics without testing. Patients with three clinical criteria can be given antibiotics either without testing or after a positive rapid antigen test or culture. Patients with two clinical criteria require a positive rapid antigen test or culture before administration of antibiotics. Patients with one criterion or none do not require testing or antibiotics. A 10-day course of oral penicillin is the treatment

of choice; erythromycin is an alternative drug for patients who are allergic to penicillin. Consider giving a single injection of intramuscular benzathine penicillin G to patients who are unlikely to complete a full 10-day course of oral therapy. Advise patients to return if their response to appropriate therapy is not prompt (within 12-24 hours) and if symptoms persist or recur within a few days.

Sinusitis

Sinusitis is an inflammation of the paranasal sinuses. In most cases the nasal mucosa are also inflamed, hence the term *rhinosinusitis*. Causes include infection, allergy, systemic disease, trauma, and noxious chemicals. Symptoms may be classified as acute (<4 weeks), subacute (4-12 weeks), or chronic (>12 weeks). Most cases of sporadic acute sinusitis are due to viral infection. Bacterial superinfection is unlikely if symptoms last for <7 days. Community-acquired bacterial infections are caused by *Streptococcus pneumoniae* or *Haemophilus influenzae*. Dental disease or instrumentation can cause anaerobic infections. Immunocompromised patients are at risk for fungal infections, and gram-negative organisms are associated with health-care associated infections. Sinus infection may spread locally (osteitis of the sinus bones, orbital cellulitis) or metastasize to the central nervous system (meningitis, brain abscess, infection of the intracranial venous sinuses).

Diagnosis

Ask about allergies, systemic diseases, trauma, and exposure to environmental toxins. A history of smoking may also predispose to sinusitis. Symptoms may include nasal congestion, purulent nasal secretions, sinus tenderness, and facial pain. Examine for rhinorrhea, pus in the nasal cavity, and local pain. Abnormal nasal sinus transillumination may also help to confirm the diagnosis when present. Patients with only one of the following have <25% (low) probability of bacterial sinusitis: symptom duration of >7 days, facial pain, and purulent nasal discharge. Diagnostic probability is >50% (high) when two or more of the above signs or symptoms are present. Avoid sinus imaging in uncomplicated acute sinusitis. Consider sinus puncture only in patients in whom precise diagnosis is needed to determine optimal therapy, such as in the immunocompromised. Patients with ophthalmic or neurologic symptoms or signs require a more detailed clinical neurologic examination and may need diagnostic imaging studies.

Therapy

Saline nasal spray or sinus irrigation may help increase mucosal moisture and remove inflammatory debris and bacteria. Avoid empirical use of antibiotics as part of initial management in low-probability patients. Use mucolytic agents (e.g., guaifenesin) to reduce viscosity of nasal secretions, topical decongestants (e.g., xylometazoline) to reduce mucosal inflammation and improve ostial drainage, and intranasal steroids to reduce inflammation. Consider immediate antibiotic therapy in patients with severe symptoms or add antibiotic therapy in patients with less severe symptoms in whom there has been no improvement after 7 to 10 days. First-line choices include amoxicillin, trimethoprim/sulfamethoxazole, or doxycycline for 10 days. Office follow-up should be considered when symptoms persist for >10 days or if new, worsening symptoms develop.

Otitis Media

Obstruction of the eustachian tube due to allergy or URI results in accumulation of middle ear secretions. Secondary bacterial or viral infection of the resulting effusion causes suppuration and features of otitis media. Risk factors for otitis media include age (younger for acute otitis media, and older for chronic otitis media), smoking, altered immune defenses, allergic rhinitis, and chronic eustachian tube dysfunction. Viruses responsible for otitis media include respiratory syncytial virus, influenza viruses, rhinoviruses, and adenoviruses. The most common bacteria include *Streptococcus pneumoniae*, *Haemophilus influenzae*, and *Moraxella catarrhalis*. Bullous myringitis is often caused by mycoplasma. Rare complications of otitis media include meningitis, epidural abscess, brain abscess, lateral sinus thrombosis, cavernous sinus thrombosis, and carotid artery thrombosis.

Diagnosis

Symptoms of otitis media include ear pain and decreased conductive hearing. Examine for fluid in the middle ear and a retracted or bulging erythematous tympanic membrane. Absent tympanic membrane mobility with pneumatic otoscopy adds additional diagnostic information (sensitivity of 89%, specificity of 80%). Tenderness to palpation over the mastoid area may indicate extension of infection into the mastoid. Chronic otitis media may be suppurative or associated with formation of a cholesteatoma (a mass of excess squamous epithelium), which can erode into surrounding structures. This may lead to otorrhea, pain, hearing loss, or neurologic symptoms.

Therapy

Consider referral for ventilation tube insertion in patients with recurrent otitis media and/or associated hearing loss. Management of acute otitis media begins with decongestant therapy and pain control. Reserve antibiotic therapy for patients with evidence of purulent otitis, or in those in whom symptoms of congestion and eustachian tube dysfunction do not respond to treatment. First-line therapy includes amoxicillin (macrolides if penicillin allergic); amoxicillin-clavulanate and cefuroxime are used in patients who do not respond to amoxicillin. Treatment duration is usually 10-14 days. Follow-up is not necessary unless symptoms persist or progress.

Book Enhancement

Go to www.acponline.org/essentials/infectious-disease-section.html to review the Centor criteria for streptococcal pharyngitis and criteria for acute sinusitis. In *MKSAP for Students 4*, assess yourself with items 7-11 in the **Infectious Disease Medicine** section.

Bibliography

American College of Physicians. Medical Knowledge Self-Assessment Program (MKSAP) 14. Philadelphia: American College of Physicians; 2006.

Harris RH. Upper Respiratory Infection. http://pier.acponline.org/physicians/diseases/d673. [Date accessed: 2008 Jan 14] In: PIER [online database]. Philadelphia: American College of Physicians; 2008.

Ioannidis J, Barza M, Lau J. Acute Sinusitis. http://pier.acponline.org/physicians/diseases/d096. [Date accessed: 2008 Jan 14] In: PIER [online database]. Philadelphia: American College of Physicians; 2008.

Stollerman G. Group A Streptococcal Pharyngitis. http://pier.acponline.org/physicians/diseases/d390. [Date accessed: 2008 Jan 14] In: PIER [online database]. Philadelphia: American College of Physicians; 2008.

Williams JW Jr, Simel DL. Does this patient have sinusitis? Diagnosing acute sinusitis by history and physical examination. JAMA. 1993; 270: 1242-6. [PMID: 8355389]

Chapter 48

Urinary Tract Infection

Irene Alexandraki, MD

The majority of acute uncomplicated urinary tract infections occur in women aged 18 to 24 years. Urinary tract infections are unusual in men aged <50 years. Approximately 10% of adult women will have at least one urinary tract infection annually. A urinary tract infection in an individual with an indwelling urinary catheter, neurogenic bladder, stones, obstruction, immunosuppression, pregnancy, renal disease, or diabetes is defined as complicated and may predispose to treatment failure or require modified approaches to management due to infection with antibiotic-resistant organisms.

Most bacteria gain access to the bladder via the urethra. Uropathogens from fecal flora can colonize the vagina and migrate to the bladder through the urethra. Pyelonephritis can develop if these organisms ascend to the kidneys via the ureters. Sexual intercourse and contraceptive use increase the risk for developing an uncomplicated urinary tract infection in women. Genetic determinants in women with recurrent urinary tract infections increase their susceptibility to vaginal colonization with uropathogenic coliforms that adhere to the uroepithelial cells. Infection of the kidney, including abscess, can occur hematogenously in patients with staphylococcal bacteremia or endocarditis.

Escherichia coli causes 80% of all infections. *Staphylococcus saprophyticus* accounts for 10%-15% of acute symptomatic urinary tract infections in young females, and *Staphylococcus aureus, Enterococcus,* and gram-negative bacilli, including *Proteus, Klebsiella, Serratia,* and *Pseudomonas,* usually cause complicated urinary tract infections. *Staphylococcus aureus* infection should arouse suspicion of hematogenously acquired infection, which most often occurs in debilitated patients.

Prevention

Asymptomatic bacteriuria is only treated in the following circumstances: in pregnant women, in patients who recently had an indwelling catheter removed, before an invasive urologic procedure, in neutropenic patients, or in patients with a urinary tract obstruction. Chronic prophylactic antibiotic therapy is beneficial in pregnant women with recurrent asymptomatic bacteriuria; if untreated, 20%-40% will progress to symptomatic urinary tract infection, including pyelonephritis. Postcoital antibiotic prophylaxis is considered in women with two or more episodes of postcoital urinary tract infection per year. Cranberry-based products may be effective in the prevention of acute cystitis in women.

Screening

Screening for asymptomatic bacteriuria is recommended before transurethral resection of the prostate, urinary tract instrumentation involving biopsy, or other tissue trauma resulting in mucosal bleeding. Screening is not recommended for simple catheter placement or cystoscopy without biopsy. Pregnant women are screened for asymptomatic bacteriuria, which is associated with low birth weight and prematurity.

Diagnosis

Symptomatic cystitis is associated with dysuria, frequency, urgency, and suprapubic pain. Abrupt symptom onset is more consistent with urinary tract infection, while gradual onset and vaginal symptoms suggest sexually transmitted disease. Specific combinations of symptoms such as dysuria and frequency without vaginal discharge or irritation, raise the probability of a urinary tract infection to more than 90% (Table 1). A history of urologic abnormalities, underlying medical conditions such as diabetes, and modifying host factors such as advanced age can predict infection with resistant organisms, delayed or incomplete response to therapy, relapse, and infectious complications (e.g., renal abscess, emphysematous pyelonephritis, perinephric abscess, sepsis).

Pyelonephritis is associated with abrupt onset of fever, chills, sweats, nausea, vomiting, diarrhea, and flank or abdominal pain; hypotension and septic shock may occur in severe cases (see Table 1). Frequency and dysuria may precede pyelonephritis. Search for complicating conditions such as recent instrumentation of the urethra and bladder, diabetes, pregnancy, or prior urinary tract infections. Infection at distant sites suggests the possibility of hematogenous pyelonephritis.

The physical examination in cystitis generally reveals only tenderness of the urethra or the suprapubic area. Fever, tachycardia, and generalized muscle tenderness may be associated with pyelonephritis, and physical examination usually reveals marked costovertebral angle tenderness; unilateral abdominal tenderness may be present. Pelvic examination might be indicated if sexually transmitted disease is suggested by history.

Obtain a urinalysis in most women to help confirm the diagnosis of urinary tract infection; pyuria is present in 91% of patients, and the diagnosis should be reconsidered if pyuria is absent. The physical examination and urinalysis can be omitted for healthy women with acute cystitis if there are no complicating factors. When the diagnosis is not clear, the urine dipstick for leukocyte esterase and/or nitrite is an acceptable screening tool but may be less sensitive than microscopic urinalysis with low-count bacteriuria.

Table 1. Differential Diagnosis of Urinary Tract Infection

Disease	Notes
Vaginitis, cervicitis, or genital herpes (see Chapter 49)	*History*: Vaginal discharge, no urinary frequency or urgency, possibly new sex partner or unprotected sexual activity; history of previous STDs, recurrent genital HSV, or vaginitis; gradual onset of symptoms (*Chlamydia*). Dysuria can result from urine coming into contact with inflamed and irritated vulvar epithelial surfaces in the absence of bacterial UTI. Women may be able to differentiate between "internal" (UTI-associated) and "external" (vulvovaginal) dysuria, which helps to guide the evaluation. *Pelvic exam*: Vulvovaginal or cervical erythema, exudate, or ulcers; cervical discharge; adnexal tenderness or mass; cervical motion tenderness. *Laboratory*: Abnormal vaginal fluid findings; viral test from vulvovaginal ulcers positive for HSV; cervical swab with PMN leukocytes (± gram-negative diplococci) on Gram stain (if done), and positive by culture (or other test) for *Chlamydia* and/or *N. gonorrhoeae* (if indicated); urinalysis with PMNs but no bacteria; urine culture negative or with low counts of non-pathogens.
Sexually transmitted urethritis (see Chapter 49)	*History*: New sex partner, unprotected sexual activity, gradual onset of symptoms (*Chlamydia*); history of previous STDs or recurrent genital HSV, ± vaginal discharge; ± urinary frequency or urgency. Inflammation of the urethra from sexually transmitted pathogens can mimic bacterial cystitis quite closely. Sexual history can suggest the diagnosis. Specific tests are needed for confirmation, in conjunction with the negative routine urine culture. *Pelvic exam*: Possible normal, or evidence of coexistent vulvovaginitis or cervicitis/salpingitis. *Laboratory*: Urinalysis with PMNs but no bacteriuria; urine culture negative or low counts of non-pathogens; urine or urethral swab positive (by culture or other specific test) for *Chlamydia* or *HSV* (or *M. genitalium* or *U. urealyticum*).
Pyelonephritis	*History*: Fever, malaise, sweats, headache; anorexia, nausea, vomiting, abdominal pain; back, flank or loin pain; ± voiding symptoms. *Exam*: Fever, tachycardia; costovertebral angle tenderness; possibly abdominal tenderness. *Laboratory*: Elevated leukocyte count, ESR, and/or C-reactive protein; urinalysis with PMNs and bacteria (as in cystitis), ± leukocyte casts; urine culture with >10^4 colony-forming units/mL of a typical uropathogen (*E. coli, Proteus*). Imaging studies (not routinely indicated for uncomplicated pyelonephritis): ultrasound, intravenous pyelogram, enhanced CT (looking for obstruction, stone).
Acute prostatitis	*History*: Spiking fever, chills, dysuria, pelvic or perineal pain, and cloudy urine; possible obstructive symptoms (dribbling, hesitancy, and anuria). *Exam*: Edematous and tender prostate. *Laboratory*: Pyuria, positive urine culture.
Chronic prostatitis	*History*: Dysuria and frequency in the absence of the signs of acute prostatitis; recurrent urinary tract infections. *Exam*: Prostate tenderness and edema, but is frequently normal. *Laboratory*: Cultures of urine or expressed prostatic secretions are almost always positive.
Painful bladder syndrome/ interstitial cystitis	*History*: Chronic bladder pain associated with bladder filling and/or emptying; urinary frequency, urgency, and nocturia. *Exam*: Diffuse tenderness in lower abdomen and pelvis. Diagnosis based upon characteristic symptoms and exclusion of other conditions.

CT = computed tomography; ESR = erythrocyte sedimentation rate; GI = gastrointestinal; HSV = herpes simplex virus; PMN = polymorphonuclear; STD = sexually transmitted disease; UTI = urinary tract infection.

Gram stain of the urine sediment increases specificity, suggests the type of microorganism, and is particularly useful in complicated urinary tract infection. Bacteriuria and pyuria are the gold standard for the diagnosis of pyelonephritis if they are associated with a suggestive history and physical findings. Leukocyte casts in the urine are specific for pyelonephritis but are uncommonly detected. In clinically ill patients obtain blood cultures.

Obtain a urine culture for women with suspected cystitis if the diagnosis is not clear from the history and physical examination; if an unusual or antimicrobial-resistant organism is suspected; if the patient is pregnant; if therapeutic options are limited because of the patient's medication intolerance history; if the episode represents a suspected relapse or treatment failure after recent treatment for urinary tract infection; and if any underlying complicating conditions are identified.

Proper specimen collection and handling is crucial. High concentrations of gram-negative bacilli (>10^3 colony-forming units/mL) may be significant in symptomatic women; high bacterial concentrations in asymptomatic women are usually irrelevant, regardless of the degree of pyuria. In complicated urinary tract infection, almost any organism can be causative and must be considered seriously if the patient is symptomatic.

Use imaging studies only if an alternative diagnosis or a urological complication is suspected. Obtain a renal and bladder ultrasound as the initial imaging study. Consider CT and MRI for patients with suggestive findings of an anatomical abnormality on ultrasound and for persistent or relapsing pyelonephritis despite a negative ultrasound.

Therapy

Treat nonpregnant women with uncomplicated cystitis empirically with trimethoprim-sulfamethoxazole (TMP-SMZ) for 3 days. If there is a high prevalence of resistance to TMP-SMZ, or intolerance to the drug, substitute nitrofurantoin, fosfomycin, or a fluoroquinolone for 3 days. Patients with underlying complicating conditions are more likely to have a drug-resistant infection, to exhibit a poor response to antimicrobial therapy even when the urine organism is susceptible, and to develop complications if initial therapy is suboptimal. In these patients, obtain a urine culture and treat empirically for 7-14 days with a fluoroquinolone or, if the organism is known to be susceptible, with TMP-SMZ. Acute cystitis in an elderly woman is not automatically considered complicated unless she has multiple co-morbidities, recent exposure to antibiotics, or is a nursing home resident. Obtain a urine culture and susceptibility testing in pregnant women with cystitis and treat for 3-7 days with an oral antimicrobial agent that is safe in pregnancy, such as amoxicillin or nitrofurantoin. Recommend alternative contraception to women with recurrent urinary tract infections who use spermicide-based contraception. Consider daily prophylaxis (one tablet of nitrofurantoin or TMP-SMZ), postcoital prophylaxis (one tablet of TMP-SMZ after coitus), or intermittent self-treatment (3 days of TMP-SMZ or a fluoroquinolone agent) with onset of symptoms in women with recurrent uncomplicated urinary tract infections. Daily topical application of intravaginal estrogen cream reduces the frequency of symptomatic urinary tract infection episodes in postmenopausal women

Administer intravenous fluids in patients with pyelonephritis who are hypotensive. If obstruction is present, catheter drainage of the bladder, replacement of existing catheters, or other drainage procedures are indicated in conjunction with antimicrobial therapy. Treat pyelonephritis with antibiotics for 7-14 days. Use parenteral therapy initially for patients who are acutely ill, nauseated, or vomiting. Consider empiric therapy with fluoroquinolones, extended-spectrum cephalosporins or penicillins, or aminoglycosides (cephalosporins or aminoglycosides alone are insufficient for *Enterococcus*). Change from parenteral to oral therapy once the patient can tolerate oral intake.

Follow-Up

Obtain urine cultures after treatment in pregnant women with acute cystitis to confirm eradication of bacteriuria. Repeat urinalyses or urine cultures at intervals to confirm sterility of the urine through the time of delivery. Perform a urine culture in nonpregnant women with complicated cystitis and confirm symptom resolution.

Confirm the eradication of bacteriuria in patients treated for pyelonephritis by repeating a urinalysis and urine culture. Treat recurrences with antimicrobial drugs based on susceptibility tests. Persistent fever and unilateral flank pain despite adequate treatment suggests perinephric or intrarenal abscess. Emphysematous and xanthogranulomatous pyelonephritis are uncommon, severe infections of the renal parenchyma occurring most commonly in patients with diabetes. Consider urologic consultation in patients with complicated kidney infections, urolithiasis, and any obstruction within the urinary tract.

Book Enhancement

Go to www.acponline.org/essentials/infectious-disease-section .html to view a table on diagnostic tests for urinary tract infection and a urinalysis showing pyuria. In *MKSAP for Students 4*, assess yourself with items 12-13 in the **Infectious Disease Medicine** section.

Bibliography

Bent S, Nallamothu BK, Simel DL, Fihn SD, Saint S. Does this woman have an acute uncomplicated urinary tract infection? JAMA. 2002; 287:2701-10. [PMID: 12020306]

Johnson JR. Urinary Tract Infection. http://pier.acponline.org/physicians/diseases/d162. [Date accessed: 2008 Jan 07] In: PIER [online database]. Philadelphia: American College of Physicians; 2008.

Nicolle LE. Uncomplicated urinary tract infection in adults including uncomplicated pyelonephritis. Urol Clin North Am. 2008;35:1-12 [PMID: 18061019]

Neal DE Jr. Complicated urinary tract infections. Urol Clin North Am. 2008;35:13-22 [PMID: 18061020]

Chapter 49

Sexually Transmitted Diseases

Sara B. Fazio, MD

Sexually transmitted diseases (STDs) are common problems in both the inpatient and the outpatient setting. Diseases characterized by urethritis and cervicitis include gonorrhea and chlamydia, while herpes simplex, primary syphilis and chancroid are the most common infectious diseases characterized by genital ulceration. Human papilloma virus (HPV) causes genital warts as well as cervical dysplasia. Human immunodeficiency virus (HIV) infection is discussed in Chapter 50.

Prevention

Key to the prevention of STDs is educating patients regarding safe sexual practices. All patients should be encouraged to use a latex condom for vaginal or anal intercourse and fellatio. Variables associated with STD acquisition include young age (<25 years), lower socioeconomic status, substance abuse, lack of or inconsistent barrier-method use, intra-uterine device use, and douching. Additionally, new or multiple sexual partners and a history of prior STD increases the risk of disease transmission. Consistent and correct use of condoms reduces transmission of all STDs and pelvic inflammatory disease (PID), chronic pelvic pain, and infertility. Many STDs are spread asymptomatically. The presence of an ulcerative genital lesion greatly increases the risk of HIV transmission, making prevention that much more critical. Partner treatment of patients diagnosed with an STD is an essential public health approach to prevention. HPV vaccination should be offered to all females between the ages of 9 and 26.

Screening

Any individual engaged in high-risk sexual behaviors should be screened for gonorrhea, chlamydia, syphilis, and HIV. All sexually active women aged <25 years should be screened routinely for chlamydia, based on evidence that screening reduces the incidence of PID by >50%. Men who have sex with men should be screened for STDs on an annual basis or more frequently based on risk behavior. Pregnant women should be offered screening for HIV, syphilis, and chlamydia at the first prenatal visit, as well as screening for gonorrhea in high-prevalence areas. A repeat test for gonorrhea should be offered in the third trimester to those at continued risk to prevent neonatal conjunctivitis (ophthalmia neonatorum). Prophylactic cesarean section is indicated in a woman with active herpes simplex virus lesions at the time of delivery to prevent infection in the newborn. The presence of one STD requires screening for other STDs. Papanicolaou (pap) smear testing to screen for HPV and cervical dysplasia is discussed in Chapter 71. While some experts recommend anal Pap smears for HIV infected homosexual men, the current Centers for Disease Control STD treatment guidelines do not recommend routine screening given the limited data available on the natural history of anal squamous intraepithelial lesions and treatment efficacy.

Diagnosis

Genital herpes is suggested by the presence of multiple painful vesicular or ulcerative lesions. The first episode of genital herpes is more severe than recurrent episodes and often involves systemic symptoms. Recurrences are often unilateral and may be preceded by a neuropathic prodrome about 24 hours before lesions develop. Diagnosis is primarily with culture; direct fluorescent antibody testing and polymerase chain reaction (PCR) testing is useful when the diagnosis is unclear. A positive HSV-2 antibody test indicates only previous infection and is not a clinically useful diagnostic test. Culture becomes less sensitive as genital lesions begin to heal. Reliance on the Tzanck test (showing multi-nucleated giant cells) is not recommended due to lack of sensitivity.

In primary syphilis, patients present with a painless ulcer with a clean base, raised indurated edges, and painless regional lymphadenopathy. Secondary syphilis is manifested by a generalized mucocutaneous rash (including the palms and soles), generalized lymphadenopathy, and constitutional symptoms. Tertiary syphilis is characterized by neurologic findings (e.g., meningitis, tabes dorsalis, Argyll Robertson pupil, and mental status changes), cardiac abnormalities, or gummatous disease. Latent syphilis is characterized by positive serology without symptoms. Diagnosis is made by dark-field microscopy or direct fluorescent antibody testing on a scraping specimen from the ulcer, or by the use of a non-treponemal serologic test (RPR or VDRL) followed by a more specific treponemal serology (FTA-ABS or TP-PA) for confirmation. Neurosyphilis requires cerebrospinal fluid examination for diagnosis. Treponemal serologies typically remain positive for life, whereas the non-treponemal serology titers regress after appropriate treatment and are used to assess disease activity.

Chancroid presents with one or more painful genital ulcers as well as frequently with unilateral suppurative inguinal lymphadenopathy. Diagnosis can be made by culture, but because this condition is relatively rare in the United States, culture medium is often not readily available and the diagnosis is often one of exclusion (Table 1).

Gonorrhea should be suspected in a man with purulent or mucopurulent urethral discharge and in women with mucopurulent cervicitis. Gonorrhea and chlamydia are also common etiologies for epididymitis in sexually active men aged <35 years, proctitis in individuals who engage in anal receptive intercourse, and

Table 1. Differential Diagnosis of Genital Ulcers

Disease	Characteristics
Syphilis (*T. pallidum*)	*Incubation*: 9-90 days. *Primary lesion*: papule. *Number of lesions*: usually 1. *Pain*: none. *Size of lesion*: 5-15 mm. *Edges*: indurated. *Base*: clean. *Depth*: moderate. *Lymph nodes*: enlarged, nontender. *U.S. epidemiology*: southeastern U.S., urban areas. The characteristics described are as seen in the classic presentation of infection. Atypical chancres may be small, nonindurated, or with unusual shapes or associated pain.
Herpes (herpes simplex virus 1 and 2)	*Incubation*: days-years. *Primary lesion*: vesicle. *Number of lesions*: multiple. *Pain*: yes. *Size of lesion*: 1-2 mm. *Edges*: flat, red. *Base*: red, exudate. *Depth*: superficial. *Lymph nodes*: enlarged, tender. *U.S. epidemiology*: most common cause of genital ulcers in U.S. Herpes ulcers differ from primary syphilis in that they are much shallower, often appear in crops, begin as a vesicle, and are painful.
Chancroid (*Haemophilus ducreyi*)	*Incubation*: 1-14 days. *Primary lesion*: pustule. *Number of lesions*: 1 or many. *Pain*: exquisite. *Size of lesion*: 5-25 mm. *Edges*: ragged, undermined. *Base*: friable, purulent exudate. *Depth*: deep, excavated. *Lymph nodes*: tender, may suppurate/form buboes. *U.S. epidemiology*: rare; occasionally seen in warmer climates in southern U.S. Many cases are imported into these areas from Mexico or the Caribbean. Chancroid differs from primary syphilis in that the ulceration is usually deeper and more destructive; the edges are ragged rather than punched out; there is significant pain and tenderness associated with it; and significant lymphadenopathy, which is also painful and tender.
Behçet's disease	A systemic disease with genital ulcers as one component of disease manifestations. Ulcers are often painful. Other manifestations include recurrent oral aphthous ulcers, uveitis, pathergy, arthritis, gastrointestinal manifestations, and central nervous system disease. In Behçet's disease, serologic tests for syphilis will be negative.
Lymphogranuloma venereum [LGV] (*Chlamydia trachomatis* serovars L1, L2, or L3)	LGV is extremely rare in the U.S. The infection can begin as a small papule, erosion, or ulcer in the genital or perineal region, which is usually asymptomatic and heals quickly without scarring. Patients with LGV rarely, if ever, present in this early ulcerative stage. Subsequently patients develop the painful lymphadenopathy and bubo formation. During this stage patients may have fever and other constitutional symptoms and develop draining fistulae. The early ulcerative lesions of LGV differ from a syphilitic chancre in that they are smaller, less destructive, and heal very promptly.
Donovanosis, also known as granuloma inguinale (*Calymmatobacterium granulomatis*)	Donovanosis is extremely rare in the U.S. Ulcers are most commonly very large, nontender, beefy red in color, and bleed easily when touched. The lesions of donovanosis differ from the syphilitic chancre in that they are larger, may be multiple in number, and usually have a very beefy red base. The ulcers do not heal spontaneously and can be present chronically.

pharyngitis. Infection at any site may be asymptomatic, most notably infection of the pharynx and rectum, allowing for unrecognized sexual transmission. Visualization of urethral discharge does not distinguish between gonococcal and chlamydial urethritis. Most endocervical infections with gonorrhea or chlamydia in women are asymptomatic, thus a high index of suspicion is necessary. Disseminated gonococcal infection is manifested by rash (Plate 36) and mono- or oligo-arthritis and tendon sheath inflammation. Diagnoses of gonorrhea and chlamydia are best made by culture or PCR nucleic acid amplification (greater sensitivity). PCR testing in men may be taken from a urine specimen; in women, PCR for chlamydia may be performed on the urine, but gonorrhea testing requires an endocervical specimen. In men with gonococcal urethritis, the organism is seen on Gram stain in 95% of cases, allowing for a rapid, specific diagnosis, but Gram stain is less sensitive in endocervical specimens in women and thus should not be used. Urethritis that does not respond to antibiotic treatment for gonorrhea and chlamydia suggests less common causes such as *Trichomonas vaginalis* or herpes simplex virus. Herpes simplex virus also causes cervicitis and proctitis.

PID is a polymicrobial infection of the endometrium, fallopian tubes, and ovaries that is diagnosed by the presence of abdominal discomfort, uterine or adnexal tenderness, or cervical motion tenderness. Other criteria include temperature >101°F (38.3°C), cervical or vaginal mucopurulent discharge, leukocytes in vaginal secretions, and documentation of gonorrhea or chlamydia infection. PID is most likely to occur within 7 days of the onset of menses. While gonorrhea and chlamydia are the primary organisms that cause PID, more recent studies have implicated "bacterial vaginosis" organisms. All women with suspected PID should be tested for gonorrhea and chlamydia and have a pregnancy test to rule out normal or ectopic implantation. In severe cases, imaging should be performed to rule out a tubo-ovarian abscess.

The majority of HPV infection is asymptomatic. Transmission of HPV can occur with skin to mucosa or skin to skin contact. Serotypes 6 and 11 are most often responsible for genital warts (condyloma acuminatum), whereas high risk HPV (serotypes 16, 18, 31, 33 and 35) are associated with cervical dysplasia and cervical cancer. Genital warts may be flat or pedunculated, and are typically diagnosed by appearance alone, though biopsy can be used if necessary.

Therapy

Counsel all patients with active symptoms to abstain from sexual contact until at least 1 week of treatment has been completed. Because herpes simplex virus persists in a dormant state, patients must be educated that treatment does not eradicate the virus and that asymptomatic shedding and transmission can occur, particularly during the first year of infection. Syphilis, gonorrhea, and chlamydia are reportable infectious diseases in every state.

Table 2. Follow-Up for Patients with Sexually Transmitted Disease

Clinical Situation	Recommended Follow-Up
Primary HSV	Counseling regarding the natural history of recurrence and use of barrier contraception.
Primary syphilis	Follow-up quantitative nontreponemal serologies performed at 6, 12, and 24 months.
Patients with tertiary syphilis; HIV patients with late latent syphilis; or treatment failure	Lumbar puncture and cerebrospinal fluid analysis for neurosyphilis.
Sexual partners of patients with syphilis	Serologic testing if >90 days from sexual contact; empiric treatment if <90 days.
Gonorrhea or chlamydia infection	Repeat diagnostic testing if symptoms persist 3-4 days after treatment.
Sexual partners of patients with gonorrhea or chlamydia	Treat all sexual contacts of the last 60 days.
Pelvic inflammatory disease	Re-evaluate within 48 to 72 hours of initiation of therapy and again at the end of antibiotic treatment. Patients not responding to therapy may require parenteral therapy or broader antibiotic coverage, additional diagnostic tests, drainage of an abscess or collection, or surgical intervention.
Any patient with an STD diagnosis	Test for other STDs, including HIV and hepatitis B virus.

HSV = herpes simplex virus; HIV = human immunodeficiency virus; STD = sexually transmitted disease.

Patients with PID can often be treated as outpatients. Hospitalize patients with PID if there is no clinical improvement after 48-72 hours of antibiotics; inability to tolerate oral antibiotics; severe illness with nausea, vomiting, or high fever; suspected intra-abdominal abscess; pregnancy; or noncompliance with outpatient therapy.

Treat primary herpes simplex virus infection with acyclovir, famciclovir, or valacyclovir for 7-10 days, and 3-5 days for recurrent disease. Treatment decreases duration of symptoms and reduces viral shedding. Suppressive therapy may be necessary to decrease the frequency of recurrences.

Chancroid is treated with a single dose of azithromycin or ceftriaxone, 3 days of ciprofloxacin, or 7 days of erythromycin base.

Primary or secondary syphilis is treated with one dose of intramuscular (IM) benzathine penicillin. Latent syphilis or tertiary non-neurosyphilis is treated with three weekly doses of IM benzathine penicillin. Doxycycline and tetracycline are alternatives for penicillin-allergic non-pregnant patients. Failure of nontreponemal serologies to decline four-fold in the 6-12 months after treatment indicates treatment failure or re-acquisition. Neurosyphilis requires intravenous penicillin or ceftriaxone; in penicillin-allergic patients, desensitization is required. The Jarisch-Herxheimer reaction is an acute febrile illness occurring within 24 hours of treatment for any stage of syphilis, and probably represents an immune response to cell wall proteins released by dying spirochetes.

Patients with documented or suspected gonorrhea, including men aged <35 years with presumed epididymitis, are treated for both gonorrhea and chlamydia, given the high frequency of co-infection. Options for gonorrhea treatment include a single dose of IM ceftriaxone or single-dose cefixime. Fluoroquinolones are no longer recommended secondary to the emergence of resistance. Chlamydia infection is effectively treated with a single dose of azithromycin, 7 days of doxycycline, or a fluoroquinolone.

In patients with suspected PID, choice of antibiotic should cover gonorrhea, chlamydia, gram-negative rods, and anaerobic bacteria. Ambulatory patients are treated with a fluoroquinolone or IM cefoxitin versus ceftriaxone and doxycycline with or without metronidazole. Duration of treatment is 14 days.

Treatment of genital warts involves removal, either by patient-applied regimens (podofilox or imiquimod) or provider administered regimens (cryotherapy, podophyllin resin, trichloracetic or bichloracetic acid) or surgical removal. Treatment may reduce, but does not eliminate, HPV.

Follow-up of patients with STDs is important in order to resolve infection and ensure adequate partner management (Table 2).

Book Enhancement

Go to www.acponline.org/essentials/infectious-disease-section .html to view examples of venereal warts, genital and perianal herpes, primary and secondary syphilis, disseminated gonorrhea, and a cervical Gram stain, and to review laboratory studies for primary syphilis and cervicitis. In *MKSAP for Students 4*, assess yourself with items 14-16 in the **Infectious Disease Medicine** section.

Bibliography

Centers for Disease Control and Prevention, Workowski KA, Berman SM. Sexually transmitted diseases treatment guidelines, 2006. MMWR Recomm Rep. 2006;55(RR-11):1-94. Erratum in: MMWR Recomm Rep. 2006;55:997. [PMID: 16888612]

Chapter 50

Human Immunodeficiency Virus Infection

Peter Gliatto, MD

The human immunodeficiency virus (HIV) slowly destroys the immune system and can lead to deadly opportunistic infections. Combination antiretroviral therapy has changed the face of HIV illness, offering for many the chance to live for decades. Despite these advances, it is sobering to remember that of the roughly 1 million persons infected with HIV in the United States, one-quarter to one-third do not know they are infected. Additionally, the effects of this disease on the developing world are devastating. All physicians must have a basic understanding of how HIV is acquired, diagnosed, and treated.

The human immunodeficiency virus enters the bloodstream via mucosal contact. It enters cells through use of an external glycoprotein, gp120, which binds to the CD4+ receptor, and a transmembrane protein, gp41. After fusion with the cell and the introduction of the viral core, the virus's RNA is reverse transcribed into DNA and incorporated into the host cell's DNA. The reverse transcriptase has a high error rate, contributing to the virus's high mutation rate, which influences its virulence and response to host defenses and drug therapy. New virions leave the cell via endocytosis to infect other cells. Infected T cells or virions enter the bloodstream, then multiply in the gastrointestinal tract, spleen, and bone marrow. With this amplification, symptoms of acute HIV infection can result. Host defenses to contain virus spread include CD8+ responses which reduce the viremia to a stable level. The virus results in a destruction of CD4+ cells over a period of years. As the CD4+ count becomes depleted, the patient becomes increasing susceptible to opportunistic infections.

Prevention

Counsel all patients about the routes of HIV transmission and risk-reduction strategies. Teach patients that all forms of sexual contact involving mucosal exposure to genital secretions or blood involve risk of HIV transmission, including oral sex. Screening for other sexually transmitted infections, particularly genital ulcer diseases, is essential, because open lesions increase likelihood of HIV transmission. Routinely offering pregnant women HIV testing is important because antiretroviral treatment administered to HIV-positive women during pregnancy can significantly reduce maternal-fetal transmission. Instruct IV-drug users on risk-reduction behaviors such as avoiding needle sharing. Educating health care workers who are at risk for occupational exposures to HIV-infected blood or bodily fluids about safety precautions (not capping used needles) and offering post-exposure treatment in appropriate circumstances (immediately after a high-risk needle-stick injury) can prevent new cases of HIV infection.

Screening

Recognition of HIV infection in earlier, asymptomatic stages facilitates effective counseling about antiretroviral therapy, monitoring of disease progression, prevention and treatment of opportunistic infections and other complications of HIV, and reduces the risk of transmission to others. Screen all Americans aged 13 to 64 years as recommended in the 2006 Centers for Disease Control (CDC) and Prevention guidelines, which eliminate the need for written consent for HIV testing. The CDC recommended the elimination of written consent in an attempt to increase the number of individuals being tested.

Diagnosis

The presentation of HIV and acquired immunodeficiency syndrome (AIDS) are protean and non-specific. It is essential to maintain a high index of suspicion based on exposures, risk factors, symptoms, and findings on physical examination and diagnostic testing.

Certain diagnoses warrant HIV testing. These include severe or treatment-refractory herpes simplex virus disease, esophageal candidiasis, *Pneumocystis jiroveci* (formerly *carinii*) pneumonitis, cryptococcal meningitis, disseminated mycobacterial infection, cytomegalovirus retinitis or gastrointestinal disease, and toxoplasmosis.

Test for HIV in any patient with signs or symptoms of immunologic dysfunction, weight loss, generalized lymphadenopathy, fever and night sweats of more than 2 weeks duration, oral thrush, severe aphthous ulcers, severe seborrheic dermatitis, or recurrent pneumonias. Unexplained hematologic abnormalities, such as anemia, leukopenia, thrombocytopenia, and polyclonal gammopathy, should prompt consideration of HIV infection.

Suspect primary HIV infection (initial, acute HIV infection) if a febrile illness occurs within several weeks of a potential exposure. Obtain a detailed sexual history and ask about other HIV risks when evaluating an unexplained acute febrile illness, especially if symptoms also include fatigue, adenopathy, pharyngitis, rash, and/or headache.

HIV testing involves a two-step approach. First is the highly sensitive enzyme-linked immunosorbent assay, which may include any one of the approved tests involving blood, oral secretions, or urine; or rapid tests, for which results may be available within an hour. All positive results of these tests require a second confirmatory test, the Western blot, which is highly specific. Seroconversion typically occurs within 6 weeks after infection. During this "window period" before seroconversion, patients have extremely high levels of circulating virus, detectable either by assays for viral nucleic acid (viral load) or viral antigen (e.g., p24 antigen). Use these tests in suspected acute HIV infection.

In patients positive for HIV, assessing the viral load and CD4 count offers important prognostic information as well as baseline values to monitor responses to therapy. The viral load is the most reliable marker for predicting the long-term risk of progression to AIDS or death. The CD4 count is the most reliable marker for the current risk of opportunistic complications of AIDS. Immunosuppression due to HIV infection can cause a number of characteristic infectious and neoplastic conditions (Table 1).

Therapy

Caution HIV-positive patients about using alcohol or other substances that may be toxic to the liver. Many of these patients are co-infected with hepatitis B or C, and drugs to treat HIV or its complications can also affect the liver and drug metabolism.

Suppressing plasma viral load slows the progression of disease, partially reconstitutes immune deficits, improves quality of life, and prolongs survival of many HIV-infected patients. Highly active antiretroviral therapy (HAART) is a drug regimen of three or more active compounds that inhibit HIV. These drugs most benefit patients with symptoms from HIV or opportunistic infections, and/or when the absolute CD4 count is suppressed and/or the viral load is relatively high (Table 2). Antiretroviral therapy for patients with earlier disease is more controversial.

Combination therapy for treatment-naïve patients usually involves a "base" that consists of a non-nucleoside reverse transcriptase inhibitor or one or two protease inhibitors (the second protease inhibitor boosts the levels of the first), combined with a "backbone" that consists of two nucleoside/nucleotide reverse transcriptase inhibitors. A third option is a regimen that consists of three different reverse transcriptase inhibitors, but this may not result in viral suppression that is as durable as with other regimens. Regimens with non-nucleoside reverse transcriptase inhibitors as

Table 1. Complications of HIV Infection

Condition	Associated CD4 Count (cells/µL)	Key Characteristics
Candidiasis	<100	Involves the oropharynx, esophagus, trachea, bronchi, or lungs.
Cryptococcosis	<100	Causes subacute meningitis; often associated with cryptococcemia.
Cryptosporidiosis	Any, but <100 with more severe disease	Persistent watery diarrhea.
Cytomegalovirus	<50	Retinitis, esophagitis, and colitis.
Kaposi's sarcoma	Any	Raised discrete red lesions, often in lower extremities; primarily in homosexual men co-infected with HHV-8.
Lymphoma	Any	β-cell lymphoma; Burkitt's, immunoblastic, or primary CNS lymphoma.
M. tuberculosis	Any	Pulmonary or extrapulmonary infection.
M. avium complex	<50	Disseminated infection, often with liver and bone marrow involvement, and diffuse adenopathy.
Pneumocystis pneumonia	<200	Typically presents with dyspnea on exertion, hypoxia, and diffuse infiltrates on chest x-ray.
Progressive multifocal leukoencephalopathy	<100	Caused by JC virus (a human polyomavirus); white matter lesions seen on imaging; presents with focal neurologic defects but preservation of mental status.
Toxoplasmosis	<100 and seropositive for toxoplasma	Fever, headache, and focal neurologic deficits; ring-enhancing lesions on imaging of CNS.

HHV-8 = human herpesvirus-8; CNS = central nervous system.

Table 2. Recommendations for Initiation of Highly Active Antiretroviral Therapy

Clinical Category	CD4 Cell Count (cells/µL)	Plasma HIV RNA (copies/mL)	Recommendations
AIDS-defining illness or severe symptoms*	Any value	Any value	Treat
Asymptomatic	<200	Any value	Treat
Asymptomatic	>200 but ≤350	Any value	Treatment should be offered after weighing the pros and cons
Asymptomatic	>350	≥100,000	Most experts recommend deferring therapy; some would treat
Asymptomatic	>350	<100,000	Defer therapy

*Constitutional symptoms, including fever, weight loss (>10% from baseline), night sweats, diarrhea.
From Department of Health and Human Services. Guidelines for the use of antiretroviral agents in HIV-1 infected adults and adolescents, October 29, 2004 (www.aidsinfo.nih.gov).

Table 3. Primary Prophylaxis Against Major Pathogens in Patients with HIV Infection

Infectious Agent	CD4 Count (cells/µL)	First-Line Therapy
Pneumocystis jiroveci	<200	Trimethoprim-sulfamethoxazole
Toxoplasmosis gondii	<100	Trimethoprim-sulfamethoxazole
Mycobacterium tuberculosis	Any; treat latent infection if PPD >5 mm and no evidence of active disease	Isoniazid (with pyridoxine)
M. avium complex	<50	Azithromycin

Adapted from Hammer SM. Clinical practice. Management of newly diagnosed HIV infection. N Engl J Med. 2005;353:1702-10. PMID: 16236741.

the base have shown favorable long-term data. Regimens that use protease inhibitors are of concern because of long-term side effects (see below). Select a combination regimen based on drug characteristics, side effect profile, and patient co-morbidities.

Drug selection for patients who have been on antiviral therapy already and who need to switch medications because of virologic failure or intolerable side effects should be based on treatment history and the pattern on virus resistance testing. Use at least two drugs that are new to the patient when changing a regimen. Fusion inhibitors are a new class of medications that target the process of the virus fusing with the cell it is targeting. Consider fusion inhibitors in patients who have been exposed to several different HIV medications and who harbor resistant viruses.

Combination therapy maximizes treatment efficacy by reducing the chances of resistance but increases the chance of drug interactions. Certain anti-retroviral drugs are associated with rare but potentially fatal hepatic steatosis, pancreatitis, myopathy, and lactic acidosis. Protease inhibitors are associated with a cluster of metabolic effects including hyperlipidemia, body fat redistribution, and insulin resistance.

Provide prophylaxis against certain opportunistic infections based on the level of immunosuppression and other clinical factors (Table 3). Vaccinate HIV patients against influenza, pneumococcal pneumonia, and, if not already immune, hepatitis A and B. Vaccination is likely more effective in patients with higher CD4 counts.

Follow-Up

The broad goal of antiretroviral therapy is to achieve the lowest possible viral load while minimizing the adverse effects of treatment. Test viral load and CD4 count four weeks after starting or changing antiretroviral therapy and every three-four months thereafter. Available evidence indicates that suppression of viral load to <5000 copies/mL is associated with improved outcomes and prolonged survival. Generally, an antiretroviral regimen should decrease viral load >1 $\log_{10}$ within 8 weeks and <50 copies/mL at 4 to 6 months. Failure to meet these criteria suggests poor adherence, poor absorption, or viral resistance.

Significant ongoing viral replication in the face of ongoing therapy may contribute to the selection of multi-drug resistance. Suspected viral resistance should prompt a complete change in the antiretroviral regimen, usually based on specific resistance testing and consultation with an expert in infectious diseases.

Regular physical exams and laboratory testing can help detect drug toxicities, opportunistic infections, and treatment failures due to resistance or non-adherence. Depending on the drug regimen, obtain complete blood count, chemistry profile, amylase or lipase values, and cholesterol and triglyceride levels every 3 to 4 months to monitor for possible drug toxicities. The physical exam should also assess for potential drug toxicities, including rashes, fat redistribution, hepatic enlargement or tenderness, muscle tenderness, and/or peripheral neuropathy. Patients infected with HIV should be tested for hepatitis B and C viruses. It is also critical for women to have regular gynecological evaluations, including Pap smears; HIV-positive women have a much higher rate of cervical cancer than uninfected individuals.

Book Enhancement

Go to www.acponline.org/essentials/infectious-disease-section.html to view examples of fat redistribution syndrome, oral hairy leukoplakia, oral candidiasis, Kaposi's sarcoma, and cytomegalovirus retinitis, and to review tables of HIV drugs and their side effects, HIV risk assessment, and HIV clinical course. In *MKSAP for Students 4*, assess yourself with items 17-21 in the **Infectious Disease Medicine** section.

Bibliography

Kilby JM. Human Immunodeficiency Virus Disease. http://pier.acponline.org/physicians/diseases/d132. [Date accessed: 2008 Jan 10] In: PIER [online database]. Philadelphia: American College of Physicians; 2008.

Simon V, Ho DD, Abdool Karim Q. HIV/AIDS epidemiology, pathogenesis, prevention, and treatment. Lancet. 2006;368:489-504. [PMID: 16890836]

Chapter 51

Health Care Associated Infections

Brijen Shah, MD

A health care associated (nosocomial) infection is a systemic or localized infection that was not present or incubating at the time of hospital admission, occurring 48 or more hours after admission to a hospital or within 48-72 hours of discharge. The most common health care associated infections in medical patients are urinary tract infections, pneumonia (including ventilator-associated pneumonia), bloodstream infections, and *Clostridium difficile* antibiotic-associated diarrhea. More than 2.1 million health care associated infections occur annually and cause significant increases in morbidity, mortality, and health care costs.

The single most important way to prevent health care associated infections is diligent hand washing or hand disinfection by each and every health care worker. In addition, infection-control programs help to prevent these infections. Infection control includes surveillance for common infections and monitoring of high-risk patients and hospital areas to identify prevalence of specific infections or organisms and setting goals for improvement. Patients with communicable diseases need to be isolated appropriately and quickly to minimize spread to other patients, visitors, and health care workers (Table 1).

Catheter-Associated Urinary Tract Infections

There are 900,000 health care associated urinary tract infections annually in the United States and most are related to the use of urinary catheters. Risk factors for development of catheter-associated urinary tract infections (CAUTIs) include advanced age, female sex, diabetes, malnutrition, renal dysfunction, and improper catheter care. Catheters increase the risk for developing a CAUTI because 1) bacteria can be inoculated directly into the bladder during insertion; 2) catheters are conduits to the bladder; 3) the glycocalyx that forms on the catheter surface protects bacteria from antibiotics and host defenses; and 4) residual urine serves as a reservoir for bacterial growth.

CAUTIs can be prevented by using a urinary catheter only when indicated and removing it as soon as possible. Hand washing and aseptic catheter placement using a closed-system catheter is the foundation for preventing infection (Table 2). Manipulation and irrigation should be minimized. Specimens should be collected using the drainage bag valve.

Patients with CAUTIs often do not experience typical signs of urinary tract infection. Nevertheless, obtain blood and urine cultures if a patient develops fever or cloudy urine, or other systemic manifestation compatible with infection. If a CAUTI is suspected, management includes removal of the catheter; catheter replacement is performed only if deemed essential. Pathogenic organisms include *E. coli, Klebsiella, Proteus, Enterococcus, Pseudomonas,* and *Staphylococcus*. Fungi (e.g., *Candida*) are most prevalent in patients with diabetes or chronic indwelling catheters. Ideally, culture results should be obtained prior to the administration of antibiotics. In general, a third-generation cephalosporin (e.g., cefotaxime, ceftriaxone) or fluoroquinolone (e.g., ciprofloxacin, levofloxacin) is used for suspected gram-negative infection and vancomycin for a suspected *Staphylococcus* or enterococcal infection (until resistance patterns are obtained). Complications from CAUTIs include pyelonephritis, sepsis, and prostatitis.

Catheter-Related Intravascular Infections

Approximately 250,000 hospital acquired bloodstream infections occur each year in the United States. The primary risk factor is

Table 1. Infection Control Precautions for Heath Care Institutions

Transmission Mode	Precautions	Patients
Airborne	Patient isolated in a private room with negative air pressure; the door must remain closed, and all entering persons wear masks with a filtering capacity of 95%. Transported patients must wear masks.	For patients with known or suspected illnesses transmitted by airborne droplet nuclei such as tuberculosis, measles, varicella, or disseminated varicella zoster virus infection.
Droplet	Patient isolated in private room and hospital personnel wear face masks when within 3 feet of the patient.	For patients with known or suspected illnesses transmitted by large-particle droplets such as *Neisseria meningitides* infections and influenza.
Contact	Patient isolated in a private room or with patients who have the same active infection. Nonsterile gloves and gowns are required for direct contact with the patient or any infective material; gowns and/or gloves are removed before exiting isolation rooms.	For patients with known or suspected illnesses transmitted by direct contact including infections due to vancomycin-resistant enterococci and methicillin-resistant *Staphylococcus aureus*.

Table 2. Best Practices to Prevent Health Care Associated Infections

Practice	Notes
Hand hygiene	• Clean hands with soap and water or waterless alcohol product before and after contact with patients or contaminated surfaces.
	• Install alcohol-based waterless cleaning products inside and outside all patient rooms and in other locations where clinical care will be provided.
	• Do not allow clinical staff to wear artificial nails.
Catheter-related bloodstream infections	• Remove unnecessary vascular lines.
	• Use recommended hand hygiene before insertion or manipulation of vascular lines.
	• Use maximal barrier precautions (gowns, gloves, masks, head covers) for insertion of vascular lines.
	• Apply appropriate skin antiseptics (chlorhexidine is the agent of choice) for insertion of vascular lines, dressing changes, and reinsertion.
	• Use the subclavian site whenever possible, because this site is associated with the lowest risk of infection.
	• Maintain clean and dry dressings.
	• Do not use prophylactic antibiotics for insertion of vascular lines.
Prevention of urinary tract infections	• Remove all unnecessary catheters.
	• Use sterile technique for insertion of catheters.
	• Do not remove urine samples from lines or open systems.
	• Do not use antibiotics prophylactically.
Prevention of ventilator-associated pneumonia	• Sterilize and maintain respiratory equipment appropriately.
	• Raise the head of the bed at a 45-degree angle (use the semi-recumbent position).
	• Use noninvasive ventilation techniques when possible.
	• Use oscillation or rotate the patient.
	• Use good oral care.
	• Use endotracheal tubes that allow for subglottic suctioning in high-risk patients.

Modified from Medical Knowledge Self-Assessment Program (MKSAP) 14. Philadelphia: American College of Physicians; 2006.

the presence of a central venous catheter; 3%-7% of these catheters become infected. Hospital acquired bloodstream infections increase morbidity, duration of hospitalization, and cost per patient.

Use of intravenous catheters should be reserved for patients with proven need, and the catheter should be removed as soon as clinically possible. Use of sterile technique and maximum sterile barriers minimize risk. Specifically, use full-body sterile drape, gown, mask, and gloves for central catheter insertion. Chlorhexidine is the most effective agent for skin decontamination before catheter insertion and is used whenever possible, instead of povidone/iodine or alcohol alone (see Table 2). The highest risk for infection is associated with femoral placement and the lowest risk is associated with subclavian placement.

The pathogenesis of central-venous catheter associated infection is contamination from skin flora, intraluminal or hub contamination, and secondary seeding from other sources. Microorganisms from patient skin or healthcare workers migrate along the catheter and cause contamination. Thrombosis, contaminated IV products, and flushing can cause contamination.

Antibiotic-coated catheters may decrease the risk of early central catheter-related infection. Because hub contamination is an important source of catheter-related infection, use of sterile technique when accessing the catheter and limiting the number of access events help prevent hub contamination. Although routine replacement of peripheral catheters may prevent infection, the same is not recommended for central venous catheters. In addition, routine changes of dressings for catheters do not seem to prevent catheter infection.

Consider catheter-related infection in any patient with fever and a central venous catheter. Purulence and cellulitis around the catheter site are more specific for catheter-related infection, but not sensitive. Clinical factors predicting catheter-related infection include placement duration >4 days, catheter thrombosis, prior positive blood cultures, respiratory infection, difficult or emergent insertion, multiple lumen catheter, immunocompromised patients, and high number of manipulations per day.

Diagnosis typically relies on culture data, because clinical features are poor predictors. Correlation of bacterial growth from tip culture with clinical features, like fever and/or positive peripheral blood culture with the same organism, are indicative of catheter-related infection. In the absence of these criteria, positive catheter cultures often represent colonization or contamination. Persistent bacteremia strongly suggests endovascular infection. Look for endocarditis in the setting of bloodstream infection and a heart murmur or previous valvular heart disease.

Remove the catheter for all catheter infections, except uncomplicated coagulase-negative staphylococcal tunneled catheter infections. Begin empirical treatment with broad-spectrum antibiotics and then narrow the regimen once culture data are obtained. Coagulase-negative staphylococci, enterococci, *S. aureus*, and gram-negative rods (*E. coli*, *Klebsiella*, and *Pseudomonas*) are the common pathogens. Use vancomycin for empiric coverage because of its activity against coagulase-negative staphylococci and *Staphylococcus aureus*. Additional empirical coverage for enteric gram-negative bacilli and *Pseudomonas aeruginosa* with the use of a third (e.g., ceftriaxone, ceftazidime) or fourth-generation cephalosporin (e.g., cefepime) may be needed for severely ill or immunocompromised patients. Use fluconazole or amphotericin for empirical treatment when fungemia is suspected. Once resistance patterns have returned, narrow to appropriate coverage. Uncomplicated infections are treated for 10-14 days for most pathogens; coagulase-negative staphylococci may be treated for 5-7 days if the infected catheter is removed.

Complications of catheter-associated blood stream infections include septic thrombosis, endocarditis, osteomyelitis, meningitis, and abscess. Patients with complicated infection require six weeks or greater of antibiotic therapy.

Hospital-Acquired and Ventilator-Associated Pneumonia

Pneumonia is the leading cause of death from hospital-acquired infection. Hospital-acquired pneumonia (HAP) is defined as occurring 48 hours or more after admission. Many cases of HAP occur outside of the intensive care unit setting, but the highest risk is in patients receiving mechanical ventilation. Ventilator-associated pneumonia (VAP) is one of the most common types of HAP, affecting 9%-27% of intubated patients, and is defined as occurring >48 hours after endotracheal intubation. The development of VAP is an independent predictor of increased mortality among critically ill patients and is associated with prolonged hospitalization and increased costs. Risk factors for VAP include nasal intubation, the presence of a nasogastric tube, supine positioning, large gastric volumes, gastric alkalinization, reintubation, malnutrition, and accumulation of circuit condensate. HAP and VAP likely occur due to micro-aspiration of organisms from the oropharynx into the lower respiratory tract, poor host immune defenses, and increased gastric pH which impacts the sterility of stomach contents.

Minimizing manipulation of the endotracheal tube and ventilator tubing and performing meticulous hand disinfection before and after any contact with the system can prevent infections. Following weaning protocols can facilitate timely extubation and reduce the risk of infection. Keeping the patient in a semi-erect position decreases aspiration of upper airway secretions and pneumonia. VAP is also increased in patients who develop sinusitis; avoiding nasal intubation and nasogastric tubes can decrease this risk. Although ventilator circuits do not need to be changed regularly, any accumulating condensate should be drained carefully into patient-specific drainage containers (Table 2).

Suspect VAP if the patient has a radiographic infiltrate that is new or progressive, along with clinical findings suggesting infection (e.g., fever, purulent sputum, leukocytosis) and decline in oxygenation. The presence of neutrophils or an organism on gram stain can refine the diagnostic accuracy for VAP.

Do not delay empiric antibiotic therapy for the purpose of performing diagnostic studies. Antibiotic selection is based on the risk for multi-drug resistant pathogens. These risk factors include prolonged duration of hospitalization (≥5 days), admission from a health care related facility, and recent prolonged antibiotic therapy. Antibiotic selection is based on local antimicrobial susceptibility and anticipated side effects and takes into consideration which antibiotics were recently administered. Common pathogens include *Enterobacter*, *Pseudomonas*, *Klebsiella*, *E. coli*, *Streptococcus*, and *S. aureus* (including MRSA). In patients with no risk factors, use ceftriaxone or levofloxacin. Patients with risk factors should be placed on antipseudomonal treatment and vancomycin. For suspected pseudomonal infections, therapy includes a β-lactam plus either an antipseudomonal quinolone or an aminoglycoside.

Clostridium difficile Antibiotic-Associated Diarrhea

Clostridium difficile antibiotic-associated diarrhea occurs in about 20% of hospitalized patients taking antibiotics. The combination of health care associated exposure to *C. difficile* and loss of normal protective colonic bacteria leads to colonization. The colitis is produced by two toxins, A and B. These have different mechanisms of action, but both cause cytotoxicity at extremely low concentrations. Risk factors include use of antibiotics, enemas, intestinal stimulants, and chemotherapeutic agents that alter the colonic flora.

Limiting unnecessary antibiotic exposure is a key factor in preventing *C. difficile* infection. Routine infection-control measures to prevent the spread of *C. difficile* include adherence to strict hand washing procedure and use of universal precautions (see Table 2). Patients with known or suspected illness should be placed under contact isolation.

Consider *C. difficile* infection in patients with diarrhea who have received antibiotic therapy in the last 2 months or have been recently hospitalized. Patients may complain of abdominal pain, fever, anorexia, malaise, or vomiting. Physical examination may demonstrate signs of volume depletion, abdominal tenderness, and, in severe cases, rigidity and rebound tenderness. Obtain an ELISA test of the stool for both toxin A and B; sensitivity is improved by serial testing. Cytotoxin assay is the gold standard for diagnosis but is not widely available. In select patients, colonoscopy may help establish diagnosis by demonstrating typical pseudomembranes. In severe cases, complications include toxic megacolon, colonic perforation, severe ileus, ascites, and death.

Metronidazole is the first-line drug therapy for *C. difficile* infection, administered orally or intravenously. Give oral vancomycin for patients with metronidazole intolerance, severe or fulminant colitis, immunosuppressed states, and recurrent infection. Treat a first relapse with a second course of the initial antibiotic used for first-line therapy.

Book Enhancement

Go to www.acponline.org/essentials/infectious-disease-section.html to view an example of *C. difficile* colitis, review the different types of intravascular catheters, and review the differential diagnosis of an intravascular catheter infection. In *MKSAP for Students 4*, assess yourself with items 22-27 in the **Infectious Disease Medicine** section.

Bibliography

American College of Physicians. Medical Knowledge Self-Assessment Program (MKSAP) 14. Philadelphia: American College of Physicians; 2006.

Klompas M. Does this patient have ventilator-associated pneumonia? JAMA 2007;297:1583-1593. [PMID: 17426278]

Mermel LA, Farr BM, Sherertz RJ, et al. Infectious Diseases Society of America; American College of Critical Care Medicine; Society for Healthcare Epidemiology of America. Guidelines for the management of intravascular catheter-related infections. Clin Infect Dis. 2001; 32: 1249-72. [PMID: 11303260]

Chapter 52

Tuberculosis

Arlina Ahluwalia, MD

Tuberculosis is a common infectious disease worldwide with mortality rates up to 80% in the untreated. Infection by *Mycobacterium tuberculosis* primarily involves the lungs but has the potential to affect nearly any organ. Initial acquisition of the infection is usually via respiratory droplets deposited in the terminal airspaces. T cells and macrophages provide the primary host response to contain the infection. Lymphatic and hematogenous dissemination, however, often results in infection in other tissues. Progression to disease may occur directly after infection, or years later through reactivation of dormant bacilli. Recent challenges to tuberculosis control in the United States include the association with HIV infection, risks of reactivation (especially in immigrants), spread of new disease, occasionally in epidemic form, and emergence of multi-drug-resistant strains. Multi-drug resistance complicates efforts to eradicate tuberculosis and constitutes a major factor in mandating lengthy 3-4–drug regimens monitored by a health care worker or public health program. Aggressive screening programs and high index of suspicion form the cornerstone of control of active tuberculosis infection and residual infection without any systemic manifestations, now called *latent tuberculosis infection* (LTBI). Treatment of LTBI decreases rates of tuberculosis reactivation.

Prevention

Implement primary prevention of tuberculosis by isolating infectious patients and promote secondary prevention by treating patients with evidence of LTBI; the risk of reactivation tuberculosis is greatest in the first 1-2 years following infection. All cases of active tuberculosis must be reported to the public health department. Hospitalized patients with suspected or confirmed active tuberculosis are isolated in a private room with negative air pressure; the door remains closed, all entering persons wear masks with a filtering capacity of 95% (different from regular surgical masks), and the hospital infection-control department must be notified.

Offer LTBI treatment to all high-risk persons with positive tuberculin skin test regardless of age unless prior treatment is documented or is medically contraindicated. Among such individuals, treatment may reduce the risk of active disease up to 90%. Bacille Calmette-Guérin (BCG) vaccine has no role in prevention of tuberculosis in the United States.

Screening

Screen high-risk individuals for LTBI with purified protein derivative (PPD) using the Mantoux skin test method. The high-risk population includes individuals who have close contact with a patient with known or suspected active tuberculosis; who were born in areas with high rates of tuberculosis infection (e.g., Asia, Africa, Latin America, Eastern Europe, Russia); who reside or are employed in high-risk congregate settings; who provide health care to high-risk persons; who are from medically underserved or low-income populations; who are of racial/ethnic minority populations with increased prevalence of tuberculosis (e.g., Asian and Pacific Islanders, Hispanics, African-Americans, Native Americans, migrant farm workers, homeless persons); or who use illicit intravenous drugs. Measurement of induration, not the size of the erythema, defines a positive screening test. Taking into account the patient's risk profile and the amount of induration increases the specificity of the skin test (Table 1).

Skin tests do not always convert after BCG vaccination, and history of vaccination alters neither testing nor consideration of treatment in most adults. Because the skin test result may not

Table 1. Criteria for Tuberculin Positivity by Risk Group

≥ 5 mm Induration	≥ 10 mm Induration	≥ 15 mm Induration
HIV-positive persons	Recent (<5 yrs) arrivals from high-prevalence countries	All others with no risk factors for TB
Recent contact with active TB case	Injection drug users	
Persons with fibrotic changes on chest x-ray consistent with old TB	Residents or employees of high-risk congregate settings: prisons and jails, nursing homes and other long-term facilities for the elderly, hospitals and other health care facilities, residential facilities for patients with AIDS, homeless shelters	
Patients with organ transplants and other immunosuppressive conditions (receiving the equivalent of ≥15 mg/d of prednisone for >4 weeks)	Mycobacteriology lab personnel	
	Persons with clinical conditions that put them at high-risk for active disease	
	Children age <4 years or exposed to adults in high-risk categories	

HIV = human immunodeficiency virus; TB = tuberculosis infection.

become positive for up to 12 weeks after an exposure to active tuberculosis, consider retesting or empiric treatment in selected high-risk individuals. Patients exposed to tuberculosis in the more distant past may have an initial negative skin test; placing a second test 7-21 days after the first may be helpful in reducing the false-negative response rate. Such two-step testing often "boosts" a negative test to positive as the immune system recalls its previous exposure, thus uncovering a true-positive result. Two-step testing may be particularly helpful in older persons and in distinguishing new from old exposures in annual employee testing programs. Another screening option is the RD1 T-cell release assay (interferon gamma assay), which is more specific than tuberculin skin testing for the diagnosis of active tuberculosis and LTBI in previously BCG-vaccinated patients. The RD1 gene is absent from the genomes of all BCG substrains and all nontuberculous mycobacteria with the exception of *M. kansasii*, *M. marinum*, and *M. szulgai*.

Diagnosis

Maintain a high level of suspicion for active tuberculosis to enable rapid diagnosis. Bacteriologic confirmation and susceptibility testing form the cornerstone of management for a patient with clinical evidence of or suspected active tuberculosis. Constitutional or pulmonary signs or symptoms, often insidious, include cough >3 weeks, chest pain, hemoptysis (more likely with cavitation and rarely on presentation), fever, chills, night sweats, easy fatigability, weight loss, and anorexia; however, often only a few cardinal symptoms are evident on presentation. Gather information about known active tuberculosis exposures, prior tuberculosis, and history of a positive skin test. The pulmonary examination is often minimally abnormal. HIV-infected or other immunocompromised patients often present without classic signs or symptoms of tuberculosis and have a greater likelihood of dissemination or extra-pulmonary infection. Table 2 summarizes a differential diagnosis for tuberculosis.

Obtain acid-fast bacilli smears and cultures (pulmonary and any suspected site of infection), chest radiograph, and skin testing in patients suspected of having active tuberculosis (Table 3). The delayed-type hypersensitivity reaction to purified protein derivative is usually positive within 48-72 hours. Remember that a false-negative skin test may occur in anergic patients and in up to 25% of active tuberculosis cases. On three separate days, send early-morning induced sputum (or early-morning gastric washings if voluntary sputum is unattainable) for rapid testing, culture, and stain (Ziehl-Neelsen or Kinyoun). Nucleic acid amplification tests of sputum may be used to exclude tuberculosis in patients with false-positive sputum (non-tuberculous mycobacteria) or to confirm the disease in some patients with false-negative smears. Patients with active disease may have only a single positive culture. For patients suspected of having pleural tuberculosis, consider thoracentesis to obtain fluid for testing or pleural biopsies. In persons not already known to be HIV-positive, test for HIV infection.

Chest x-ray abnormalities of reactivation tuberculosis classically include lesions in the apical-posterior segments of the upper lung and superior segments of the lower lobe. Primary progressive tuberculosis may manifest as hilar adenopathy or infiltrates in any part of the lung similar to bacterial pneumonia. Atypical or absent radiologic findings commonly occur in immunocompromised patients but may also be the case for immunocompetent patients. Bronchoscopy may aid diagnosis in certain circumstances.

Therapy

LTBI is treated with isoniazid for nine months, or alternatively, rifampin for four months, though cases must be individualized. Before treatment is initiated, exclude active tuberculosis and HIV infection.

Table 2. Differential Diagnosis of Tuberculosis (TB)

Disease	Notes
Nontuberculous mycobacterium	Signs and symptoms may be the same as for *M. tuberculosis*. Usually less fever and weight loss than in patients with *M. tuberculosis*. Presence of multiple nodules with bronchiectasis on computed tomography of the lung was highly specific for *M. avium* complex in one study.
Sarcoidosis (see Chapter 79)	Dyspnea and cough. Chest x-ray: diffuse infiltrative lung disease with bilateral hilar adenopathy. Noncaseating granulomas on biopsy. Diagnosis made after exclusion of other possibilities.
Aspiration pneumonia	May have indolent course. Radiologic infiltrates are more common in dependent areas. Patient may have decrease in mental status or evidence of reduced gag reflex.
Lung abscess	Frequently in posterior upper segment of upper lobes. May be acute or indolent. Patient usually has very foul-smelling sputum.
Histoplasmosis or coccidioidomycosis	Patient may have fever, cough, night sweats. These diseases are usually geographically specific (histoplasmosis, Midwest; coccidiomycosis, Southwest). Chest x-rays may be miliary (histoplasmosis) or cavitary.
Wegener's granulomatosis (see Chapter 90)	Patients have fever and cough. Necrotizing granulomas in the lung and necrotizing glomerulonephritis. Chest x-ray shows a cavitary lesion up to 70% of the time.
Actinomycosis	Cough, hemoptysis, and eventually draining sinuses are characteristic. Indolent course; may have respiratory symptoms up to 5 months before diagnosis. Sulphur granules are seen in stain of draining sinuses.
Neoplasm (see Chapter 69)	Patients may have same symptoms as TB (i.e., weight loss and cough). Primary lung cancer, lymphoma, metastasis. Cytology or biopsy to rule out. Patients may have neoplasm and *M. tuberculosis* infection.

Table 3. Laboratory and Other Studies for Tuberculosis (TB)

Test	Notes
Complete blood count	Anemia present in 10%, particularly if disseminated infection; leukocytosis present in 10%.
Electrolytes	Hyponatremia in up to 11% of patients.
Chest x-ray	Lesions in the apical-posterior segments of the upper lung and superior segments of the lower lobe are the classic appearance of reactivation TB. May be normal in patients with endobronchial disease, peribronchial node with fistula, or symptomatic HIV patients with active TB. In disseminated disease, 50%-90% have a miliary pattern on chest x-ray.
Tuberculin skin test (PPD)	Sensitivity, 59%-100%; specificity, 44%-100%. Sensitivity and specificity change with risk factor of patient and established cut-off point for that risk factor (see Table 1). Positive test may be indication of latent TB. False-positive results can occur with exposure to, or disease of, nontuberculous mycobacteria. False-negative results occur in anergic patients and in up to 25% of active cases.
RD1 T-cell-based assays	More specific than tuberculin skin testing in the setting of previous Calmette-Guérin bacillus vaccination; may be more sensitive in cases of immune deficiency. Cannot distinguish between LTBI and active infection.
Smear of sputum for acid-fast bacilli	Sensitivity, 50%-80% (with multiple specimens up to 96%). At least 5000 to 10,000 organisms should be present for a smear to be positive. The more acid-fast bacilli seen, the more infectious is the patient. Induced sputum or gastric washings may be obtained if patient does not have a productive cough. Nontuberculous mycobacteria may produce positive smears. Nocardia are acid fast on the modified acid-fast stain.
Culture of sputum for acid-fast bacilli	Sensitivity, 67%-82%; specificity, 99%-100%. Solid media cultures in conjunction with liquid media are frequently the gold standard used for diagnosis. The only false-positive results that occur are as a result of laboratory error or other contamination of specimen. False-negative results do occur and are often due to nontuberculous mycobacterial overgrowth and antibiotic treatment.
Nucleic acid amplification of smear-positive sputum	Sensitivity, 95%; specificity, 98%. Rapid test; results available in a few hours. False-positive result only if laboratory contamination, although test does not indicate if bacteria are alive or dead (i.e., the test may remain positive for some time after treatment).

HIV = human immunodeficiency virus; LTBI = latent tuberculosis infection; PPD = purified protein derivative.

At least 6 months of 3-4–drug treatment is standard for suspected or confirmed active tuberculosis, ideally using directly observed therapy. These approaches decrease acquired drug resistance, relapse, reactivation, and transmission. Initial treatment of patients with documented absence of resistance usually consists of isoniazid, rifampin, pyrazinamide, and possibly ethambutol. Repeated sputum smear and culture after the initial 2-month phase of therapy may aid in determining whether the continuation phase of treatment requires 4 or 7 months of therapy, especially in cavitary disease. Multi-drug-resistant (MDR) tuberculosis is resistant to at least isoniazid and rifampin, and possibly to other chemotherapeutic agents. Extensively drug-resistant tuberculosis (XDR) is resistant to at least isoniazid, rifampin, fluoroquinolones, and either aminoglycosides or capreomycin, or both. Treatment of MDR or XDR tuberculosis requires an individualized regimen in consultation with an expert based on comprehensive drug susceptibility testing.

Obtain baseline blood tests specific to potential drug toxicity before starting therapy to detect abnormalities that might complicate therapy (e.g., hepatic dysfunction complicated by isoniazid, pyrazinamide, or rifampin). Audiometry (streptomycin toxicity) or visual testing (ethambutol toxicity) may also be required for baseline or follow-up.

Hospitalization of all patients suspected of having active tuberculosis is not required, but is appropriate in cases of respiratory distress, marked hemoptysis, other indicators of systemic disease requiring hospital support, or an unstable housing situation. Consider maintenance of isolation in MDR tuberculosis until the patient is culture-negative. Surgical resection of diseased tissue is rarely required but may be considered in certain circumstances (e.g., bronchopleural fistula, lack of response in MDR tuberculosis).

Follow-Up

Ensure careful monitoring for treatment compliance for active tuberculosis or LTBI. Consider monthly sputum cultures to monitor treatment response, and adjust the drug regimen based on susceptibilities and length of therapy. A tuberculosis expert should be consulted if the sputum culture remains positive or if the patient has not improved clinically after 3 months of therapy. Periodic (monthly) assessments for adverse reactions in patients on treatment, including hepatitis, anemia, thrombocytopenia, visual changes, and gout, should focus on symptom surveillance rather than scheduled laboratory testing. Periodic laboratory monitoring in patients at higher risk for hepatitis (e.g., elderly, history of alcohol abuse, viral hepatitis, HIV) is reasonable. Ensure that household members and other close contacts of infectious tuberculosis patients are tested for LTBI.

Book Enhancement

Go to www.acponline.org/essentials/infectious-disease-section.html to view an x-ray of reactivation tuberculosis and a positive Mantoux skin test and to review a list of persons at higher risk for active tuberculosis once infected. In *MKSAP for Students 4*, assess yourself with items 28-34 in the **Infectious Disease Medicine** section.

Bibliography

American Thoracic Society; Centers for Disease Control and Prevention; Infectious Diseases Society of America. Controlling tuberculosis in the United States. Am J Respir Crit Care Med. 2005;172:1169-227. [PMID: 16249321]

Webb R, Feldman S. Tuberculosis. http://pier.acponline.org/physicians/diseases/ d273. [Date accessed: 2008 Feb 4] In: PIER [online database]. Philadelphia: American College of Physicians; 2008.

Chapter 53

Community-Acquired Pneumonia

Irene Alexandraki, MD

Community-acquired pneumonia (CAP) affects 4 million adults per year in the United States, 20% of whom will require hospitalization. CAP is the leading cause of death from infectious disease in the United States and the sixth-leading cause of death overall.

Host defense mechanisms keep the lower airways sterile. Pneumonia develops when there is a defect in host defenses, exposure to a particularly virulent organism, or an overwhelming inoculum. The pathogens descend from the oropharynx to the lower respiratory tract (90% of cases) or are acquired through inhalation (viruses), hematogenously (*Staphylococcus*), or directly from a contiguous infected site. Alterations in anatomical barriers and impairment in the immune system, including humoral or cell-mediated immunity, or phagocytic function are risk factors for pneumonia.

Streptococcus pneumoniae is the most common pathogen isolated from patients with CAP. Drug-resistant *S. pneumoniae* accounts for up to 40% of isolates. Other common bacterial pathogens include *H. influenzae* and atypical pathogens, such as *M. pneumoniae*, *C. pneumoniae*, and *Legionella*. Gram-negative bacterial pneumonia may be present in patients with medical comorbidities such as chronic cardiopulmonary disease, recent antibiotic therapy, or residents of nursing homes. *Klebsiella pneumoniae* causes severe pneumonia in alcoholic patients. *Pseudomonas aeruginosa* is more common with structural lung disease such as bronchiectasis. Viral pathogens, including influenza, parainfluenza, adenovirus, and respiratory syncytial virus also cause CAP. Prior influenza infection increases susceptibility to a secondary bacterial pulmonary infection, resulting in increased morbidity and mortality during influenza epidemics and pandemics.

Prevention

Influenza vaccine prevents or attenuates illness due to influenza and reduces pneumonia-related mortality during influenza season by 27% to 50%. Administer influenza vaccine yearly between early September and mid-November to patients at increased risk for influenza complications and persons who can transmit the infection to high-risk patients and other special groups. Consider empiric use of oseltamivir and zanamivir against influenza A or B, in unvaccinated, high-risk patients during an epidemic.

Administer pneumococcal vaccine to all patients aged ≥65 years and to all persons aged <65 years who live in long-term care facilities or have coronary artery disease, heart failure, chronic obstructive pulmonary disease, diabetes mellitus, alcoholism, cirrhosis, cerebrospinal fluid leaks, and asplenia. Immunize immunocompromised persons aged <65 years, including patients with HIV infection, malignancies, multiple myeloma, leukemia, lymphoma, Hodgkin's disease, chronic renal disease, or nephrotic syndrome. Vaccinate Alaskan natives and American Indian populations because they have rates that are three to four times higher than the baseline population at any age. Revaccinate immunocompromised patients once, 5 years after initial vaccination. The current pneumococcal vaccine contains purified, capsular polysaccharide from 23 serotypes that cause 85% to 90% of invasive pneumonia in adults and children and is effective in preventing pneumococcal bacteremia and meningitis.

Review the vaccination status and risk factors in all patients aged >50 years and revaccinate (once) anyone aged ≥65 years who was vaccinated initially before age 65. Consider giving the vaccine to any hospitalized patient before discharge.

Diagnosis

Consider pneumonia in a patient with cough, sputum, fever, chills, or dyspnea. Ask about pleuritic chest pain, duration of symptoms, night sweats, and weight loss. Symptoms may gradually worsen over days or develop abruptly. Patients with chronic illnesses with pneumonia may present with nonrespiratory symptoms or deterioration of their illness. Elderly patients may have confusion, weakness, lethargy, poor oral intake, or complaints of falling; they may be afebrile and remain undiagnosed until late in the course of illness.

Ask the patient about chronic heart and lung disease (at risk for pneumococcus, enteric gram-negative bacteria, and *H. influenzae*), travel to the southwest United States (coccidioidomycosis) or Southeast Asia (tuberculosis), alcohol abuse (anaerobes, *K. pneumoniae*), injection-drug use (*S. aureus*, anaerobes, *M. tuberculosis*), or exposure to farm animals (*Coxiella burnetii*), birds (*Chlamydia psittaci, Cryptococcus, Histoplasma*), and bats (*Histoplasma*). Assess risk of aspiration, such as history of stroke, seizures, alcoholism, or poor dentition (anaerobes). Obtain information about residence and recent antibiotic therapy, which may help predict likely etiologic pathogens.

Look for tachypnea, crackles, bronchial breath sounds, egophony, and dullness to percussion with reduced breath sounds. Respiratory rate >30/min, systolic blood pressure <90 mm Hg, diastolic blood pressure <60 mm Hg, heart rate >125 bpm, and temperature <35°C (95°F) or >40°C (104°F) are associated with increased likelihood of a poor outcome, and the presence of any of these is an indication for prompt hospitalization. Also consider hospitalization for those who have failed outpatient therapy, have decompensated comorbid illness, have complex social needs, or require intravenous antibiotics or oxygen.

Obtain a chest x-ray in patients with clinical features suggesting CAP. A chest x-ray documents the presence of pneumonia and complications such as pleural effusion, cavitation, and multilobar illness. Obtain a chest CT scan if loculated pleural effusion or cavitation is suspected or to evaluate nonresponding patients. Limit laboratory testing in outpatients to chest x-ray, and pulse oximetry to assess oxygenation.

For hospitalized patients, obtain chest x-ray, blood cultures, routine metabolic panel, pulse oximetry, and complete blood count. Obtain an arterial blood gas when carbon dioxide retention is suspected, such as in patients with chronic obstructive pulmonary disease. Obtain a sputum culture in any patient at risk for infection with drug-resistant or unusual pathogens and to correlate with sputum Gram stain results. Consider testing concentrated urine for *Legionella* and pneumococcal antigens.

Consider unusual pathogens, including *M. tuberculosis*, fungi, and viruses, or *Pneumocystis* in patients who do not respond to empiric therapy within 48-72 hours. Also consider empyema, lung abscess, metastatic infectious complications (e.g., endocarditis), and noninfectious processes (Table 1). In such circumstances, consider additional diagnostic testing such as chest CT scan, pulmonary angiography, or bronchoscopy.

Therapy

Administer oxygen to hospitalized patients, titrating to an oxygen saturation level of ≥90%. Monitor oxygen therapy carefully in patients with chronic obstructive pulmonary disease because they may further retain carbon dioxide. Provide intravenous hydration to inpatients with signs of dehydration and chest physiotherapy to patients with large volumes of respiratory secretions, and mechanically ventilate those with respiratory failure.

Treat outpatients without cardiopulmonary disease or other comorbidities with a macrolide (azithromycin or clarithromycin) or doxycycline. For outpatients with cardiopulmonary disease or modifying factors (Table 2), use an antipneumococcal quinolone (levofloxacin, gatifloxacin, moxifloxacin), or a combination of a β-lactam (cefuroxime, cefpodoxime, amoxicillin/clavulanate, or high-dose amoxicillin) with a macrolide, if no risk factors for enteric gram-negative bacteria. Both macrolides and quinolones will provide coverage of atypical organisms.

In hospitalized patients, do not delay therapy while awaiting sputum sampling for culture. Give intravenous antibiotics within 8 hours of the patient's arrival to the hospital after rapid assessment of oxygenation and collection of routine blood work and blood cultures. Treat inpatients based on the presence of cardiopulmonary disease or modifying factors with either an intravenous antipneumococcal quinolone or a combination of a β-lactam (e.g., cefotaxime, ceftriaxone, ampicillin/sulbactam) and a macrolide.

Patients with at least two of the following have an increased risk of death: respiratory rate ≥30/min, diastolic blood pressure ≤60 mm Hg, BUN >19 mg/dL, or confusion; these patients require intensive care unit (ICU) admission. Any patient requiring mechanical ventilation or who has septic shock or hypotension with multilobar infiltrates requires ICU admission. ICU patients without any risk factors for *P. aeruginosa* are treated with a β-lactam (i.e., ceftriaxone or cefotaxime) and azithromycin or a respiratory quinolone (i.e., ciprofloxacin or levofloxacin). If *Pseudomonas* infection is a possibility, select either an antipseudomonal β-lactam (e.g., piperacillin-tazobactam, cefepime,

Table 1. Differential Diagnosis of Community-Acquired Pneumonia (CAP)

Disease	Notes
Bronchiolitis obliterans with organizing pneumonia	Subacute illness (4-6 weeks), with alveolar infiltrates (often peripheral), fever. Diagnose with transbronchial or open lung biopsy, or a characteristic clinical picture and response to steroids.
Bronchogenic carcinoma (see Chapter 69)	May cause postobstructive pneumonia, and not present as a mass on chest x-ray. Suspect in cigarette smokers, especially with hemoptysis and radiographic evidence of volume loss or a mass effect.
Eosinophilic pneumonia (see Chapter 79)	Presents as an acute illness, with the radiographic "photo negative" of pulmonary edema, usually with peripheral eosinophilia. Biopsy may not be needed with a classic presentation.
Hypersensitivity pneumonitis (see Chapter 79)	Recurrent episodes of fever and dyspnea, with rapid resolution of infiltrates; chronic infiltrates after multiple episodes. Diagnose with precipitating antibodies to the antigen (molds etc.), characteristic history, or open lung biopsy.
Interstitial pneumonia (see Chapter 79)	Nonspecific radiographic pattern that can result from infection (viral, atypical pathogen), inflammation (usual interstitial pneumonia), or from drug toxicity (amiodarone). Careful exposure history and duration of illness can help distinguish between several possibilities, but open lung biopsy may be required to diagnose definitively.
Pulmonary embolus (see Chapter 80)	If infarction is present, the patient may have fever, lung infiltrate, dyspnea, and hemoptysis. Suspect with appropriate risk factors of immobilization, heart failure, or recent surgery. The infiltrate of infarction may "melt away" rapidly.
Sarcoidosis (see Chapter 79)	Can present as lung infiltrates of any type, with or without mediastinal adenopathy. Should be suspected if the radiographic abnormalities in the lung parenchyma are extensive and the patient is not as ill as suggested by the radiographic pattern. Serum ACE level can enhance suspicion if elevated. Can be diagnosed usually by transbronchial lung biopsy.
Wegener's granulomatosis (see Chapter 90)	Characteristic nodular and cavitary infiltrates, with hemoptysis, otitis media. Can be limited to lung or also can involve the kidneys as rapidly progressive glomerulonephritis. In general, diagnose with characteristic clinical picture and positive c-ANCA, negative p-ANCA. If uncertain, open lung biopsy to document vasculitis.

ACE = angiotensin-converting enzyme; c-ANCA = cytoplasmic antineutrophil cytoplasmic antibody; p-ANCA = perinuclear antineutrophil cytoplasmic antibody.

Table 2. Modifying Factors that Increase the Risk of Infection with Specific Pathogens

Modifying Factor Putting Patient at Risk	Pathogen
Age >65 years; β-lactam therapy within the past 3 months; alcoholism; immune-suppressive illness (including corticosteroids); multiple medical comorbidities; exposure to a child in a day care center	Penicillin-resistant and drug-resistant pneumococci
Residence in a nursing home; underlying cardiopulmonary disease; multiple medical comorbidities; recent antibiotic therapy	Enteric gram-negative bacteria
Structural lung disease (e.g., bronchiectasis); corticosteroid therapy (prednisone, >10 mg/d); broad-spectrum antibiotic therapy for >7 days in the past month; malnutrition	*Pseudomonas aeruginosa*
Endobronchial obstruction (e.g., tumor)	Anaerobes, *S. pneumoniae, H. influenzae, S. aureus*
Intravenous drug use	*S. aureus*, anaerobes, *M. tuberculosis, S. pneumoniae*
Influenza epidemic in the community	Influenza, *S. pneumoniae, S. aureus, H. influenzae*
Chronic obstructive pulmonary disease; smoking history	*S. pneumoniae, H. influenzae, M. catarrhalis, P. aeruginosa*, legionella species, *Chlamydia pneumoniae*
Poor dental hygiene; aspiration; presence of a lung abscess	Oral anaerobes
Animal exposure	Farm animals (*Coxiella burnetii*), birds (*Chlamydia psittaci, Cryptococcus, Histoplasma*), bats (*Histoplasma*)

imipenem, meropenem) and a respiratory quinolone, or a combination of an antipseudomonal β-lactam with an aminoglycoside and either azithromycin or an antipneumococcal quinolone. If community-acquired methicillin-resistant *S. aureus* is a consideration, add vancomycin or linezolid. In the ICU, it is important that empiric therapy be active against *Legionella*; observational evidence suggests quinolones may be more effective than macrolides.

Switch patients to oral antibiotic therapy once they have improvement in symptoms, no fever on two occasions 8 hours apart, and are able to take medications by mouth. Treat patients with mild-to-moderate CAP for 7 days or less if there is a good clinical response, no fever for 48-72 hours, and no sign of extrapulmonary infection. Treat patients with *Legionella* infection for 5-10 days when a quinolone is used. Treat patients with severe illness, empyema, lung abscess, meningitis, or documented infection with pathogens such as *P. aeruginosa* or *S. aureus* for 10 days or longer. Patients with bacteremic *S. aureus* pneumonia need 4-6 weeks of therapy and testing to rule out endocarditis, whereas patients with uncomplicated bacteremic pneumococcal pneumonia may need only a 7- to 10-day course of therapy if they have a good clinical response.

Follow-Up

Follow-up is necessary to assure the pneumonia has resolved, exclude other existing pulmonary disease, and focus on prevention of future episodes. If the patient has clinical response to therapy, obtain a chest x-ray 4-6 weeks after initial therapy. Radiographic resolution lags behind clinical resolution, taking as long as 6-8 weeks. Lung cancer, inflammatory disease, or infection with unusual or resistant pathogens may be present if the x-ray fails to resolve.

Book Enhancement

Go to www.acponline.org/essentials/infectious-disease-section .html to view an x-ray of a right middle lobe pneumonia and sputum Gram stains and to review tables of patient and epidemiological risk factors that are associated with specific pathogens. In *MKSAP for Students 4*, assess yourself with items 35-40 in the **Infectious Disease Medicine** section.

Bibliography

Mandell LA, Wunderink RG, Anzueto A, et al; Infectious Diseases Society of America; American Thoracic Society. Infectious Diseases Society of America/American Thoracic Society consensus guidelines on the management of community-acquired pneumonia in adults. Clin Infect Dis. 2007;44:S27-72. [PMID: 17278083]

Niederman MS. Community Acquired Pneumonia. http://pier.acponline .org/physicians/diseases/d104. [Date accessed: 2008 Jan 7] In: PIER [online database]. Philadelphia: American College of Physicians; 2008

Chapter 54

Infective Endocarditis

Fred A. Lopez, MD

Most patients with infective endocarditis (IE) have an underlying cardiac lesion. Endothelial damage created by turbulent blood flow in this setting is the inciting event for formation of a nonbacterial thrombotic endocarditis (NBTE), which consists of fibrin, platelets, and other coagulation-associated proteins. Bacteria with adherence properties colonize NBTE during episodes of transient bacteremia, forming a vegetation. Bacteremia results from disruption of a mucosal surface such as in the oropharynx or dental-associated gingival crevice, resulting from daily activities such as flossing and brushing of teeth as well as certain dental procedures. The ability of bacteria to avoid host-associated immune defenses by enveloping themselves within the vegetation contributes to the propagation and persistence of infection.

Staphylococci (*S. aureus*, coagulase-negative staphylococci), streptococci (particularly *S. viridans*), and enterococci are the most common organisms causing native valve infective endocarditis. Prosthetic valve infective endocarditis is categorized according to its temporal relationship to surgery. Infections within the first 2 months are most frequently due to coagulase-negative staphylococci; afterwards, the microbiology is similar to native-valve infective endocarditis. Due to virulence factors that facilitate adherence, colonization, persistence, tissue invasion, abscess formation, and dissemination, *S. aureus* can cause infective endocarditis in normal cardiac valves. It is also the most common cause of infective endocarditis in intravenous drug users, usually involving the tricuspid valve, and in hemodialysis patients. Nosocomial infective endocarditis is usually secondary to staphylococci and enterococci and is often associated with vascular catheters or invasive procedures.

Suspect endocarditis when blood culture results are positive in a patient with valvular disease and in anyone with an unexplained febrile or chronic illness. The mortality rate is approximately 10% for streptococcal endocarditis, 35% for staphylococcal endocarditis, and 25%-50% for prosthetic valve endocarditis.

Prevention

Do not recommend antibiotic prophylaxis in patients with low-risk and moderate-risk cardiac conditions undergoing any type of procedure, and do not offer antibiotic prophylaxis to patients undergoing low-risk procedures, regardless of their cardiac condition. Offer antibiotic prophylaxis to patients with both an increased risk of infection and an increased risk of adverse outcome should IE develop (Table 1). The goal is to create high enough serum antibiotic concentrations in order to prevent attachment and growth of bacteria on predisposed cardiac structures. The choice of antibiotics is based on the predicted type of bacteremia. Because certain dental or respiratory tract procedures result in viridans group streptococcal bacteremia, a single dose of oral amoxicillin is given 30 to 60 minutes before the procedure. Clindamycin or azithromycin is used in individuals with a history of anaphylaxis, angioedema, or urticaria with penicillins or ampicillin. Dental procedures for which prophylaxis is indicated include those in which there is perforation of the oral mucosa or manipulation of the periapical region of the teeth or gingival tissue. Exact recommendations for infective endocarditis prophylaxis are available in guidelines published by the American Heart Association.

Diagnosis

Establishing the diagnosis of infective endocarditis includes applying specific clinical criteria or obtaining definitive histopathologic confirmation from involved valves. Risk factors for infective endocarditis include intravenous drug use, recent procedures associated with risk of transient bacteremia, presence of a prosthetic valve, and certain cardiac abnormalities (Table 1).

Fever, malaise, and fatigue are sensitive but non-specific symptoms associated with infective endocarditis. Physical examination findings suggestive of infective endocarditis include a new cardiac murmur, new-onset cardiac failure, focal neurologic signs, splenomegaly, and cutaneous manifestations such as petechiae, and splinter hemorrhages. The presence of Osler's nodes (violaceous, circumscribed, painful nodules found in the pulp of the fingers and toes) or Janeway lesions (painless, erythematous, macular lesions found on the soles and palms) is highly suggestive of infective endocarditis.

Nonspecific laboratory abnormalities of infective endocarditis include leukocytosis, normocytic normochromic anemia, electrocardiographic conduction abnormalities (e.g., atrioventricular block from extension of infection into the conduction system), hematuria and low serum complement levels (glomerulonephritis), and radiographic abnormalities suggesting heart failure or

Table 1. Indications for Bacterial Endocarditis Antibiotic Prophylaxis

- Prosthetic heart valve
- Prior endocarditis
- Heart transplant recipient with valvulopathy
- Uncorrected complex cyanotic congenital heart disease
- Corrected complex congenital heart disease (receive prophylaxis for 6 months following correction)

septic emboli from right-sided endocarditis (multiple bilateral small nodules on chest x-ray).

Obtain an echocardiogram to detect valvular abnormalities, particularly in bacteremic patients with underlying valvular disease, history of previous infective endocarditis, history of intravenous drug use, or an unrecognized source of bacteremia. Transthoracic echocardiography is noninvasive and the initial diagnostic test of choice, but it has a sensitivity of only 50%-80% for detection of valvular vegetations. Use of transesophageal echocardiography increases both the sensitivity and specificity to detect vegetations to approximately 95%. Transesophageal echocardiography is particularly useful to better delineate native valvular anatomy and is essential to more accurately identify paravalvular abscesses and evaluate prosthetic valves.

Obtain blood cultures to identify the microbiologic cause of infective endocarditis. Additional serologic tests for *Coxiella burnetii* (Q fever), *Bartonella* spp., *Legionella* spp., *Brucella* spp., *Mycoplasma* spp., and *Chlamydia* spp. can be obtained when there is a high clinical suspicion of infective endocarditis but blood cultures are negative in the absence of antibiotic therapy. Additional causes of culture-negative endocarditis include a group of gram-negative pathogens constituting the HACEK group, nutritionally variant streptococci such as *Abiotrophia* spp., *Trophermyma whippleii*, and fungi such as *Aspergillus* spp. and *Histoplasma capsulatum*.

Local extension of infection can result in paravalvular abscesses, heart failure due to valvular damage, pericarditis, and myocardial infarction from vegetation-associated emboli. Neurologic complications include stroke (embolic or hemorrhagic), brain abscess, and meningitis. Emboli can result in renal and splenic infarction and abscesses and vertebral osteomyelitis. Mycotic aneurysm, an infection-induced dilatation of an artery, can occur anywhere in the vascular system. Right-sided infective endocarditis can result in pulmonary artery occlusion or multiple bilateral pulmonary abscesses. Immunologic-induced glomerulonephritis

is suspected in patients with low complement levels and hematuria, red blood cell casts, or proteinuria.

The Duke criteria are a set of validated clinical and laboratory criteria for the diagnosis of infective endocarditis with a sensitivity >80% (Table 2). Consider other medical conditions that can mimic the syndrome of IE, especially when patients with negative blood cultures do not respond to empiric antibiotic therapy or when TEE is unrevealing (Table 3).

Therapy

A distinct trend of improved outcome has been documented if the infected valve is resected in selected individuals with infective endocarditis. Absolute indications for surgical intervention of native valve infective endocarditis include valvular dysfunction with heart failure or infection refractory to antibiotic therapy. Relative indications include onset of atrioventricular block, extension of infection into perivalvular tissue, fungal endocarditis, relapse after prolonged antibiotic therapy, recurrent emboli despite antibiotic therapy, or persistent fever during empiric antibiotic therapy of culture-negative infective endocarditis. In prosthetic valve endocarditis, relapse after prolonged therapy and the presence of *S. aureus* are indications for surgery.

Begin empiric antibiotics in proven or suspected infective endocarditis after at least three sets of blood cultures are obtained from separate sites. Empiric therapy for community-acquired native valve infective endocarditis includes vancomycin and gentamicin for streptococci (especially *S. viridans* and *S. bovis*), staphylococci (particularly in intravenous drug users and those with indwelling vascular catheters), and enterococci. Empiric therapy for early prosthetic valve infective endocarditis includes vancomycin, gentamicin, and rifampin for multi-drug-resistant bacteria, particularly coagulase-negative staphylococci. Pathogen-directed therapy is instituted once the microbiologic cause has been identified and recommended regimens are published in a scientific statement developed by the American Heart Association.

Table 2. Modified Duke Criteria for the Diagnosis of Infective Endocarditis

Definite endocarditis = either 2 major, 1 major and 3 minor, or 5 minor criteria
Possible endocarditis = either 1 major and 1 minor or 3 minor criteria

Major criteria	1. Microbiologic (any of the following):
	Typical microorganisms (including *Staphylococcus aureus*) grown from 2 blood cultures
	A microorganism grown from persistently positive blood cultures
	Positive serological test or single positive blood culture for *Coxiella burnetii*
	2. Evidence of endocardial involvement (either of the following):
	Echocardiogram: oscillating intracardiac mass, abscess, or new partial dehiscence of a prosthetic valve
	Physical examination: new valvular regurgitation (changes in pre-existing murmur is not sufficient)
Minor criteria	1. Predisposing heart condition or injection drug use
	2. Fever >38.0°C (100.4°F)
	3. Vascular phenomena: major arterial emboli, septic pulmonary infarcts, mycotic aneurysm, intracranial hemorrhage, conjunctival hemorrhage, or Janeway lesions
	4. Immunological phenomena: glomerulonephritis, Osler's nodes, Roth spots, positive rheumatoid factor
	5. Microbiological: serological evidence of infection or positive blood cultures not meeting the major criteria (a single blood culture for coagulase-negative staphylococci is not sufficient)

Adapted from Li JS, Sexton DJ, Mick N, et al. Proposed modifications to the Duke criteria for the diagnosis of infective endocarditis. Clin Infect Dis.2000;30:633-8. PMID: 10770721

Table 3. Differential Diagnosis of Infective Endocarditis (IE)

Disease	Notes
Pulmonary embolus (see Chapter 80)	Low-grade fever with pulmonary symptoms. Diagnosed by clinical algorithms using radiological/nuclear medicine studies.
Bacteremic infections	Disseminated infection from a focal source. TEE is negative.
Acute leukemia (see Chapter 43)	Fever, systemic symptoms, splenomegaly. CBC and bone marrow examination are diagnostic.
Malignancy with metastases	Low-grade fever and systemic symptoms associated with known primary neoplasm. Imaging studies and biopsy are diagnostic.
Collagen vascular disease with angiitis (see Chapter 90)	Low-grade fever, systemic symptoms, positive rheumatoid factor. Similar symptoms and a false-positive RF may be seen in IE. Specific immunologic tests help in diagnosis.
Atrial myxoma	Low-grade fever, embolic phenomena, specific imaging characteristics on echocardiogram. Blood cultures are negative.
Nonbacterial thrombotic endocarditis (see Chapter 89)	Fever and emboli. Blood cultures are negative.
Cerebrovascular accident (see Chapter 65)	Acute loss of motor function, speech or mental status changes. Patients are afebrile, echocardiogram is normal; blood cultures are negative.

CBC = complete blood count; RF = rheumatoid factor; TEE = transesophageal echocardiography.

Intravenous antibiotics are usually administered for at least 4-6 weeks. Oral antibiotics are not recommended due to unreliable absorption and are used only when patients refuse parenteral therapy or when parenteral therapy is not possible.

Follow-Up

Most patients with infective endocarditis will be cured. With the exception of infection with *S. aureus*, fever resolves after 3-5 days of antimicrobial therapy. Outpatient treatment can be considered if vital signs are stable, symptoms are improving, and therapy is tolerated. Monitoring for refractory infection, development of heart failure, and antibiotic toxicity is important. An echocardiogram is obtained at the completion of therapy in order to establish a new baseline, because there is an increased risk for recurrent infective endocarditis. Valve replacement may be required months or years after successful medical therapy. All patients will require antibiotic prophylaxis for certain bacteremia-associated procedures (see Prevention above).

Book Enhancement

Go to www.acponline.org/essentials/infectious-disease-section .html to access a table on drug therapy and the revised prevention guidelines and to view a patient with splinter hemorrhages. In *MKSAP for Students 4*, assess yourself with items 41-44 in the **Infectious Disease Medicine** section.

Bibliography

American College of Physicians. Medical Knowledge Self-Assessment Program (MKSAP) 14. Philadelphia: American College of Physicians; 2006.

Baddour LM, Wilson WR, Bayer AS, et al. Infective endocarditis: diagnosis, antimicrobial therapy, and management of complications: a statement for healthcare professionals from the Committee on Rheumatic Fever, Endocarditis, and Kawasaki Disease, Council on Cardiovascular Disease in the Young, and the Councils on Clinical Cardiology, Stroke, and Cardiovascular Surgery and Anesthesia, American Heart Association: endorsed by the Infectious Diseases Society of America. Circulation. 2005;111:394-434. [Erratum in: Circulation. 2005;112:2373.] [PMID: 15956145]

Butt AA, Baddour LM, Yu VL. Infective Endocarditis. http://pier .acponline.org/ physicians/diseases/d821. [Date accessed: 2008 Jan 30] In: PIER [online database]. Philadelphia: American College of Physicians; 2008.

Moreillon P, Que YA. Infective endocarditis. Lancet. 2004; 363:139-49. [PMID: 14726169]

Wilson W, Taubert KA, Gewitz M, et al. Prevention of infective endocarditis. Guidelines from the American Heart Association. A guideline from the American Heart Association Rheumatic Fever, Endocarditis, and Kawasaki Disease Committee, Council on Cardiovascular Disease in the Young, and the Council on Clinical Cardiology, Council on Cardiovascular Surgery and Anesthesia, and the Quality of Care and Outcomes Research Interdisciplinary Working Group. Circulation. 2007;116:1736-54. [PMID: 17446442]

Chapter 55

Osteomyelitis

David C. Tompkins, MD

Osteomyelitis is an infection of bone caused by a variety of bacteria and, less commonly, mycobacteria and fungi. Normal bone is highly resistant to infection, and the development of osteomyelitis often requires trauma, the presence of a foreign body, or inoculation with particular pathogens. *Staphylococcus aureus*, for example, expresses a number of receptors for bone components (e.g., fibronectin, laminin, collagen) that allow adherence to bone and the establishment of infection.

Osteomyelitis can be characterized by the duration of illness (acute or chronic), mechanism of infection (hematogenous, extension from a contiguous focus, direct contamination), affected bone, physiologic status of the host, and presence of orthopedic hardware. The clinical presentation and treatment vary depending on the type of osteomyelitis.

Acute hematogenous osteomyelitis occurs most often in children and the elderly. In children osteomyelitis frequently occurs in the metaphysis of the femur, tibia, and humerus. In adults, the intervertebral disc space and two adjacent vertebrae are the most common sites of hematogenous osteomyelitis. Only one microorganism is usually isolated in patients with hematogenous osteomyelitis; 40%-60% of cases are caused by *S. aureus*.

Spread from a contiguous focus of infection to bone is much more common in adults, particularly in persons aged >50 years who have diabetes or peripheral vascular disease. Patients with osteomyelitis from contiguous spread usually have a polymicrobial infection. Direct contamination of bone exposed by an open fracture or by surgery may lead to osteomyelitis depending on the degree of contamination and associated soft tissue injury. Table 1 summarizes clinical risk factors and associated organisms for osteomyelitis.

Prevention

Patients with diabetes or peripheral vascular disease are at increased risk for osteomyelitis, particularly involving the small bones of the feet. These patients should be educated about the importance of meticulous attention to foot care and proper management of minor foot injuries. In addition, patients with diabetes should have a yearly foot exam by a health care provider and custom-made footwear to accommodate foot deformities.

Hematogenous seeding of orthopedic implants can occur following dental and other invasive procedures. The administration of antimicrobials before an invasive procedure can reduce the risk of transient bacteremia and seeding of an orthopedic implant. Consider antimicrobial prophylaxis prior to high-risk dental procedures in high-risk patients, such as those with a joint replacement within 2 years or prior prosthetic joint infection. Administering a single antibiotic dose with activity against staphylococci and streptococci (e.g., amoxicillin, cephalexin, or cephradine) within 60 minutes of the procedure is recommended for such patients.

Diagnosis

Look for predisposing factors (e.g., diabetes, prior surgery, rheumatoid arthritis, peripheral vascular disease), as well as causes of bacteremia (e.g., recent infections, illicit intravenous drug use, long-term intravenous catheters). The clinical hallmarks of osteomyelitis are local pain and fever, particularly in patients with acute hematogenous osteomyelitis, but these may be absent in chronic and contiguous osteomyelitis. The presence of a sinus tract

Table 1. Clinical Risk Factors and Associated Bacterial Agents Causing Osteomyelitis

Risk Factor	Possible Organisms
Contiguous infection (e.g., diabetic foot, wound)	Polymicrobial infection; most commonly *S. aureus* and coagulase-negative staphylococci. May also include streptococci, enterococci, gram-negative bacilli (e.g., *Pseudomonas* sp., *Enterobacter* sp., *E. coli*, *Serratia* sp.) and anaerobes (e.g., *Peptostreptococcus*, *Clostridium* sp., *Bacteroids fragilis*)
Contaminated open fracture	*Staphylococcus* sp., aerobic gram-negative bacilli (e.g., *Pseudomonas* sp., *Enterobacter* sp., *E. coli*, *Serratia* sp.)
Dog bite, cat bite	*Pasteurella multocida*
Foot puncture wound (wearing sneakers)	*Pseudomonas aeruginosa*
Hematogenous (e.g., bacteremia)	*Staphylococcus aureus*
Illicit intravenous drug use	Varies in different communities but typically includes *S. aureus* and gram-negative bacilli.
Sickle cell disease	*Salmonella* sp.
Hemodialysis	*Staphylococcus* sp., *P. aeruginosa*

(a fistula draining pus from a deep tissue infection to the skin) overlying a bone structure and palpation of bone when using a sterile, blunt, stainless steel probe in the depth of a foot ulcer are almost always associated with osteomyelitis. Table 2 summarizes a differential diagnosis for osteomyelitis.

Patients who have undergone total joint arthroplasty and have joint pain since surgery are more likely to have a prosthetic infection when compared with patients who are pain-free. Prosthetic loosening in the first 2 years after arthroplasty raises the index of suspicion for a prosthetic joint infection.

Antimicrobial therapy is ideally based on the identification of the infecting organism(s) and the *in vitro* sensitivities. Blood cultures are obtained when signs and symptoms of infection are present. Superficial cultures obtained from drainage sites are usually contaminated with skin flora and correlate poorly with deep cultures. Therefore, obtain deep surgical cultures, if possible, prior to the initiation of antibiotics. Biopsy material should be incubated in anaerobic and aerobic media. Table 3 summarizes laboratory and other studies useful in the diagnosis of osteomyelitis.

Therapy

Surgical debridement is usually warranted in cases of chronic osteomyelitis, contiguous osteomyelitis, and orthopedic implant-associated osteomyelitis. Complete drainage and debridement of all necrotic soft tissue and resection of dead and infected bone is required. Failure to remove an infected orthopedic implant allows the offending micro-organisms to form a biofilm and therefore escape the effect of antimicrobials. In patients with peripheral vascular disease, revascularization is extremely important to allow adequate oxygenation of soft tissues, promote bone healing, and allow access of antibiotics and the host humoral response to the infected area.

Antibiotic treatment is typically begun immediately after appropriate cultures are obtained. The optimal duration of antibiotic therapy in osteomyelitis is not clear; however, animal models and clinical experience have demonstrated a higher failure rate with shorter (<4 weeks) duration of therapy. Children with acute hematogenous osteomyelitis can be successfully treated with 3 weeks of antibiotics. Adult patients with uncomplicated acute hematogenous vertebral osteomyelitis are treated with 4-6 weeks

Table 2. Differential Diagnosis of Osteomyelitis

Disease	Notes
Soft tissue infection	Imaging studies show sparing of the bone. Probe to bone test is negative.
Infectious arthritis (see Chapter 88)	Severe functional limitation and joint swelling on exam is often present. Bone is not infected early in the disease course.
Metastatic malignancy to the bone	Usually associated with a primary lesion: breast, prostate, and lung. Metastasis usually multifocal; tends to remain isolated to one vertebral body, whereas osteomyelitis often crosses the end plate.
Neuropathic arthropathy in diabetes	Radiologic features should be suggestive. Absence of systemic signs and symptoms of infection. May be difficult to distinguish from infection.
Osteoarthritis	Radiologic features should be suggestive. Absence of systemic signs and symptoms of infection. CRP level, ESR, and leukocyte count normal.

CRP = C-reactive protein; ESR = erythrocyte sedimentation rate.

Table 3. Laboratory and Other Studies for Osteomyelitis

Test	Notes
Leukocyte count	Absence of leukocytosis cannot be used as evidence against the diagnosis of infection (sensitivity 26%).
Erythrocyte sedimentation rate and C-reactive protein	Most sensitive in acute hematogenous osteomyelitis but often normal in early disease (sensitivity 50%-90%).
Sinus tract culture	Correlation is best for *S. aureus* (sensitivity 80%). The association is poor for other microorganisms (sensitivity <40%).
Blood cultures	Obtain in patients with fever or systemic signs of sepsis. Less sensitive in chronic osteomyelitis or implant-associated osteomyelitis (sensitivity <20%).
Plain bone x-ray	Obtain in all patients. Soft-tissue swelling and subperiosteal elevation are the earliest abnormalities; they may not be seen for several weeks (sensitivity 62%).
Technetium (^{99m}Tc) methylene diphosphonate scan	Radionuclide scanning may be helpful early in the course, but usefulness is limited by a lack of specificity (sensitivity 70%-100%; specificity 38%-82%).
Magnetic resonance imaging (MRI)	MRI is excellent in distinguishing soft-tissue infection from osteomyelitis; it is more sensitive than plain x-rays and allows better identification of optimal areas for needle aspiration or biopsy (sensitivity 91%-95%).
Fluorodeoxyglucose positron emission tomography (PET scan)	PET has the highest diagnostic accuracy of imaging tests for confirming or excluding the diagnosis of chronic osteomyelitis (sensitivity 69%-100%).
Percutaneous bone biopsy	Not as invasive as an open biopsy. Mainly used in disc space infection or diabetic foot infection (sensitivity 87%).
Surgical bone biopsy	The gold standard for diagnosing osteomyelitis (sensitivity 100%, specificity 100%).

of antimicrobial therapy. Initial intravenous antimicrobial therapy is directed against the most common bacteria responsible for hematogenous osteomyelitis, including *S. aureus*. A reasonable empiric antibiotic includes nafcillin, cefazolin, or vancomycin. Patients with sickle cell disease have an increased risk of salmonella as well as streptococcal infection; illicit intravenous drug users are at increased risk for gram-negative infections. For both of these groups, levofloxacin plus either nafcillin/oxacillin or vancomycin is a reasonable choice for empiric coverage. Surgical intervention should be considered in patients with acute hematogenous osteomyelitis when there is involvement of the femoral head, failure to make a specific microbiologic diagnosis with noninvasive techniques, neurologic complications, fragments of dead bone (sequestra), and failure to improve while on appropriate antimicrobial therapy.

In patients with chronic osteomyelitis without acute soft tissue infection or sepsis syndrome, withhold antimicrobial therapy until deep bone cultures have been obtained. Patients with chronic or contiguous osteomyelitis usually require a combination of surgical debridement and extended antimicrobial therapy based upon culture results. Antimicrobials should be administered for 4-6 weeks in order to allow the débrided bone to be covered by vascularized soft tissue and to reduce the high relapse rate.

The duration of antimicrobial therapy in implant-related osteomyelitis is adjusted according to the surgical therapeutic modality. Following removal of all hardware and infected bone, administer 4-6 weeks of antimicrobial therapy. Antibiotic-impregnated polymethylmethacrylate can deliver high local levels of antimicrobials and is sometimes used at the time of surgical debridement. If removal of a foreign body is not possible (mechanical instability or contraindications to surgery), initial parenteral therapy is followed by prolonged suppression using an oral antimicrobial agent.

Follow-Up

Patients receiving treatment for osteomyelitis require regular follow-up to monitor for drug-related toxicity, vascular-access complications, and disease recurrence. Persistent elevation of erythrocyte sedimentation rate or C-reactive protein levels despite appropriate antibiotic therapy may reflect the presence of a persistent focus of infection. Interpretation of imaging studies is often difficult, particularly following surgical therapy of osteomyelitis; therefore, follow-up images are not routinely obtained.

Book Enhancement

Go to www.acponline.org/essentials/infectious-disease-section.html to view MRI and CT scans of vertebral osteomyelitis and the clinical appearance of osteomyelitis involving the digit. In *MKSAP for Students 4*, assess yourself with items 45-48 in the **Infectious Disease Medicine** section.

Bibliography

Berbari EF, Osmon DR, Steckelberg JM. Osteomyelitis. http://pier.acponline.org/physicians/diseases/d592. [Date accessed: 2008 Feb 11] In: PIER [online database]. Philadelphia: American College of Physicians; 2008.

Butalia S, Palda VA, Sargeant RJ, et al. Does this patient with diabetes have osteomyelitis of the lower extremity? JAMA. 2008;299:806-13. [PMID: 18285592]

Lew DP, Waldvogel FA. Osteomyelitis. Lancet. 2004;364:369-79. [PMID: 15276398]

Section VII
Nephrology

Chapter 56

Acute Kidney Injury

Harold M. Szerlip, MD

To better reflect the range of structural and functional changes that occur during acute injury to the kidney, the term *acute kidney injury* (AKI) is preferred over the older term *acute renal failure*. AKI is defined as an abrupt elevation in the serum creatinine concentration or a decrease in urine output. AKI can be divided into three stages (Table 1). The etiology may be secondary to decreased perfusion from prerenal causes; ischemic renal parenchymal disease, toxins, tubular obstruction, immunologic events or allergic reactions; or post-renal obstruction of urine outflow. Because both renal hypoperfusion and urinary outflow obstruction can lead to renal parenchymal injury, it is paramount to promptly diagnose and correct these disorders.

Because the blood perfusing the corticomedullary portion of the kidney has a low oxygen content, those parts of the nephron that reside within this area, the straight segment of the proximal tubule and the ascending loop of Henle, function under near-hypoxic conditions. Insults that decrease renal perfusion or toxins that interfere with tubular cell energetics will cause oxygen demand to exceed oxygen delivery. The resultant ischemia and subsequent reperfusion activate numerous cellular processes that produce both tubular cell apoptosis and necrosis. The loss of polarity of the tubular epithelial cells interferes with the vectorial transport of electrolytes out of the lumen back into the renal interstitium. The sloughing of these cells into the tubular lumen causes obstruction.

Prevention

AKI is associated with a marked increase in morbidity and mortality; therefore it is important to prevent its occurrence. This is best accomplished by identifying patients who are at risk. AKI is most likely to occur in patients who already have decreased renal function or whose intravascular volume is depleted. Patients with hypertension or diabetes or who are elderly are especially at risk.

The use of nonsteroidal anti-inflammatory drugs (NSAIDs), which can compromise renal hemodynamics, also places patients at risk. Routinely estimate glomerular filtration in patients at risk for AKI. Serum creatinine concentration alone is a poor indicator of renal function: estimate glomerular filtration by using the Cockroft-Gault equation or the Modification of Diet in Renal Disease (MDRD) equation (Table 2). A glomerular filtration rate of <60 mL/min/1.73 m^2 represents significant renal dysfunction.

In at-risk individuals, avoid, if possible, the use of nephrotoxins such as iodinated contrast or aminoglycosides and stop NSAIDs. In high-risk patients requiring imaging with contrast, use the smallest possible dose of a low osmolar or isoosmolar contrast agent and treat with isotonic saline or bicarbonate prior to and immediately after the procedure. The use of *N*-acetylcysteine may also be beneficial. All patients at high risk for renal failure and any patient requiring a nephrotoxic drug should have an estimated glomerular filtration rate calculated. When prescribing aminoglycosides, consider once-daily dosing or follow peak and trough levels and discontinue their use as early as possible. Avoid over-diuresis in patients with heart failure, nephrotic syndrome, or cirrhosis. Patients who rely upon an activated renin-angiotensin axis to maintain glomerular filtration are especially prone to develop renal failure when angiotensin-converting enzyme (ACE) inhibitors and angiotensin receptor blockers (ARBs) are added. This includes patients who are volume depleted from over-diuresis, have decompensated heart failure, chronic kidney disease, are using NSAIDs, or have renal artery stenosis. In high-risk patients with poor oral intake or who are having excessive fluid losses (e.g., diarrhea, vomiting, burns) maintain intravascular volume using intravenous fluids.

Diagnosis

The diagnosis of AKI is made when there is an abrupt increase in serum creatinine concentration or a decrease in urine volume

Table 1. Stages of Acute Kidney Injury (AKI)

Stage	Serum Creatinine Criteria	Urine Output Criteria
1 (risk)	Increase of ≥150%-200%	<0.5 mL/kg/h for >6 h
2 (injury)	Increase of ≥200%-300%	<0.5 mL/kg/h for >12 h
3 (failure)	Increase of >300% or >4 mg/dL with acute increase ≥0.5 mg/dL	<0.5 mL/kg/h for >24 h or anuria for 12 h

Table 2. Formulas for Estimating Glomerular Filtration (GFR)

Modification of Diet in Renal Disease (MDRD)	GFR (mL/min/1.73 m^2) = 186 × [serum creatinine]$^{-1.154}$ × (age)$^{-0.203}$ × 0.742 (if female) × 1.21 (if black)
Cockroft-Gault	Creatinine clearance (mL/min) = [(140−age) × (body weight in kg)]/(72 × serum creatinine) × 0.85 (if female)

(see Table 1). After establishing the presence of AKI, it is essential to determine the etiology. Intrinsic AKI is divided into oliguric (≤400 mL/24 hr) and non-oliguric (>400 mL/24 hr) forms; the lower the urine output, the worse is the prognosis. Pre-renal and post-renal causes must be distinguished from intrinsic renal parenchymal disease because they are often rapidly reversible (Table 3).

Important historical clues to pre-renal causes include a history of volume loss (e.g., nausea, vomiting, diarrhea), feeling lightheaded on standing, decreased urine volume, or urine that appears more concentrated. After abdominal surgery, patients may sequester large amounts of fluid within tissues and have reduced effective circulating volume. Look for a history of heart failure, liver disease, and nephrotic syndrome, which are other conditions associated with decreased effective circulating volume. Obtain a complete list of all medications, especially NSAIDs, diuretics, and ACE inhibitors or ARBs.

Post-renal causes occur most commonly in elderly males with prostatic hypertrophy, in children with a history of congenital urinary tract abnormalities, and in patients with a history of pelvic malignancy. Other causes include renal stone disease, especially if there is a solitary kidney, and neuropathic conditions affecting bladder emptying such as diabetic neuropathy. Historical clues may include difficulty passing urine, lower abdominal or flank pain, dysuria, or hematuria.

Renal parenchymal disease is divided into processes that affect the tubules (acute tubular necrosis), the interstitium (interstitial nephritis), glomerulae (glomerulonephritis), or vasculature (renal artery stenosis, vasculitis). Look for possible renal toxins such as aminoglycosides, amphotericin, *cis*-platinum, and intravenous contrast. Review over-the-counter medications such as NSAIDs and illicit drug use. Patients using cocaine or who are found comatose from drug ingestions may develop rhabdomyolysis, resulting in release of myoglobin, a renal tubular toxin. For hospitalized patients, review the blood pressure records for evidence of prolonged hypotension, particularly in surgical patients. Know about recent invasive vascular procedures that may result in atheroemboli, such as angiography, aortic stenting, or aneurysm repair. Ask about symptoms related to underlying systemic disease such as fever, joint pain, fatigue, rashes, or jaundice. The antiviral drugs acyclovir and indinavir can precipitate in the renal tubules and cause obstruction.

Renal tubule obstruction and AKI can also occur in patients with lymphoma or leukemia who develop tumor lysis following chemotherapy, resulting in significant elevations of serum and urine uric acid concentration. Patients with multiple myeloma can precipitate immunoglobulin light chains within the tubules.

Findings on physical examination that suggest volume depletion include tachycardia, or a postural pulse increment of >30/min, dry axilla, flat neck veins, and dry oral mucosa. Elevated jugular venous pressure, an S_3 gallop, and crackles on lung exam suggest decreased renal perfusion from heart failure. Spider telangiectasia, jaundice, and ascites support a diagnosis of liver disease. Prostate enlargement, suprapubic fullness, or abdominal and pelvic masses suggest urinary obstruction. Clues to vasculitis include palpable purpura (Plate 47), petechiae, joint swelling, and skin rashes. The presence of a fine red to purple "star-burst"

Table 3. Differential Diagnosis of Acute Kidney Injury (AKI)

Disease	Notes
Prerenal	BUN/creatinine ratio >15; urine sodium <10 or FENa <1%; bland urinary sediment and urine specific gravity >1.018. Occurs in the setting of volume depletion, cirrhosis (including HRS), heart failure, sepsis, or impaired renal autoregulation.
Intra-renal	
Renal artery occlusive disease	Mild proteinuria, occasionally erythrocytes; atheroembolic disease characterized by urinary eosinophils; associated with recent manipulation of the aorta, atrial fibrillation, or recent myocardial infarction.
Intrarenal vascular disease	Hematuria with erythrocyte or granular casts, mild proteinuria, leukocytes. Consider vasculitis (i.e., PAN), malignant hypertension, or TTP-HUS.
Acute glomerulonephritis	Hematuria with erythrocyte casts, mild or nephritic-range proteinuria. FENa >1%. SLE, IgA nephropathy, postinfectious, anti-GBM disease, Wegener's granulomatosis.
Acute tubular necrosis (ATN)	Muddy brown casts, tubular epithelial cell casts, FENa >1%. Consider radiocontrast agents; drugs including aminoglycosides, amphotericin B; episodes of hypotension. Aside from prerenal AKI, ATN is the most common cause of AKI in the hospital setting.
Acute interstitial nephritis (AIN)	Pyuria, leukocyte casts, urinary eosinophils; nephrotic proteinuria in the case of drug- or NSAID-induced minimal change disease. Drug history (methicillin, NSAIDs, but can include nearly any drug), rash. Discontinue any unnecessary or suspect medications.
Intrarenal tubular obstruction	Coarse tubular casts, including muddy brown granular casts, crystalluria, urinary light chains. Consider rhabdomyolysis, tumor lysis syndrome, crystalluria, multiple myeloma.
Renal vein obstruction	Hematuria, nephrotic range proteinuria. Consider nephrotic syndrome (membranous nephropathy), clotting disorders, malignancy, trauma, compression.
Postrenal (urinary tract obstruction)	Micro or macroscopic hematuria, bacteriuria, pyuria, crystal deposition. Urinalysis can also be normal. Consider nephrolithiasis, tumors, granuloma, pregnancy, hematomas, radiation, neurogenic bladder, benign prostatic hypertrophy, retroperitoneal fibrosis

BUN = blood urea nitrogen; FENa = fractional excretion of sodium; GBM = glomerular basement membrane; HRS = hepatorenal syndrome; NSAID = nonsteroidal anti-inflammatory drug; PAN = polyarteritis nodosa; SLE = systemic lupus erythematosus; TTP-HUS = thrombotic thrombocytopenic purpura-hemolytic uremic syndrome.

reticular rash (livedo reticularis) or blue toes (the "blue toe syndrome") suggests atheroembolic disease.

Examine the urine for casts, cells, and crystals (Table 4). Muddy brown granular casts (Plate 37) are consistent with renal injury secondary to tubular necrosis; red blood cell casts (Plate 38) and proteinuria of greater than 3 g/day are pathognomonic for glomerular diseases; and leukocytes, leukocyte casts, and, rarely, eosinophils are associated with acute interstitial nephritis. Pre-renal disease is associated with a normal urinalysis. Blood on a urine dipstick without red blood cells detected on the microscopic examination suggests the presence of myoglobin and supports a diagnosis of rhabdomyolysis; obtain a serum creatine phosphokinase concentration to confirm the diagnosis.

Measure serum electrolytes, BUN, creatinine, calcium, phosphorous, uric acid, glucose, and albumin concentrations and a complete blood count with differential in all patients with AKI. Measure urine sodium and creatinine concentrations and urine osmolality. Low urine flow is associated with reabsorption of urea along the nephron, and patients with pre-renal failure frequently have a BUN to creatinine ratio of >20:1. Volume depletion leads to activation of hormonal systems aimed at conserving salt and water and is characterized by high urine osmolality and low urine sodium with a fractional excretion of sodium of <1%. Acute glomerular disease can produce the same findings but is also associated with proteinuria, microscopic hematuria, and red blood cell casts in the urine.

The first imaging test of choice is a renal ultrasound, which can show hydronephrosis from obstruction and demonstrate increased echogenicity or loss of size associated with chronic kidney disease. If the history and physical exam suggest an underlying thrombotic or vasculitic process or the urinalysis shows red cells, red cell casts, or proteinuria suggesting glomerular disease, obtain an antinuclear antibody, C- and P-antineutrophil cytoplasmic antibodies, anti-glomerular basement membrane antibodies, hepatitis B surface antigen, hepatitis C antibodies, complement levels, and anti-double-stranded deoxyribonucleic acid antibodies. Look for schistocytes and decreased platelets on peripheral smear, which imply a thrombotic microangiopathy such as hemolytic uremic syndrome or thrombotic thrombocytopenia purpura. If present, confirm hemolysis with a serum lactate dehydrogenase and haptoglobin concentrations. A renal biopsy will diagnose acute glomerulonephritis and should be performed in patients with normal-appearing kidneys on renal imaging who do not improve with conservative therapy.

Therapy

In patients with AKI, non-drug therapy is aimed at increasing renal perfusion and relieving obstruction. Treat volume depletion with normal saline; if severe anemia is present, transfuse packed red blood cells. If the serum albumin is extremely low, or in patients with portal hypertension and ascites, albumin may be beneficial as a volume expander. In patients with rhabdomyolysis, intravenous

Table 4. Laboratory and Other Studies for Acute Kidney Injury (AKI)

Test	Notes
Urinalysis with microscopic exam	Significant proteinuria; glomerular disease. Dipstick hematuria without erythrocytes; rhabdomyolysis. Dysmorphic erythrocytes; acute glomerulonephritis.
BUN/Creatinine	>20:1 BUN/creatinine ratio suggests prerenal azotemia.
Fractional excretion of sodium (FENa)	>1: acute tubular necrosis (ATN); ≤1 suggests prerenal azotemia (when oliguria present), and acute glomerulonephritis.
Spot urine sodium	<10 meq/L suggests prerenal azotemia.
Serum phosphorus	Severe hyperphosphatemia suggests acute rhabdomyolysis, tumor lysis syndrome.
Serum calcium	Hypercalcemia can cause AKI via several mechanisms.
Uric acid	>15 mg/dL suggests rhabdomyolysis, tumor lysis syndrome.
ANA	Antinuclear antibody (ANA) indicated in acute nephritis/systemic disease.
ANCA (antineutrophil cytoplasmic antibody)	c-ANCA (anti-PR3) more specific for Wegener's; p-ANCA (anti-MPO) specific for microscopic polyangiitis or pauci-immune glomerulonephritis.
Anti-GBM	Positive in 90% of Goodpasture syndrome patients.
Complete blood count	Anemia can occur with severe AKI; decreased platelets suggest HUS-TTP.
Complement (C3)	Depressed C3 in 60%-70% of type I/II MPGN. Serial values needed for diagnosis of SLE.
Cryoglobulins	Especially for AKI in setting of hepatitis C.
Ds-DNA	Double stranded-DNA (Ds-DNA) sensitivity 75% in SLE.
Hepatitis serology	Acute glomerulonephritis, hepatorenal syndrome.
Renal biopsy	Indicated when there is evidence of intrinsic renal disease, and results will affect management strategy or clarify diagnosis.
Serum and urine protein electrophoresis	Obtain in setting of AKI, anemia, hypercalcemia, especially in patients >60 or when serum anion gap is low to diagnose multiple myeloma.
Urine eosinophils	Suggests acute interstitial nephritis or atheroembolic disease.
Renal ultrasound	Sensitivity, 93%-98% for acute obstruction.

GBM = glomerular basement membrane; MPGN = mesangioproliferative glomerulonephritis; PAN = polyarteritis nodosa; SLE = systemic lupus erythematosus; TTP-HUS = thrombotic thrombocytopenic purpura-hemolytic uremic syndrome.

normal saline may prevent renal toxicity from myoglobin. If there is evidence of urinary obstruction, place a catheter in the bladder to relieve bladder outlet obstruction; if the obstruction is above the bladder, either retrograde or antegrade nephrostomies will be necessary.

Discontinue all drugs that decrease renal perfusion, such as NSAIDs, and stop all diuretics in volume-depleted patients. Reduce the dose or discontinue ACE inhibitors and ARBs if the serum creatinine elevation is >50%. Discontinue all nephrotoxins such as aminoglycosides, *cis*-platinum, and amphotericin unless absolutely necessary. In all patients with uremic signs or symptoms (nausea, vomiting, change in mental status, seizures, pericarditis), or who have hyperkalemia, metabolic acidosis, or volume overload that cannot be easily managed with medication, begin renal replacement therapy (dialysis). In patients who are critically ill and oliguric, or in non-oliguric patients whose creatinine continues to rise without a readily reversible cause, begin renal replacement therapy before symptoms or laboratory findings make it mandatory.

Whenever possible identify and specifically treat the underlying cause of AKI. This may include treating collagen vascular diseases, vasculitides, and pulmonary-renal syndromes such as Goodpasture's syndrome and Wegener's granulomatosis with cytotoxic and immunosuppressant drugs and, depending on the disease, plasmapheresis.

Most complications associated with AKI can be managed with dialysis; however, in patients who do not yet require dialysis, or when dialysis is not promptly available, drug therapy is required. The treatment of metabolic acidosis is controversial, but many experts use sodium bicarbonate when the pH is <7.0. Immediately treat hyperkalemia with electrocardiographic changes with intravenous calcium gluconate to stabilize the myocardium. Shift potassium from the extracellular to the intracellular space with intravenous regular insulin and glucose; inhaled nebulized albuterol may be added if necessary. In patients with underlying metabolic acidosis, intravenous administration of sodium bicarbonate will also shift potassium into cells. These short-term measures must be followed by removal of potassium from the body. If the patient has a normal intravascular volume and is making urine, the administration of a loop diuretic will help with potassium excretion; otherwise, give a cation exchange resin (sodium polystyrene sulfonate with sorbitol) by mouth. If these measures are not successful in reducing the serum potassium concentration, initiate emergency hemodialysis. In patients who develop hyperphosphatemia, begin phosphate binders such as calcium carbonate, calcium acetate, aluminum hydroxide, lanthanum carbonate, or sevelamer hydrochloride.

Avoid overly aggressive treatment of hypertension. In patients with extremely elevated blood pressure, use intravenous nitroprusside, nitroglycerine, labetalol, fenoldopam, or nicardipine to lower the mean arterial blood pressure by 10%-15%. If there is evidence of volume overload, use loop diuretics. Avoid the use of ACE inhibitors or ARBs. When initiating or switching to oral medications for blood pressure control, use short-acting β-blockers such as metoprolol, calcium-channel blockers, centrally-acting α-blockers, or vasodilators such as hydralazine.

Adjust the dose of all medications that are excreted by the kidney. In patients with a rising serum creatinine, assume a glomerular filtration rate of <10 mL/min; glomerular filtration rate cannot be measured in non-steady state conditions using any formulas. Confirm correct drug dosage by measuring drug levels if possible. Avoid drugs that have no proven benefit for the prevention or treatment of AKI, including loop diuretics, unless clinically volume overloaded, mannitol, and dopamine.

Book Enhancement

Go to www.acponline.org/essentials/nephrology-section.html to view findings in the microscopic urinalysis including fat droplets, muddy brown and red cell casts; to view clinical examples of livedo reticularis and the blue toe syndrome; and to access a table of laboratory tests useful in the evaluation of acute renal failure. In *MKSAP for Students 4*, assess yourself with items 2-17 in the **Nephrology** section.

Bibliography

Abuelo JG. Normotensive ischemic acute renal failure. N Engl J Med. 2007;357:797-805. [PMID: 17715412]

Kumar V. Acute Renal Failure. http://pier.acponline.org/physicians/diseases/d639. [Date accessed: 2008 Jan 8] In: PIER [online database]. Philadelphia: American College of Physicians; 2008.

Chapter 57

Chronic Kidney Disease

John Jason White, MD

Chronic kidney disease (CKD) is a worldwide epidemic with increasing incidence and prevalence. Diabetes mellitus and hypertension are the leading causes of CKD in the United States. Hyperglycemia leads to pathological changes in the kidney that usually follow a characteristic clinical course manifested at first by microalbuminuria, then by clinical proteinuria, and ultimately by loss of kidney function. Hypertensive nephropathy is characterized by long-standing hypertension, left ventricular hypertrophy, minimal proteinuria, and progressive kidney failure.

Prevention

To prevent CKD, the causative diseases need to be aggressively managed. Treatment goals for patients with diabetes include a target HbA_{1C} of <7% and blood pressure of <130/80 mm Hg. Target blood pressure for patients without diabetes or pre-existing renal disease is <140/90 mm Hg.

Screening

Screen "high-risk" patients for CKD, including the elderly, patients with diseases associated with CKD (e.g., hypertension, diabetes, and systemic lupus erythematosus), African Americans, Native Americans, Hispanics, Asians, or Pacific Islanders. Measure the serum creatinine and estimate the glomerular filtration rate (GFR) using the Modification of Diet in Renal Disease (MDRD) or Cockroft-Gault equation and classify the stage of CKD (Table 1).

Measure the blood pressure in all patients. Check patients with diabetes for microalbuminuria with a spot urine sample (abnormal = 30-299 mg/g creatinine). Screen patients with type 1 diabetes beginning 5 years after diagnosis and yearly thereafter, and screen patients with type 2 diabetes at the time of diagnosis then yearly.

Diagnosis

Focus the history on clues related to possible etiologies of renal disease. Ask about diabetes, hypertension, and high-risk behaviors predisposing to infectious diseases associated with CKD and proteinuria (e.g., HIV, hepatitis B and C, and syphilis). Ask about a family history of kidney disease (e.g., polycystic kidney disease and Alport's syndrome). Inquire about symptoms of urinary obstruction and urinary tract infection. Obtain a detailed medication history; many medications may contribute to the development of CKD and many require dose-adjustment based on the estimated glomerular filtration rate. Specifically ask about nonsteroidal anti-inflammatory drugs, phenacetin, acetaminophen, and herbal preparations. When GFR declines <20 mL/min, "uremic" symptoms such as anorexia, nausea, vomiting, weight loss, or itching may develop and the patient may develop symptoms of fluid retention.

Although many patients with early CKD have unremarkable physical findings, a thorough exam may identify important clinical consequences and comorbidities. Look for hypertension and signs of volume overload, including elevated central venous pressure, pulmonary crackles, S_3 gallop, or edema. Examine the optic fundi for evidence of hypertensive or diabetic retinopathy and check for signs of uremia such as asterixis or pericardial rub.

CKD is defined as the presence of decreased kidney function (GFR <60 mL/min) or kidney damage that persists ≥3 months. To evaluate for kidney damage, obtain a spot urine for protein and creatinine to estimate the protein-to-creatinine ratio (abnormal >200 mg/g) and a urinalysis to look for red cells, white cells, and

Table 1. Stages of Chronic Kidney Disease

Stage	Description	GFR* (mL/min/1.73 m²)	Action
1	Kidney damage with normal GFR	≥90	Treatment of comorbid conditions, interventions to slow disease progression, reduction of risk factors for cardiovascular disease.
2	Kidney damage with mildly decreased GFR	60-89	Estimate disease progression.
3	Moderately decreased GFR	30-59	Evaluation and treatment of disease complications (e.g., anemia, renal osteodystrophy).
4	Severely decreased GFR	15-29	Preparation for kidney replacement therapy (dialysis, transplantation).
5	Kidney failure	<15 (or dialysis)	Kidney replacement therapy if uremia is present.

*MDRD equation: GFR (mL/min/1.73 m²) = 186 × [serum creatinine]$^{-1.154}$ × (age)$^{-0.203}$ × 0.742 (if female) × 1.21 (if black); GRF = glomerular filtration rate.

Table 2. Laboratory and Other Studies for Chronic Kidney Disease (CKD)

Test	Notes
Spot urine protein-creatinine ratio	The preferred quantitative measure for diagnosing proteinuria. 24-hour urine collections are inaccurate and not recommended. Urine dipsticks can be used to screen non-diabetic patients, but positive results should be followed with a quantitative measurement. Normal ratio is <200 mg/g. First-morning specimens are preferred, but random specimens are acceptable. Patients with two or more positive quantitative test results spaced by 1 to 2 weeks are diagnosed with persistent proteinuria and must undergo further evaluation and management.
Spot urine albumin-creatinine ratio	Normal ratio is <30 mg/g; 30-300 mg/g is defined as microalbuminuria. In adults, albuminuria is a more sensitive marker than total protein for CKD due to diabetes, hypertension, and glomerular diseases.
Urinalysis	Hematuria, proteinuria, casts, and white cells are some of the abnormalities seen in CKD. The presence of dysmorphic red cells suggests active glomerular disease.
Electrolytes	Hyperkalemia and metabolic acidosis often develops in CKD; hyponatremia may occur in edematous states associated with CKD.
Calcium	Hypocalcemia can be seen in patients with CKD. Corrected total calcium (mg/dL) = total calcium (mg/dL) + 0.8 × [4 − serum albumin (g/dL)].
Phosphorus	Phosphate retention is common and leads to development of secondary hyperparathyroidism.
Intact parathyroid hormone	Used to detect secondary hyperparathyroidism. Should be measured in CKD stage 3 and higher.
Albumin	A marker of nutritional status and an independent predictor of mortality in dialysis patients.
Lipid profile	Patients with CKD are at high risk for cardiovascular disease.
Complete blood count	If hemoglobin <11, check red blood cell indices, iron stores, reticulocyte count, and stool occult blood to evaluate need for iron replacement or erythropoiesis stimulating agent.
Renal ultrasound	Hydronephrosis may be found on ultrasound examination in patients with urinary tract obstruction or vesicoureteral reflux. The presence of multiple discrete macroscopic cysts suggests autosomal dominant or recessive polycystic kidney disease. Increased cortical echogenicity and small kidney size are nonspecific indicators of CKD.
Other imaging studies	IVP, CT, MRI, or nuclear medicine scanning can be used for specific situations such as stone disease, renal artery stenosis, or obstruction.

CT = computed tomography; IVP = intravenous pyelogram; MRI = magnetic resonance imaging.

casts. Also obtain a complete blood count; serum electrolytes; a fasting lipid profile; an ultrasound of the kidneys; and in patients with CKD stage 3 or higher, serum albumin and intact parathyroid hormone levels (Table 2).

Once the diagnosis of CKD is established, classify it as diabetic, non-diabetic, or transplant-related kidney disease (Table 3). In diabetic patients, the existence of retinopathy suggests diabetes as the cause of nephropathy; however, only 50% of type 2 diabetic patients with CKD have coexisting retinopathy. In non-diabetic kidney disease the differential is broad and includes glomerular (nephritic or nephrotic syndromes), tubulointerstitial, vascular, and cystic diseases; a kidney biopsy is often required to diagnose non-diabetic kidney diseases. CKD in transplant patients may be caused by chronic rejection, drug toxicity, or recurrence of original kidney disease.

Therapy

Patients with CKD require dietary modification and maintenance of ideal body weight. CKD is associated with sodium retention, inability to excrete daily potassium load, and retention of phosphorus. Refer patients with CKD stage 4 or higher to a renal dietitian. CKD patients have salt-sensitive hypertension; sodium restriction <2.4 g/day is crucial in these patients. Recommend potassium restriction to <2 g/day for patients with hyperkalemia and restrict dietary phosphorus to <1 g/day when serum phosphorus is >4.6 mg/dL. Recommend a low-protein diet (0.6 g/kg/day) for patients with stages 4 and 5, provided caloric intake

can be maintained at 35 kcal/kg/d. Counsel patients about the importance of smoking cessation, limiting alcohol consumption, and exercise.

Use angiotensin-converting enzyme (ACE) inhibitors or angiotensin receptor blockers (ARB) as first-line therapy in diabetics with hypertension or in any patient with proteinuria. If the baseline creatinine is <2.0 mg/dL, an increase in serum creatinine of <0.5 mg/dL after initiating therapy is acceptable; if the baseline creatinine is >2.0 mg/dL, an increase up to 1.0 mg/dL is acceptable. Use diuretics as second-line agents in diabetics and first-line therapy in non-diabetics without proteinuria. Use thiazide diuretics when estimated glomerular filtration rate is >30 mL/min and loop diuretics when <30 mL/min. Use other medications as needed to titrate blood pressure <130/80 mm Hg.

Proteinuria is associated with a progressive decline in renal function and an increase in cardiovascular disease; reduction in proteinuria is associated with slower progression of CKD. Initiate ACE inhibitors or ARB therapy to lower the protein-to-creatinine ratio to <500-1000 mg/g. If proteinuria persists, combine ACE inhibitors and ARBs as tolerated by blood pressure and serum potassium levels. Add non-dihydropyridine calcium-channel blockers as second-line therapy to further lower blood pressure and reduce proteinuria. In diabetic patients, maintain hemoglobin HbA_{1C} at <7% to slow progression of CKD.

As GFR declines, erythropoietin production in the kidney diminishes and anemia ultimately results. Use erythropoiesis stimulating agents to correct anemia to maintain target hemoglobin levels of 10-12 g/dL. Higher hemoglobin levels may increase the

Table 3. Differential Diagnosis of Chronic Kidney Disease (CKD)

Disease	Notes
Diabetic kidney disease (see Chapter 8)	Diabetic kidney disease is #1 cause of CKD in the United States. Diabetic kidney disease, particularly type 1, usually follows a characteristic course, first manifested by microalbuminuria, then clinical proteinuria, hypertension, and declining GFR. Diabetic nephropathy is often accompanied by diabetic retinopathy, particularly in type 1 DM. In patients with type 2 DM, the presence of retinopathy strongly suggests coexisting diabetic nephropathy. Even in the absence of retinopathy, diabetic nephropathy is likely, but an evaluation for other causes of proteinuria is reasonable.
Nondiabetic kidney disease	
Glomerular disease	May present with "nephritic" picture with hematuria, variable proteinuria, and hypertension, often with other systemic manifestations. Common causes include post-infectious glomerulonephritis, IgA nephropathy, and membrano-proliferative glomerulonephritis. "Nephrotic" syndrome refers to high-grade proteinuria (often >3 g/24h), hypoalbuminemia, and edema. Common causes include minimal change disease, focal glomerulosclerosis, membranous nephropathy, and amyloidosis. SLE commonly affects the kidney and may cause nephritic or nephritic syndrome. A kidney biopsy is often needed to make specific a diagnosis and to guide therapy.
Tubulointerstitial	Patients generally have "bland" or relatively normal urinalyses but may have proteinuria, a concentrating defect, pyuria, casts or radiologic abnormalities. Analgesic nephropathy, lead nephropathy, chronic obstruction and reflux nephropathy are examples.
Vascular (see Chapter 90)	The clinical presentation depends on the type of blood vessels involved (small, medium, or large). Patients with small vessel disease often have hematuria, proteinuria, and an associated systemic illness. Patients with vasculitis can present with a rapidly progressive glomerulonephritis. Hypertension is an example of medium vessel disease and is the #2 cause of CKD in the US. Hypertensive disease is generally slowly progressive leading to Stage 5 CKD in the minority of patients. African-Americans have more aggressive CKD caused by hypertension. Renal artery stenosis is an example of large vessel disease.
Cystic	Patients can have normal urinalyses findings. Diagnosis is usually made by imaging techniques and family history. Simple renal cysts are common, particularly in older persons. Autosomal dominant polycystic disease type I and II are the most common forms.
Transplant	CKD in the renal transplant recipient may be due to chronic rejection, drug toxicity, or recurrence of native renal disease. A careful history, serum drug levels, and often kidney biopsy is required for diagnosis.

DM = diabetes; GFR = glomerular filtration rate; SLE = systemic lupus erythematosus.

risk of death and serious cardiovascular complications and is avoided. Use iron to maintain iron stores (transferrin saturation >20% and ferritin >200 ng/mL). Evaluate and rule out other causes of anemia.

Alterations in bone mineral metabolism develops in Stage ≥3 CKD due to phosphorus retention, hypocalcemia (from 1, 25-OH vitamin D deficiency), and secondary hyperparathyroidism and can result in renal osteodystrophy and increased morbidity and mortality. When phosphorus levels remain elevated despite dietary restriction, treat with dietary phosphate binders. Calcium salts such as calcium carbonate and calcium gluconate can be used to maintain serum phosphorus between 2.7 and 4.6 mg/dL. When calcium levels are elevated, use non-calcium containing phosphate binders (e.g., lanthanum carbonate and sevelamer). Use of aluminum containing antacids should be avoided due to the risk of aluminum toxicity. Use 1, 25 vitamin D or vitamin D analogs to maintain serum calcium within the normal range and to suppress elevated parathyroid hormone levels. Parathyroid hormone suppression is indicated when >70 pg/mL in Stage 3 CKD and >110 pg/mL in Stage 4 CKD. 25-OH Vitamin D insufficiency/deficiency is also common in patients with CKD and is treated with vitamin D_2 (ergocalciferol).

Metabolic acidosis commonly develops in advanced CKD, accelerating renal osteodystrophy, suppressing albumin synthesis, and is associated with malnutrition. Use sodium bicarbonate to maintain serum bicarbonate within the 20 to 26 meq/L range.

Hyperkalemia may develop in advanced CKD and in certain forms of renal tubular acidosis. Restrict dietary potassium and use sodium polystyrene sulfonate to maintain potassium within normal levels. Severe hyperkalemia (>6.0 meq/L) is associated with life-threatening cardiac dysrhythmias; these patients require hospitalization and referral to a nephrologist.

Follow-Up

Patients with CKD require close follow-up with laboratory measurements initially every 3 to 4 months and more frequently in advanced CKD. Consult a nephrologist for patients with CKD before GFR <30 mL/min. Because CKD is a cardiovascular disease risk equivalent, patients with CKD are more likely to die of cardiovascular disease than to reach Stage 5 CKD. Therefore, treatment goals for cardiac risk factors are the same as for established coronary artery disease.

Avoid use of radiocontrast agents and known nephrotoxic agents as much as possible. Ensure medications are dosed appropriately for GFR. Limit the amount of gadolinium used for magnetic resonance imaging in Stage 3 CKD and avoid completely when GFR <30 mL/min to prevent nephrogenic systemic fibrosis.

Patients reaching Stage 5 CKD often become uremic and require renal replacement therapy. Treatment of uremia in the United States is dominated by hemodialysis. Hemodialysis is predominantly performed at outpatient centers 3 sessions per week for approximately 3.5 hours. Other treatment options include home hemodialysis, peritoneal dialysis, and renal transplantation. Transplantation is the preeminent treatment for uremia; however, the short supply of donor organs dictates that hemodialysis will remain the primary treatment of uremia. Immunosuppression and prevention of graft rejection are the primary challenges in renal transplant patients.

Book Enhancement

Go to www.acponline.org/essentials/nephrology-section.html to access a tutorial on the detection of microalbuminuria, tables on the interpretation of urinary sediment and risk factors for chronic kidney disease, and to learn more about nephrogenic systemic fibrosis. In *MKSAP for Students 4*, assess yourself with items 18-19 in the **Nephrology** section.

Bibliography

Levey AS, Coresh J, Balk E, et al. National Kidney Foundation practice guidelines for chronic kidney disease: evaluation, classification, and stratification. Ann Intern Med. 2003;139:137-47. [PMID: 12859163]

Meyer TW, Hostetter TH. Uremia. N Engl J Med. 2007;357:1316-25. [PMID: 17898101]

Rahman M. Chronic Kidney Disease. http://pier.acponline.org/physicians/diseases/d938. [Date accessed: 2008 Jan 7] In: PIER [online database]. Philadelphia: American College of Physicians; 2008.

Chapter 58

Acid-Base Disorders

Tomoko Tanabe, MD

A systematic approach to acid-base problem solving involves answering five questions:

- Is the patient acidemic or alkalemic?
- Is the acid-base disorder primarily metabolic or respiratory?
- What is the anion gap?
- If a metabolic acidosis exists, is there an appropriate respiratory compensation?
- If an anion-gap acidemia is present, is there a complicating metabolic disturbance?

Case 1—A 47-year-old man with a 3-day history of severe diarrhea is evaluated because of weakness and dizziness. Laboratory studies show serum sodium, 130 meq/L; serum potassium, 3.2 meq/L; serum chloride, 100 meq/L; and serum bicarbonate, 10 meq/L. Arterial blood gas studies on room air reveal pH, 7.24; $PaCO_2$, 23 mm Hg; and bicarbonate, 9 meq/L.

Comment—The low pH and low HCO_3^- concentration indicate a primary metabolic acidosis. In contrast, a high $PaCO_2$ would have indicated a primary respiratory acidosis. If the pH were elevated, this would indicate an alkalosis; a high bicarbonate concentration indicates metabolic alkalosis, whereas a low $PaCO_2$ indicates respiratory alkalosis.

The anion gap is calculated regardless of the primary disturbance. The equation is:

$$\text{Anion gap} = [Na^+] - ([Cl^-] + [HCO_3^-])$$

In Case 1, the anion gap = $(130 - [100 + 10] = 20)$, indicating an anion gap metabolic acidosis. If the primary disturbance is a condition other than metabolic acidosis, the presence of an anion gap reveals a "hidden" metabolic acidosis.

Negative charges on proteins account for the missing unmeasured anions. The presence of either a low albumin level (an anion) or an unmeasured cationic light chain (e.g., multiple myeloma) results in a low anion gap. When the primary disturbance is a metabolic acidosis, the anion gap helps narrow the diagnostic possibilities to an anion gap acidosis or a non-anion gap acidosis. Healthy individuals have an anion gap of 12 ± 2 meq/L.

The compensatory response to a primary disturbance is predictable and brings the pH toward normal (Table 1). Compensation may be appropriate even if the pH is abnormal. Assessment of compensation helps detect mixed respiratory and metabolic acid-base disturbances. In Case 1, the expected $PaCO_2$ = $[(1.5 \times 10) + 8] = 23 (\pm 2)$. Because the measured $PaCO_2$ is 23 mm Hg and within the predicted range, respiratory compensation is appropriate. If the $PaCO_2$ is lower than expected, a complicating respiratory alkalosis is diagnosed; if the $PaCO_2$ is higher than expected, a complicating respiratory acidosis is diagnosed.

The process for diagnosing a complicating metabolic disturbance involves calculating the "corrected HCO_3^-." If the corrected HCO_3^- is <24 ± 2 meq/L, a co-existing non-anion gap metabolic acidosis is present; if the corrected HCO_3^- is >24 ± 2 meq/L, a co-existing metabolic alkalosis is present. The equation is:

$$\text{Corrected } HCO_3^- = [\text{measured } HCO_3^-] + ([\text{measured anion-gap}] - 12)$$

This formula is based upon the assumption that the measured anion-gap represents in part the bicarbonate that was consumed compensating for the acidosis. If the anion gap is added to the measured bicarbonate concentration and the "normal" anion-gap of 12 is subtracted, the result represents the bicarbonate concentration if the anion gap acidosis was not present.

Anion Gap Metabolic Acidosis

Anion gap metabolic acidosis results when acids associated with an unmeasured anion (the conjugate base of the acid, such as lactate) are produced or exogenously gained. Common causes of high anion-gap metabolic acidosis include lactic acidosis, ketoacidosis (ethanol, starvation, and diabetes), uremia, methanol, ethylene glycol, and aspirin poisonings. A decrease in bicarbonate concentration and resultant anion-gap metabolic acidosis occur when lactic acid accumulates, as seen most commonly in states of tissue hypoperfusion. Drug-induced mitochondrial dysfunction, as seen with nucleoside therapy in treatment of AIDS, can lead to lactic acidosis in the absence of obvious tissue hypoxia. Tonic-clonic seizures, which are associated with an increased metabolic rate, result in a lactic acidosis that quickly reverses.

Ethylene glycol poisoning causes an anion-gap acidosis and acute renal failure. Clinical clues include an osmolal gap and urinary calcium oxalate crystals. Methanol poisoning also causes an anion-gap acidosis, osmolal gap, and optic nerve toxicity. Isopropyl alcohol poisoning causes an osmolal gap but no acid-base disturbance. An osmolal gap is present when the measured plasma osmolality exceeds the calculated plasma osmolality by >10 mOsm/kg. The equation is:

$$\text{Plasma osmolality} = (2 \times [Na^+]) + ([\text{glucose}]/18) + ([\text{blood urea nitrogen}]/2.8)$$

When glucose is in short supply or cannot be utilized, the liver converts free fatty acids into ketones to be used as an alternative energy source. In diabetic ketoacidosis, decreased insulin activity and increased glucagon activity lead to formation of acetoacetic acid and β-hydroxybutyric acid. The presence of these ketoacids decreases the serum bicarbonate concentration and increases the anion gap.

The key to treatment of anion gap metabolic acidosis is reversing the condition that led to excess acid production. Treatment with bicarbonate is unnecessary, except in extreme cases of acidosis when the pH is <7.1-7.2, a level at which dysrhythmia becomes more likely and cardiac contractility and responsiveness to catecholamines are impaired.

Non-Anion Gap Metabolic Acidosis

A non-anion gap metabolic acidosis is a hyperchloremic metabolic acidosis that develops because either fluids containing sodium bicarbonate (or potential sodium bicarbonate) are lost or hydrogen chloride (or potential hydrogen chloride) is added to the extracellular fluid. The ensuing hyperchloremic metabolic acidosis will not change the anion gap, because the reduction in the bicarbonate concentration is offset by the increase in chloride.

The most common cause of non-anion gap metabolic acidosis is severe diarrhea. Diarrhea leads to loss of bicarbonate because the intestinal fluid below the stomach is relatively alkaline. All types of renal tubular acidosis (RTA) cause hyperchloremic metabolic acidosis. Proximal (type 2) renal tubular acidosis is caused by a reduced capacity of the kidney to reabsorb bicarbonate. Distal (type 1) renal tubular acidosis results from an inability of the renal tubules to generate or maintain a normal pH gradient (normal minimal urinary pH is <5.5). Type 4 renal tubular acidosis, commonly associated with diabetes, is a hyperkalemic hyperchloremic metabolic acidosis that is due to hypoaldosteronism or an inadequate renal tubular response to aldosterone. This leads to a reduction in urinary excretion of potassium and hyperkalemia, which interferes with renal production of NH_4^+. This, along with inhibition of renal hydrogen ion excretion caused by aldosterone deficiency, leads to development of metabolic acidosis.

Bicarbonate therapy is generally indicated in non–anion gap acidosis, whereas correction of the underlying cause is the primary concern in anion gap acidosis. Oral bicarbonate (or oral citrate solutions) is the preferred agent for chronic therapy for non–anion gap acidosis. The preferred bicarbonate salt in hypokalemic RTA is potassium bicarbonate or potassium citrate. For acute presentations, especially in patients with concomitant impaired respiratory function, intravenous bicarbonate therapy is indicated.

Case 2—A 36-year-old woman is evaluated because of generalized weakness. Laboratory studies show blood urea nitrogen, 40 mg/dL; serum creatinine, 1.9 mg/dL; serum sodium, 130 meq/L; serum potassium, 3.0 meq/L; serum chloride, 85 meq/L; and serum bicarbonate, 36 meq/L. Arterial blood gas studies on room air reveal pH of 7.58 and $PaCO_2$ of 42 mm Hg. The urinary sodium concentration is 50 meq/L; potassium concentration is 30 meq/L; and chloride concentration is 2 meq/L.

Comment—The elevated arterial pH and HCO_3^- are consistent with a primary metabolic alkalosis. The anion gap is normal (10 meq/L). The arterial $PaCO_2$ is inappropriately low for the degree of metabolic alkalosis (Table 1). Therefore, both metabolic alkalosis and respiratory alkalosis are present.

Metabolic Alkalosis

A primary increase in HCO_3^- concentration can result from loss of hydrogen chloride or, less commonly, addition of bicarbonate. Once generated, the metabolic alkalosis is corrected through urinary excretion of the excess bicarbonate. Alkalosis is maintained only when renal bicarbonate excretion is limited owing to a reduction in renal function or stimulation of renal tubule bicarbonate reabsorption. Increased reabsorption is caused by extracellular fluid volume contraction, chloride depletion, hypokalemia, or elevated mineralocorticoid activity.

The most common causes of metabolic alkalosis are vomiting, nasogastric suction, and diuretic therapy. In these cases, which are classified as chloride responsive, administration of sodium chloride fluid reverses the alkalosis by expanding the intravascular

Table 1. Compensatory Response to a Primary Acid-Base Disturbance

Condition	Expected Compensation
Metabolic acidosis	• Acute: $\Delta PaCO_2 = (1.5) [HCO_3] + 8$ • Chronic: $\Delta PaCO_2 = [HCO_3] + 15$ • Failure of the $PaCO_2$ to decrease to expected value = complicating respiratory acidosis; excessive decrease of the $PaCO_2$ = complicating respiratory alkalosis
Respiratory acidosis	• Acute: 1 meq/L ↑ $[HCO_3]$ for each 10 mm Hg ↑ in $PaCO_2$ • Chronic: 3.5 meq/L ↑ $[HCO_3]$ for each 10 mm Hg ↑ in $PaCO_2$ • Failure of the $[HCO_3]$ to increase to the expected value = complicating metabolic acidosis; excessive increase in $[HCO_3]$ = complicating metabolic alkalosis
Metabolic alkalosis	• 0.7 mm Hg ↑ in $PaCO_2$ for each ↑ 1 meq/L $[HCO_3]$ • The response is limited by hypoxemia
Respiratory alkalosis	• Acute: 2 meq/L ↓ $[HCO_3]$ for each 10 mm Hg ↓ in $PaCO_2$ • Chronic: 4 meq/L ↓ $[HCO_3]$ for each 10 mm Hg ↓ in $PaCO_2$ • Failure of the $[HCO_3]$ to decrease to the expected value = complicating metabolic alkalosis; excessive decrease in $[HCO_3]$ = complicating metabolic acidosis

volume and reducing the activity of the renin-angiotensin-aldosterone axis. Persistent delivery of sodium chloride to the distal tubule in the presence of aldosterone results in urinary loss of potassium and hydrogen. This process generates hypokalemia, maintaining the metabolic alkalosis. The very low urinary chloride concentration in Case 2 suggests vomiting or remote diuretic ingestion and that sodium chloride volume expansion will correct the alkalosis.

Less commonly, metabolic alkalosis is maintained in the absence of volume depletion. This condition is recognized by a high urinary chloride level (>20 meq/L) related to elevated mineralocorticoid effect and does not correct with sodium chloride volume replacement. Consequently, these disorders are also called *chloride-unresponsive* or *chloride-resistant metabolic alkaloses*. Examples are primary hyperaldosteronism and Cushing's syndrome.

H_2 blockers and proton pump inhibitors may help to decrease losses of H^+ in patients with prolonged gastric aspiration or chronic vomiting. Potassium chloride is almost always indicated in hypokalemia, although potassium concentrations may increase as the alkalosis is corrected. In very severe metabolic alkalosis (pH >7.6), hemodialysis is the preferred treatment, and use of acidic solutions is rarely indicated.

Respiratory Acidosis

Respiratory acidosis is due to a primary increase in arterial $PaCO_2$, which accumulates when ventilation is inadequate. Hypoventilation can result from neurological disorders (stroke) or medications (narcotics) that affect the central nervous system respiratory center, respiratory muscle weakness (e.g., myasthenia gravis or Guillain-Barré syndrome) or chest wall deformity (severe kyphoscoliosis), obstruction of airways (chronic obstructive pulmonary disease), or ventilation-perfusion mismatch (venous thromboembolism). Table 1 shows the expected level of metabolic compensation.

Treatment of respiratory acidosis should focus on treating the underlying disorder. In patients with acute respiratory acidosis and hypoxemia, supplemental oxygen may be administered. However, to treat the hypercapnia, an increase in effective alveolar ventilation through reversal of the underlying cause or endotracheal intubation and mechanical ventilation is indicated.

Respiratory Alkalosis

Hyperventilation reduces the arterial $PaCO_2$, which increases the pH, causing respiratory alkalosis. Common causes of respiratory alkalosis can be sorted by conditions involving the pulmonary vasculature (e.g., pulmonary hypertension and venous thromboembolism), pulmonary parenchyma (e.g., pulmonary fibrosis, heart failure, and pneumonia), pulmonary airways (asthma), and conditions affecting ventilatory control (e.g., anxiety, aspirin toxicity, sepsis, hypoxia, and pregnancy). The expected compensatory responses for acute and chronic respiratory alkalosis are shown in Table 1.

The underlying cause for respiratory alkalosis should always be pursued. In psychogenic hyperventilation, rebreathing air using a bag increases the systemic $PaCO_2$. This method also may help to rapidly reduce the pH in patients with mixed, severe alkalosis (pH ~ 7.7).

Book Enhancement

Go to www.acponline.org/essentials/nephrology-section.html to view a differential diagnosis of acid-base disorders, additional acid-base equations, and an algorithmic approach to metabolic acidosis. In *MKSAP for Students 4*, assess yourself with items 20-27 in the **Nephrology** section.

Bibliography

Adrogué HJ, Madias NE. Management of life-threatening acid-base disorders. First of two parts. N Engl J Med. 1998;338:26-34. Erratum in: N Engl J Med 1999;340:247. [PMID: 9414329]

Adrogué HJ, Madias NE. Management of life-threatening acid-base disorders. Second of two parts. N Engl J Med. 1998;338:107-11. [PMID: 9420343]

American College of Physicians. Medical Knowledge Self-Assessment Program 14. Philadelphia: American College of Physicians; 2006.

Chapter 59

Fluid and Electrolyte Disorders

Mary Jane Barchman, MD

Total body water (TBW) constitutes approximately 60% of body weight in males and 50% in females. Two-thirds of TBW is intracellular fluid and one-third is extracellular fluid. The extracellular fluid is distributed 25% as intravascular volume and 75% as interstitial volume. Osmolality of the various compartments is similar, but the solutes dictating the osmolarity are not; the main extracellular osmole is sodium and the primary intracellular osmoles are potassium and phosphates. Plasma osmolality (P_{osm}) is calculated as:

$$P_{osm} = 2[Na^+] + ([BUN]/2.8) + ([glucose]/18)$$

Water Metabolism

Normal plasma osmolality (285-295 mOsm/L) is maintained by thirst, renal handling of water, and antidiuretic hormone (ADH). The thirst center is located in the hypothalamus and is stimulated or suppressed by changes in plasma osmolality and effective intravascular volume. Water is filtered at the glomerulus, and 80% is absorbed isotonically in the proximal tubule. Water is then passively reabsorbed throughout the descending loop of Henle in response to the increasing osmolarity in the medullary interstitium; this segment of the tubule is impermeable to sodium chloride. The ascending limb of Henle constitutes the diluting segment of the nephron since sodium chloride is reabsorbed to maintain the medullary gradient but water is retained, resulting in a minimum urine osmolality of 50-100 mOsm/L. Water is reabsorbed in the distal tubule and cortical collecting duct under the influence of ADH. The hypothalamic osmostat has projections to the posterior pituitary gland, which stimulate or inhibit ADH release based on plasma osmolality and effective intravascular volume. Pain, nausea, emotional stress, psychosis, and a number of drugs also increase ADH levels. When hypoosmolality and hypovolemia occur together, low-volume stimulus overrides the inhibitory effect of the hypoosmolality, and ADH secretion increases to protect volume preferentially.

Hyponatremia

Hyponatremia (serum sodium < 136 meq/L) can be associated with high, normal, or low plasma osmolality. Hyponatremia with high plasma osmolality occurs with accumulation of solutes in the extracellular fluid, which in turn causes movement of water from the intracellular space to the extracellular space. Hyperglycemia is the most common cause of high solute load, but mannitol, radiologic contrast, sorbitol, or glycine can also be culprits. Treatment is directed toward removal of the solute (e.g., insulin for hyperglycemia).

Hyponatremia with normal plasma osmolality (pseudohyponatremia) is characterized by low sodium concentration due to measurement in a falsely large volume; an interfering substance displaces water in the sample like ice cubes in a pitcher. The most common space-occupying substances are lipids and paraproteins as in hyperlipidemia and multiple myeloma.

Evaluation of volume status is the first step in determining the cause of hyponatremia with hypoosmolality (Figure 1). The most common category is volume overload (e.g., heart failure, cirrhosis, nephrotic syndrome, and renal failure). In each of these edematous states, the kidney is conserving both salt and water because renal perfusion is compromised by poor cardiac output, arteriovenous shunting, or decreased intravascular oncotic pressure. Renal conservation of salt and water is documented by a low urine sodium concentration (U_{Na}< 10 meq/L) and highly concentrated urine (>450 mOsm/L). This results in water overload greater than sodium overload, but both are present. Symptomatic hyponatremia is uncommon, and aggressive treatment to raise the serum sodium is usually unnecessary. The general approach to treatment is to treat the underlying cause, restriction of sodium (2-3 g/day) and water (1-1.5 L/day), and adjunctive use of loop diuretics.

Hypoosmolal hyponatremia associated with volume depletion is manifested by dry mucous membranes, hypotension, and tachycardia. Volume loss can be gastrointestinal, renal, or "third spacing" of fluids. The urine indices reflect renal sodium (<10 meq/L) and water conservation (>450 mOsm/L). If volume loss is due to vomiting, a low urine chloride concentration is corroborative. Treatment is intravenous normal saline as well as managing the condition that precipitated the volume loss. Hypertonic saline is reserved for symptomatic hyponatremia. As volume is restored, the stimulus for ADH release will decrease, potentially leading to correction of the sodium concentration too quickly; consequently, serum sodium levels must be monitored closely. Correcting hyponatremia too rapidly can lead to central pontine myelinolysis characterized by flaccid paralysis, dysarthria, and dysphagia. The rate of sodium correction must be no greater than 0.3-0.5 meq/L/h.

Hypoosmolal hyponatremia with euvolemia is caused either by massive intake of water or inability of the kidney to excrete a free water load. The normal renal capacity for water excretion is approximately 15 L/day. Massive increase in water intake occurs in psychogenic polydipsia or rarely in hypothalamic diseases. Urine indices are compatible with adequate intravascular volume

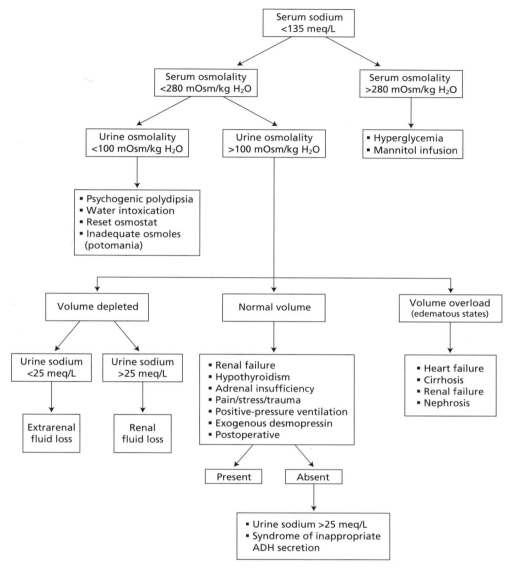

Figure 1 Diagnostic approach to hyponatremia. (ADH = antidiuretic hormone.) (Modified from Medical Knowledge Self-Assessment Program (MKSAP) 14. Philadelphia: American College of Physicians; 2006.)

(U_{Na} > 20 meq/L), and the urine is maximally dilute (50-100 mOsm/L). The treatment is water restriction.

Hypothyroidism, adrenal insufficiency, reset osmostat, inadequate osmoles, and syndrome of inappropriate ADH (SIADH) secretion are all associated with hyponatremia due to a renal defect in excreting free water. Thyroid and cortisol deficiencies lead to increased ADH release. The most common physiologic stimulus for reset osmostat is pregnancy, which contributes to the increase in plasma volume. At least 50 mOsm are needed to excrete 1 liter of water; malnourished patients may not have adequate osmoles to excrete excess free water. The treatment is water restriction until nutrition can be corrected. SIADH is always associated with hyponatremia but is a diagnosis of exclusion. Urine indices are compatible with euvolemia (U_{Na} > 20 meq/L), but the urine is inappropriately concentrated in the face of plasma hypo-osmolality. SIADH is frequently accompanied by very low uric acid and

blood urea nitrogen levels, which help differentiate it from other causes of hyponatremia. Causes of SIADH include malignancy (e.g., small cell carcinoma of the lung), intracranial pathology, and pulmonary diseases, especially those that increase intrathoracic pressure and decrease venous return to the heart.

Symptoms occur below a sodium level of 110 meq/L and include obtundation, coma, seizures, and death if untreated. In general, symptoms tend to be worse in situations where the hyponatremia developed quickly. Serum sodium levels should be corrected to 120 meq/L at a rate of 1-2 meq/L/h, and once this level is achieved the rate of correction is slowed to 0.3-0.5 meq/L/h. The quantity of sodium chloride required to increase the serum sodium is calculated as:

$$\text{meq sodium required} = \text{TBW (liters)} \times (\text{desired increase in serum } [\text{Na}^+])$$

where the desired increase in serum sodium equals:

$$120 \text{ meq/L} - \text{current } [Na^+]$$

Hypernatremia

Hypernatremia is serum sodium >145 meq/L. All hypernatremia is associated with intracellular fluid contraction, and both thirst and ADH levels should be elevated. Therefore, severe hypernatremia indicates a defective thirst mechanism, inadequate access to water, and/or a renal concentrating defect. The brain generates idiogenic osmoles to protect intracellular volume within 4 hours of development of hypernatremia, and the process stabilizes by 4-7 days. Hypernatremia associated with volume overload is unusual and often iatrogenic (i.e., administration of saline or excessive dosing of sodium bicarbonate). Rarely, mild hypernatremia and volume overload occurs with Cushing's syndrome or primary hyperaldosteronism. Symptoms of hypernatremia include weakness, lethargy, seizures, and coma. Spontaneous diuresis often self-corrects volume overload hypernatremia, but when needed, therapy includes diuretics or dialysis while simultaneously replacing free water.

Most commonly, hypernatremia is due to loss of hypotonic fluids with inadequate water replacement. Hypernatremia associated with volume depletion occurs with gastrointestinal, renal, cutaneous, or pulmonary losses. Therapy is directed at sodium chloride replacement, free water replacement, and correction of the underlying problem leading to hypotonic fluid loss. The water deficit is estimated by the formula:

$$\text{Water deficit} = TBW - (\text{desired } [Na^+]/\text{current } [Na^+]) \times TBW$$

Because of the presence of idiogenic osmoles created by the brain to protect intracellular fluid volume, correcting hypernatremia too quickly can lead to cerebral edema. Extreme care must be taken to correct sodium concentration at a rate no greater than 1meq/L/h with a goal of 50% correction at 24-36 hours and complete correction in 3-7 days.

Central diabetes insipidus is a partial or complete deficiency of ADH production and/or release resulting in inadequate concentration of the urine. Provided the patient has access to water, the serum sodium concentration is normal. The presence of hypernatremia indicates loss of free water, and treatment is water replacement and administration of ADH (dDAVP, vasopressin). Nephrogenic diabetes insipidus is an insensitivity of the cortical collecting duct to circulating ADH and can be caused by drugs (e.g., lithium and foscarnet), hypokalemia, hypercalcemia, sickle cell disease and trait, and amyloidosis. Treatment requires adequate water intake, salt restriction, and in some cases, a thiazide diuretic. Thiazide diuretics effectively block sodium reabsorption in the distal renal tubule, thereby causing natriuresis. Patients with an intact thirst mechanism do not develop significant hypernatremia unless their access to water is interrupted by unconsciousness, immobility, or altered mental status.

Potassium Metabolism

Serum potassium concentration is tightly regulated. Most of the body's potassium is intracellular and is maintained by the integrity of the cell membrane and Na^+/K^+ ATPase. Because potassium is a steady-state ion, intake must equal output in order to maintain balance. Typical dietary intake of potassium is 50-100 meq/day, and renal excretion can be up to 1000 meq/day. Potassium is excreted primarily by the kidneys (90%). Normal renal handling of potassium depends on adequate glomerular filtration, aldosterone, intact distal tubular function, distal tubular flow, distal tubular sodium delivery, acid-base status, and intracellular potassium stores. Intracellular potassium balance is further affected by shifting between the intracellular and extracellular fluid due to circulating insulin, catecholamines, acid-base status, and plasma osmolality.

Hypokalemia

Hypokalemia (<3.5 meq/L) can result from potassium loss or intracellular shift but rarely from inadequate potassium intake. The most common causes for potassium loss are gastrointestinal and renal (diuretics). Rare causes include primary aldosteronism, Bartter's syndrome, Gitelman's syndrome, and periodic paralysis.

Manifestations of hypokalemia are ileus, muscle cramps, paralysis, rhabdomyolysis, impaired insulin secretion, and cardiac arrhythmias. Electrocardiographic findings of hypokalemia include U waves and flat or inverted T waves. Hypomagnesemia should always be suspected in hypokalemic patients because these ions are often lost together and magnesium is necessary for renal conservation of potassium.

Hypokalemia is treated with either oral or intravenous potassium salts. In severe cases, potassium is given intravenously at a rate not >20-40 meq/h and at a concentration not >40 meq/L. Although total potassium deficits are difficult to predict, a serum level of 3 meq/L is equivalent to a deficit of 200-400 meq and a serum level of 2 meq/L is equivalent to a 400-800 meq deficit.

Hyperkalemia

Excessive dietary intake of potassium is rarely a cause for hyperkalemia unless there is coexisting renal insufficiency. Potassium may shift out of cells secondary to tissue injury (e.g., rhabdomyolysis or hemolysis), hyperosmolality, insulin deficiency, β-adrenergic blockade, metabolic acidosis, or poisoning of the Na^+/K^+ ATPase (i.e., digoxin toxicity) and cause hyperkalemia. Decreased renal potassium excretion occurs if there is reduced glomerular filtration, poor distal tubular urine flow (e.g., hypovolemia or reduced effective circulating volume), aldosterone deficiency, or tubulointerstitial disease leading to aldosterone unresponsiveness. Medications such as angiotensin-converting enzyme inhibitors, angiotensin receptor blockers, nonsteroidal anti-inflammatory drugs, and β- blockers all decrease aldosterone production by decreasing angiotensin II levels. Heparin and cyclosporine decrease aldosterone production. Potassium-sparing diuretics that inhibit aldosterone effect (spironolactone) or block sodium channels in the collecting duct (triamterene, amiloride) can lead to

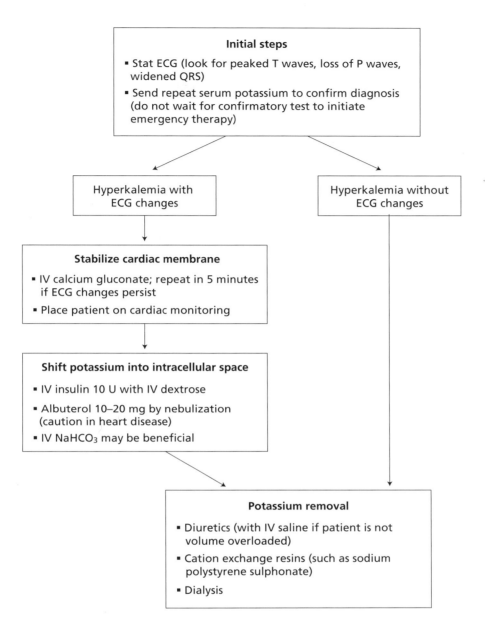

Figure 2 Management approach to hyperkalemia. (ECG = electrocardiogram; IV = intravenous.) (Modified from Medical Knowledge Self-Assessment Program (MKSAP) 14. Philadelphia: American College of Physicians; 2006.)

hyperkalemia. Trimethoprim and pentamidine similarly block sodium channels and can cause hyperkalemia.

Hyporeninemic hypoaldosteronism commonly causes mild hyperkalemia and is characterized by deficient angiotensin II production due to both decreased renin production and an intra-adrenal defect leading to aldosterone deficiency. This syndrome is most commonly associated with diabetic nephropathy but also by chronic interstitial nephritis, renal transplant recipients taking cyclosporine, HIV patients, and use of nonsteroidal anti-inflammatory drugs. Severe hyperkalemia is uncommon unless there is also renal insufficiency.

Acute hyperkalemia causes muscle weakness or flaccid paralysis. The cardiac toxicity is manifest by peaked T waves, flattened P waves, and widened QRS complexes on electrocardiography.

Ventricular arrhythmias result from an increased resting membrane potential and are managed acutely with intravenous calcium, which raises the threshold for depolarization. Other measures include shifting potassium into cells with sodium bicarbonate, β-adrenergic agonists, and insulin and glucose, or augmenting excretion of potassium with loop diuretics, cation exchange resins, or dialysis (Figure 2). Chronic hyperkalemia is managed with a low potassium diet, loop diuretics, and avoidance of drugs known to increase potassium levels.

Book Enhancement

Go to www.acponline.org/essentials/nephrology-section.html to view the electrocardiographic manifestations of hyperkalemia and hypokalemia, access tables on common causes of hypokalemia, hyperkalemia, SIADH, and a differential diagnosis of hyponatremia. In *MKSAP for Students 4*, assess yourself with items 28-32 in the **Nephrology** section.

Bibliography

American College of Physicians. Medical Knowledge Self-Assessment Program (MKSAP) 14. Philadelphia: American College of Physicians; 2006.

Ellison DH, Berl T. The syndrome of inappropriate antidiuresis. N Engl J Med 2007;356:2064-2072. [PMID: 17507705]

Gennari FJ. Disorders of potassium homeostasis. Hypokalemia and hyperkalemia. Crit Care Clin. 2002;18:273-88. [PMID: 12053834]

Lien YH, Shapiro JI. Hyponatremia: clinical diagnosis and management. Am J Med. 2007;120:653-8. [PMID: 17679119]

Chapter 60

Calcium and Phosphorus Metabolism

Mary Jane Barchman, MD

Calcium is a vital regulator of numerous cellular functions. Ionized or free calcium is the metabolically active fraction and is tightly regulated by a dynamic balance between bone, gastrointestinal absorption, and renal excretion under the influence of parathyroid hormone and $1,25\text{-}(OH)_2$ vitamin D. Calcium in the extracellular fluid exists as ionized calcium, protein bound (primarily to albumin), and complexed to organic ions. The protein-bound calcium fraction increases with alkalosis and decreases with acidosis. Phosphorus is a critical component of cellular energy metabolism and bone formation. Major regulators of phosphorus include parathyroid hormone, which increases renal excretion; vitamin D, which increases intestinal absorption; insulin, which shifts phosphorus intracellularly; and renal function and dietary intake.

Hypocalcemia

Acute hypocalcemia leads to neuromuscular irritability (e.g., cramps, paresthesias, tetany, seizures, laryngospasm, and prolonged QT intervals). Mild hypocalcemia is well tolerated, especially if the fall in ionized calcium has been gradual. Precipitous development of hypocalcemia is more likely to result in symptoms and may be detected by positive Chvostek's sign (unilateral contraction of the facial muscles when the facial nerve is tapped just in front of the ear) and Trousseau's sign (carpal spasm after occluding the brachial artery with inflated blood pressure cuff).

Most cases of low total calcium are due to low albumin levels; the ionized calcium concentration is normal. In general, total calcium declines by 0.8 mg/dL for each 1 g/dL decrement in plasma albumin concentration. The most common cause of acquired hypocalcemia is surgical excision or vascular injury to the parathyroid glands. Other causes include autoimmune destruction and infiltrative diseases. Hypomagnesemia can cause hypocalcemia by impairing the release and activity of parathyroid hormone. Patients who undergo subtotal parathyroidectomy may develop "hungry bone" syndrome, postoperatively characterized by hypocalcemia and hypophosphatemia. Disorders of vitamin D can cause mild hypocalcemia. Hyperphosphatemia due to renal failure, rhabdomyolysis, or tumor lysis syndrome may result in hypocalcemia caused by formation and deposition of calcium-phosphate complexes. Hypocalcemia may also complicate pancreatitis when ionized calcium complexes with the free fatty acids are liberated by the action of pancreatic enzymes.

In patients with symptomatic hypocalcemia, treatment includes intravenous 10% calcium gluconate or calcium chloride. In less severe cases, calcium is replaced orally with vitamin D; magnesium must also be replenished if serum values are low.

Hypercalcemia

Causes for hypercalcemia are divided into parathyroid hormone-mediated and non-parathyroid hormone-mediated (Table 1). Primary hyperparathyroidism is the most common cause of hypercalcemia in outpatients. Effects of parathyroid hormone excess include increase in $1,25\text{-}(OH)_2$ vitamin D levels, stimulation of osteoclastic bone resorption, enhanced distal tubular reabsorption of calcium, decreased proximal tubular reabsorption of phosphorus, hypercalcemia, and hypophosphatemia, and increased urinary phosphate and calcium. Primary hyperparathyroidism is most commonly caused by a single parathyroid adenoma, and, less commonly, hyperplasia of the parathyroid glands. Secondary hyperparathyroidism is a normal physiologic response to chronically low calcium levels caused by renal failure, vitamin D deficiency, or gastrointestinal malabsorption; parathyroid hormone is elevated but calcium levels are low to low-normal.

Non-parathyroid hormone-mediated hypercalcemia is present when parathyroid hormone levels are suppressed (<20 pg/mL). Malignancy is the most common cause and is responsible for most cases of hypercalcemia in hospitalized patients. The mechanism of hypercalcemia is related to humoral factors (parathyroid hormone-related protein) or local osteolysis of bone. Granulomatous tissue (e.g., sarcoidosis) can produce excess active vitamin D leading to hypercalcemia.

Symptoms of hypercalcemia vary depending on the severity of hypercalcemia and the rate at which it developed. Mild hypercalcemia (10-11.5 mg/dL) is usually well tolerated and asymptomatic. As serum calcium levels increase, more progressive symptoms occur, such as fatigue, weakness, polyuria, anorexia, nausea, vomiting, abdominal pain, constipation, lethargy and even coma. Serious cardiac dysrhythmias may occur when serum calcium levels are >14 mg/dL.

Hypercalcemia requiring acute intervention is most common in the setting of malignancy. Therapy is directed at maximizing renal clearance of calcium and attenuating calcium efflux from bone lesions. Due to the vasoconstrictive effects of calcium and a tendency toward nephrogenic diabetes insipidus with hypercalcemia, these patients are usually hypovolemic and require resuscitation with normal saline. Improved intravascular volume leads to improved glomerular filtration and increased sodium delivery to more distal nephron segments where calcium can be excreted. After generous volume resuscitation, calcium excretion can be

Table 1. Differential Diagnosis of Hypercalcemia

Disease	Notes
Primary hyperparathyroidism	Often an incidental finding. Calcium elevated, phosphate low; PTH normal (20%) or elevated (80%); calcitriol normal or elevated; alkaline phosphatase normal or elevated; urine calcium normal or elevated.
Humoral hypercalcemia of malignancy	Most common cause of hypercalcemia in patients with cancer, even in those with skeletal metastases. Calcium elevated; phosphate normal or low (elevated if GFR <35 mL/min); PTH suppressed; PTHrP normal or elevated but not needed for diagnosis; calcitriol normal or low; alkaline phosphatase normal or elevated; urine calcium increased.
Metastatic bone disease	Hypercalciuria without hypercalcemia most common. Calcium elevated; phosphate normal or elevated; alkaline phosphatase usually elevated; PTH suppressed; PTHrP low, normal, or elevated; calcitriol low.
Multiple myeloma	Common cause of hypercalcemia in patients with decreased GFR and anemia. Calcium elevated; phosphate elevated; alkaline phosphatase normal; PTH suppressed; PTHrP normal or low; serum protein immunoelectrophoresis abnormal.
Granulomatous disease (e.g., sarcoidosis and tuberculosis)	Calcium elevated; phosphate elevated; alkaline phosphatase elevated but may not be of skeletal origin; urine calcium elevated; calcitriol elevated (particularly in sarcoidosis); PTH suppressed.
Milk-alkali syndrome	Consider in healthy people in whom primary hyperparathyroidism has been excluded. Excessive ingestion of calcium containing antacids present. Calcium elevated; phosphate elevated; creatinine elevated; alkaline phosphatase normal; bicarbonate elevated; PTH suppressed; calcitriol normal or low; urine calcium variable.
Benign familial hypocalciuric hypercalcemia	Constitutive over-expression of the calcium sensing receptor gene. Calcium elevated; phosphate low; PTH normal; (urine calcium ÷ serum calcium) × (serum creatinine ÷ urine creatinine) = calcium to creatinine clearance ratio <0.01 in familial hypocalciuric hypercalcemia. Hypercalcemia without elevated PTH in other family members.
Immobilization	Occurs in persons with high bone turnover before immobilizing event (untreated primary hyperparathyroidism, hyperthyroidism, Paget's disease of bone). Calcium elevated; phosphate elevated; alkaline phosphatase elevated; PTH suppressed; urine calcium elevated.
Hyperthyroidism	A frequent incidental finding in hyperthyroidism. Results from direct stimulation of osteoclasts by thyroxine or tri-iodothyronine.

GFR = glomerular filtration rate; PTH = parathyroid hormone; PTHrP = parathyroid hormone-related protein.

further augmented by the addition of a loop diuretic. Bisphosphonates, given intravenously, may be used to decrease bone resorption and may have a prolonged effect. If the neoplastic or granulomatous process results in increased active vitamin D levels, oral corticosteroid therapy may be beneficial. In secondary hyperparathyroidism due to renal failure, a combination of calcitriol and phosphorus binder therapy is used to suppress PTH concentration to no more than 3-4 times normal. Tertiary hyperparathyroidism occasionally develops in these patients and is characterized by elevated PTH concentration despite elevated serum calcium levels. Cinacalcet is new agent for the treatment of secondary or tertiary hyperparathyroidism that suppresses parathyroid hormone secretion by acting primarily on the calcium-sensing receptor in the parathyroid glands. Cinacalcet may retard the development of renal bone disease while resulting in significantly less elevation in serum calcium and phosphorus levels.

Hyperphosphatemia

Hyperphosphatemia is most often due to renal failure with phosphate retention but can also occur with hypoparathyroidism, rhabdomyolysis, tumor lysis syndrome, acidosis, and overzealous phosphate administration. The symptoms of hyperphosphatemia are attributable to the attendant hypocalcemia. Most hyperphosphatemia is transient unless related to renal failure. The treatment for hyperphosphatemia of renal failure is phosphorus-restricted diet, oral phosphate binders, saline diuresis, or dialysis.

Hypophosphatemia

Hypophosphatemia may result from impaired gastrointestinal absorption, increased renal excretion, or intracellular shift. Severe hypophosphatemia (<1 mg/dL) usually indicates total body phosphate depletion and is characterized by muscle weakness, rhabdomyolysis, respiratory failure, heart failure, seizures, and coma; rarely, hemolysis, platelet dysfunction and metabolic acidosis can occur. Moderate hypophosphatemia (1.0-2.5 mg/dL) is common in hospitalized patients but may not necessarily reflect total body phosphorus depletion. For example, insulin treatment of hyperglycemia will shift phosphate intracellularly. Persistent, moderate hypophosphatemia is treated with oral phosphorus replacement. Severe hypophosphatemia is treated with intravenous potassium phosphate or sodium phosphate. Hypophosphatemic patients frequently have associated hypokalemia and hypomagnesemia, which requires correction.

Book Enhancement

Go to www.acponline.org/essentials/nephrology-section.html to access an algorithm for the diagnosis of hypercalcemia, a differential diagnosis of hypophosphatemia, and to view x-rays of patients with osteitis fibrosa cystica and nephrocalcinosis. In *MKSAP for Students 4*, assess yourself with items 33-37 in the **Nephrology** section.

Bibliography

American College of Physicians. Medical Knowledge Self-Assessment Program 14. Philadelphia: American College of Physicians; 2006

Inzucchi SE. Management of hypercalcemia. Diagnostic workup, therapeutic options for hyperparathyroidism and other common causes. Postgrad Med. 2004;115:27-36. [PMID: 15171076]

Stewart AF. Clinical practice. Hypercalcemia associated with cancer. N Engl J Med. 2005;352:373-9. [PMID: 15673803]

Section VIII
Neurology

Chapter 61

Approach to the Altered Mental State

Robert W. Neilson Jr., MD

Normal consciousness is a state of awareness of self and the environment and the ability to interact with the environment. This requires an intact and functioning brainstem reticular activating system and its cortical projections. Alterations in mental status may range from an agitated, confused state (delirium) to an unarousable, unresponsive state (coma). Delirium is an acute state of confusion. It may manifest as a reduced level of consciousness, cognitive abnormalities, perceptual disturbances, and emotional disturbances. Because delirium is most common in the elderly, care should be taken not to confuse delirium with dementia. Coma is a sleeplike state in that the eyes are closed and the patient is unarousable even when vigorously stimulated. Whether it is delirium, coma, or some state in between, each represents a different stage of the same disease process and is investigated in the same manner. The potential causes are broad and diverse; major categories include metabolic derangement, toxin exposure, structural lesion, vascular insult, seizure, infection, and withdrawal syndromes.

Differential Diagnosis

Metabolic derangements may include disorders of temperature, electrolytes, glucose, hormones, or vitamins. Both hyperthermia and hypothermia can cause alteration of mental status. Electrolyte disorders include hypernatremia or hyponatremia and hypercalcemia. Hyperosmolar nonketotic syndrome is seen in patients with severe hyperglycemia. Hypoglycemia occurs commonly in the treatment of diabetes mellitus. Severe untreated hypothyroidism can result in myxedema coma. Thyrotoxic crisis, or "thyroid storm," is a life-threatening complication of hyperthyroidism characterized by marked agitation, restlessness, delirium, or coma. Acute hemorrhage or infarction of the pituitary gland can lead to pituitary apoplexy. Lastly, thiamine deficiency in alcoholics or the malnourished may lead to Wernicke's encephalopathy.

Toxins can arise from exogenous or endogenous sources. Exogenous sources include illicit and prescription drugs, alcohol, and noxious fumes. Endogenous sources usually arise from organ system failure. Examples include liver failure (hepatic encephalopathy), kidney failure (uremic encephalopathy), and cardiopulmonary insufficiency (hypoxia and/or hypercapnia).

Structural lesions can cause coma through diffuse insult to the cerebral hemispheres, damage to the reticular activating system in the brainstem, or interruption of the connections between the two. Hemispheric mass lesions result in coma either by expanding across the midline laterally to compromise both cerebral hemispheres (lateral herniation) or by impinging on the brainstem to

compress the rostral reticular formation (transtentorial herniation). Brainstem mass lesions produce coma by directly affecting the reticular formation. Because the pathways for lateral eye movements traverse the reticular activating system, impairment of reflex eye movements is often the critical element of diagnosis. Types of mass-occupying lesions include neoplasms (primary or metastatic), intracranial hemorrhage, and infection.

Vascular insults include hemorrhagic or ischemic phenomenon, inflammation, and hypertension. Subarachnoid hemorrhage and hemorrhagic stroke cause intracerebral hemorrhage, and cerebral ischemia can result from thrombotic or embolic occlusion of a major vessel. Unilateral hemispheric lesions from stroke can blunt awareness but do not result in coma unless edema and mass effect cause downward compression upon the reticular activating system. Global cerebral ischemia, usually resulting from cardiac arrest or ventricular fibrillation, may cause coma. Vasculitis of the central nervous system may also cause alteration of mental status, as well as other systemic signs and symptoms. Malignant hypertension can lead to stroke or hypertensive encephalopathy.

Patients with complex partial seizures are awake but exhibit decreased responsiveness and awareness of self and surroundings. Generalized seizures are characterized by loss of consciousness at the onset. Seizures are followed by a postictal recovery period that may last seconds or hours and can include a period of deep sleep, confusion, and headache. In the late stages of status epilepticus, the patient is unconscious but motor movements may be subtle even though seizure activity is continuing throughout the brain.

Central nervous system infection also adversely affects mental status. Examples include meningitis, encephalitis, and subdural empyema. Infection may also travel from a distant site, such as septic emboli from endocarditis. Moreover, infection or fever from any source can cause delirium in the elderly.

Alcohol withdrawal may be complicated by delirium tremens. It occurs most often in chronic heavy abusers with underlying neurologic damage. Delirium tremens is characterized by hallucinations, disorientation, tachycardia, hypertension, low-grade fever, agitation, and diaphoresis.

Evaluation

Coma is a medical emergency and requires rapid assessment and treatment. Cerebrovascular disease accounts for about half of cases of medical coma; hypoxic injury accounts for another 20%; and the remainder are due to toxic, metabolic, and infectious causes. All patients require the emergency ABCs of resuscitation and a focused history from family or bystanders. Patients with witnessed cardiac arrest and resuscitation may have a hypoxic or ischemic insult to the brain. Exclude cervical spine injury by history or imaging. Treat patients with unexplained coma with intravenous glucose (unless rapid finger stick determines normoglycemia) and thiamine for possible Wernicke's encephalopathy. Administer naloxone if opiate overdose is a possibility.

All patients should have a full laboratory evaluation to assess for toxic and metabolic abnormalities, infection, or drug intoxication. Evaluation should include arterial blood gases, complete metabolic panel, complete blood count with differential, ammonia level, and drug and alcohol screen. More focused testing for salicylates, acetaminophen, or other specific drugs such as tricyclic antidepressants depends on the history and clinical suspicion.

The physical exam should address three main issues: 1) does the patient have meningitis; 2) are signs of a mass lesion present; and 3) is this a diffuse syndrome of exogenous or endogenous metabolic cause? The neurological examination should focus on whether there are lateralizing signs suggesting a focal lesion or signs of meningismus and fever suggesting infection. Key physical examination features are pupil size and reactivity, ocular motility, motor activity (including posturing), and respiratory patterns. Coma without focal signs, fever, or meningismus suggests a diffuse insult such as hypoxia or a metabolic, toxic, drug-induced, infectious, or postictal state. In the case of coma after cardiac arrest, patients who lack papillary and corneal reflexes at 24 hours and have no motor response at 72 hours have little chance of meaningful recovery. Coma without focal signs but with meningismus, with or without fever, suggests meningitis, meningoencephalitis, or subarachnoid hemorrhage. Coma with focal signs implies a structural lesion such as stroke, hemorrhage, tumor, or abscess.

Patients with focal findings on examination or unexplained coma should have emergent imaging to exclude hemorrhage or mass lesion. Lumbar puncture is indicated when meningitis or subarachnoid hemorrhage is suspected but neuroimaging is normal. The possibility of nonconvulsive status epilepticus should be evaluated by emergent electroencephalogram.

Delirium may predispose patients to prolonged hospitalization, more frequent impairment of physical function, and increased rates of institutionalization. Therefore, rapid detection, evaluation, and intervention are essential. Diagnosis of delirium is based upon clinical information. The Confusion Assessment Method (CAM) algorithm (Table 1) is a useful tool in diagnosing delirium. There are no laboratory tests, imaging studies, or other tests that can provide greater accuracy than the CAM algorithm (sensitivity 94%-100%; specificity, 90%-95%). Diagnosis requires that the patient show an acute change in mental status with a fluctuating course, inattention, and either disorganized thinking or an altered level of consciousness.

Look for the time course of mental status changes, association of mental status changes with other events (e.g., medication changes or development of physical symptoms), presence of sensory deprivation (absence of glasses or hearing aids), and presence of uncontrolled pain. Take a medication history with particular attention to sedative-hypnotics, barbiturates, alcohol, antidepressants, anticholinergics, opioid analgesics, antipsychotics, anticonvulsants, antihistamines, and anti-Parkinsonian agents; the more medications taken, the greater the likelihood that medication is causing or contributing to the delirium.

Perform a complete mental status, neurological, and medical examination. Look for signs of infection, heart failure, myocardial ischemia, dehydration, malnutrition, urinary retention, and fecal impaction.

Tailor laboratory evaluation to the specific clinical situation (Table 2). The yield of tests and procedures is low when the pretest probability is low. Cerebral imaging, although commonly used, is usually not helpful in the diagnosis of delirium unless there is a history of fall or evidence of focal neurologic impairment.

Attempt to reduce the incidence of delirium by targeting intervention to the individual's risk factors, such as cognitive impairment, sleep deprivation, immobility, visual and hearing impairment, and dehydration. Delirium often results from both underlying vulnerability and acute precipitating factors (Table 3). Amelioration of underlying vulnerability and prevention of acute precipitants will reduce delirium's incidence.

Use of physical restraints is generally avoided because they can increase agitation and the risk for patient injury. However, if other measures to control a patient's behavior are ineffective and it seems likely that the patient, if unrestrained, may cause personal injury or injure others, restraints can be used with caution.

Table 1. Confusion Assessment Method (CAM) for the Diagnosis of Delirium*

Feature	Assessment
1. Acute onset and fluctuating course	Usually obtained from a family member or nurse and shown by positive responses to the following questions: "Is there evidence of an acute change in mental status from the patient's baseline?"; "Did the abnormal behavior fluctuate during the day, that is, tend to come and go, or increase and decrease in severity?"
2. Inattention	Shown by a positive response to the following: "Did the patient have difficulty focusing attention, for example, being easily distracted or having difficulty keeping track of what was being said?"
3. Disorganized thinking	Shown by a positive response to the following: "Was the patient's thinking disorganized or incoherent, such as rambling or irrelevant conversation, unclear or illogical flow of ideas, or unpredictable switching from subject to subject?"
4. Altered level of consciousness	Shown by any answer other than "alert" to the following: "Overall, how would you rate this patient's level of consciousness?" Normal = alert; Hyperalert = vigilant; Drowsy, easily aroused = lethargic; Difficult to arouse = stupor; Unarousable = coma.

*The diagnosis of delirium requires the presence of features 1 and 2 plus either 3 or 4.
Adapted from Inouye SK, van Dyck CH, Alessi CA, et al. Clarifying confusion: the confusion assessment method. A new method for detection of delirium. Ann Intern Med. 1990;113:941-8. PMID: 2240918.

Table 2. Laboratory and Other Studies for the Evaluation of Delirium

Test	Notes
Complete blood count	Screen for infection and anemia (hematocrit <30%), both of which may be associated with delirium.
Serum electrolytes, especially sodium	Screen for hypernatremia and hyponatremia, which frequently present with delirium.
BUN, creatinine	Screen for dehydration (common) and renal failure (rare).
Glucose	Screen for hypoglycemia (especially in diabetics) and severe hyperglycemia or hyperosmolar state.
Liver failure tests: albumin, bilirubin, PT	Only if liver failure and hepatic encephalopathy are suspected.
Urinalysis, culture	Screen for urinary tract infection, which commonly manifests as delirium in the frail elderly.
Chest x-ray	Pneumonia can cause delirium. A chest x-ray is also helpful when evaluating delirium with no obvious cause.
Electrocardiogram	Myocardial infarction and arrhythmia may produce delirium.
Arterial blood gases	Helpful in patients with chronic obstructive pulmonary disease if hypercapnia is suspected, even with a normal oxygen saturation level.
Drug levels, toxic screen	Delirium can occur with "normal" serum levels of some drugs. Toxic screening is only helpful if ingestion is suspected.
Cerebral imaging: CT/MRI	Reserved for cases of high suspicion, new focal abnormalities on neurologic examination, or no found cause after assessing other causes.
Lumbar puncture	Rarely helpful in the absence of high suspicion of meningitis or subarachnoid bleed.
Electroencephalography	Rarely assists in the evaluation unless nonconvulsive status epilepticus is suspected.

BUN = blood urea nitrogen; CT = computed tomography; PT = prothrombin time; MRI = magnetic resonance imaging.

Table 3. Predisposing and Precipitating Factors for Delirium

Predisposing	Precipitating
Older age	>6 total medications
Cognitive impairment	>3 new inpatient medications
Increased comorbidity	Psychotropic medication
Male gender	Infection
Depression	Intensive care unit admission
Alcohol abuse	Hip fracture
Sensory impairment	Dehydration
	Environmental change
	Restraint use
	Malnutrition
	Urinary catheter use
	Iatrogenic event (e.g., medication error)

Use of sedating agents may worsen or prolong delirium. Antipsychotics or anxiolytics should only be used in life-threatening circumstances (such as in the ICU) or when behavioral measures have been ineffective. Low-dose haloperidol, risperidone, and olanzapine are equally effective in treating agitation associated with delirium. Attempt to use the lowest dose of the least toxic agent that successfully controls the agitation.

Book Enhancement

Go to www.acponline.org/essentials/neurology-section.html to review the CAM assessment tool, the clinical features of alcohol withdrawal, and a list of medications to avoid when managing delirium. In *MKSAP for Students 4*, assess yourself with items 1-3 in the **Neurology** section.

Bibliography

Booth CM, Boone RH, Tomlinson G, Detsky AS. Is this patient dead, vegetative, or severely neurologically impaired? Assessing outcome for comatose survivors of cardiac arrest. JAMA. 2004;291:870-9. [PMID: 14970067]

Marcantonio ER. Delirium. http://pier.acponline.org/physicians/diseases/d169. [Date accessed: 2008 Jan 29] In: PIER [online database]. Philadelphia: American College of Physicians; 2008.

Chapter 62

Headache

Eyad Al-Hibi, MD

The art of diagnosing and managing headaches depends on four cornerstones: 1) recognizing typical features, patterns, and prevalence of various headache syndromes; 2) attending to "red flags" in the history or physical examination; 3) using diagnostic studies wisely; and 4) developing an evidence-based strategy for treatment.

Over 90% of headaches are primary headaches, including migraine, tension-type headaches, and cluster headaches. Secondary headache disorders account for a small but important minority of diagnoses, including sinusitis, subarachnoid hemorrhage, meningitis, encephalitis, brain tumor, and benign intracranial hypertension (Table 1).

Evaluation

Identify the pattern of headache and seek any "red flags" suggesting an underlying serious condition such as tumor, aneurysm, or infection (Table 2). The odds of a significant abnormality on neuroimaging are increased if the patient reports rapidly increasing headache frequency, dizziness or lack of coordination, tingling,

or awakening from sleep due to headache. A neurological abnormality on physical examination or any red flag symptom is an indication for neuroimaging. Noncontrast computed tomography of the head is the procedure of choice when acute, sudden, severe headache suggests subarachnoid hemorrhage. A lumbar puncture is indicated if meningitis (fever and neck stiffness) or encephalitis (focal neurological signs, confusion, altered mental status) or if subarachnoid hemorrhage is suspected but imaging studies are normal. Lumbar puncture is diagnostic for benign intracranial hypertension.

Migraine

While tension headache is the most common type of headache reported in community-based surveys, migraine is the most common headache disorder seen in clinical practice and is frequently missed or misdiagnosed as another type of headache (i.e., tension-type or sinus headache). The criteria for diagnosis are well established and can be recalled with the mnemonic POUND: Pulsatile quality; One-day's duration (between 4 and 72 hours); Unilateral

Table 1. Differential Diagnosis of Headache

Disease	Notes
Tension-type headache	Lasts from 30 minutes to 7 days; typically has bilateral location, has a nonpulsating pressing or tightening quality, is mild-to-moderate in intensity, and does not prohibit activity. There is no aggravation of headache by using stairs or by doing any similar routine activity; not associated with nausea or vomiting.
Migraine headache	Lasts from 4 to 72 hours, may be unilateral, pulsating quality, moderate-to-severe in intensity; associated with nausea or vomiting, photophobia, and phonophobia.
Cluster headache	Onset is sudden; duration, minutes to hours, sometimes several times per day, which migraines almost never are; repeats over a course of weeks, then disappears for months or years; often associated with unilateral tearing and nasal congestion or rhinitis; pain is severe and unilateral, periorbital. More common in men but relatively uncommon overall (<1.0% prevalence).
Frontal sinusitis	Usually worse when lying down; associated with nasal congestion; tenderness overlies affected sinus.
Medication-overuse headache	Chronic headache with few features of migraine; tends to occur daily in patients who frequently use headache medications.
Subarachnoid hemorrhage (see Chapter 65)	Sudden, explosive onset of severe headache ("worst headache of my life"); sometimes preceded by "sentinel" headaches (10%).
Meningitis (see Chapter 64)	Meningitis is associated with fever and meningeal signs. Encephalitis is associated with neurologic abnormalities, confusion, altered mental state, or change in level of consciousness.
Benign intracranial hypertension (pseudotumor cerebri)	Often abrupt onset, associated with nausea, vomiting, dizziness, blurred vision, papilledema; neurologic exam is normal but may have CN VI palsy; headache aggravated by coughing, straining, or changing position.
Intracranial neoplasms	Worse on awakening, generally progressive; headache aggravated by coughing straining or changing position.
Temporal arteritis (see Chapter 90)	Occurs almost exclusively in patients >50 years; associated with tenderness of scalp and temporal artery, jaw claudication, and visual changes.

Table 2. Items of a Detailed Headache History

Element	Notes
Date, circumstances, and suddenness of onset of headache disorder	How long have you been having headaches? Did anything unusual happen around the time your headaches began? An injury? A fever? An illness? Starting a new medication? An emotionally significant event (e.g., death, divorce)? Did your headaches begin suddenly or increase gradually over time?
Frequency of headaches	How often have you had headaches during the past month? During the past 6 months? Has there been any change in the frequency of your headaches over time? If so, over what period of time?
Duration of individual attacks	How long do your headaches typically last if untreated? How long do they usually last when treated?
Location of pain	Where do you feel pain during a headache? If the pain is only on one side, is it always on the same side? Does the pain spread or change location in the course of an attack? Is the pain superficial or deep?
Severity and course of pain	During a typical headache attack, are you able to perform your usual daily activities or do you have to restrict your activities? Describe the restrictions your headache imposes. How does your pain change in intensity over the course of a typical attack? Have your headaches become more severe over time? If so, over what period of time?
Quality of pain	Can you describe the kind of pain you feel during an attack? Is it throbbing/pulsating? Pressure-like/constricting? None of the above?
Pattern of occurrence	Do your headaches occur in any regular pattern? On weekends? During vacations? At a particular point in your menstrual cycle? During or after especially stressful times?
Precipitating or aggravating factors	Can you identify anything (e.g., foods, substances, situations, activities) that seem to trigger your headaches? Can you identify anything that aggravates your headache once it has started?
Ameliorating factors	Aside from taking medication, what do you do to relieve your headache once it has started?
Associated features	Do you usually know when you're about to get a headache? How? Do you regularly experience any symptoms other than head pain during an attack? Nausea? Vomiting? Sensitivity to light or sound? How do you feel once the head pain has stopped?
Family history	Does anyone else in your (extended) family suffer from any sort of recurring headaches?
Past and current headache treatments	What medications (prescription and nonprescription) have you tried for your headaches? At what dose and for how long? Were any of them effective? What other sorts of treatment (apart from drugs) have you tried? For how long? Were any of them effective?
Diagnostic studies	Have you ever had a CT or MRI scan or any other diagnostic studies in connection with your headaches? If so, when and where? What were you told about the results?

CT = computed tomography; MRI = magnetic resonance imaging.

in location; Nausea or vomiting; Disabling intensity (goes to bed); >3 features are 90% predictive of migraine headache in patients consulting a physician for headache. Aura occurs in only 15% to 20% of patients with migraine.

Effective non-drug strategies include avoidance of triggers, biofeedback, cognitive behavioral therapy, stress management, and relaxation therapy. Specific dietary triggers are associated with migraines in many individuals and elimination diets decreased migraine symptoms substantially in some individuals. Common dietary triggers include caffeine; nitrates or nitrites in preserved meats; phenylethylamine, tyramine and xanthine in aged cheese, red wine, beer, champagne, and chocolate; monosodium glutamate (Asian and prepared foods); dairy products; and fatty foods. Relaxation training, thermal biofeedback with relaxation training, electromyogram (EMG) biofeedback, and cognitive behavior therapy reduce migraine frequency by 30%-50%.

For acute attacks, treat as soon as possible to maximize the likelihood of rapid and sustained relief and to minimize the need for back-up and rescue medication and subsequent emergency department visits.

The treatment approach depends on several factors, including headache severity and frequency, associated symptoms (such as nausea and vomiting), and co-existing medical conditions. Intranasal and parenteral routes of drug administration should be used in patients with severe nausea or vomiting. Mild attacks are effectively treated with nonsteroidal anti-inflammatory drugs, acetaminophen, or aspirin. More severe attacks are treated with triptans, which have the highest overall efficacy rates for moderate to severe migraine headaches. Triptans are contraindicated in the presence of cardiovascular disease. Dihydroergotamine is an alternative to triptans for migraine-specific treatment but may not be as effective and is contraindicated in coronary artery disease and pregnancy. Dihydroergotamine should not be used concomitantly with a triptan. Acute therapies are limited to no more than 2 to 3 days per week to avoid medication-induced (rebound) headaches. Consider daily preventive drug therapy with non-selective β-blockers (e.g., propranolol) for frequent, severe, or disabling migraine attacks (>3/month). Anticonvulsants, antidepressants, or calcium-channel blockers can also be used but have less evidence supporting their efficacy.

Tension-Type Headaches

Tension-type headaches have a 1-year prevalence of approximately 40%. Tension-type headaches may last minutes to days. Patients describe bilateral, pressing pain of mild to moderate intensity not aggravated by physical activities and without nausea. Chronic tension-type headache is present at least 50% of days and has a significant impact on the individual's daily life. Non-drug approaches include biofeedback training and cognitive-behavioral therapy. Treatment usually begins with nonsteroidal anti-inflammatory drugs, and prophylaxis, often with a tricyclic antidepressant, may be needed.

Chronic Daily Headache

Chronic daily headache of long duration refers to headache disorders that occur daily or near daily and last 4 or more hours. The most common diagnoses are chronic tension-type headache and chronic (transformed) migraine. The latter usually evolves in patients with several years' history of episodic migraine. For most of these patients, the daily, moderate headache does not always have migraine features; however, several times per month migraine headaches are superimposed on the baseline headache. Individuals usually have significant disability secondary to pain, and many have depression, anxiety, panic disorder, and sleep disturbance requiring identification and treatment.

Analgesic Rebound Headache

Another condition that can produce frequent headache is medication overuse (analgesic rebound). Use of analgesic medication more than 2 to 3 days per week may result in headache occurring 15 or more days each month. When the offending medication is withheld, "withdrawal" headaches ensue. There is agreement that opioids, butalbital combinations, isometheptene combinations, over-the-counter analgesic combinations, decongestants, ergotamine, and triptans can result in this pattern. Treatment is withdrawal of medication.

Cluster Headaches

Cluster headaches are much less common than migraine or tension headache and are characterized by unilateral severe and "boring" pain. Onset to peak intensity is usually minutes and the pain is usually orbital, supraorbital, and temporal in location, lasting 15 minutes to 3 hours. Frequency ranges from one every other day to eight per day. Accompanying autonomic symptoms include lacrimation, nasal congestion, rhinorrhea, miosis, ptosis, and conjunctival injection. The attacks occur in clusters that last weeks to months, with remissions lasting months to years. Oxygen inhalation via a non-rebreathing facial mask at a flow rate of 7 L/min is often effective in terminating the attack. Subcutaneous sumatriptan is the other mainstay of acute therapy.

Book Enhancement

Go to www.acponline.org/essentials/neurology-section.html to review a table of headache "red flags", to calculate the probability of a migraine headache, to use an algorithm to manage an acute migraine headache, and to view an MRI scan of a brain tumor. In *MKSAP for Students 4*, assess yourself with items 4-9 in the **Neurology** section.

Bibliography

American College of Physicians. Medical Knowledge Self-Assessment Program 14. Philadelphia: American College of Physicians; 2006.

Detsky ME, McDonald DR, Baerlocher MO, et al. Does this patient with headache have a migraine or need neuroimaging? JAMA. 2006;296: 1274-83. [PMID: 16968852]

Chapter 63

Dementia

Mark Allee, MD

Dementia is an acquired, persistent impairment of intellectual function with compromise in at least three of the following spheres of mental activity: language, memory, visuospatial skills, emotion or personality, and cognition (abstraction, calculation, judgment, and executive function). This loss of function must be of sufficient severity to cause social or occupational disability. Advancing age is the major risk factor for dementia. Common causes include Alzheimer's disease (50%-75%), vascular dementia (10%-20%), Lewy body dementia (10%-15%), and frontotemporal dementia (5%-15%). Important conditions in the differential diagnosis are listed in Table 1. Dementia is the result of structural neuronal changes from inclusion of foreign material or remodeling secondary to vascular insult. Patients with Alzheimer's disease have a normal neurologic examination except for characteristic broad-based cognitive and prominent recent memory impairment. Vascular dementia is causally related to cerebrovascular disease. In practice, at least one third of patients with vascular dementia experience an insidious disease onset and gradual decline. A number of these patients also have an absence of both a clear history of stroke and focal neurologic signs on examination. Dementia with Lewy bodies is characterized by parkinsonism responsive to

dopaminergic therapy, visual hallucinations, and/or fluctuating cognition. Patients with frontotemporal dementia demonstrate early executive and personality changes.

The signature pathologic feature of Alzheimer's disease is the deposition of insoluble, neurotoxic β-amyloid protein in extracellular parenchymal plaques. Another characteristic finding is the intracellular accumulation of neurofibrillary tangles. These tangles are composed of abnormal microtubule-associated tau protein and are quantitatively associated with the severity of dementia. The central cholinergic deficit associated with Alzheimer's disease results from early degeneration of the basal forebrain and is the rationale behind cholinergic augmentation. Causes for vascular dementia include large-vessel occlusions, multiple small-vessel occlusions, or primary hemorrhagic processes. Among these, small-vessel cerebrovascular disease is the most common. Dementia with Lewy bodies is a degenerative condition characterized by intraneuronal Lewy body inclusions in the cerebral cortex. Frontotemporal dementia is found in a variety of diseases associated with disproportionate atrophy of the frontal and anterior temporal brain regions, including Pick's disease, and, occasionally, motor neuron disease. Many of these conditions are associated

Table 1. Important Conditions in the Differential Diagnosis of Dementia

Disease	Characteristics
Alzheimer's disease	Gradual memory loss, preserved level of consciousness. Seizure, falls, tremor, weakness, or reflex abnormalities are not typical early in the disease course. As the illness progresses, other cortical deficits such as aphasia, apraxia, agnosia, inattention, and left-right confusion develop.
Creutzfeldt-Jakob disease	Rapid progression, early age of onset, prominent myoclonus, characteristic EEG pattern of triphasic sharp waves. CSF protein 14-3-3 has good specificity for Creutzfeldt-Jakob disease, but diffusion-weighted MRI may be more sensitive and specific.
Delirium	Altered level of alertness and attention often in conjunction with globally impaired cognition. Onset may be abrupt, and fluctuating level of alertness is common.
Dementia with Lewy bodies	Mild parkinsonism, hallucinations, and delusions early in the illness course.
Depression	Low mood, reduced enjoyment of activities, diminished sense of self-worth or confidence, hopelessness, decreased appetite, libido, and disturbed sleep. May have increased somatic complaints, irritability, and wishes for death.
Frontotemporal dementia (including Pick disease)	Onset often <60 years. Language difficulties are common, as are behavioral disturbances, worsened impulsivity or aggression, or apathy. Functional neuroimaging often shows diminished function in frontal and/or temporal lobes.
Mild cognitive impairment	Objective memory impairment in the absence of other cognitive deficits and intact ADL. Patients with mild cognitive impairment progress to dementia at a rate of about 12%-15% per year.
Normal pressure hydrocephalus	Triad of dementia, gait abnormality, and urinary incontinence associated with psychomotor slowing and apathy. Ventriculo-peritoneal shunting can be curative in some patients.
Vascular dementia	Loss of function should be correlated temporally with cerebrovascular events. May be associated with "silent" strokes, multiple small strokes, or patients with cerebrovascular risk factors, even if a neurologic exam does not suggest a stroke.

ADL = activities of daily living; CSF = cerebral spinal fluid; EEG = electroencephalogram.

with the deposition of tau-positive inclusions in affected neurons; however, the cause of these tau deposits is not known.

Prevention

Treatment and control of hypertension, hyperlipidemia, and diabetes mellitus reduces the incidence of dementia. The treatment of elevated homocysteine with folate is safe, inexpensive, and may reduce the risk of dementia. Specific lifestyle modifications, such as smoking cessation, regular physical exercise, and avoidance of head trauma, may also be beneficial.

Screening

Although there is insufficient evidence for dementia screening in the general population, consider screening patients aged >70 years and younger patients with risk factors for cerebrovascular disease, a history of stroke, or other neurologic conditions. If screening is undertaken, use a standardized cognitive screening test and interview a family member or caregiver. The Mini-Mental State Examination is the most well known and validated screening test; it has a sensitivity of 87% and a specificity of 82% in discriminating patients with Alzheimer's disease from normal controls. The exam is sensitive to cognitive change over time, but it may be insensitive for mild dementia.

Diagnosis

Specifically inquire about memory loss, getting lost, word-finding difficulties, and difficulties with dressing, grooming, and housework. Changes in the patient's emotional state could indicate underlying depression. Perform a comprehensive neurologic exam to look for concurrent central nervous system disease. Look for evidence of gait abnormalities, falls, weakness, clumsiness, sensory abnormalities, incontinence, and rigidity. Perform a mental status exam to evaluate level of alertness, orientation, concentration, abstract reasoning, memory, and mood.

Diagnostic testing may disclose a reversible cause of the dementia (Table 2). Obtain a CT or MRI of the head in all patients. Symptoms that may indicate a radiographic abnormality include symptoms of <3 years' duration, rapid progression, early age of onset, focal neurologic deficits, cerebrovascular disease risk factors, recent history of head trauma or central nervous system infection, and clinical features atypical for Alzheimer's disease. Consider other studies such as lumbar puncture, electroencephalogram, and neuropsychological testing only when the clinical picture suggests a specific underlying disease or unusual clinical course.

Therapy

There is no specific chronologic age that defines a person as elderly. However, people older than 50 years are at increased risk for conditions that may limit their functional status, and the risk for those conditions continues to increase with age. Functional status refers to a person's ability to function independently in the physical, mental, and social realms of life. Adopt a proactive approach to maximize functional status of the patient by assessing and treating psychiatric and behavioral symptoms with non-drug interventions. Educate patients and their caregivers about sleep hygiene, specifically addressing sleep scheduling, nap restriction, daily physical activity, reduction of caffeine intake, and evaluation of nocturia. Local and national organizations may be useful to clinicians and families, including the Alzheimer's Association (www.alz.org).

Table 2. Laboratory and Other Studies for Dementia

Test	Notes
Recommended Studies in All Patients	
MRI or CT scan	Numerous expert consensus statements recommend neuroimaging to discover unsuspected structural lesions.
Complete blood count	Leukocytosis, anemia, or thrombocytopenia may indicate a condition related to cognitive problems.
Metabolic profile	Abnormal sodium, calcium, glucose, and liver or renal function can be related to cognitive problems.
TSH	Thyroid disease can cause cognitive problems.
Vitamin B$_{12}$	If low normal, measure methylmalonic acid and homocysteine (see Chapter 38).
RPR	Tertiary syphilis can cause dementia.
Suggested Studies in Selected Patients	
HIV antibody	Advanced HIV disease can lead to dementia.
Toxicology screen	Screen for benzodiazepines
Erythrocyte sedimentation rate	Consider vasculitis and systemic rheumatologic diseases, including lupus erythematosus.
Heavy metals	Useful when there is environmental exposure.
Folate	Consider in the setting of very poor nutrition.
Urinalysis	Look for infection, malignancy, or other systemic diseases.
Lumbar puncture	Consider when there is a reactive RPR; patient aged <55; rapidly progressive dementia; immunosuppression; suspicion of CNS metastatic cancer, infection, vasculitis, or hydrocephalus; suspicion of Creutzfeldt-Jakob disease.
Electroencephalogram	In the setting of delirium, seizures, encephalitis, or possible Creutzfeldt-Jakob disease.
Neuropsychologic testing	May be helpful in the differential diagnosis of Alzheimer disease from frontotemporal dementia, major depression, mild cognitive impairment, or normal aging.

CNS = central nervous system; HIV = human immunodeficiency virus; RPR = rapid plasma regain; TSH = thyroid stimulating hormone.

The major goal of pharmacotherapy is to delay cognitive and functional decline and to treat symptoms. Acetylcholinesterase inhibitors are indicated for Alzheimer's disease, dementia with Lewy bodies, and mixed Alzheimer's disease and vascular dementia. Commonly used inhibitors include donepezil, galanthamine and rivastigmine. These medications are initiated once the diagnosis has been made and the patient is medically and psychiatrically stable. The treatment must be continuous and without lengthy interruptions. Memantine, a noncompetitive NMDA (N-methyl-D-aspartate) receptor antagonist, can be added to patients on a stable dose of a cholinesterase inhibitor. In patients with vascular dementia, aggressively control hypertension, hyperlipidemia, hypothyroidism, vitamin B_{12} deficiency, and diabetes mellitus. Aspirin may help to stabilize or improve cognition in patients with vascular dementia by preventing further cerebrovascular events.

Treat concomitant depression but avoid antidepressants with anticholinergic side effects, such as tricyclic antidepressants (e.g., amitriptyline and nortriptyline). Consider using an antipsychotic medication in the treatment of hallucinations and delusions or behavioral disturbances (e.g., aggression, severe irritability, agitation, explosiveness) if there is risk of harm to the patient or others, or if patient distress is significant and non-drug treatments have been ineffective. Atypical neuroleptics, such as risperidone, olanzapine, and quetiapine, may be beneficial and should be initiated at low doses. The FDA has issued a black box warning for all six atypical antipsychotics. This warning is in response to an increased risk of mortality due to cardiovascular events or infections, usually respiratory. Clinicians need to weigh the potential benefits of drug treatment, including the suffering and morbidity due to untreated psychosis and behavioral disturbances.

Avoid the use of sedative-hypnotics, antihistamines, or benzodiazepines for sleep induction in patients with dementia due to side effects and potential hazards, including exacerbation of delirium. Consider consultation with a geriatric psychiatrist in patients with difficult-to-treat symptoms or the development of polypharmacy.

Follow-Up

Each visit should include the evaluation of general health and hygiene and the driving ability of the patient. Inquire about dental or denture care, bathing and skin care, sensory aids (glasses, hearing aids), sleep hygiene, eating routine, and scheduled toileting. Inquire about motor vehicle accidents or near accidents, and changes in driving habits or patterns. Patients who show driving impairment must no longer drive. Patients who have received the diagnosis of dementia but have not yet shown any difficulties with driving should undergo a driving evaluation and refrain from driving before completion of the evaluation.

Book Enhancement

Go to www.acponline.org/essentials/neurology-section.html to access a Mini-Mental State Examination tutorial, to review the diagnostic criteria for vascular dementia, and to view MRI scans of patients with Alzheimer's disease, vascular dementia, and normal pressure hydrocephalus. In *MKSAP for Students 4*, assess yourself with items 10-14 in the **Neurology** section.

Bibliography

Blass DM, Rabins PV. Dementia. http://pier.acponline.org/physicians/diseases/d224. [Date accessed: 2008 Jan 24] In: PIER [online database]. Philadelphia: American College of Physicians; 2008.

Joshi S, Morley JE. Cognitive impairment. Med Clin North Am. 2006; 90:769-87. [PMID: 16962841]

Qaseem A, Snow V, Cross JT Jr, et al. Current pharmacologic treatment of dementia: a clinical practice guideline from the American College of Physicians and the American Academy of Family Physicians. Ann Intern Med. 2008;148:370-8. [PMID: 18316755]

Chapter 64

Approach to Meningitis and Encephalitis

Fred A. Lopez, MD

Central nervous system infections are medical emergencies classified by anatomical location and include the syndromes of meningitis (infection of tissues surrounding the cerebral cortex) and encephalitis (infection of the cerebral cortex). Bacterial meningitis requires early clinical recognition, an understanding of microbial causes, and an expedient diagnostic and therapeutic approach. Encephalitis is almost always caused by viral infection. Approximately 20,000 cases of encephalitis occur in the United States each year, with the predominant endemic cause being herpes simplex virus (HSV).

Bacterial Meningitis

More than 75% of cases of bacterial meningitis are due to either *Streptococcus pneumoniae* or *Neisseria meningitidis*. *Streptococcus pneumoniae* is the most common etiologic agent of bacterial meningitis and may occur in patients with other foci of infection (e.g., pneumonia, otitis media, mastoiditis, sinusitis, and endocarditis) or following head trauma with leak of cerebrospinal fluid. The pneumococcal conjugate vaccine (children) and the pneumococcal polyvalent polysaccharide vaccine (adults) are effective in prevention of invasive disease.

Neisseria meningitidis is the second most common etiologic agent of bacterial meningitis in the United States, occurring primarily in children and young adults. Patients with deficiencies in the terminal complement components (C5-C9) are predisposed to infection with *N. meningitidis*. An unconjugated polysaccharide meningococcal vaccine against serogroups A, C, Y, and W-135 is available, and in 2005 a meningococcal polysaccharide diphtheria toxoid conjugate vaccine was approved by the FDA. Neither vaccine affords protection against serogroup B, the causative agent in up to one-third of US cases.

Meningitis caused by *Listeria monocytogenes* is associated with extremes of age (neonates and persons age >50 years), alcoholism, malignancy, immunosuppression, diabetes mellitus, hepatic failure, renal failure, iron overload, collagen vascular disorders, and HIV infection. Group B streptococcal meningitis, an important cause of infection in neonates, is seen in adults with underlying conditions such as diabetes mellitus, pregnancy, cardiac disease, malignancy, collagen vascular disorders, alcoholism, hepatic failure, renal failure, corticosteroid use, and HIV infection. Aerobic gram-negative bacilli (*Klebsiella* species, *Escherichia coli*, *Serratia marcescens*, *Pseudomonas aeruginosa*), *Staphylococcus aureus,* and *Staphylococcus epidermidis* may cause meningitis in patients with head trauma, following neurosurgical procedures, or with cerebrospinal fluid shunts. The differential diagnosis of bacterial meningitis is broad and includes other microbial agents (Table 1).

Diagnosis

Look for fever, headache, neck stiffness, and altered mental status; the absence of these findings essentially rules out the diagnosis. Jolt accentuation of the headache elicited with horizontal movement of the head is more sensitive for the diagnosis of meningitis than the Kernig or Brudzinski signs.

The clinical presentations of viral and bacterial meningitis are similar. The diagnosis is established by cerebrospinal fluid (CSF) analysis (Table 2). Although some clinicians routinely perform CT scanning prior to doing a lumbar puncture in suspected bacterial meningitis in order to reduce the risk of brain herniation, this procedure should not delay empiric antibiotic therapy based on the patient's age and underlying condition. A CSF white cell count ≥500/µL, a CSF lactate acid ≥3.5 mmol/L, or a CSF-serum glucose ratio ≤0.4 are highly predictive of bacterial meningitis. Consider CSF PCR for enterovirus (echovirus, Coxsackie, non-polio enteroviruses) and herpes simplex virus as well as arboviral IgM antibody capture enzyme-linked immunosorbent assay testing (West Nile virus, St. Louis encephalitis virus, California encephalitis virus, Eastern equine encephalitis) in patients with CSF evaluation consistent with aseptic meningitis (meningeal inflammation with negative bacterial cultures), encephalitis, or both when no bacterial agents are identified on Gram stain. Fungal, mycobacterial, HIV and spirochetal testing should be performed when clinically indicated (e.g., immunosuppression, exposure history).

Treatment

If cerebrospinal fluid examination reveals purulent meningitis and a positive Gram stain suggests a specific etiology, targeted antimicrobial therapy is initiated. If the Gram stain is negative, empiric antibiotic therapy is initiated, based upon the patient's age and underlying conditions (Table 3). Administer dexamethasone concomitant with or just prior to the first dose of antimicrobial therapy because this attenuates the inflammatory response following antimicrobial-induced lysis of meningeal pathogens.

Table 1. Differential Diagnosis of Meningitis

Disease	Notes
Bacterial meningitis	Fever, severe headache, stiff neck, photophobia, drowsiness or confusion, and nausea and vomiting and CSF polymorphonucleocyte predominance.
Enterovirus	Fever, severe headache, stiff neck, photophobia, drowsiness or confusion, and nausea and vomiting with a lymphocytic predominance on CSF evaluation. Most cases occur in the summer and early fall. Children are the most often affected. Most frequently identified cause of aseptic meningitis. Primarily echovirus and coxsackievirus. PCR for enterovirus is available.
Arboviruses	Most often present as encephalitis but can present as meningitis or meningoencephalitis. Seen in patients living or traveling to areas where there is arboviral activity or epidemic. St. Louis encephalitis virus, California encephalitis virus, and West Nile virus are the most common. They occur most frequently in warmer months and when contact with mosquito vectors is most likely.
Herpes simplex virus	HSV-1 most often presents as temporal lobe encephalitis and HSV-2 causes aseptic meningitis. HSV meningitis often associated with primary genital infection. HSV accounts for approximately 0.5%-3% of all cases of aseptic meningitis. HSV meningitis often is self-limiting and does not require antiviral treatment. HSV encephalitis does require antiviral treatment.
HIV disease	HIV-associated aseptic meningitis generally follows a mononucleosis-like syndrome. Most commonly seen in acute HIV infection. Viral load should be obtained to exclude acute HIV. Always a consideration in young adults and patients with high-risk behaviors.
Tuberculous meningitis	Headache, nausea, vomiting, fever, mental status changes lasting more than 2 weeks. CSF abnormalities are nonspecific and generally show normal to slightly decreased glucose, elevated protein, and moderate pleocytosis with variable differential. CSF culture for *M. tuberculosis* is low yield and may take several weeks to become positive. A negative TB PCR result on the CSF does not exclude the diagnosis of tuberculous meningitis.
Borrelia burgdorferi (Lyme disease)	Associated with a rash (erythema migrans) early in the disease followed by aseptic meningitis approximately 4 weeks after the initial signs of disease. Vector tick is endemic to the northeastern U.S. and Great Lakes area. Occurs most frequently in the summer and autumn seasons.
Cryptococcal meningitis	Subacute or chronic presentation. 50% of cases occur in patients who are HIV negative. CSF pleocytosis of 40-400 cells/μl with lymphocyte predominance and slightly low glucose is typical. India ink stain of the CSF has limited sensitivity. CSF is positive for cryptococcal polysaccharide antigen in 90% of patients.

CSF = cerebrospinal fluid; HIV = human immunodeficiency virus; HSV = herpes simplex virus; HSV-1 = oral herpes simplex virus; HSV-2 = genital herpes simplex virus; PCR = polymerase chain reaction; TB = tuberculosis.

Table 2. Cerebrospinal Fluid (CSF) Findings in Meningitis

CSF Parameter	Bacterial Meningitis	Viral Meningitis[a]	Tuberculous Meningitis	Cryptococcal Meningitis
Opening pressure (mm H_2O)	200–500[b]	≤250	180–300	>200
Leukocyte count (cells/μL)	1000–5000[c]	50–1000	50–300	20–500[d]
Leukocyte count differential	Neutrophils	Lymphocytes[e]	Lymphocytes[f]	Lymphocytes
Glucose (mg/dL)	<40[g]	>45	≤45	<40[h]
Protein (mg/dL)	100–500	<200	50–300	>45
Gram stain	Positive in 60%–90%[i]	Negative	Negative	Negative
Acid-fast smear	Negative	Negative	Positive in <25%	Negative
India ink preparation	Negative	Negative	Negative	Positive in ≥60%[j]
Cryptococcal antigen	Negative	Negative	Negative	Positive in >85%[k]
Culture	Positive in 70%–85%	Negative	Positive in 25%–86%	Positive in ≥95%

[a] Primarily echoviruses and coxsackieviruses.

[b] Values >600 mm H_2O suggest cerebral edema, intracranial abscess, or communicating hydrocephalus.

[c] Range <100 to >10,000 cells/μL.

[d] Only 13%–31% of AIDS patients have >20 cells/μL.

[e] May have a neutrophil predominance early but changes to lymphocyte predominance after 6–48 hours.

[f] With antituberculous therapy, an initial lymphocyte predominance may become neutrophilic.

[g] CSF:plasma glucose ratio is ≤0.40 in most patients.

[h] Only one third of AIDS patients have a CSF glucose <40 mg/dL.

[i] Likelihood of a positive Gram stain correlates with the number of bacteria in the CSF.

[j] 72%–88% in AIDS patients.

[k] 91%–100% in AIDS patients.

Modified from Medical Knowledge Self-Assessment Program (MKSAP) 14. Philadelphia: American College of Physicians; 2006.

Table 3. Empiric Antimicrobial Therapy for Purulent Meningitis

Predisposing Factor	Common Bacterial Pathogens	Antimicrobial Agents
Age 0–4 weeks	Streptococcus agalactiae, Escherichia coli, Listeria monocytogenes, Klebsiella species	Ampicillin + cefotaxime; or ampicillin + an aminoglycoside
Age 1–23 months	Streptococcus pneumoniae, Haemophilus influenzae, S. agalactiae, Neisseria meningitidis, E. coli	Vancomycin + a third-generation cephalosporin[a,b,c]
Age 2–50 years	S. pneumoniae, N. meningitidis	Vancomycin + a third-generation cephalosporin[a,b,c]
Age >50 years	S. pneumoniae, N. meningitidis, L. monocytogenes, aerobic gram-negative bacilli	Vancomycin + ampicillin + a third-generation cephalosporin[a,b]
Basilar skull fracture	S. pneumoniae, H. influenzae, group A β-hemolytic streptococci	Vancomycin + a third-generation cephalosporin[a]
Postneurosurgery or head trauma	Staphylococcus aureus, coagulase-negative staphylococci (especially Staphylococcus epidermidis), aerobic gram-negative bacilli (including Pseudomonas aeruginosa)	Vancomycin + either ceftazidime or cefepime or meropenem
Cerebrospinal fluid shunt	S. aureus, coagulase-negative staphylococci (especially S. epidermidis), aerobic gram-negative bacilli (including P. aeruginosa), diphtheroids (including Propionibacterium acnes)	Vancomycin + either ceftazidime or cefepime or meropenem

[a] Cefotaxime or ceftriaxone.
[b] Some experts would add rifampin if dexamethasone is given.
[c] Add ampicillin if the patient has risk factors for Listeria monocytogenes infection or if infection with L. monocytogenes is suspected.
Modified from Medical Knowledge Self-Assessment Program (MKSAP) 14. Philadelphia: American College of Physicians; 2006.

Viral Encephalitis

Viral encephalitis presents as an acute-onset, febrile illness associated with headache, altered level of consciousness, and, occasionally, focal neurologic signs. While the clinical presentation of encephalitis is similar to meningitis, the two syndromes differ in that meningitis is not characterized by focal neurologic signs. Arboviral diseases such as Eastern equine encephalitis, St. Louis encephalitis, and others have occurred in humans in the United States for years. Although these viral infections may be fatal or have significant morbidity, the prevalence in humans has been low, and effective treatments and vaccines have not been developed. Lack of attention changed in 1999 when the first cases of West Nile virus encephalitis occurred in the United States. The virus spread throughout the United States and is now diagnosed in thousands of patients annually. West Nile virus encephalitis is most severe in older age groups, and the highest mortality and morbidity rates occur in those ≥65 years of age. The most common manifestations are encephalitis, meningitis, flaccid paralysis, and fever.

The most common cause of nonepidemic sporadic focal encephalitis in the United States is herpes simplex virus (HSV-1), with one-third of cases occurring at age <20 years and one-half occurring at age >50 years. The encephalitis results from reactivation of the latent virus in the trigeminal ganglion, which leads to inflammatory necrotic lesions in the temporal cortex and limbic system. Most cases occur in the absence of an antecedent illness.

Diagnosis

Obtain CSF analysis (including polymerase chain reaction for herpes simplex virus and arboviral-associated IgM antibody capture ELISA), MRI, and electroencephalogram. CSF analysis usually reveals an increased opening pressure, a lymphocytic pleocytosis, a modestly elevated protein level, and a normal or slightly low glucose level. CSF cultures for HSV-1 and arboviruses are usually negative, but sensitivity of the polymerase chain reaction for HSV and arboviral IgM antibody capture ELISA exceeds 90%.

In HSV encephalitis, MRI demonstrates unilateral or bilateral abnormalities in the medial and inferior temporal lobes, which may extend into the frontal lobe. The electroencephalogram findings include focal delta activity over the temporal lobes; periodic lateralizing epileptiform discharges (PLEDs) also may be noted. Brain biopsy is reserved for patients who do not respond to acyclovir.

Treatment

The diagnosis of HSV-1 encephalitis is critical because it is the only central nervous system viral infection for which antiviral therapy (i.e., acyclovir) is proven effective. In HSV encephalitis, prompt acyclovir reduces mortality to approximately 25% in adults and older children. Over 50% of patients who survive will have neurologic sequelae.

Book Enhancement

Go to www.acponline.org/essentials/neurology-section.html for a diagnostic algorithm, to review the differential diagnosis and laboratory studies for meningitis, and view a cerebrospinal fluid Gram stain. In MKSAP for Students 4, assess yourself with items 15-17 in the Neurology section.

Bibliography

American College of Physicians. Medical Knowledge Self-Assessment Program 14. Philadelphia: American College of Physicians; 2006.

Attia J, Hatala R, Cook DJ, Wong JG. The rational clinical examination. Does this adult patient have acute meningitis? JAMA. 1999;282:175-81. [PMID: 10411200]

Fitch MT, van de Beek D. Emergency diagnosis and treatment of adult meningitis. Lancet Infectious Diseases. 2007;7:191-200.

Straus SE, Thorpe KE, Holroyd-Leduc J. How do I perform a lumbar puncture and analyze the results to diagnose bacterial meningitis? JAMA. 2006;296:2012-22. [PMID: 17062865]

Chapter 65

Stroke and Transient Ischemic Attack

Jane P. Gagliardi, MD

Stroke, irreversible neurological symptoms caused by disrupted cerebral blood flow and cerebral ischemia, is the third leading cause of death in the United States and an important cause of disability. Most strokes are ischemic, resulting from thrombosis, embolism, or hypertensive vasospasm. Hemorrhagic stroke results from rupture of a blood vessel. Transient ischemic attack (TIA) results from temporary disruption of cerebral blood flow and mimics stroke but most resolve within 30 minutes; attacks lasting longer than one hour are most often associated with brain infarction. Up to 40% of patients with TIA will eventually have a stroke; up to 20% will have a stroke within 90 days. Stroke is a time-critical medical emergency. Within the first minutes to hours after the onset of cerebral ischemia, an infarct core, which is an area of brain that is irreversibly damaged, develops. The ischemic penumbra, which is potentially viable brain tissue, surrounds this area and will eventually become part of the infarct core if blood flow is not restored quickly. The time course of this process is poorly defined. Substantial volumes of brain potentially remain viable for up to 24 hours after stroke in extreme cases, but most damage occurs in the first 3 to 6 hours post stroke. Therefore, the penumbra is the target of acute ischemic stroke therapy. The differential diagnosis of stroke includes seizure, hypoglycemia, metabolic abnormalities, complicated migraine, rapidly growing mass or brain tumor, and functional illness (Table 1).

Prevention

Educate patients and families about symptoms of stroke and the critical need to be evaluated immediately if they occur. Address modifiable risk factors by encouraging smoking cessation, controlling blood pressure (preferably with an angiotensin-converting enzyme inhibitor), and controlling cholesterol with statins. Discontinue hormone replacement therapy in post-menopausal women and consider low-dose every-other-day aspirin therapy in women >45 years old. Begin anticoagulation for atrial fibrillation unless bleeding risks outweigh potential benefits; in those patients, start antiplatelet therapy. Asymptomatic carotid bruits are common and their prevalence increases with age. The presence of a carotid bruit cannot be used to rule in, nor can its absence rule out, surgically amenable carotid artery stenosis. Among patients <75 years with >60% carotid stenosis, carotid endarterectomy performed by a surgeon with low surgical morbidity (i.e., <3% perioperative stroke or mortality rate) can reduce annual stroke risk by half.

Diagnosis

Treatment requires rapid recognition and diagnosis. The abrupt or sudden onset of focal neurologic symptoms is a possible indicator of ischemic stroke or intracerebral hemorrhage, whereas a

Table 1. Differential Diagnosis of Stroke and Transient Ischemic Attack

Disease	Notes
Stroke	Abrupt onset; fixed focal findings referable to arterial distribution (i.e., hemiparesis of face, arm, or leg ± aphasia). Cannot distinguish stroke subtypes or infarct from hemorrhage without brain imaging.
TIA	Same as for stroke but lasting <24 hours (usually <30 minutes).
Seizure	Abrupt onset and termination of ictus; usually decreased responsiveness during ictus; often involuntary movements during ictus; usually postictal lethargy or confusion; sometimes postictal focal findings that resolve over 24 hours. May accompany stroke.
Hypoglycemia	May look like stroke or TIA; almost always in diabetic patients taking hypoglycemic medications; may or may not be accompanied by seizure.
Complicated migraine (see Chapter 62)	Similar onset and focal findings as stroke; usually severe headache preceding or following attack; sensory and visual disturbances often prominent; sensory symptoms often spread over affected area. Suspect in younger patients, more often women with history of severe headache; MRI usually normal; stroke may accompany migraine.
Mass lesion (tumor, abscess, subdural hematoma)	Focal symptoms occur over days, not minutes; may not be in one vascular territory; primary cancer, fever, immunosuppression, and history of trauma often present. Can be distinguished from stroke by brain imaging.
Encephalitis (see Chapter 64)	Onset over days, not minutes. Fever, followed by headache, possibly meningeal signs, and photophobia, and with structural involvement suggested by mental status change.
Functional	May look like stroke, but findings nonanatomical or inconsistent; MRI normal.

CT = computed tomography; MRI = magnetic resonance imaging; TIA = transient ischemic attack.

thunderclap headache ("worst headache of my life") suggests subarachnoid hemorrhage. A thorough neurological examination is performed to localize the ischemic region (Table 2). The presence of facial paresis, arm drift, or abnormal speech is highly suggestive of stroke. Small, deep penetrating arteries that arise from the larger vessels also may be affected by stroke. Occlusion of these vessels may cause small infarctions with stereotypical clinical "lacunar" syndromes, such as pure motor hemiparesis, pure sensory stroke, clumsy hand–dysarthria syndrome, and ataxic hemiparesis. Neuroimaging is essential to rule out hemorrhage and plan appropriate treatment. Obtain cranial CT or MRI within 30 minutes of arrival. Perform carotid imaging (to assess for stenosis warranting consideration for carotid endarterectomy) and echocardiography (to assess for thrombus, ejection fraction, and patent foramen ovale) within the first 2 days. Obtain laboratory values to define potential underlying conditions as dictated by the history and physical examination (Table 3).

Therapy

Hospitalize all patients with suspected stroke, high risk for stroke, or TIA lasting >10 minutes, preferably in a dedicated stroke unit (intensive care, if warranted) with a multidisciplinary stroke team. Stroke patients treated in specialized stroke units have less mortality and morbidity than patients treated in conventional ward settings. Initiate cardiac monitoring, frequent vital signs, and blood glucose and oxygen monitoring. Hold antihypertensive agents unless systolic blood pressure is >200 mm Hg or there is cardiac ischemia, renal insufficiency, aortic dissection, intracranial hemorrhage, or planned thrombolytic therapy; in these cases, gradually lower blood pressure in 10 to 15 mm Hg decrements with intravenous nicardipine or labetalol.

The thrombolytic agent rt-PA (alteplase) increases chances of recovery when administered intravenously within 3 hours of symptom onset to patients with ischemic stroke. Brain imaging must be negative for hemorrhage. Thrombolysis is contraindicated in patients with mean arterial pressure >130 mm Hg, systolic blood pressure >185 mm Hg, diastolic blood pressure >110 mm Hg, or intracerebral hemorrhage. If administered after 3 hours, risk of hemorrhage and death increases. Withhold aspirin and anticoagulants for 24 hours after rt-PA.

Antiplatelet therapy (aspirin or dipyridamole/aspirin) should be initiated within 48 hours for stroke and TIA to reduce subsequent stroke risk. Clopidogrel is an alternative for patients who cannot tolerate aspirin; routine combination of clopidogrel and aspirin is not recommended due to increased risk of major bleeding. Anticoagulation is not recommended for stroke patients unless cerebral venous thrombosis, basilar occlusion/stenosis, or extracranial arterial dissection is suspected. Consider anticoagulation in patients with possible causes of embolic stroke, including

Table 2. Cerebrovascular Territories and Syndromes

Artery	Major Clinical Features
Anterior cerebral artery	Contralateral leg weakness
Middle cerebral artery	Contralateral face and arm weakness greater than leg weakness; sensory loss, field cut, aphasia or neglect (depending on side)
Posterior cerebral artery	Contralateral field cut
Deep/"lacunar"	Contralateral motor or sensory deficit without cortical signs (e.g., aphasia, apraxia, neglect, and higher cognitive functions)
Basilar artery	Oculomotor deficits and/or ataxia with "crossed" sensory/motor deficits. Crossed signs include sensory or motor deficit on one side of the face and the opposite side of the body.
Vertebral artery	Lower cranial nerve deficits (e.g., dysphagia, dysarthria, and tongue or palate deviation) and/or ataxia with crossed sensory deficits

Modified from Medical Knowledge Self-Assessment Program (MKSAP) 14. Philadelphia: American College of Physicians; 2006.

Table 3. Laboratory Studies for Transient Ischemic Attack and Stroke

Test	Rationale
Complete blood count	Ensure adequate oxygen-carrying capacity.
Prothrombin time and partial thromboplastin time	Baseline studies in anticipation of possible anticoagulation.
Lupus anticoagulant, anticardiolipin antibodies, factor V Leiden, protein C and S, antithrombin III (selected patients)	Screening for hypercoagulable states.
Blood glucose, creatinine, and lipid profile	Define underlying risk factors.
Blood cultures (selected patients)	Obtain blood cultures if patient is febrile, especially if endocarditis is suspected.
Antinuclear antibody and related serologic studies, erythrocyte sedimentation rate, RPR or VDRL (selected patients)	Obtain if vasculitis is suspected. Neurosyphilis may present as acute stroke.
Hemoglobin electrophoresis (selected patients)	Identify hemoglobinopathies causing stroke.
Serum protein electrophoresis (selected patients)	Useful in defining lymphoproliferative diseases predisposing to brain hemorrhage.

RPR = rapid plasma reagin.

atrial fibrillation, intracardiac thrombus, or dilated cardiomyopathy with significantly reduced ejection fraction.

Use antipyretics to keep core body temperature at <38°C (100.4°F). Use supplemental oxygen to maintain oxygen saturations at >95%. Monitor blood glucose and use insulin, if necessary, to achieve blood glucose of <150 mg/dL in an effort to prevent post-stroke complications. Prevent decubitus ulcers and deep venous thrombosis through frequent repositioning and use of subcutaneous heparin or graduated or pneumatic compression stockings. Hold oral nutrition until swallowing is evaluated and consider early nasogastric tube feeding if risk for aspiration is suspected or confirmed.

Consult with physical, occupational, and speech therapists. Consider referring patients with >70% carotid stenosis for carotid endarterectomy to decrease the risk of recurrent stroke. In one study, 2-year stroke risk decreased from 26% to 9% in stroke patients with symptomatic >70% carotid stenosis who underwent carotid endarterectomy. There may be some benefit from carotid endarterectomy among selected patients (e.g., those expected to live more than 5 years) with symptomatic 50%-69% carotid stenosis; there is no clear benefit from carotid endarterectomy in patients with less than 50% carotid stenosis.

Follow-Up Issues

Follow post-stroke patients with a goal of maximizing function and preventing recurrence. Refer patients for intensive rehabilitation (at home or in a facility) to improve function. Recognize and treat post-stroke depression, which is common and can contribute to cognitive, functional, and social difficulties that impair rehabilitative efforts. Fracture risk increases seven-fold after stroke; consider B_{12}, folic acid, and bisphosphonates, which are associated with improved bone mineralization and decreased fracture rates post-stroke.

Book Enhancement

Go to www.acponline.org/essentials/neurology-section.html to view a Hollenhorst plaque and CT scans showing ischemic and hemorrhagic strokes and subarachnoid hemorrhage, an echocardiogram showing a left atrial thrombus, and to review inclusion and exclusion criteria for thrombolytic therapy. In *MKSAP for Students 4*, assess yourself with items 18-24 in the **Neurology** section.

Bibliography

Goldstein LB, Simel DL. Is this patient having a stroke? JAMA. 2005; 293:2391-402. [PMID: 15900010]

Grotte JC. Stroke and Transient Ischemic Attack. http://pier.acponline .org/physicians/diseases/d114. [Date accessed: 2008 Jan 16] In: PIER [online database]. Philadelphia: American College of Physicians; 2008.

Sauvé JS, Laupacis A, Ostbye T, Feagan B, Sackett DL. The rational clinical examination. Does this patient have a clinically important carotid bruit? JAMA. 1993;270:2843-5. [PMID: 8133624]

van der Worp HB, van Gijn J. Clinical practice. Acute ischemic stroke. N Engl J Med. 2007;357:572-9. [PMID: 17687132]

Chapter 66

Peripheral Neuropathy

Christopher A. Klipstein, MD

Peripheral neuropathy is a general term for any disorder affecting the peripheral nerves. Clinical manifestations include various combinations of altered sensation, pain, muscle weakness, and autonomic dysfunction. The history, exam, and electrodiagnostic studies can be used to determine the type of neuropathy present, thereby narrowing the list of possible etiologies.

Differential Diagnosis

Peripheral neuropathies may be divided into disorders producing focal or widespread nerve dysfunction. Mononeuropathies are isolated disorders affecting a single peripheral nerve. They are most frequently caused by nerve entrapment or compression (e.g., carpal tunnel syndrome). When multiple noncontiguous peripheral nerves are involved, the term mononeuropathy multiplex is used. Mononeuropathy multiplex is often the result of a systemic disease (e.g., diabetes mellitus, amyloidosis, or sarcoidosis) where the mechanism of nerve injury may be a combination of compressive, ischemic, metabolic, and inflammatory factors. When successive acute involvement of individual nerves is accompanied by pain, suspect a vasculitis as the cause.

Peripheral polyneuropathy refers to diffuse, generalized, usually symmetric involvement of the peripheral nerves. Polyneuropathy is often a manifestation of systemic disease or exposure to a toxin or medication. Patients with polyneuropathies present in variable ways based upon the pathophysiology of the underlying etiology. Polyneuropathies can be characterized as axonal or demyelinating. Axonal polyneuropathies result from dysfunction of peripheral nerve cells and their axons, usually from metabolic or toxic causes (e.g., diabetes, alcohol). Demyelinating polyneuropathies are due to dysfunction of the peripheral nerve myelin that encases many peripheral nerves.

Axonal polyneuropathies typically present with symmetric distal sensory loss, with or without burning, tingling, or muscle weakness. Because the longest nerves are affected earliest and most severely, initial symptoms are usually in the feet, beginning with numbness and paresthesias in the toes that gradually proceed up the limb, eventually resulting in depressed ankle jerks and atrophy of the intrinsic foot muscles. As the sensory symptoms ascend, the fingers and hands become involved, resulting in the classic "stocking-glove" pattern of sensory loss. Common etiologies for axonal polyneuropathies include diabetes, alcoholism, vitamin B_{12} deficiency, and uremia.

In contrast, most patients with a demyelinating polyneuropathy present initially with motor symptoms. Symmetric proximal weakness suggests a myopathy (muscle disease) or an acquired demyelinating polyneuropathy like Guillain-Barré syndrome or chronic inflammatory demyelinating polyneuropathy. Guillain-Barré syndrome is caused by an immune-mediated attack directed toward a component of peripheral nerve myelin. The syndrome is characterized by rapid-onset symmetric weakness in all limbs progressing over several days to weeks, with diminished or absent deep tendon reflexes. Patients usually note weakness in the legs first, more often proximal than distal, and symptoms spread in an ascending fashion. Although patients frequently report paresthesias with onset of symptoms, objective sensory loss is unusual. Acute illness (usually an infection) precedes the onset of neurologic symptoms in about two thirds of patients. Patients with chronic inflammatory demyelinating polyneuropathy present with slowly progressive, relatively symmetric limb weakness and sensory disturbances. The symptoms typically progress for several months, and symptom severity can fluctuate over many years.

Evaluation

For patients with a peripheral neuropathy, use the distribution of symptoms, combined with the characterization of the pathology (axonal or demyelinating), to identify potential etiologies (Table 1). Patients with severe or rapidly progressive symptoms or with no clear etiology warrant prompt evaluation. Despite extensive diagnostic evaluation, no etiology is found in approximately 20% of cases of polyneuropathy.

Focus the initial history on the distribution, time course, and nature of the deficit (sensory or motor, or both). In addition, ask about symptoms of systemic diseases that are associated with neuropathy (e.g., diabetes, uremia), exposure to medications (Table 2) or toxins (e.g., alcohol, heavy metals) that can cause a peripheral neuropathy, and any family history of neuropathy. In the appropriate clinical context, inquire about recent viral illnesses, HIV risk factors, foreign travel (leprosy), and the possibility of a tick bite (Lyme disease). Utilize the review of systems to look for evidence of other organ involvement and symptoms of an underlying malignancy.

Use the physical exam to confirm the distribution of nerve involvement and to determine the extent of motor and/or sensory involvement. Abnormalities detected in the distribution of a single nerve indicate a mononeuropathy. Measure strength in all major muscle groups and test all sensory modalities (i.e., light touch, pin prick, temperature, vibration, and proprioception). Assess deep tendon reflexes; remember that hyporeflexia suggests peripheral pathology while hyperactive reflexes imply a central

Table 1. Classification of Peripheral Neuropathies

Category	Distribution/Pattern	Examples	Mechanism
Mononeuropathy	Focal (single nerve)	Carpal tunnel syndrome	Entrapment
Mononeuropathies multiplex	Asymmetric, multifocal (several noncontiguous nerves)	Vasculitis, diabetes mellitus, lymphoma, amyloidosis, sarcoidosis, Lyme disease, acute HIV infection, leprosy	Ischemia, infiltration, inflammation
Axonal polyneuropathies	Symmetric, distal, predominantly sensory symptoms, sometimes also motor symptoms	Alcohol, drugs, chronic arsenic exposure, diabetes mellitus, uremia, low B_{12} or folate, hypothyroidism, paraproteinemias, paraneoplastic, chronic HIV infection, Charcot-Marie-Tooth disease	Toxic, metabolic, oncologic, inflammation, hereditary
Demyelinating polyneuropathies	Symmetric, often proximal, predominantly motor symptoms, spreading in ascending fashion	Acute arsenic toxicity, Guillain-Barré syndrome, chronic inflammatory demyelinating polyneuropathy, paraproteinemias	Toxic, immunologic, oncologic

Table 2. Drugs Associated with Peripheral Neuropathies

- Amiodarone
- Cisplatin
- Colchicine
- Dapsone
- HIV drugs:
  —Didanosine (ddI)
  —Zalcitabine (ddC)
  —Stavudine (d4T)
- Hydralazine
- Isoniazid
- Metronidazole
- Nitrofurantoin
- Paclitaxel
- Phenytoin
- Vincristine

cause. Observe the gait and perform a Romberg test. In addition, look for evidence of systemic disease (e.g., lymphadenopathy, organomegaly, rashes, and arthritis).

Electromyography and nerve conduction studies are often the most useful tests in the evaluation of peripheral neuropathies. They augment the ability of the history and physical examination to distinguish neuropathies from myopathies and to differentiate mononeuropathies from polyneuropathies. For patients with polyneuropathies, these tests provide information as to the type of fibers involved (motor, sensory, or both) and characterize the pathologic process as primarily axonal or demyelinating.

Laboratory evaluation for the most common etiologies of an axonal polyneuropathy (causing distal, symmetric, sensorimotor symptoms) often includes fasting blood glucose, glycosylated hemoglobin, blood urea nitrogen, serum creatinine, complete blood count, erythrocyte sedimentation rate, serum protein electrophoresis, urinalysis, thyroid stimulating hormone, and vitamin B_{12} and folate levels. In specific clinical contexts, other studies are potentially useful, including an antinuclear antibody test, HIV test, Lyme titer, and heavy metal screen.

When electromyography and nerve conduction findings suggest an acquired demyelinating neuropathy, the two most common etiologies are Guillain-Barré syndrome and chronic inflammatory demyelinating polyneuropathy. Diagnosis is based on clinical recognition of progressive muscle weakness and reduced deep tendon reflexes combined with abnormal electrodiagnostic studies and a high protein level with few or no leukocytes in cerebrospinal fluid (albuminocytologic dissociation).

Nerve biopsy (usually sural nerve) is only indicated to investigate for possible vasculitis, amyloidosis, sarcoidosis, leprosy, or tumor infiltration. Molecular genetic tests are commercially available for a number of hereditary neuropathies.

Therapy

Treatment of axonal polyneuropathies is centered on removal of the toxic agent (e.g., alcohol) or improvement of the underlying metabolic condition (e.g., diabetes, vitamin B_{12} deficiency). This will often halt the progression of symptoms. Treat pain and dysesthesias symptomatically using agents such as tricyclic antidepressants, gabapentin, pregabalin or duloxetine. Educate patients with diminished distal sensation about appropriate foot care to decrease risk of foot ulcers and infections.

Vasculitic mononeuropathies and acute demyelinating polyneuropathies require prompt recognition and treatment with immunomodulating agents. Treat nonambulatory patients with Guillain-Barré syndrome with plasmapheresis or intravenous immune globulin. There is no evidence that corticosteroids shorten the course or reduce residual deficits in Guillain-Barré syndrome. Ventilatory support (needed in up to 30% of cases), infection surveillance, prophylaxis of venous thrombosis, pain management, and nutritional and psychologic support contribute to reduced morbidity and mortality.

In addition to plasmapheresis and intravenous immune globulin, corticosteroids are effective for chronic inflammatory demyelinating polyneuropathy. Most patients need long-term serial treatment with plasmapheresis or intravenous immune globulin every 4 to 6 weeks to prevent relapse.

Book Enhancement

Go to www.acponline.org/essentials/neurology-section.html to review an approach to the diagnosis of peripheral neuropathy, to review salient features of the history and physical examination, and to review a differential diagnosis of distal sensory polyneuropathy.

In *MKSAP for Students 4*, assess yourself with items 25-26 in the **Neurology** section.

Bibliography

American College of Physicians. Medical Knowledge Self-Assessment Program 14. Philadelphia: American College of Physicians; 2006.

England JD, Asbury AK. Peripheral neuropathy. Lancet. 2004;363:2151-61. [PMID: 15220040]

Section IX
Oncology

Chapter 67

Breast Cancer

Kathleen F. Ryan, MD

Breast cancer is the most frequently diagnosed cancer and the second most common cause of cancer death in women. More than 200,000 new cases of invasive breast cancer are diagnosed annually and, of these cases, >40,000 people will die. Most cases will affect women, but nearly 2000 cases will be in men. The main risk factor for women is age. Other important risk factors are genetic mutations (*BRCA-1* and *2*), personal or family history (especially first-degree relatives) of breast cancer, prior biopsy showing atypical ductal or lobar hyperplasia, and prolonged estrogen exposure (early menarche, late menopause, or nulliparity). Only age shows a strong enough correlation to target women for screening. Women with strong family histories of breast or ovarian cancer should be screened for *BRCA* mutations. *BRCA-1* and *2* are highly associated with cancer risk (>60% by age 50), including a small percentage of all breast cancers (<5%).

Prevention

Prevention strategies are available for women at high risk for breast cancer (5-year risk ≥1.7%). One option is a 5-year course of anti-estrogen medications, tamoxifen or raloxifene, to reduce the risk of developing estrogen receptor–positive cancer. The risks of these medications are not insignificant: they include thrombosis, endometrial cancer, and annoying symptoms like hot flashes. Due to these possible side effects, cancer risk must be calculated to determine whether the benefits outweigh the risks of treatment. The Gail Model was developed to give a quantitative cancer risk. The National Cancer Institute Web site (http://bcra.nci.nih.gov/brc/) has a risk calculator based upon this model which looks at factors such as current age, age of menarche, age at first live birth, breast cancer in first-degree relatives, previous breast biopsy, and ethnicity. Consider offering anti-estrogen therapy to women between the ages of 35 and 60 with a breast cancer risk of ≥1.7 % in the next 5 years based upon the Gail Model.

Prophylactic mastectomy is another option for women at increased risk for breast cancer; especially women found to have a genetic predisposition. Women with a known *BRCA-1* or *BRCA-2* mutation should be referred for evaluation by a genetics counselor who can educate them about the benefits of prophylactic oophorectomy.

Screening

The American Cancer Society recommends all women age ≥20 years be taught and encouraged to perform breast self-examination (BSE) and report any breast changes to their health professional. Women between the ages of 20 and 39 should have clinical breast examinations (CBE) done by a health professional every 3 years and annually after age 40. BSE does not improve cancer-specific or all-cause mortality. The sensitivity of CBE is directly related to the time taken to perform the examination.

Annual screening mammograms begin at age 40. In women 50-69 years of age, screening decreases cancer mortality by one-third. There is no consensus on what age to stop screening. Woman ≥35 years with a ≥1.7% risk should have CBE every 6-12 months and yearly mammography. For women with known *BRCA-1* and *BRCA-2* mutations, consider starting screening around age 25. Specialized imaging such as ultrasonography, scintigraphy with sestamibi, or MRI should be reserved for the small group of women with abnormal or inconclusive mammograms or clinical exams.

Diagnosis

Women reporting new breast symptoms or new abnormalities on examination should be carefully evaluated. History focusing on age, family history of breast or ovarian cancer, and use of hormone replacement or oral contraceptives should be elicited. Age of menarche, number of pregnancies, and menopausal status is also important. Inquire about breast pain, nipple discharge, abdominal discomfort, bone pain, and respiratory or neurological symptoms. Knowing the results of prior imaging studies or biopsies is important.

Physical examination should focus on detailed examination of both breasts and full evaluation of lymph nodes. Usually breast cancer presents as a new lump, nipple discharge, or retraction with skin dimpling. Erythema, scaliness, and peau d'orange (skin edema with enlargement of pores and change in color) are signs of inflammatory breast cancer, which is often misdiagnosed as mastitis. Younger women may have denser breasts which make mass detection more challenging as compared to older women with more fat content in their breasts. Standardization of the CBE improves examiner accuracy. Four variables important for proper examination of the breast are: proper positioning of the patient, accurate identification of breast boundaries, finger position and palpation pressure, and duration of the examination. Axillary adenopathy may indicate more advanced disease, whereas supraclavicular or cervical adenopathy usually means metastatic disease.

For nipple discharge, cytology is an excellent diagnostic tool. Mammography or ultrasonography should be done on all patients with new breast symptoms or abnormal examination findings. Women <40 years are likely to have benign findings; following the abnormality through one menstrual cycle instead of immediate imaging is a reasonable option. Obtain a tissue diagnosis in women with a persistent suspicious abnormality on mammogram or in all women with a suspicious palpable mass, even if an imaging study is not abnormal (Table 1). If surgery is planned, a preoperative evaluation consisting of bilateral mammography, chest x-ray, and laboratory studies based upon age and comorbid illnesses is performed. The differential diagnosis of breast masses is summarized in Table 2. Evaluation of estrogen/progesterone (ER/PR) receptor status is important as it predicts benefit from hormonal therapy. HER1-4 is a family of membrane bound proteins with tyrosine kinase activity that act as epidermal growth factors. Over expression of HER2 occurs in up to 40% of breast cancers and is associated with poorer prognosis.

Staging of breast cancer is based upon the TNM staging system: using tumor size (T), axillary node status (N), and presence or absence of metastatic disease can determine therapy options.

The two most prognostic factors are tumor size and axillary node status. As it evolves, genomic testing may replace staging systems.

Therapy

Surgery is a mainstay treatment for breast cancer. Lumpectomy (breast conservation surgery) followed by radiation is an option for patients with focal disease (tumor <5 cm) or ductal carcinoma *in situ*; survival rates are similar to mastectomy. For more extensive ductal carcinoma, modified radical mastectomy with radiation is the best option to lower recurrence rates. For very large tumors or contraindication to radiation (e.g., prior radiation) mastectomy is needed. Radiation does carry the risk of future cardiovascular damage and lymphoma. For metastatic disease surgery is used only as palliation, for example, to prevent complications such as infection.

Table 1. Evaluation of Clinical Breast Abnormalities

Breast Abnormality	Diagnostic Test
Palpable lump or mass and age <30	Ultrasound: Consider observation to assess resolution within 1 or 2 menstrual cycles. If persistent, do ultrasonography. If asymptomatic and cystic on ultrasonography, observe. If symptomatic or not clearly cystic on ultrasonography, aspirate. If aspirate fluid is bloody or a mass persists following aspiration, biopsy or excise for diagnosis. If solid on ultrasonography, do mammogram and obtain tissue diagnosis (fine-needle aspiration, core biopsy, or surgical excision). If not visualized on ultrasonography, obtain mammogram and obtain tissue diagnosis.
Palpable lump or mass and age ≥30	Mammogram: If BI-RADS category 1-3,* obtain ultrasound and follow protocol above. If BI-RADS category 4-5, obtain tissue diagnosis.
Nipple discharge, no mass, any age	Bilateral, milky: Pregnancy test (if negative, endocrine evaluation). Persistent, spontaneous, unilateral, one duct, or serous/bloody: Cytology optional, obtain mammogram and surgical referral for duct exploration.
Thickening or asymmetry and age <30	Consider unilateral mammogram; if normal, reassess in 3-6 months; if abnormal, obtain tissue diagnosis.
Thickening or asymmetry and age ≥30	Obtain bilateral mammogram; if normal, reassess in 3-6 months; if abnormal, obtain tissue diagnosis.
Skin changes (e.g., erythema, peau d'orange, scaling, nipple excoriation, eczema) and age <30	Consider mastitis and treat with antibiotics if appropriate and reevaluate in 2 weeks. Otherwise, evaluate as below.
Skin changes (e.g., erythema, peau d'orange, scaling, nipple excoriation, eczema) and age ≥30	Obtain bilateral mammogram; if normal, obtain skin biopsy; if abnormal or indeterminate, obtain needle biopsy or excision (also consider skin punch biopsy).

* Breast Imaging Reporting and Data System. BI-RADS 1: negative; BI-RADS 2: benign finding; BI-RADS 3: probably benign finding; short-interval follow-up suggested; BI-RADS 4: suspicious abnormality; consider biopsy; BI-RADS 5: highly suggests malignancy; take appropriate action.

Table 2. Differential Diagnosis of Breast Mass

Disease	Characteristics
Fibrocystic changes of the breast	Excessive nodularity and general lumpiness; pain may be exacerbated premenstrually.
Fibroadenoma	Tender, discrete, mobile, well-circumscribed mass. Confirmed by exam, ultrasonography, and fine-needle aspiration.
Breast cyst	Severe localized pain associated with rapid expansion of a cyst. Ultrasonography usually diagnostic; the test of choice in women aged <40 years.
Breast hematoma	Tender mass, usually in association with breast trauma or after biopsy.
Breast cancer	Pain in 5% to 20% of patients. Firm, irregular mass and axillary nodes may be present. Skin thickening and erythema suggest an underlying neoplasm or inflammation. Examination, mammography, ultrasonography, and fine-needle aspiration are indicated. Associated bloody discharge more suggestive of cancer.
Breast abscess	Erythema, pain, and fever; more common in lactating breast.
Ductal papilloma	Unilateral bloody discharge; mass may not be detectable. Refer for duct exploration.

Sampling of the lymph nodes is done as part of staging. Because aggressive removal of all axillary nodes does not improve survival and leads to limb lymphedema, sentinel node dissection technique is often used instead. Dye or tracer is injected into the tumor and the first draining lymph node is biopsied and examined for tumor. If tumor is absent, no further dissection is needed; if tumor is noted, further lymph node dissection is done.

Estrogen/progesterone (ER/PR) receptor status predicts benefit from hormonal therapy. A 5-year course of adjuvant tamoxifen or raloxifene is generally prescribed for women with ER/PR receptor positive tumors following lumpectomy and radiation therapy unless contraindicated.

Aromatase inhibitors (anastrozole, letrozole, exemestane) also offer risk reduction for new breast cancer events. They block final conversion in adipose tissue of adrenal steroidal precursors to estradiol in women.

The decision to use systemic chemotherapy is based upon risk of recurrent disease. Presence of invasive disease within the biopsy is the most powerful prognostic factor for recurrence. Typical chemotherapy regimens usually include methotrexate, cyclophosphamide, doxorubicin or epirubicin, and 5-fluorouracil. For patients with HER2 positive breast cancer, a monoclonal antibody, trastuzumab, is used as adjuvant therapy.

For patients with metastatic disease, therapy is palliative. ER/PR receptor positive patients who have bone or visceral disease are initially treated with tamoxifen. For tamoxifen-resistant disease, aromatase inhibitors are used in postmenopausal women. For patients with lytic bone disease, radiation therapy is used to reduce pain or prevent pathologic fractures. Pamidronate is used to treat hypercalcemia from bone involvement. Control of pain and sensitivity to psychosocial issues is important and involvement in hospice can be beneficial to patients and their families.

Follow-Up

Breast cancer survivors should undergo annual mammography of the preserved and contralateral breast. In absence of specific symptoms, routine blood tests or imaging procedures looking for metastatic disease should not be done.

Book Enhancement

Go to www.acponline.org/essentials/oncology-section.html to see an example of Paget's disease of the breast, the clinical appearance of peau d'orange, and the most common anatomical locations of breast cancer. Use the Gail Model to estimate the risk of breast cancer based upon historical data. In *MKSAP for Students 4*, assess yourself with items 6-8 in the **Oncology** section.

Bibliography

Barton MB, Harris R, Fletcher SW. The rational clinical examination. Does this patient have breast cancer? The screening clinical breast examination: should it be done? How? JAMA. 1999;282:1270-80. [PMID: 10517431]

Qaseem A, Snow V, Sherif K, Aronson M, Weiss KB, Owens DK; Clinical Efficacy Assessment Subcommittee of the American College of Physicians. Screening mammography for women 40 to 49 years of age: a clinical practice guideline from the American College of Physicians. Ann Intern Med. 2007;146:511-5. [PMID: 17404353]

Wolff AC. Breast Cancer. http://pier.acponline.org/physicians/diseases/d192. [Date accessed: 2008 Jan 8] In: PIER [online database]. Philadelphia: American College of Physicians; 2008.

Chapter 68

Colon Cancer

Kathleen F. Ryan, MD

Colon cancer is the second leading cause of cancer death in the United States. Over 153,000 new cases of colon cancer are diagnosed annually, and more than 52,000 people will die. Death is preventable by using effective, safe, and relatively inexpensive screening methods.

Colon cancer arises from adenomatous polyps, and their removal reduces the risk of colon cancer. The main risk factors for malignant transformation are polyp size (>1.0 cm), number, and histological type.

Genetic mutations are the basis for inherited colon cancer syndromes. Genes implicated in the development of colorectal cancer fall into three categories: oncogenes, tumor suppressor genes, and DNA nucleotide mismatch repair genes. Hereditary syndromes include autosomal dominant familial adenomatous polyposis and its variants (1% of all colorectal cancers); autosomal dominant hereditary nonpolyposis colorectal cancer (5% to 10%); and the very rare autosomal dominant hamartomatous polyposis syndromes (Peutz-Jegher's syndrome and juvenile polyposis). Approximately 75% of colorectal cancers arise in individuals who have no obvious cancer risk.

Although the precise pathologic mechanisms of colon cancer have not been identified, dietary and lifestyle factors, including physical inactivity, calcium deficiency, excess body weight, and excessive consumption of alcohol—likely in conjunction with a diet low in folic acid and methionine—and smoking at an early age, are associated with an increased risk for developing colorectal cancer.

Prevention

Diet and exercise have been shown to reduce the risk of colon cancer. Consumption of fresh fruits and high fiber foods (e.g., vegetables and whole grains) and moderate intake of red meats and fat is recommended. A regular program of physical exercise will help maintain normal body weight. Patients should avoid excess alcohol intake and not smoke. Some studies show a reduction in recurrent polyps with aspirin, but aspirin is not recommended for prevention of colon cancer or polyps.

Screening

Screening recommendations are based upon risk. All adults age >50 years at average risk for colon cancer can be screened by any one of a number of acceptable methods (Table 1). Patients at high risk are screened more intensely with colonoscopy, usually beginning at age 40 years and repeated every 5 years (Table 2). High risk is defined as having multiple first-degree relatives with colon cancer or a first-degree relative diagnosed with colonic adenomatous polyps or colon cancer at age ≤60 years. Patients with a personal history of an adenomatous polyp of >1.0 cm require a repeat colonoscopy within 3 years. Serum carcinoembryonic antigen (CEA) should not be used as a screening test for colon cancer due to its poor sensitivity and specificity. CT colonoscopy (virtual colonoscopy) is a new screening modality which uses helical CT to capture 2D axial images that can be converted into a 3D view. Studies are underway to determine its effectiveness in screening populations.

Diagnosis

Common signs and symptoms of colorectal cancer are influenced by the site of the primary tumor and may include a change in bowel habits, diarrhea, constipation, a feeling that the bowel does not empty completely, bright-red blood in the stool or melanotic

Table 1. Average-Risk Screening for Colorectal Cancer

Screening Tool	US Preventive Services Task Force (2002)	American Cancer Society (2006)
FOBT	Recommended annually.	Recommended annually.
FIT	No recommendation.	Recommended annually in lieu of FOBT.
Sigmoidoscopy	Recommended, "periodicity unspecified."	Recommended every 5 years.
FOBT or FIT combined with sigmoidoscopy	FOBT with sigmoidoscopy recommended as an option.	Recommended every 5 years; combination preferred over either option alone.
Double-contrast barium enema	"Insufficient evidence to recommend either for or against."	Recommended as an option every 5 years.
Colonoscopy	"Insufficient evidence to recommend either for or against."	Recommended as an option every 10 years.

FOBT = fecal occult blood test; FIT = fecal immunochemical test.

Table 2. Screening Recommendations if Family History is Positive for Colon Cancer

Familial Risk Category	Recommendation
Second- or third-degree relatives with colorectal cancer	Same as average risk.
First-degree relative with colon cancer or adenomatous polyps at age ≥60 years	Same as average risk, beginning at age 40.
Two or more first-degree relatives with colon cancer, or one first-degree relative with colon cancer or adenomatous polyps at age <60 years	Colonoscopy every 5 years, beginning at age 40 or 10 years younger than the earliest diagnosis in the family, whichever comes first; double-contrast barium enema may be substituted, but colonoscopy is preferred.

Table 3. Differential Diagnosis of Colorectal Cancer

Disease	Notes
Hematochezia (see Chapter 20)	Blood on the tissue and stool characterizes hemorrhoids; diverticulosis and arteriovenous malformations usually exhibit massive bleeding. These nonmalignant conditions account for more than 95% of visible rectal bleeding, although evaluation to rule out cancer is always necessary.
Positive FOBT	Approximately 3%-5% of persons with a positive FOBT finding will have colon cancer. Up to 50% will have polyps (at least half of these are serendipitous rather than bleeding). The remainder are from NSAIDs, upper GI lesions, or are false-positive results.
Iron deficiency anemia (see Chapter 38)	Menstrual blood is a frequent cause of iron loss in women of childbearing age but should not be presumed to be the diagnosis. Other causes include IBD, GERD and causes listed above (positive FOBT). Sprue, in particular, causes iron malabsorption and is characterized by loose or diarrheal stools and fat malabsorption. A substantial fraction of persons over age 50 with iron deficiency anemia will be found to have colon cancer.
Change in bowel habits (see Chapter 13)	IBS is characterized by abdominal pain, diarrhea or constipation, or both. Changes in diet, such as amount of fiber or calcium, may alter bowel frequency. Bed rest may decrease bowel frequency. Many medications affect bowel frequency. Colon cancer accounts for <5% of cases, even in older individuals. Cancer must nonetheless be considered.
Abdominal mass or hepatomegaly	Abdominal masses on physical exam can arise from many different problems. Abdominal and bowel imaging are the next steps. These findings are extremely rare presentations of colon cancer, although a rectal mass on rectal exam is quite specific for colon cancer or polyp.
Hypogastric abdominal pain (see Chapter 13)	IBS, diverticulitis, IBD, ischemic colitis, colonic volvulus, uterine or ovarian disease all have symptom patterns suggesting each of the diseases listed. Bowel, abdominal, and genitourinary imaging should follow physical exam for evaluating these possible conditions and for ruling out colon cancer. Colon cancer will account for abdominal pain in <5% of patients.

FOBT = fecal occult blood test; GERD = gastroesophageal reflux disease; GI = gastrointestinal; IBD = inflammatory bowel disease; IBS = irritable bowel syndrome; NSAID = nonsteroidal anti-inflammatory drug.

stools, and stools that are narrower in caliber than usual. Other signs include general abdominal discomfort (frequent gas pains, bloating, fullness, or cramps), weight loss for no known reason, fatigue, and vomiting. Findings of iron deficiency anemia in patients age >40 years require careful evaluation for colon cancer (Table 3). Colonoscopy is performed when colon cancer is suspected. The sensitivity and specificity of colonoscopy are each >95%, and colonoscopy is the reference standard for detecting cancer or polyps. If colonoscopy is unavailable, a double-contrast barium enema can be used; sensitivity and specificity are 85% and 80%, respectively, for detecting cancer, but it is much less sensitive in detecting polyps. If an inherited colon cancer syndrome is suspected when there is a dominant pattern of cancer occurrence in family members, both patient and family members should be referred for genetic testing. Also suspect an inherited syndrome if hamartomatous polyps or more than 10 adenomatous polyps are found on colonoscopy.

Therapy

Surgery is an integral therapy in treating colorectal cancer. Surgery is usually followed by chemotherapy in patients with advanced stage colon and most rectal cancers. There is debate over the usefulness of preoperative staging, but many experts agree that a complete blood count, serum carcinoembryonic antigen, aminotransaminase levels, chest x-ray, and abdominal and pelvic CT scan should be part of the initial evaluation. In rectal cancer, an endoscopic ultrasound is done to determine depth of tumor invasion.

In early stage colon cancer (I and II), resection of the tumor for cure is performed (Table 4). For later stages (III), the cancer is resected and adjuvant chemotherapy is initiated. For advanced stage metastatic disease (IV), removal of the primary tumor is indicated for palliative relief of obstruction or to stop bleeding. Isolated hepatic metastasis can be resected, depending upon the patient's overall functional status.

For rectal cancers beyond stage I, radiation therapy in addition to surgery (with or without chemotherapy) is first-line treatment. The addition of radiation therapy to surgery and chemotherapy has been shown to decrease recurrence and death.

Chemotherapy is used as both adjuvant and palliative therapy in colon and rectal cancer after surgery to decrease relapses and increase survival. First-line agents for stage III colorectal cancer include 5-fluorouracil, leucovorin, and possibly oxaliplatin. In metastatic colorectal cancer, multi-agent chemotherapy increases

Table 4. Staging, Treatment, and Survival for Colon Cancer

AJCC* Stage	Definition	Treatment	5-Year Survival (%)
I	Confined to muscularis propria	Resection for cure	92
II	Extends into subserosa or directly invades other structures	Resection for cure	73
III	Metastatic to regional lymph nodes	Resection and adjuvant chemotherapy	56
IV	Distant metastases	Palliative resection, multi-agent chemotherapy	8

* Modified from the American Joint Committee on Cancer; with permission.

median survival compared with standard chemotherapy. Agents include oxaliplatin or irinotecan combined with a fluoropyrimidine. The addition of bevacizumab, an anti-angiogenesis monoclonal antibody, further increases the efficacy of chemotherapy. The monoclonal antibodies cetuximab and panitumumab are epidermal growth factor receptor inhibitors which have been approved to treat metastatic colon cancer.

Follow-Up

Colon cancer survivors are at increased risk for future adenomatous polyps and new colon cancers. The most common sites of recurrence of colon cancer are the site of initial removal as well as liver, bone, and brain. Follow-up exams allow removal of polyps and prevention of cancer. If removal of a (noninvasive) cancerous polyp was performed, follow-up colonoscopies are recommended at 3 and 6 months, 1 year, and 2 years. If a resection for invasive cancer was done, repeat colonoscopy at 3 years is performed to examine the anastomotic site, as well as to look for new neoplasms.

Five to twenty percent of patients with stages I or II colon cancer will develop metastases. Some metastatic disease can be surgically resected (salvage surgery), resulting in a substantial cure rate. When a curative approach is not appropriate, palliative care is instituted. Patients with stage III disease are followed for both recurrence of the tumor and adverse effects of the chemotherapy. Periodic measurements of aminotransaminase levels, chest x-ray, and carcinoembryonic antigen level are often done but have not been shown to improve survival.

Book Enhancement

Go to www.acponline.org/essentials/oncology-section.html to review inherited colon cancer syndromes, review the TNM staging system for colorectal cancer, view the results of a virtual colonoscopy, and view a rectal cancer identified during colonoscopy. In *MKSAP for Students 4*, assess yourself with items 14-16 in the **Oncology** section.

Bibliography

Ballinger AB, Anggiansah C. Colorectal cancer. BMJ. 2007;335:715-8. [PMID: 17916855]

Lieberman D. Screening for colorectal cancer in average-risk populations. Am J Med. 2006;119:728-35. [PMID: 16945604]

Chapter 69

Lung Cancer

Cynthia H. Ledford, MD

Lung cancer is the leading cause of cancer-related death in both men and women in the United States. Despite the greater prevalence of the three most common cancers, breast, prostate, and colon cancer, the total number of deaths due to these cancers combined does not exceed the number of deaths due to lung cancer. Lung cancer mortality correlates with prevalence of cigarette smoking, and lung cancer will occur in 15% of lifetime smokers.

Prevention

Abstinence from smoking is the best method of preventing lung cancer. All patients should be screened for current and past smoking and encouraged to stop smoking; smoking cessation could prevent up to 90% of all lung cancers. Retinol (vitamin A), β-carotene, *N*-acetylcysteine, and selenium supplementation do not prevent lung cancer.

Screening

There is no proven role for routine screening for lung cancer. Recent high survival rates for computed tomography (CT) screen-detected lung cancer appear promising; however, results may be due to lead-time bias and screening with CT scanning is not currently recommended.

Diagnosis

Carefully evaluate new pulmonary or chest complaints, particularly in smokers or former smokers. Ask about symptoms of primary tumor such as hemoptysis, pulmonary infections, shortness of breath, cough, or chest pain. Patients with small-cell lung cancer often present with symptoms of metastatic disease and paraneoplastic syndromes (Table 1).

In patients with new or persistent pulmonary symptoms, look for examination findings suggestive of primary tumor (abnormal lung findings), intrathoracic spread (hoarse voice, Horner's syndrome, brachial plexopathy, chest wall tenderness), extrathoracic spread (wasting, lymphadenopathy, focal neurological findings, bone tenderness, skin nodules, hepatomegaly), and paraneoplastic syndromes. Obtain a chest x-ray to look for mass, lymphadenopathy, and pleural effusion. Small lung cancers may require computed tomography for detection.

Histological confirmation is necessary for diagnosis and can be obtained by percutaneous lung biopsy, peripheral lymph node biopsy, pleural cytology, or transbronchial biopsy. Sputum cytology is reserved for patients with poor pulmonary function who cannot tolerate invasive procedures. Treatment and prognosis vary based upon whether the patient has non-small-cell lung cancer (adenocarcinoma, large-cell carcinoma, or squamous cell carcinoma) or small-cell lung cancer.

In staging non-small-cell lung cancer, the task is to find evidence of metastatic disease, which eliminates surgery as a therapeutic option. Perform a staging evaluation with chest and upper abdomen CT scan, plus a positron emission tomography (PET) scan to assess for mediastinal adenopathy. Complete blood count, calcium, alkaline phosphatase, and aminotransferase levels can detect more advanced disease. A bone scan is only indicated if there is bony pain or elevated calcium or alkaline phosphatase levels; a brain CT or MRI is indicated only in the presence of neurological signs or symptoms (Table 2).

Table 1. Paraneoplastic and Other Syndromes Associated with Lung Cancer

Syndrome	Mechanism
Acromegaly	Growth-hormone-releasing hormone (small-cell carcinoma)
Cushing's syndrome	Adrenocorticotrophic hormone (small-cell carcinoma)
Eaton-Lambert	Proximal limb weakness and fatigue due to antibodies to voltage-gated calcium channels (small-cell carcinoma)
Hypercalcemia	Parathyroid-hormone-related hormone (small-cell carcinoma)
Hypertrophic pulmonary osteoarthropathy	Painful, new periosteal bone growth and clubbing (most common with adenocarcinoma)
Hyponatremia	Arginine vasopressin and atrial natriuretic peptide (small cell carcinoma)
Pancoast's syndrome	Shoulder pain, lower brachial plexopathy, and Horner's syndrome from apical lung tumor
Superior vena cava syndrome	External compression of superior vena cava causing face and arm swelling
Trousseau's syndrome	Hypercoagulable state (most common with adenocarcinoma)
Vocal cord paralysis	Entrapment of recurrent laryngeal nerve

Table 2. Staging, Treatment and Prognosis for Non-Small-Cell Lung Cancer

Stage	Definition	Treatment	Prognosis
I	Tumor surrounded by lung or pleura, more than 2 cm from carina	Surgery and adjuvant chemotherapy; radiotherapy if not a surgical candidate; intent is cure	50%-70% long-term disease-free survival
II	Locally advanced disease, without mediastinal involvement	Surgery and adjuvant chemotherapy; radiotherapy if not a surgical candidate; intent is cure	20%-40% long-term disease-free survival
III	Mediastinal involvement	Combined modalities of chemotherapy, radiotherapy, and/or surgery	5%-20% long-term disease-free survival
IV	Distant metastases	Palliative intent	—

Small-cell lung cancer is generally viewed as a systemic (metastatic) disease at the time of diagnosis; the majority of patients have obvious extensive disease. Metastases from small-cell lung cancer involve the liver, bone, bone marrow, brain, adrenals, retroperitoneal lymph nodes, pancreas, and subcutaneous soft tissues. In all patients who are eligible for treatment, perform a chest x-ray, CT scan of chest and abdomen, MRI of the brain, and bone scan. Look for abnormal electrolytes, calcium, aminotransferase and serum lactic dehydrogenase levels. Further exhaustive search for metastases is not needed once the patient is found to have unequivocal evidence of distant metastases.

A patient may present with a pulmonary nodule, a discrete radiographic density <3 cm that is completely surrounded by aerated lung. Two characteristics distinguish benign pulmonary nodules: no growth in 2 years and calcification in a diffuse, central, or laminar pattern. Malignant nodules are typically >2 cm, have speculated edges, and are located in the upper lobes. Characteristics that increase the probability of malignancy are aged >40 years, past or current smoker, and, previous diagnosis of cancer. There is no single guideline for management of pulmonary nodules, but the general approach is to determine behavior over time and stratify risk. Obtain old chest x-rays or CT scans to determine stability over time. If unavailable, solid nodules <4-5 mm or non-solid nodules 5-9 mm in low-risk patients are followed with a repeat CT in 1 year. Solid nodules ≥1.5-2 cm in high-risk patients require immediate biopsy.

Therapy

Prognosis and management of non-small-cell lung cancer depends upon tumor staging. Tumor size (T), mediastinal nodal status (N), and presence or absence of metastatic disease (M) is used to assign patients to a stage of 1 to 4 (Table 2). Consult a medical oncologist, radiation therapist, and thoracic surgeon for patients with stage III disease regarding a combined modality approach, consisting of chemotherapy and either surgery or radiation therapy. Encourage all patients to quit smoking before surgery or high-dose radiation to improve lung function and reduce therapeutic morbidity.

Inoperable or metastatic non-small-cell lung cancer necessitates a combined approach or chemotherapy. Consult a medical and radiation oncologist for patients with stage IIIB disease for specifics of chemotherapy and radiation therapy regimens. Patients with a good performance status who have failed one chemotherapy regimen may benefit from repeat treatment with single-agent regimens. Treatment is not shown to be beneficial in patients with poor performance status (e.g., bed bound, weight loss >10%, severe symptoms).

The mainstay of treatment for small-cell lung cancer is chemotherapy with a combination of a platinum agent (carboplatin or cisplatin) and etoposide or irinotecan. Chemotherapy markedly improves the survival of patients, even elderly patients with poor performance status who can tolerate standard chemotherapy regimens. Unfortunately, despite impressive initial responses, resistance to chemotherapy soon ensues and most patients relapse and die of their disease.

High-dose chemotherapy with autologous hematopoietic stem cell transplantation is not recommended for patients with small-cell lung cancer outside of a clinical trial because substantial toxicity may negate benefits. Consider second-line chemotherapy for patients with recurrent small-cell lung cancer with good performance status if they relapse late (>3 months). Early relapses (<3 months) are considered "chemorefractory" because they rarely respond to chemotherapy. Although selected patients with relapse may benefit from second-line chemotherapy, responses are often short-term.

Palliative treatment is important in even advanced disease. Use corticosteroids and radiation therapy for patients with brain metastases. Select thoracic radiation for pulmonary airway obstruction, superior vena cava syndrome, and spinal cord metastases. Use radiation therapy to relieve pain, particularly bony pain, visceral pain secondary to capsular distension, or pain due to nerve compression. Treat symptomatic pleural effusions with thoracentesis and pleurodesis to obliterate the pleural space, if necessary.

Assess patients on a regular basis for pain; make pain management a high priority and treat it aggressively. Severe pain usually requires opioid analgesics. Pain is better controlled if pain medications are administered on a scheduled basis. Manage constipation with prophylactic laxatives or stool softeners begun at the same time as the narcotic medication regimen. Use anti-depressants for depression, bisphosphonates for lytic bone disease, erythropoietin to treat anemia, megestrol for cachexia and anorexia, and home oxygen for hypoxia.

Follow-Up

Continue comprehensive, ongoing follow-up of patients for recurrence, for management of disease and treatment complications, and for palliation of symptoms. Most patients with lung cancer will develop recurrent disease. In long-term survivors, surveillance may lead to the detection of a second primary tumor, most commonly of the lung. Schedule follow-up at frequent intervals and evaluate for recurrent disease using clinical examination and laboratory testing. Address the need for additional radiotherapy or chemotherapy for recurrent disease. Patients with advanced, metastatic disease should be seen every month to assess new symptoms, particularly pain, anorexia, fatigue, and dyspnea.

Book Enhancement

Go to www.acponline.org/essentials/oncology-section.html to view a CT scan of the chest showing locally advanced lung cancer, a CT of the liver showing liver metastases, a chest x-ray showing a pulmonary nodule, and a clinical photograph of a patient with the superior vena cava syndrome. In *MKSAP for Students 4*, assess yourself with items 17-19 in the **Oncology** section.

Bibliography

Argiris A. Lung Cancer (Small-Cell). http://pier.acponline.org/physicians/diseases/d665. [Date accessed: 2008 Jan 24] In: PIER [online database]. Philadelphia: American College of Physicians; 2008.

Collins LG, Haines C, Perkel R, Enck RE. Lung cancer: diagnosis and management. Am Fam Physician. 2007;75:56-63. [PMID: 17225705]

Schiller J. Lung Cancer (Non-Small Cell). http://pier.acponline.org/physicians/diseases/d203. [Date accessed: 2008 Jan 24] In: PIER [online database]. Philadelphia: American College of Physicians; 2008.

Chapter 70

Prostate Cancer

Eric H. Green, MD

Prostate cancer is the most common cancer in men and second only to lung cancer in causing cancer-related deaths. Tumor growth can be slow or moderate in pace, but occasionally is quite rapid. Prostate cancer is strongly associated with age, its incidence rising from near zero in patients younger than 40 years to 1 in 100 men in their seventies. In addition, it is more common in black men and men with a family history of prostate cancer. Given the older age at which many patients are diagnosed and the slowly progressive nature of low-grade tumors, many patients with prostate cancer die of other illnesses.

Prevention

Because prostate cancer is common, slow-growing, and usually dependent on testosterone for growth, it is a potentially good target for chemoprophylaxis. Prophylactic use of finasteride, an alpha-reductase inhibitor, does reduce the incidence of prostate cancer, but the cancers that do develop seem to be of a higher grade. Because the Gleason scoring system was not developed for men receiving androgen-inhibitor therapy, the implications of the tumor grading for men taking finasteride is uncertain. The overall prostate cancer mortality is unchanged with finasteride; therefore, finasteride should not be used for cancer prevention.

Screening

Prostate cancer screening tests are imperfect, and evidence of screening benefit is insufficient. Screening should only be done after a detailed discussion with the patient outlining both the potential benefits of screening and its known harms. Inform patients of the indolent nature of many prostate cancers, suggesting that early detection may not change outcomes; the low specificity and positive predictive value of current tests; the likely need for a multiple biopsies after an abnormal test; and the morbidity associated with current treatment.

Patients who elect screening receive both a serum prostate-specific antigen (PSA) measurement and a digital rectal examination. Screening, if done, starts at age 50 (or age 45 if black or positive family history of prostate cancer) and continues until age 70 or stops when the patient has a life expectancy of <10 years.

Diagnosis

Early prostate cancer is usually asymptomatic, although some patients may present with hematospermia, painful ejaculation, or symptoms of bladder outlet obstruction such as urinary hesitancy and frequency. Patients with metastatic disease may present with bone pain, back pain, weight loss, or fatigue. Men with metastatic disease from an unknown primary should be evaluated for the possibility of prostate cancer. Digital rectal examination can be used to detect prostate cancer. Although it has low sensitivity, digital rectal examination is inexpensive, without risk, and easy to perform. Any abnormality on digital rectal examination requires biopsy, regardless of PSA level. More advanced disease may present with signs of metastatic spread, including pelvic lymphadenopathy, bone tenderness, or signs of spinal cord compression, including leg weakness and poor rectal tone. Table 1 describes important conditions in the differential diagnosis of prostate cancer.

Serum PSA measurement is the best available non-invasive test to diagnose prostate cancer. The normal range of PSA varies with age and race, with older men and white men having higher PSA values. PSA testing is avoided immediately after a urinary tract infection or prostatitis; both can raise PSA levels for up to 4-8 weeks. Although digital rectal exam can also elevate PSA, this change is rarely clinically significant. PSA values >4.0 ng/mL are generally considered abnormal. However, only 25% of men with PSA's between 4.0 and 10.0 ng/mL have prostate cancer although most of these cancers are early stage and therefore potentially curable. Further, approximately 20% of patients with a PSA <4.0 will have prostate cancer. Because PSA rises very slowly over time, a rise in PSA >0.75 ng/mL in 1 year, regardless of initial value, is considered abnormal.

Refer any patient with an abnormal PSA for transrectal ultrasound-guided prostate biopsies. This outpatient procedure usually consists of six random needle biopsies. Random biopsies have a high false-positive rate and often need to be repeated if negative. Tumors detected on these biopsies are further classified according to their histology using the Gleason score. In the Gleason histologic scoring system, tumors are graded from 1 to 5 based on the degree of glandular differentiation and structural architecture. The composite Gleason score is derived by adding together the two most prevalent differentiation patterns (a primary and a secondary grade) and is the best predictor of the biology of the tumor. Patients with a Gleason score >7, PSA >15, large tumors, or the presence of bone pain requires a bone scan and CT scan of the abdomen and pelvis to evaluate for metastatic disease. Table 2 reviews laboratory and other studies for prostate cancer.

Therapy

Three major treatment strategies exist for localized prostate cancer: surgery, radiation therapy, and active surveillance. To date,

Table 1. Differential Diagnosis of Prostate Cancer

Disease	Notes
Abnormal Findings on Prostate Examination	
Benign prostatic hyperplasia (BPH)	Characterized by symptoms of urinary outflow obstruction, including nocturia, urinary urgency and hesitancy. May also cause elevation of serum PSA test level. Prostate cancer and BPH can coexist but there is no causal association between the two diseases. BPH results in a generalized and typically symmetric enlargement of the gland, whereas prostate cancer may manifest as a palpable lump, as induration, or as asymmetrical enlargement. Biopsy distinguishes between the two entities.
Acute prostatitis	Can result in elevated serum PSA levels but also spiking fever, chills, dysuria, pelvic or perineal pain, and possible obstructive symptoms (dribbling, hesitancy, and anuria). DRE reveals edematous and tender prostate; pyuria; positive urine culture.
Metastatic Skeletal Disease	
Osteomyelitis	Osteomyelitis results in increased uptake on bone scans and can be confused with metastatic disease. Osteomyelitis is not associated with an elevated PSA level, and metastatic prostate cancer in the context of a normal PSA level is very unusual. Metastatic prostate cancer tends to be multifocal, whereas osteomyelitis tends to be unifocal. Prostate cancer and osteomyelitis have very different appearances on CT and MRI scans.
Paget's disease	Paget's disease of the bone can look like sclerotic bone metastases. Paget's disease is not associated with an elevated PSA level, whereas metastatic prostate cancer is.
Other cancers	Many other cancers spread to the pelvic and retroperitoneal lymph nodes and the bones, including bladder cancer, colorectal cancer, testicular cancer, renal cell carcinoma, urothelial carcinomas of the ureter and renal pelvis, and penile cancer. Prostate cancer can generally be distinguished from other malignancies on the basis of histopathologic examination of biopsy specimens.

CT = computed tomography; DRE = digital rectal examination; MRI = magnetic resonance imaging; PSA = prostate-specific antigen.

Table 2. Laboratory and Other Studies for Prostate Cancer

Test	Notes
Prostate-specific antigen	The PPV of a serum PSA level >4.0 ng/mL is ~30%-37%. Most men with PSA level between 4-10 ng/mL do not have prostate cancer. BPH, prostatitis, urinary tract infections, prostatic stones, manipulation of the prostate or lower urinary tract, and ejaculation can result in elevation of the serum PSA level. The initial serum PSA level carries important prognostic information with lower levels predicting localized and less aggressive tumors. PSA level >50 ng/mL has a PPV for prostate cancer of 98%-99%.
Bone alkaline phosphatase	Not used in diagnosing prostate cancer. Elevated levels in patients with prostate cancer suggest bone metastases.
Transrectal ultrasound	PPV=7%-34%; NPV=85%. Transrectal ultrasound is used to guide prostate biopsies. It is not used for screening or staging prostate cancer.
Prostate biopsy	The only way to definitively diagnose prostate cancer.
CBC	Metastatic cancer to the bone marrow is common and can result in anemia.
CT scan of abdomen and pelvis	Helpful in evaluating for pelvic or retroperitoneal lymph node metastases or bone metastases in the pelvis and lower spine. Bone or lymph node metastases are rare in men with PSA levels <20 ng/mL, especially if the Gleason score is <8.
Bone scan	Bone scans are useful for detecting metastatic prostate cancer, and bone is the most common site of metastatic prostate cancer. Osteoarthritis, other degenerative changes, trauma or fractures, osteomyelitis, and Paget's disease can all result in increased uptake on bone scans. Ambiguous bone scan results often lead to additional bone-imaging studies such as plain films, CT or MRI scans. A biopsy is performed for ambiguous radiologic imaging results.

CBC = complete blood count; CT = computed tomography; NPV = negative predictive value; PPV = positive predictive value; PSA = prostate-specific antigen.

the optimal treatment is not defined. Most men with >10 year life expectancy undergo either radical prostatectomy or some form of radiation therapy. Radical prostatectomy is curative in patients with disease confined to the prostate (T0-T2) who lack high-risk features such as a high PSA or Gleason score. Although radical prostatectomy has a relatively low rate of perioperative complications, up to 60%-80% of patients will have post-operative erectile dysfunction and some will develop urinary incontinence.

Radiation therapy can be delivered using either external beam radiation or by implanting radioactive "seeds" around the prostate (brachytherapy). Brachytherapy is used in patients with low-risk local disease and is associated with low rates of impotence; however, it can lead to urinary obstruction. External beam radiation is effective in both localized and locally advanced therapy. When it is used for locally advanced disease (defined by tumor size, a high PSA, or high Gleason scores), it is often combined with androgen deprivation therapy. Although external beam radiation therapy can result in impotence or urinary incontinence, the rates are less than with radical prostatectomy. Both forms of radiation therapy can lead to radiation proctitis. Palliative external beam radiation is effective for painful bony metastases.

Active surveillance without immediate therapy is a reasonable treatment modality for some patients, especially older patients with low-grade prostate-confined disease, and patients with multiple co-morbidities and a limited life expectancy. This treatment strategy capitalizes on the slow-growing nature of most prostate cancers and produces reasonable rates of 5 and 10-year survival.

Prostate cancers are dependent on testosterone for growth; thus, androgen deprivation therapy is often used to treat higher-risk localized cancers, advanced disease, and local treatment failures (defined by a rise in PSA after surgical or radiation therapy). Commonly used androgen deprivation therapies are the luteinizing hormone-releasing hormone (LHRH) analogues, leuprolide, or goserelin. When these agents are initiated, there is often a transient testosterone surge with an increase in symptoms. To minimize the flair in symptoms from this surge, many patients need short-term androgen blockade with bicalutamide or flutamide. Androgen blockade is always used when initiating LHRH analogs in patients with epidural or painful bone metastases. Long-term androgen blockade is also recommended for progressive disease treated with LHRH analogues. Androgen blockade has significant side-effects, including hot flashes, loss of libido, gynecomastia, impotence, and osteoporosis. If diethylstilbestrol is used as an androgen deprivation therapy, it has the added side effect of an increased risk of thrombosis. In some patients, orchiectomy is used in place of medications for androgen deprivation. In patients whose disease progresses despite androgen deprivation therapy, chemotherapy is often used. In patients with prostate cancer metastatic to bone, annual infusions of the bisphosphonate zoledronate can decrease the risk for skeletal-related complications.

Follow-Up

Patients are monitored at least annually for recurrent disease after definitive local therapy with serum PSA levels and an interval history and examination to evaluate for signs or symptoms of relapse. In patients undergoing active surveillance, re-evaluation is done more frequently, with PSA measurements sometimes done at 3 month intervals. Digital rectal exam or imaging studies such as a bone scan or CT scan are not routinely performed unless specifically indicated by signs or symptoms of recurrence. Consider obtaining a bone density scan on men who are receiving long-term androgen deprivation; bisphosphonates can be used in patients who develop osteoporosis. The primary complication of prostate cancer is metastatic spread, most commonly to regional lymph nodes and bone. Bone metastases can cause severe pain as well as spinal cord compression. Back pain in a patient with prostate cancer may represent the first sign of spinal cord compression from epidural metastases and requires urgent evaluation with a spine MRI.

Book Enhancement

Go to www.acponline.org/essentials/oncology-section.html to review the TMN classification of prostate cancer, see an illustration of the prostate cancer stages and a transrectal biopsy. In *MKSAP for Students 4*, assess yourself with items 20-21 in the **Oncology** section.

Bibliography

Gilligan T, Oh W. Prostate Cancer. http://pier.acponline.org/physicians/ diseases/ d188. [Date accessed: 2008 Jan 15] In: PIER [online database]. Philadelphia: American College of Physicians; 2008.

Walsh PC, DeWeese TL, Eisenberger MA. Clinical practice. Localized prostate cancer. N Engl J Med. 2007;357:2696-705. [PMID: 18160689]

Chapter 71

Cervical Cancer

Asra R. Khan, MD

Cervical cancer is the most common cancer in women worldwide and the seventh most common in the United States. Women in their teens to age 30 years typically present with dysplasia, while invasive cancer is more commonly seen after age 45 years. Persistent infection with high-risk human papillomavirus (HPV) subtypes (16 and 18) can cause cervical dysplasia and subsequently cancer. Dysplastic lesions can progress into cellular intraepithelial neoplasia, which in turn can evolve into well-differentiated low-grade lesions and then undifferentiated high-grade lesions. These precancerous lesions may regress spontaneously at any point in this progression or progress to invasive cancer.

Prevention

HPV infection is sexually transmitted and can cause cervical dysplasia and cervical cancer. Having multiple sexual partners increases exposure to HPV, and intercourse at an early age exposes the cervix to HPV when it is most vulnerable to infection. Using condoms helps decrease exposure to HPV. Therefore, patients should be advised to limit their number of sexual partners, avoid intercourse at an early age (age <13-15 years), and use condoms to decrease the risk of acquiring HPV infection. Patients should also be advised on smoking cessation; women who smoke have an increased risk of developing cervical dysplasia and cancer because of the carcinogenic and immunosuppressive effect of smoking.

A vaccine against high-risk HPV has been approved for females aged 9-26 years and is recommended for 11-12 year old girls or females between 13-26 years of age who have not received or completed the vaccine series. Ideally, it should be administered prior to onset of sexual activity. The vaccine consists of three doses; the second is given 2 months after the initial dose and the third dose 6 months after the initial dose.

The vaccine is very effective against HPV 16 and 18; however, it does not protect against all types of HPV. It also does not treat existing HPV-related infections, warts or precancers. Roughly 30% of cervical cancers will not be prevented by the vaccine, so women should continue to get regular Pap smears. Moreover, the length of immunity is not yet known, so a booster may be needed.

Screening

Annual Pap smears decrease the risk of dying from cervical cancer by 95%. Screening is initiated within 3 years after the onset of vaginal intercourse and no later than age 21. The screening interval may be decreased to every 2-3 years in women aged >30 years with three consecutive satisfactory, normal smears unless there is a history of diethylstilbestrol exposure (DES), the patient is HIV positive, or is immunocompromised. Alternatively, women 30 years and above can be screened with combined Pap smear and HPV DNA testing (Table 1). If both HPV DNA testing and pap smear are negative, the screening interval can be increased to 3 years. If the cytology is negative, but high-risk HPV DNA testing is positive, both tests should be repeated at 6-12 months. Discontinue screening at age 65 to 70 if the patient was adequately screened, had normal pap smears, and has no other risk factors. Also, discontinue screening patients who have had a total hysterectomy (with removal of the cervix) for a benign disease.

If Pap smear results are unsatisfactory, it should be repeated. If the cytology result is atypical squamous cells of undetermined significance (ASCUS), test for HPV infection. If positive for high-risk HPV, refer for colposcopy. If results are negative for the

Table 1. Laboratory and Other Studies for Cervical Cancer

Test	Notes
Pap smear	Annual Pap smears reduce the risk of dying from cervical cancer by 95%.
HPV DNA	Testing for high-risk HPV DNA identifies more women with high-grade dysplasia than does Pap smear.
Colposcopy	Used to direct cervical biopsies after Pap smear that shows high-grade squamous intraepithelial lesion or cancer.
Cervical biopsy	Helps differentiate cervical dysplasia from microinvasive and invasive cancer.
Chest x-ray	In staging to detect asymptomatic lung metastasis (1%).
IVP	In staging to determine hydroureter, which would mean the tumor is stage 3B.
Renal ultrasound	May be used as a substitute for IVP in apparent early cancers.
CT scan of abdomen and pelvis	May be used to help direct therapy but is not used as a part of staging.
Exam under anesthesia with cystoscopy and proctoscopy	Used to help determine stage to detect regional spread.

CT = computed tomography; IVP = intravenous pyelogram.

Table 2. Differential Diagnosis of Cervical Cancer*

Disease	Notes
Dysplasia	Abnormal Pap test result. Needs colposcopy and biopsy.
Nabothian cysts	Nabothian cysts are formed when glandular tissue is covered by squamous epithelium. Nabothian cysts are common and can become quite large. If diagnosis is questionable, needs biopsy.
Cervicitis (see Chapter 49)	Postcoital bleeding. There are no discrete lesions on the cervix, but rather the cervix is red and inflamed. Needs biopsy if Pap smear result is abnormal.
Cervical ectopy	Presence of columnar epithelium on the ectocervix is a normal variant appearing as a red, beefy area; occasionally mistaken for cervicitis. Close inspection reveals the demarcation where the squamous epithelium begins.
Cervical atrophy	Postcoital bleeding. Vagina and cervix tend to be pale and atrophic. Obtain Pap smear.
Cervical polyp	Finger-like mass protruding from os. Needs biopsy or excision.
Cervical cysts	Tend to be well-circumscribed bubble-like lesions on the cervix. If diagnosis is questionable, needs biopsy.

* Go to www.acponline.org/essentials/oncology-section to see images of these findings.

high-risk subtypes, repeat the Pap smear in 1 year. For high-grade squamous intraepithelial lesion, squamous cell cancer, or atypical glandular cells, refer for colposcopy.

Diagnosis

Symptoms of cervical cancer may include post-coital bleeding, foul smelling vaginal discharge, change in urinary or bowel habits, right upper quadrant abdominal pain, back pain, or leg swelling. The first symptom is frequently bleeding after intercourse. Large exophytic tumors and large ulcerative lesions can become necrotic and produce a foul-smelling vaginal discharge. Advanced cervical cancer may impinge on the urinary bladder, ureters, or rectosigmoid causing change in urinary or bowel habits. Cancer can invade through the parametrium to the pelvic sidewall and obstruct the ureter, infiltrate nerves along the uterosacral ligament and sacrum, and compress the iliac vessels. The "terrible triad" of advanced cervical cancer is sciatic back pain, hydroureter, and leg swelling.

On physical examination look for an exophytic or ulcerative lesion on the cervix, foul-smelling vaginal discharge, firmness in the parametrium, leg swelling, and supraclavicular lymphadenopathy (Virchow's node). See Table 2 for a differential diagnosis of cervical lesions. Metastatic disease to the liver may present with right upper quadrant abdominal mass and tenderness.

A Pap smear can detect cervical dysplasia, microinvasive and small invasive cancers of the cervix, and is indicated for any patient with postcoital bleeding. Cervical dysplasia and some early cancers are not visible to the naked eye and require colposcopic examination of the cervix for detection. The colposcope is a low-powered magnification device that permits the identification of mucosal abnormalities characteristic of dysplasia or invasive cancer. Biopsies are taken of any grossly visible abnormality of the cervix to determine the histologic diagnosis and to exclude invasive cancer.

On all patients with cervical cancer the following tests should be obtained: chest x-ray, abdominal and pelvic CT scan, and pelvic examination under anesthesia with cystoscopy and proctoscopy (Table 1). Proper staging helps with prognosis and tailoring of treatment and gives a small survival advantage.

Therapy

Stage 1A1 cancers have a small chance of recurrence and lymph node metastasis; younger women with this diagnosis wishing fertility may be treated with loop electrosurgical excision procedure (LEEP) or conization instead of hysterectomy to preserve childbearing. Patients who have finished childbearing may undergo vaginal, abdominal, or modified radical hysterectomy to decrease the chance of recurrence. Once cervical cancer has extended to stage 1A2 or beyond, LEEP, conization, or abdominal or vaginal hysterectomy alone cannot cure the patient; these patients require modified radical hysterectomy. If a tumor has become grossly invasive (stage 1B or 2A), a radical hysterectomy is required to ensure that the tumor is removed en bloc with an adequate margin and regional lymph nodes.

Patients with early cervical cancer who are not surgical candidates or who do not wish surgery may undergo primary radiation therapy. Once a tumor has grown into the parametrium or lower vagina (stages 2B to 4A), adequate margins cannot be obtained by surgery and patients require radiotherapy. Pelvic exenteration consists of resection of the uterus, vagina, bladder, and rectosigmoid and is reserved for patients with recurrent or persistent cancer after radiation therapy provided they are good surgical candidates with no evidence of metastatic disease. Chemotherapy is not effective following high-dose radiation because radiation fibrosis prevents adequate drug delivery.

Of cancers occurring during pregnancy, cervical cancer is one of the most common. Treatment is based on stage, but the timing of treatment is influenced by the duration of the pregnancy.

Radiation-sensitizing chemotherapy increases the response to radiation by facilitating additional tumor cell killing. Because of the direct killing of tumor cells by the chemotherapy, the tumor tends to shrink more rapidly, and thus the hypoxic tumor cells (which are relatively resistant to radiation) receive more blood supply and oxygenation, becoming more sensitive to radiation. Radiation-sensitizing chemotherapy is not regarded as an adequate systemic chemotherapy because the drugs are given in too low a dose and over too short a time period.

Once cervical cancer has spread from the pelvis, pelvic surgery and radiation are no longer options and chemotherapy is needed to treat distant disease. Cisplatin is the most active chemotherapeutic agent with which to treat cervical cancer.

Follow-Up

Routine examination may allow for early detection of recurrence. At follow-up visits, include history, physical examination, and vaginal cuff Pap smear. Patients with advanced disease may require chest x-rays and abdominal and pelvic CT scans.

Book Enhancement

Go to www.acponline.org/essentials/oncology-section.html to view a normal nulliparous cervix, nabothian cysts, cervical polyp, cervical ectopy, cervical warts, invasive cancer, cervical cancer histology, and a table to review the staging of cervical cancer. In *MKSAP for Students 4*, assess yourself with item 22 in the **Oncology** section.

Bibliography

Fanning J. Cervical Cancer. http://pier.acponline.org/physicians/diseases/d643. [Date accessed: 2008 Jan 8] In: PIER [online database]. Philadelphia: American College of Physicians; 2008.

Spitzer M, Apgar BS, Brotzman GL. Management of histologic abnormalities of the cervix. Am Fam Physician. 2006;73:105-12. [PMID: 16417073]

Chapter 72

Skin Cancer

Cynthia H. Ledford, MD

More than 1 million cases of the most common skin cancers (basal cell cancer and squamous cell cancer) are diagnosed annually in the United States. The incidence of melanoma, the most serious form of skin cancer, has increased almost 3 percent per year since 1981. The incidence of melanoma is increasing worldwide at a rate faster than any other cancer with the exception of lung cancer in women. Melanoma is the most common cancer among people 25 to 29 years old.

Prevention

Sunlight is the most important environmental factor in skin cancer. Children and adults should avoid excessive sun exposure and sunburn by using protective clothing, avoiding exposure during peak hours, and wearing sunscreen with SPF 15 or greater. Studies suggest that sunscreen has a direct protective effect against acute ultraviolet damage and non-melanotic skin cancer.

Screening

Patients can examine their own skin for changes in moles and have regular clinical examinations. Individuals at high risk for melanoma benefit most from screening exams. Risk factors for melanoma include large number of nevi (benign or dysplastic), blistering sunburns, poor tanning ability, and personal or family history of melanoma. A nonfamilial melanoma occurs in the setting of a preexisting dysplastic nevus in 30%-50% of cases; dysplastic nevi are acquired pigmented lesions that are larger than typical nevi (>5 mm), have irregular margins, or have color variation.

Patients are at increased risk for basal cell carcinoma if they are organ transplant recipients, survivors of childhood leukemia, recipients of radiation treatment, have had previous basal cell carcinoma, or are elderly whites with a history of excessive sun exposure. Actinic keratoses are precursors of squamous cell carcinoma. Actinic keratoses present as 1-3-mm tan to red, raised, scaling 'rough spots' on sun-exposed areas such as the forearms or forehead. Patients with risk factors, sun-damaged skin, and actinic keratoses should be screened for basal cell carcinoma and squamous cell carcinoma.

The US Preventive Services Task Force has not found sufficient evidence to recommend for or against screening by clinical examination or counseling to prevent skin cancer.

Diagnosis

Diagnose melanoma by carefully evaluating any skin lesions that are new or have changed in size, shape, or color (Table 1 and Plate 39). Review the history of the lesion and the patient's risk factors for melanoma, perform a complete skin exam, and evaluate lymph nodes. Change in a skin lesion is the most important clue in the diagnosis of melanoma.

Biopsy is the gold standard to diagnose melanoma and to distinguish it from other pigmented lesions (Table 2). The biopsy must include sufficient tissue to allow accurate assessment of thickness, extension (Clark's level), ulceration, and adequacy of surgical margins. An excisional biopsy is preferred; incisional biopsy is an alternative if excision biopsy would be disfiguring. For undiagnosed pigmented lesions, destruction or superficial shave biopsies are inappropriate because the ability to diagnose and stage a potentially lethal skin cancer is lost. After diagnosis of melanoma, staging work-up, emphasizing complete skin and regional node exam, determine the extent of disease and risk of recurrence.

Assess lymph nodes in patients with primary melanomas >1mm thick or if other poor prognostic factors are present such as extension (Clark's level IV) or ulceration. Sentinel node involvement is a powerful prognostic indicator and stratifies patients for trials of adjuvant therapy. In patients with more advanced disease, such as node involvement, evaluation includes CBC, liver chemistry studies, and serum lactate dehydrogenase level, chest x-ray, and CT scans of chest and abdomen, although the yield of routine imaging is low. Staging is based on tumor thickness (T), node involvement (N), and metastases (M).

In assessing potential basal cell or squamous carcinomas, ask about nonhealing skin lesions, bleeding, slow tumor growth, itching, and pain. Basal cell carcinoma can appear as a translucent

Table 1. ABCDs of Melanoma
A symmetry: a lesion that is not regularly round or oval.
B order irregularity: a lesion with notching, scalloping, or poorly defined margins.
C olor variegation: a lesion with shades of brown, tan, red, white, or blue-black, or combinations thereof.
D iameter: a lesion >6 mm diameter. Although a high level of suspicion exists for a lesion >6 mm in diameter, early melanomas may be diagnosed at a smaller size.

Table 2. Differential Diagnosis of Melanoma*

Disease	Notes
Common nevi (moles)	Tend to be small macules or papules, most are <5 mm, border is regular, smooth and well defined, coloration is homogeneous, usually no more than 2 shades of brown, any site affected.
Dysplastic nevi	Occur predominantly on the trunk, usually >5 mm, with a flat component, border is characteristically fuzzy and ill defined. The shape can be round, oval, or asymmetric. The color is usually brown but can be mottled with dark brown, pink, and tan colors. Some individuals have only 1-5 lesions, whereas others have more than 100 lesions. Some of the clinical features of dysplastic nevi are similar to melanoma. Significant asymmetry and heterogeneity of color should prompt a biopsy to rule out melanoma.
Melanoma	The border is more irregular, often >10 mm, color with significant heterogeneity ranging from tan-brown, dark brown, black, pink, red, gray, blue, white. Often raised. Can be located at any site, but particularly lower legs in females.

* Go to the Web enhancement for Skin Cancer at http://www.acponline.org/essentials/oncology-section.html to see clinical photographs of the these conditions.

Table 3. Differential Diagnosis of Basal Cell Carcinoma (BCC)*

Disease	Notes
Nodular BCC	A skin-toned to pink pearly translucent, *firm* papule with telangiectasias. It may have rolled borders and a central depression with ulceration. Is often found on the head and neck.
Superficial BCC	Well-defined erythematous scaling plaque or occasional papules with a thin pearly border. Larger lesions often have hemorrhagic crusts and occur predominately on the trunk. Total cutaneous examination to find other similar plaques may help distinguish the solitary lesion of superficial BCC from psoriasis.
Morpheaform BCC	A skin-colored waxy scar-like area that develops on the head and neck of an older person. Morpheaform BCC is so named because it resembles morphea (scleroderma).
Common nevi (moles)	Nevi can become elevated and may be irritated by clothing, causing inflammation and bleeding. The nevi also undergo progressive loss of color over time. By age 60, nevi may be flesh-colored, dome-shaped *soft* papules. Even inflamed nevi do not have overlying telangiectasia.
Sebaceous hyperplasia	Benign, 2-4 mm papules with a characteristic yellow color and central umbilication. Occurs in clusters on the face *without* telangiectasia and bleeding.
Actinic keratosis	Early lesions 1-3 mm often felt, not seen, having a rough sandpaper texture. Color ranges from skin-colored to pink to erythematous to brown. Early superficial BCC may look like early actinic keratoses. With time, superficial BCC develops a rolled border and actinic keratoses get a thicker keratotic scale.
Bowen's disease (SCC in situ)	A solitary sharply demarcated, pink to fiery red scaly plaque that resembles superficial BCC, psoriasis or eczema. Most common in sun-exposed regions.
Psoriasis	In the early phase, the sharply demarcated erythematous plaques with slight scale may resemble superficial BCC. As the psoriatic area matures, a silvery-white scale develops that has characteristic pinpoint bleeding when removed.
Nummular eczema	Round, 1-3 cm well-demarcated eczematous patches found on the extremities. Pruritus may be intense, which results in scratching. The scratch marks may be the best way to discriminate it from superficial BCC.
Tinea	Scaly patch with central clearing and an active border of erythema, papules, and vesicles. Tinea is more erythematous than BCC and usually has a larger area of central clearing.

* Go to the Web enhancement for Skin Cancer at http://www.acponline.org/essentials/oncology-section.html to see images of these conditions.
SCC = squamous cell carcinoma.

nodule (Plate 40) with telangiectasia on the face (nodular), pink scaly flat lesions with pearly edge on the trunk or limbs (superficial), or a slowly enlarging skin-colored "scar" (morphea) (Table 3). Change in a skin lesion associated with spontaneous bleeding is the most readily recognized clue in the diagnosis of basal cell carcinoma. Actinic keratoses can progress to squamous cell carcinoma. Cutaneous squamous cell carcinoma presents as scaly, keratotic macule or patch, commonly on scalp, neck, pinnae, or lip (Plate 41). Biopsy confirms the diagnosis of basal cell or squamous cell carcinoma. Basal cell carcinoma cell type, location, and size determine treatment. The thickness of squamous cell carcinoma is an important prognostic indicator.

Therapy

Surgery is the mainstay of therapy for patients with melanoma. Because melanoma tumor cells extend beyond the visible borders of the melanoma, wide excision is necessary to ensure that all melanoma is removed. The extent of surgery depends upon the thickness of the primary melanoma. Eighty percent of patients with melanoma are cured with wide-margin surgical resection.

Node dissection is performed in patients with clinically palpable regional lymph nodes. Patients with stage III melanoma (node positive) have potentially curable melanoma and should be treated aggressively with surgery. Surgical resection of solitary metastases in skin, lung, gastrointestinal tract, and brain is beneficial in patients without evidence of other metastases. Surgery can also acheive excellent palliation in selected patients with symptomatic metastatic disease.

Surgery is the mainstay of therapy for basal cell and squamous cell carcinoma. The goal of primary treatment in low-risk basal cell carcinoma is cure of the tumor with maximal preservation of function and appearance. Treatment decisions are influenced by the patient's age and underlying health. High-risk or recurrent basal cell carcinoma may be treated with Mohs surgery, which offers the best cure, or radiation. Mohs micrographic surgery involves careful excision with use of markers and immediate preparation of tissue to allow immediate histological examination to ensure that all margins are clear of tumor. Electrodessication or curettage can treat small squamous cell carcinoma; larger tumors require excision. Squamous cell carcinoma penetrating the dermis may be treated with radiation.

Recommendations for chemotherapy, immunotherapy, or both for melanoma depend on the patient's stage of disease. Many patients with melanoma are at low risk for recurrence and therefore do not require postsurgical treatment. Adjuvant treatment with high-dose interferon therapy is beneficial in patients with thick primary melanoma (>4-mm) or positive nodes, but toxicity is considerable. Interferon is the only treatment that is FDA approved for the treatment of high-risk patients to prevent recurrence of disease and possibly improve overall survival rates.

Widely metastatic melanoma is an incurable disease, and there is no evidence that treatment prolongs overall survival. Palliation of symptoms may be possible with chemotherapy or immunotherapy with interferon or interleukin-2.

The main drug modality used to destroy multiple actinic keratoses, low-risk squamous cell carcinoma, and superficial basal cell carcinoma is topical 5-fluorouracil or topical imiquimod. Treatment is often painful and unsightly. In patients with small nodular or superficial basal cell carcinoma who cannot tolerate local anesthesia or whose tumor is located in an area likely to form a keloidal scar, photodynamic therapy with topical methyl aminolevulinate acid and red light is an option.

Follow-Up

Due to increased risk of second primary melanoma, provide careful lifelong surveillance in patients with a history of melanoma. Early detection of asymptomatic metastatic melanoma does not improve survival; therefore, extensive follow-up with x-rays and laboratory studies is not indicated. Most recurrences of melanoma occur within 10 years.

Following treatment, the majority of recurrences of squamous cell carcinoma occur within the first 2 years and nearly all within 5 years. Most basal cell carcinoma recurrences occur in the first 3 years after treatment. As with melanoma, patients with squamous cell and basal cell carcinoma are at lifelong risk of second skin cancers.

Book Enhancement

Go to www.acponline.org/essentials/oncology-section.html to view images of a common nevus; nodular, superficial, and morpheaform varieties of basal cell carcinoma; malignant melanoma, nodular melanoma, and dysplastic nevi; squamous cell carcinoma, Bowen's disease, and actinic keratosis. In *MKSAP for Students 4*, assess yourself with items 23-25 in the **Oncology** section.

Bibliography

Schuchter L. Melanoma. http://pier.acponline.org/physicians/diseases/d313. [Date accessed: 2008 Jan 10] In: PIER [online database]. Philadelphia: American College of Physicians; 2008.

Tsao H, Atkins MB, Sober AJ. Management of cutaneous melanoma. N Engl J Med. 2004;351:998-1012. Erratum in: N Engl J Med. 2004; 351:2461. [PMID: 15342808]

Chapter 73

Pain Management

Patrick C. Alguire, MD

An accepted definition of pain is "an unpleasant sensory and emotional experience associated with actual or potential tissue damage or described in terms of such damage." Pain is classified as *nociceptive* (somatic and visceral), resulting from the stimulation of specialized receptors, or *neuropathic*, based on a primary dysfunction of the peripheral or central nervous system. Acute pain originates from the specialized nociceptive nerve endings and is protective by warning of potential or actual injury. Chronic pain is defined as pain that persists for 1 month beyond the normal time of healing.

Assessing Pain

Because pain is subjective, physicians must listen to and believe a patient's report of pain. When assessing chronic pain, remember that autonomic responses (e.g., tachycardia, hypertension, and diaphoresis) are not reliable indicators of pain. They may be entirely absent despite the presence of pain, particularly chronic pain.

Determine the site of pain, its onset, temporal pattern, exacerbating and relieving factors, and associated symptoms. Learn how much the pain is interfering with daily activities or affecting the patient's psychological state. To help patients quantify their pain, use a number of pain-intensity assessment tools, including the universal pain assessment tool (www.anes.ucla.edu/pain/FacesScale1.jpg) or quantify on a scale of 1 (minimum) to 10 (maximum).

Physical examination must focus close attention to the painful and related areas. Laboratory, x-ray, CT, and other imaging studies may be necessary for proper evaluation. Ongoing reassessment of the patient's response to therapy helps determine if the therapeutic regimen has been a success.

Treating Pain

On the 0-10 pain intensity scale, levels 1–3 are equated with mild pain. Mild pain can usually be adequately treated with aspirin, acetaminophen, and nonsteroidal anti-inflammatory drugs (NSAIDs). These drugs differ from opioids in two important ways: there is a ceiling effect to the analgesia (more drug is not associated with greater pain control); and they do not produce tolerance or physical dependence. Unless contraindicated, management of all levels of pain includes one of these drugs.

On the 0-10 pain intensity scale, 4-6 equals moderate pain. In the treatment of moderate pain, low-dose opioid drugs are added to aspirin, acetaminophen, or NSAIDS. For patient convenience, many opioids are marketed as combination products containing one of these agents. It is the daily cumulative acetaminophen dose (4 grams) that limits the dosing of the opioid in combination medications. For this reason, separate dosing of the opioid and acetaminophen is preferred.

On the 0-10 pain intensity scale, 7-10 equals severe pain. The treatment of severe pain requires higher-dose opioid drugs and continuation of aspirin, acetaminophen, or NSAIDs.

Adjuvant Therapy

There are a number of drug and non-drug therapies that can enhance the effects of nonopioid and opioid analgesics. At the top of the list are tricyclic antidepressants. Studies have confirmed their effectiveness in diabetic neuropathy and postherpetic neuralgia and are frequently used for neuropathic pain from other sources. Anticonvulsants are used to relieve the shooting, electrical pains of peripheral nerve dysfunction. Clinical trials have demonstrated their effectiveness in diabetic neuropathy, postherpetic neuralgia, and trigeminal neuralgia. Corticosteroids can reduce edema and lyse certain tumors and thereby enhance the analgesic effect of nonopioid and opioid drugs. They are effective in the management of malignant infiltration of the brachial and lumbar plexus and spinal cord compression as well as headache pain due to brain tumors.

Anatomic interventions include epidural and intrathecal administration of opioids and sympathetic plexus nerve block for visceral pain. Neurolytic celiac plexus block appears to be superior to systemic opioids for the treatment of pain from pancreatic cancer.

Routes of Opioid Administration

Oral administration is the preferred route for opioid analgesics because of its convenience, low cost, and ability to produce stable opioid blood levels. For most immediate release opioids, peak blood levels are reached in about 1 hour. Therefore, if pain is not adequately relieved after 1 hour, and side effects are not a limiting factor, a second dose can be safely consumed.

Intramuscular injections are not recommended because of the associated pain, unreliable absorption, and relatively long interval to peak drug concentrations. If a parenteral route is needed, intravenous or subcutaneous administration is preferred.

Intravenous administration is associated with the most rapid onset of analgesia but also the shortest duration of action. For initial intravenous dosing in opioid-naïve patients, one-half the recommended dose is advised. The time to peak effect of intravenous opioids varies with the drug and ranges from 5 to 30 minutes. If severe pain persists but side effects are minimal at the time of the peak effect, a repeat dose is given. Repeated intravenous doses are administered in this fashion to titrate to the point of adequate pain relief followed by a constant intravenous infusion of a maintenance dose.

Continuous intravenous dosing is associated with steady blood levels of the opioid and provides the best analgesic control with the fewest side effects. Subcutaneous constant infusion is an alternative to intravenous infusion.

For patients receiving parenteral opioids, patient-controlled analgesia is a useful modality to help maintain patient independence and control by matching drug delivery to analgesic need. The opioid may be administered via a portable pump to deliver the drug intravenously or subcutaneously.

A transdermal opioid patch is available for the treatment of chronic pain. The opioid fentanyl is absorbed through the skin to provide a continuous infusion of drug using a 72-hour reservoir. Fentanyl is also available as a solid sweetened lozenge and mucosal patch.

All patients taking parenteral or sustained-release opioids need access to a short-acting opioid preparation to manage breakthrough pain. The dose of the immediate-release opioid for breakthrough pain is calculated as 10% (5%-15%) of the total daily opioid dose.

Common Side Effects of Opioids

Constipation is an almost inevitable side effect of long-term opioid therapy and should be anticipated. An example of a constipation-prevention regimen includes docusate, bisacodyl, or senna concentrate, and a hyperosmotic agent such as milk of magnesia or lactulose.

Opioid-related nausea and vomiting are managed with a phenothiazine antiemetic, transdermal scopolamine, or hydroxyzine. Some patients will experience less nausea if the opioid blood level remains constant throughout the day rather than experiencing period peaks. Changing the dosing interval of an immediate-release preparation from every 4 hours to a smaller dose every 3 hours may even out the blood level and reduce nausea and vomiting. Changing to a sustained-release opioid or the transdermal route also produces more constant opioid blood levels and may be helpful.

Opioid-related itching and urticaria are due to the release of histamine. For these patients, an antihistamine is useful. Oxymorphone and fentanyl are two opioids that do not release histamine, and switching to these opioids can be considered.

Opioid-naïve patients are more susceptible to respiratory depression than are patients receiving long-term opioids. When rapid reversal of opiate depression is indicated, naloxone can be administered in small increments to improve respiratory function without totally reversing analgesia.

Meperidine and Mixed Agonist-Antagonist Analgesics

After repeated doses of meperidine, the toxic metabolite normeperidine accumulates and can produce anxiety, tremors, myoclonus, and seizures. Because the metabolite is excreted by the kidneys, patients with renal insufficiency are at particularly high risk for this complication. Meperidine should not be dosed beyond 48 hours and is not indicated in the management of chronic pain. Mixed agonist-antagonist drugs offer no advantages over morphine-like drugs and are capable of precipitating opioid withdrawal symptoms when given to patients taking chronic morphine-like opioids.

Tolerance, Dependence, and Addiction

Tolerance is the need for an increased amount of drug to achieve the same analgesic effect. This is a common and expected occurrence in individuals who take opioids chronically. The first sign of tolerance may be a decrease in the duration of effective pain relief with the usual dose of opioid. To treat tolerance, increase the current opioid dose by 10%-15%.

Physical dependence is a physiological state marked by the development of withdrawal symptoms when medications are discontinued abruptly. The appearance of anxiety, irritability, excessive salivation, tearing, runny nose, sweating, nausea, vomiting, and insomnia signal the withdrawal syndrome. Prevent opioid withdrawal by slowly tapering chronically used opioids, and by avoiding opioid antagonists and mixed agonists-antagonists in patients on chronic opioid therapy.

Addiction is an abnormal behavioral condition in which a person develops an overwhelming involvement in acquiring and using a drug despite adverse social, psychological, or physical consequences. Tolerance and physical dependence are not equivalent to addiction. Addiction is relatively rare and occurs in a small percentage of patients taking opioids as prescribed to control pain.

Book Enhancement

Go to www.acponline.org/essentials/oncology-section.html to use the equianalgesic conversion table, fentanyl conversion table, access pain assessment tools, review pain management quick tips and the WHO analgesic ladder, and complete a self-assessment quiz on opioid conversions. In *MKSAP for Students 4*, assess yourself with item 26 in the **Oncology** section.

Bibliography

Woolf CJ, American College of Physicians, American Physiological Society. Pain: moving from symptom control toward mechanism-specific pharmacologic management. Ann Intern Med. 2004;140:441-51. [PMID: 15023710]

Section X
Pulmonary Medicine

Chapter 74

Approach to Dyspnea

Mark D. Holden, MD

Dyspnea may be either acute or chronic. Primary causes related to the cardiovascular system are associated with a decreased cardiac output, elevated left atrial pressure, increased pulmonary capillary pressure or poor oxygen delivery. Respiratory system causes are related to the central control of respiration, abnormalities of the ventilatory pump, pleural disease, and disturbance of airflow or the gas exchange process. Anemia can also cause dyspnea due to reduced oxygen content.

The pathophysiology of dyspnea is complex and incompletely understood. The brainstem and higher brain centers receive afferent sensory information from a variety of chemoreceptors and mechanoreceptors. Central and peripheral chemoreceptors sense changes in Pco_2 and Po_2. Mechanoreceptors, such as pulmonary stretch receptors, muscle spindles, and diaphragmatic tendon organs sense expansion of the lungs and chest wall, contraction of respiratory muscles, and airway flow. Information from these receptors is integrated by the central nervous system to modulate the perception of dyspnea. Efferent impulses from the medullary respiratory center to the ventilatory muscles also signal higher cortical centers, providing awareness of respiratory drive. Dyspnea is associated with increased efferent output to respiratory muscles, impaired chest expansion, bronchoconstriction, and stimulation of pulmonary vagal receptors. The sensation of dyspnea may also occur when there is an imbalance of efferent respiratory motor signals and resultant afferent receptor responses reflecting the ineffectiveness of ventilation.

Acute Dyspnea

Acute dyspnea arises rapidly over minutes to 24 hours and has a limited differential diagnosis. Cardiovascular causes are related to acute decreases in left ventricular ejection or any event that increases pulmonary capillary pressure (e.g., acute coronary syndrome, tachycardia, cardiac tamponade). Respiratory causes are related to airway dysfunction (bronchospasm, aspiration, and obstruction), disruption of the gas exchange system by parenchymal disease (e.g., pneumonia, acute respiratory distress syndrome), vascular disease (pulmonary embolism), and disturbances of the ventilatory pump (e.g., pleural effusion, pneumothorax, respiratory muscle weakness).

The history and physical exam provide important clues to the differential diagnosis of dyspnea, which is summarized in Table 1. Look for fever and cough suggesting pneumonia; intermittent wheezing suggests asthma, whereas wheezing following allergen exposure (food, insect sting, medication) or associated with urticaria is more typical of anaphylaxis; a history of acute pleuritic chest pain suggests pneumothorax or pulmonary embolism; stridor suggests upper airway obstruction; and a history of recent trauma suggests pneumothorax or hemothorax. Paroxysmal nocturnal dyspnea (positive likelihood ratio = 2.6) and a history of heart failure (positive likelihood ratio = 5.8) increase the probability of heart failure as the cause of dyspnea.

On physical examination, look for signs supporting pneumonia such as crackles, dullness to percussion, or egophony; hyperresonance and absent breath sounds suggest pneumothorax; dullness to percussion, absent breath sounds, and diminished tactile fremitus suggest pleural effusion; wheezing indicates airflow through narrowed airways; the presence of an S_3 strongly supports the diagnosis of heart failure (positive likelihood ratio = 11) as do elevated central venous pressure and basilar crackles. Pulse oximetry should be routinely used to assess oxygen saturation. Low oxygen saturation suggests a problem with respiratory gas exchange and points to processes such as asthma or acute exacerbation of chronic obstructive pulmonary disease, acute respiratory distress syndrome, heart failure, pulmonary fibrosis, or pulmonary vascular disease.

Chest x-ray is the key diagnostic tool. Look for focal infiltrates (pneumonia), atelectasis, air or fluid in the pleural space; vascular congestion (positive likelihood ratio = 12) and cardiomegaly support heart failure. Depending upon the clinical situation, other helpful diagnostic tests may include spiral computed tomography of the chest, ventilation-perfusion scan or pulmonary angiography to diagnose pulmonary embolism. High-resolution computed tomography might be useful when chest radiography is normal but suspicion for an infiltrative lung disease is high. An electrocardiogram showing atrial fibrillation supports heart failure (positive likelihood ratio = 3.8), and a serum B-type natriuretic peptide (BNP) <100 pg/mL helps exclude heart failure (negative likelihood ratio = 0.11). Bronchoscopy can be useful in the diagnosis of suspected foreign body aspiration, airway obstruction, and in certain cases of pneumonia.

Chronic Dyspnea

Dyspnea becomes chronic when symptoms persist >1 month. In two-thirds of patients, chronic dyspnea results from chronic obstructive pulmonary disease (COPD), asthma, interstitial lung disease, or heart failure. Less common causes include valvular and pericardial heart disease (Table 1).

The history should include detailed exploration of the quality and severity of the dyspnea, precipitating and positional factors, timing of symptoms, associated features, and cardiopulmonary risk factors. Patients with dyspnea due to heart failure tend to

Table 1. Differential Diagnosis of Dyspnea

Condition	Notes
Anemia (see Chapter 38)	Conjunctival rim and palmar crease pallor; known blood loss.
Asthma (see Chapter 76)	Known asthma; wheezing; improvement with inhaled β-agonist.
COPD (see Chapter 77)	Known COPD; smoking >40 pack/year; age ≥45 years; maximum laryngeal height ≤4 cm; barrel chest; distant breath sounds; B-type natriuretic peptide (BNP) <100 pg/mL.
Heart failure (see Chapter 6)	History of heart failure; paroxysmal nocturnal dyspnea; S_3; jugular venous distention; atrial fibrillation; pulmonary congestion on x-ray.
Interstitial pulmonary fibrosis (see Chapter 79)	Diffuse late crackles; low diffusing capacity; abnormal chest x-ray or CT scan.
Neuromuscular weakness	Focal weakness; neurologic symptoms.
Pericardial tamponade or constriction	Hepatojugular reflux, peripheral edema, increased central venous pressure, pulsus paradoxus; abnormal echocardiogram.
Pleural effusion (see Chapter 75)	Dullness to percussion; diminished breath sounds; abnormal chest-x-ray.
Pneumonia (see Chapter 53)	Fever, cough, sputum, tachycardia; localized crackles; abnormal chest x-ray.
Pneumothorax	Sudden onset, pleuritic pain, decreased breath sounds, hyper-resonance to percussion, shifted trachea; abnormal chest x-ray.
Psychogenic	Poor exercise tolerance and evidence of anxiety.
Pulmonary embolism (see Chapter 80)	Sudden onset dyspnea; pleuritic chest pain (30%); syncope, hypotension, elevated neck veins; ECG evidence of right heart strain with large, central pulmonary emboli.
Pulmonary hypertension	Increased P_2; persistently split S_2, right sternal heave; tricuspid insufficiency murmur; electrocardiographic changes of RVH.
Systemic sclerosis	Typical joint and skin findings; esophageal dysmotility; pulmonary hypertension or interstitial pulmonary fibrosis.
Valvular heart disease (see Chapter 7)	Aortic stenosis: chest pain, heart failure, syncope, long, late-peaking systolic murmur radiating to the neck. Mitral stenosis: dyspnea onset often during pregnancy, mid-diastolic rumbling murmur. Aortic regurgitation: early diastolic murmur at base, rapidly collapsing pulse. Mitral regurgitation: holosystolic murmur, S_3, displaced apex beat.

COPD = chronic obstructive pulmonary disease; ECG = electrocardiogram; RVH = right ventricular hypertrophy.

characterize their dyspnea as air hunger or suffocating, while those with asthma often describe chest tightness. The history must also include a detailed review of medical problems, prescription and non-prescription medications, substance use, hobbies, and occupational/environmental exposures.

The findings from the history and physical exam direct the selection of diagnostic testing, which may include chest x-ray, electrocardiogram, pulmonary function testing, and echocardiography. Laboratory testing should include a complete blood count and assessment of thyroid function. The results of these initial tests may suggest further investigation with computed tomography. Lung biopsy may be necessary if parenchymal lung disease of uncertain etiology is found.

Supportive evidence for COPD includes smoking >40 years (positive likelihood ratio = 8.3), self-reported history of COPD (positive likelihood ratio = 7.3), laryngeal height (distance from sternal notch to top of thyroid cartilage) ≤4 cm (positive likelihood ratio = 2.8), and age ≥45 years (positive likelihood ratio = 1.3). Presence of all four signs is associated with a positive likelihood ratio of 220. Physical findings of advanced disease include hyperresonance to percussion, decreased breath sounds, prolonged expiration, and wheezes. Common, but non-specific, radiographic signs of emphysema are flattening of the diaphragms, irregular lung lucency, and reduction or absence of vasculature. Pulmonary function testing demonstrates airflow obstruction with an FEV_1/FVC (forced expiratory volume in 1 second/forced vital capacity) ratio <0.70. Consider other causes of chronic airway obstruction including bronchiectasis and cystic fibrosis, particularly if symptoms include voluminous sputum production with frequent purulent exacerbations (bronchiectasis) or chronic obstructive pulmonary symptoms beginning at an early age and in the absence of a smoking history (cystic fibrosis).

Patients with asthma have intermittent dyspnea with episodic airway obstruction. A personal or family history of atopic diseases may be present. Patients may describe exacerbations with exercise or exposure to airway irritants or cold, chest tightness, wheezing, sputum production or dry cough. Physical examination during exacerbations may reveal diminished breath sounds, wheezes, and prolonged expiration. Chest x-ray is frequently normal but may show hyperinflation. Spirometry during an attack will show obstruction that typically improves following bronchodilator administration, but normal spirometry does not exclude asthma. Asthma that is suspected despite normal spirometry may require provocative testing with methacholine to establish the diagnosis.

Rare mimics of asthma include upper airway obstruction due to vocal cord paralysis, tumors of the trachea, tracheal stenosis, tracheomalacia, and vocal cord dysfunction (paradoxical adduction during inspiration). The flow-volume curve usually shows a characteristic expiratory or inspiratory plateau or both. Diagnosis usually requires computed tomography, MRI scan or direct endoscopic visualization of the airway, depending upon the suspected nature of the diagnosis.

Interstitial lung disease presents with progressive dyspnea on exertion and cough but may include other symptoms related to the specific etiology. The history may identify occupational or environmental exposures or symptoms of systemic disease. Physical examination findings are often non-specific and may include dry, basilar crackles. The exam should include a careful search for extra-pulmonary involvement (e.g., skin, joint, and neurologic findings), suggesting an underlying systemic illness. The chest x-ray may be normal or show reticular, nodular, or alveolar infiltrates, or pleural effusion. High-resolution computed tomography may provide evidence of interstitial disease when the chest x-ray is normal. In the appropriate clinical setting, specific radiographic patterns may indicate specific diagnoses. Pulmonary function testing typically shows evidence of restriction and decreased DLco. Characteristically, arterial blood gas abnormalities include resting hypoxemia or hypoxemia on exercise testing. Specialized procedures such as bronchoalveolar lavage, transbronchial lung biopsy via bronchoscopy, video-assisted thoracoscopic lung biopsy, or open lung biopsy may be necessary to confirm a diagnosis.

Patients with neuromuscular disease may present with dyspnea as well as other extra-pulmonary symptoms including difficulty rising from a chair or climbing stairs (proximal muscle weakness), diplopia (myasthenia gravis), and muscle fasciculations (amyotrophic lateral sclerosis). Cardiopulmonary examination is typically normal early in the course of these diseases. Pulmonary function testing may indicate inspiratory muscle weakness, with inability to generate a maximum inspiratory pressure more negative than −60 mm Hg.

Dyspnea of Obscure Cause

When no diagnosis can be made after evaluation for cardiac, pulmonary, or neuromuscular disorders, cardiopulmonary exercise testing can be used to evaluate cardiac performance, ventilatory capacity, and gas exchange during exercise. Cardiopulmonary exercise testing quantifies the patient's exercise tolerance and provides evidence of abnormal cardiac or pulmonary responses to exercise that may suggest a diagnosis. While the patient exercises on a treadmill or stationary bicycle, exhaled gases are collected and continuous oximetry and electrocardiography are performed. An indwelling arterial line can be placed for arterial blood gas measurements. Low maximal oxygen uptake in the absence of an identifiable abnormality often indicates deconditioning.

Panic disorder and hyperventilation syndrome are relatively uncommon causes of chronic dyspnea and are usually associated with other, extra-pulmonary symptoms.

Book Enhancement

Go to www.acponline.org/essentials/pulmonary-section.html to view x-rays and CT scans of heart failure, pneumothorax, pulmonary fibrosis, and emphysema. In *MKSAP for Students 4*, assess yourself with items 3-8 in the **Pulmonary Medicine** section.

Bibliography

American Thoracic Society. Dyspnea. Mechanisms, assessment, and management: a consensus statement. Am J Respir Crit Care Med. 1999;159:321-40. [PMID: 9872857]

Straus SE, McAlister FA, Sackett DL, Deeks JJ. The accuracy of patient history, wheezing, and laryngeal measurements in diagnosing obstructive airway disease. CARE-COAD1 Group. Clinical Assessment of the Reliability of the Examination-Chronic Obstructive Airways Disease. JAMA. 2000;283:1853-7. Erratum in: JAMA 2000;284:181. [PMID: 10770147]

Wang CS, FitzGerald JM, Schulzer M, et al. Does this dyspneic patient in the emergency department have congestive heart failure? JAMA. 2005;294:1944-56. [PMID: 16234501]

Chapter 75

Pleural Effusion

Dario M. Torre, MD

A pleural effusion is created by an imbalance between the production and removal of fluid from the pleural space. Two major mechanisms lead to the accumulation of excessive fluid in the pleural space: increased capillary hydrostatic pressure (e.g., heart failure, superior vena cava syndrome, constrictive pericarditis) and/or decreased plasma oncotic pressure (e.g., cirrhosis, nephrotic syndrome, hypoalbuminemia). Pleural effusions may be caused by a wide variety of disease processes including heart failure, cirrhosis, nephrosis, infection, cancer, trauma, collagen vascular disease, venous thromboembolism, or aortic rupture.

The evaluation of a pleural effusion requires a systematic history, physical examination, and pertinent laboratory and imaging tests. The leading causes of pleural effusion in the United States are heart failure, pneumonia, and cancer.

Diagnosis

Pleural effusions may present with symptoms such as fever, dyspnea, and chest pain. Fever suggests an underlying infection, malignancy, or associated collagen vascular disease. Chest pain and dyspnea may be caused by the space-occupying effect of a large effusion or associated parenchymal lung disease. Small pleural effusions, such as those caused by nephrotic syndrome or rheumatoid arthritis, are often asymptomatic. Large fluid accumulation in the pleural space blocks transmission of sound between the lung and the chest wall; percussion over an effusion is dull and tactile (vocal) fremitus is diminished or absent. On auscultation, the most common findings are decreased to absent breath sounds over the effusion and bronchial breath sounds towards the top of the effusion. A pleural friction rub, a harsh, rubbing, scratchy sound heard predominantly during expiration may be auscultated.

Chest radiography is the first diagnostic test for pleural effusion (Figure 1); it can identify and quantify the amount of fluid and may demonstrate underlying diseases responsible for the effusion such as pneumonia or cancer, or suggest aortic dissection (widened mediastinum). Approximately 250 mL of pleural fluid is needed to blunt the costophrenic angle on chest x-ray; greater amounts of fluid opacify the lower thorax and create a "meniscus sign."

After documenting the presence of an effusion, obtain decubitus films to evaluate whether the effusion is free-flowing

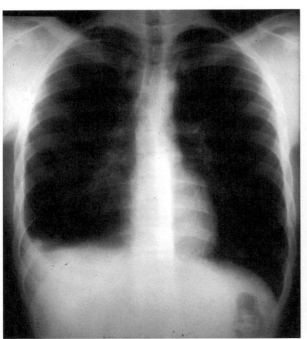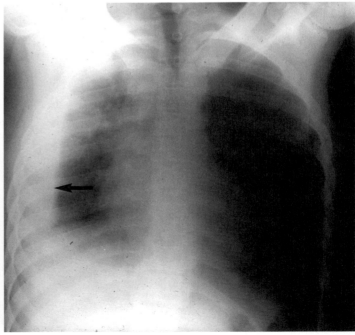

Figure 1 Chest x-ray showing a right-sided pleural effusion (*left panel*) that layers out along the right thorax when the x-ray is repeated with the patient in the right lateral decubitus position (*right panel*).

or loculated and whether a sufficient quantity of fluid is present to perform a thoracentesis. A 1-cm distance measured from the pleural fluid line to the chest wall on a decubitus x-ray is indicative of enough pleural fluid to perform a thoracentesis. Chest CT scan is an extremely valuable adjunct to chest radiography because it can more effectively define size and location of the pleural effusion and distinguish parenchymal from pleural disease. A helical chest CT with contrast is highly sensitive for pulmonary embolus and may be indicated if the pretest probability of pulmonary embolism is moderate to high. Ultrasound can be used to detect loculations, guide thoracentesis, and detect pleural abnormalities that are not apparent on chest x-ray.

A massive effusion, occupying the entire hemithorax, increases the likelihood of an underlying lung cancer or pleural mesothelioma. Bilateral transudative effusions are commonly associated with heart or liver failure. Bilateral exudative effusions suggest malignancy but are also found in patients with pleuritis due to systemic lupus erythematosus and other collagen vascular diseases. An empyema is suggested by the presence of a non-free-flowing effusion on upright and decubitus chest x-rays or obvious loculation by chest CT scan.

An electrocardiogram and echocardiogram can be useful to exclude pericardial disease or right ventricular strain and dilation caused by a moderate- to large-size pulmonary embolism. Antinuclear antibody, rheumatoid factor, erythrocyte sedimentation rate, and complement levels may be useful if other signs and symptoms suggest collagen vascular disease.

Obtain a thoracentesis in all patients with a newly discovered pleural effusion to assist in diagnosis and management. Most pleural fluid analyses narrow the diagnostic possibilities but are not definitive by themselves. Pleural fluid evaluation should include pH, glucose, lactate dehydrogenase (LDH), protein, and bacterial and acid-fast bacillus stains and culture. If tuberculosis is suspected, adenosine deaminase activity and the polymerase chain reaction can be useful adjuncts to diagnosis. Gross pus in the pleural space is diagnostic of empyema.

Exudative pleural effusions are predominantly caused by inflammatory, infectious, and malignant conditions and less commonly by collagen vascular disease, intra-abdominal processes, and hypothyroidism. Venous thromboembolic disease may cause either an exudative (particularly in the case of pulmonary infarction) or, less commonly, a transudative effusion. Transudative pleural effusions are more commonly associated with heart failure and cirrhosis and less commonly with nephrotic syndrome and constrictive pericarditis. Differentiation of an exudate from a transudate is made with greatest confidence when pleural fluid test results are well above or below the designated cut off points

(Table 1). Fluid with borderline test results can be either a transudate or an exudate.

The most likely diagnoses associated with a pleural fluid leukocyte cell count >10,000/μL include parapneumonic effusion, acute pancreatitis, splenic infarction, and subphrenic, hepatic, and splenic abscesses. A pleural fluid leukocyte cell count >50,000/μL is always associated with complicated parapneumonic effusions and empyema but occasionally occurs with acute pancreatitis and pulmonary infarction. Malignant disease and tuberculosis typically present with a lymphocyte-predominant exudate.

Normal pleural fluid pH is 7.60 to 7.66. Transudates have a pleural fluid pH of 7.45 to 7.55. There are a limited number of diagnoses associated with a pleural fluid pH <7.30; the most common causes are complicated parapneumonic effusion or empyema, esophageal rupture, rheumatoid pleural disease, and malignancy.

Pleural fluid amylase should be measured only when pancreatic disease, esophageal rupture, or malignancy is considered. A chylous effusion (milky white appearing fluid) is highly likely if the triglyceride level is >110 mg/dL. A chylous effusion is commonly caused by leakage of lymph, rich in triglycerides, from the thoracic duct due to trauma or obstruction (e.g., lymphoma). Pleural fluid cytology has a variable diagnostic yield for malignancy, ranging from 40%-90%. When malignancy is suspected but a first thoracentesis is non-diagnostic, submission of a second large-volume fluid sample to the laboratory may be helpful. Figure 2 and Table 2 summarize a diagnostic approach and ancillary tests used to evaluate the causes of pleural effusion.

Approximately 25% of pleural effusions remain undiagnosed after analysis of one or more pleural fluid samples. Additional diagnostic evaluations are undertaken if the effusion is persistently symptomatic or if a progressive disease is suspected, such as malignancy, tuberculosis, or pulmonary embolism.

Therapy

Treatment of pleural effusions is dictated by the underlying cause. However, large effusions should be evacuated. For massive effusions associated with mediastinal shift, 2 L or more can be removed safely in one setting. Otherwise, therapeutic thoracentesis is limited to 1-1.5 L at a time to minimize the likelihood of re-expansion pulmonary edema.

In pleural effusions associated with pneumonia, the presence of loculated pleural fluid, pleural fluid pH <7.20, pleural fluid glucose <60 mg/dL, positive pleural fluid Gram stain or culture, or the presence of gross pus in the pleural space predict a poor response to antibiotics alone; such pleural effusions are treated

Table 1. Light's Criteria for the Characterization of Pleural Effusions

Pleural effusions are defined as being exudative if they demonstrate any one of the following criteria:*

- Pleural fluid to serum total protein ratio >0.5.
- Pleural fluid to serum LDH (lactic dehydrogenase) ratio >0.6.
- Pleural fluid LDH value >2/3 of the upper limit of normal for serum LDH.

* Pleural fluid parameters may assume exudative characteristics in patients with heart failure who are receiving diuretics. In cases where Light's criteria suggests the presence of a pleural exudate but the clinical picture suggests the presence of a transudate, measurement of a serum to pleural fluid albumin gradient of >1.2 g/dL supports the diagnosis of a transudative effusion. A pleural fluid cholesterol level of <60 mg/dL also suggests the presence of a pleural transudate.

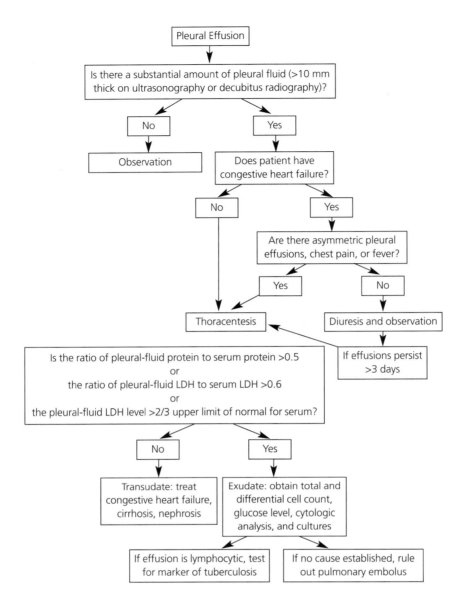

Figure 2 Evaluation of patient with pleural effusion. (From Light RW. Clinical practice. Pleural effusion. N Engl J Med. 2002;346:1971-7; with permission. Copyright © 2002 Massachusetts Medical Society.)

Table 2. Additional Pleural Fluid Tests

Test	Notes
Erythrocyte count	>100,000/μL; malignancy, trauma, parapneumonic, pulmonary embolism
Leukocyte count	>10,000/μL; empyema
Neutrophils	>50%; parapneumonic, pulmonary embolism, abdominal diseases
Lymphocytes	>50%; malignancy, tuberculosis, pulmonary embolism, coronary artery bypass surgery
pH	<7.2; complicated parapneumonic or empyema, malignancy (<10%), tuberculosis (<10%), esophageal rupture
Glucose	<60 mg/dL; complicated parapneumonic or empyema, tuberculosis (20%), malignancy (<10%), rheumatoid arthritis
Adenosine deaminase	>40 U/L; tuberculosis (>90%), complicated parapneumonic (30%) or empyema (60%), malignancy (5%)
Cytology	Present; malignancy
Culture	Positive; infection
Useful in Certain Circumstances	
Hematocrit fluid/blood ratio	≥0.5; hemothorax
Amylase	Greater than upper limit of normal for serum; malignancy, pancreatic disease, esophageal rupture
Triglycerides	>110 mg/dL; chylothorax

with drainage of the fluid through a catheter or chest tube. Recurrent symptomatic pleural effusions are challenging to treat. Recurrent symptomatic malignant pleural effusion are often treated with pleurodesis, the instillation of a chemotherapeutic agent or talc through a chest tube into the pleural space causing adhesion between the parietal and visceral pleura. Alternatively, adhesions are formed by physical abrasion of the pleural surface under thorascopic guidance or through a small thoracotomy incision.

Book Enhancement

Go to www.acponline.org/essentials/pulmonary-section.html to access a table on causes of transudative and exudative pleural effusions, test characteristics of common pleural fluid tests, and diagnoses that can be established by pleural fluid analysis; to view images of a thoracentesis, and to view x-rays of a pneumothorax, hydropneumothorax, and trapped lung. In *MKSAP for Students 4*, assess yourself with items 9-11 in the **Pulmonary Medicine** section.

Bibliography

American College of Physicians. Medical Knowledge Self-Assessment Program 14. Philadelphia: American College of Physicians; 2006.

Heffner JE, Brown LK, Barbieri CA. Diagnostic value of tests that discriminate between exudative and transudative pleural effusions. Primary Study Investigators. Chest. 1997;111:970-80. [PMID: 9106577]

Light RW. Clinical practice. Pleural effusion. N Engl J Med. 2002; 346:1971-7. [PMID: 12075059]

Chapter 76

Asthma

Patricia Short, MD

Asthma is a disease of intermittent and reversible airway obstruction associated with chronic inflammation and a disordered immune response affecting 5%-10% of the U.S. population with a steadily increasing prevalence. The underlying cause of asthma remains unknown. Eosinophils are increased in the airway of patients with asthma, especially those with active disease. Neutrophils are also increased during exacerbations and in severe disease; their role in the pathogenesis remains unclear. T-helper 2 (Th2) cells, a subtype of CD4 T cells, appear to play a central role in activation of the inflammatory response in asthma. Airway inflammation contributes to airway hyper-responsiveness and narrowing. Structural alterations occur in the lungs of some patients consisting of subepithelial fibrosis, increased smooth muscle mass, angiogenesis, and hyperplasia of mucous gland and goblet cells, a process known as airway remodeling. Effective management involves use of objective measures of lung function to assess severity and to monitor therapeutic efficacy, identification and avoidance of environmental triggers that exacerbate symptoms, long-term use of medications that decrease airway inflammation, and use of medications to treat acute exacerbations.

Diagnosis

The diagnosis of asthma is based on episodic symptoms of airflow limitation and/or airway inflammation, evidence of reversible airflow obstruction, and exclusion of alternative diagnoses. Episodic symptoms of airflow obstruction include wheezing, dyspnea, cough, and chest tightness. Symptoms that worsen in the presence of aeroallergens, irritants, or exercise are typical, as are early morning or late evening symptoms that awaken the patient from sleep. The diagnosis of asthma should be considered in all patients with a chronic cough, especially if the cough is nocturnal, seasonal, or related to a workplace or activity; coughing may be the only manifestation of asthma. A history of atopic dermatitis, eczema, or family history of asthma are additional risk factors for development of the disease.

Physical examination findings of asthma include wheezing during normal breathing or with forced expiration, chest hyperexpansion, and prolonged expiratory phase. Accessory muscle use may be seen during an acute exacerbation. Additional findings may include nasal mucosal thickening, nasal polyps, or rhinitis manifested by cobblestoning of the oropharynx. Patients may also have evidence of atopic dermatitis or eczema on skin examination.

Perform spirometry in all patients suspected of having asthma (Table 1). Spirometric measurements, including forced expiratory volume in 1 second (FEV_1) and forced vital capacity (FVC),

are taken before and after bronchodilator use. A reduced FEV_1 or a reduced FEV_1/FVC ratio documents airflow obstruction. An increase in FEV_1 of >12% and a minimum of 200 mL increase in FEV_1 after bronchodilator use establishes the presence of airflow reversibility and the diagnosis of asthma. However, normal spirometry does not exclude the diagnosis. Patients suspected of having asthma who have normal spirometry should proceed with a bronchoprovocation test such as a methacholine challenge. The lower the concentration of inhaled methacholine needed to cause a 20% drop in FEV_1, the more likely the patient has asthma. Methacholine challenge has a high sensitivity and high negative predictive value for the diagnosis of asthma. Other bronchoprovocation tests include histamine and exercise.

For patients with a smoking history who present with respiratory complaints consistent with asthma, consider obtaining diffusing capacity for carbon monoxide (DLco) to differentiate between asthma and chronic obstructive pulmonary disease (e.g., chronic bronchitis, emphysema). The DLco is normal to increased in asthma and decreased in chronic obstructive pulmonary disease.

Alternative diagnoses should be considered when asthma is difficult to control or if signs and symptoms are atypical. Vocal cord dysfunction, chronic obstructive pulmonary disease, heart failure, interstitial lung disease, pulmonary hypertension, cystic fibrosis, Churg-Strauss syndrome, allergic bronchopulmonary aspergillosis, mechanical obstruction of the airway (e.g., endobronchial tumor or foreign body), and medication-induced symptoms are in the differential diagnosis of asthma (Table 2).

Therapy

Encourage patients with asthma to reduce exposures to factors that worsen their asthma. Advise dust mite-allergic individuals to use physical measures to reduce mite allergen exposure. Other measures include use of air conditioning to maintain humidity at less than 50%, removing carpets, reducing the use of fabric in items such as upholstered furniture, drapes, and soft toys. Covering mattresses and pillows and laundering all bedding materials weekly in hot water (≥130°F) can also help reduce exposure. Sensitive individuals may also benefit from other environmental control measures such as reduction of cockroach exposure through extermination and control of potential reservoirs of allergen through cleaning, removing cats from the home, and reducing dampness in the home. Other irritants to avoid include perfume, cleaning agents, sprays, dust, and vapors.

Advise patients to minimize exposure to tobacco smoke, wood-burning stoves, fireplaces, and unvented gas stoves. Aspirin

Table 1. Laboratory and Other Studies for Asthma

Test	Notes
Spirometry	Abnormal spirometry (reversible obstruction) can help to confirm an asthma diagnosis, but normal spirometry does not exclude asthma.
Peak flow variability	A patient with normal spirometry but marked diurnal variability (based on a peak flow diary kept for >2 weeks) may have asthma, and warrant an empiric trial of anti-asthma medications or testing with bronchoprovocation.
Bronchoprovocation test	In a patient with a highly suggestive history of asthma and normal baseline spirometry, a low PC_{20} (the concentration of inhaled methacholine needed to cause a 20% drop in the FEV_1) on methacholine challenge testing supports a diagnosis of asthma. Cold air, exercise, and histamine are other types of provocative tests used. A normal bronchoprovocation test will nearly rule out a diagnosis of asthma.
Chest x-ray	Chest x-ray may be needed to exclude other diagnoses, but it is not recommended as a routine test in the initial evaluation of asthma.
CBC with differential	A CBC is not helpful in the diagnosis of asthma.
Sputum evaluation	Routine sputum evaluation is not helpful in the diagnosis of asthma.
IgE	Routine serum IgE is not helpful in the diagnosis of asthma.
Quantitative IgE antibody assays	Specific IgE immunoassays (e.g., RAST) are not useful in the diagnosis of asthma.
Skin testing	There is a strong association between allergen sensitization, exposure, and asthma. Allergy testing is the only reliable way to detect the presence of specific IgE to allergens. Skin testing (or in vitro testing) may be indicated to guide the management of asthma in selected patients, but results are not useful in establishing the diagnosis of asthma.

CBC = complete blood count; FEV_1 = forced expiratory volume in 1 second; IgE = immunoglobulin E; RAST = radioallergosorbent test.

Table 2. Differential Diagnosis of Asthma

Condition	Notes
COPD (see Chapter 77)	Less reversibility of airflow obstruction; associated with a history of tobacco use. May coexist with asthma in adults.
Vocal cord dysfunction	Abrupt onset of severe symptoms, often with rapid improvement. Monophonic wheeze heard loudest during either inspiration or expiration. The preferred diagnostic test is direct visualization of the vocal cords during symptoms. May closely mimic asthma, particularly in young adults.
Heart failure (see Chapter 6)	Spirometry may or may not be normal. Wheezing may be a sentinel manifestation of HF. Consider HF when there is not prompt improvement with asthma therapy. Always a consideration for persons with underlying cardiac disease.
Medications	Chronic cough in persons on selected medications (e.g., ACE inhibitors).
Bronchiectasis	Voluminous sputum production, often purulent, sometimes blood tinged. Suspect when physical exam shows crackles with wheeze, clubbing, or with peribronchial thickening on chest x-ray.
Pulmonary infiltration with eosinophilia syndromes (ABPA, Churg-Strauss, Loeffler's syndrome, Carrington's pneumonia)	Wheezing may be seen in ABPA, eosinophilic pneumonia, and Churg-Strauss angiitis. Note that in uncomplicated asthma, chest x-ray is normal. Findings of infiltrates, striking peripheral blood eosinophilia, and constitutional symptoms, such as fever and weight loss suggest chronic eosinophilic pneumonia. Asthma with eosinophilia, markedly high serum IgE levels, and intermittent pulmonary infiltrates is characteristic of ABPA. Upper airway and sinus disease, difficult-to-treat asthma, and multisystem organ dysfunction suggests Churg-Strauss angiitis.
Obstructive sleep apnea (see Chapter 78)	Excessive snoring and daytime fatigue. More commonly seen in obese patients. Patient's sleep partner may offer history of noisy, labored, or erratic breathing.
Mechanical airway obstruction	Respiratory noises may be more pronounced in the inspiratory or expiratory phase of respiration, depending on location of obstruction. Diagnosed via the flow-volume loop.
Cystic fibrosis	Associated with thick, purulent sputum containing bacteria and GI symptoms due to pancreatic insufficiency. Recurrent respiratory infections may be present without GI or other system involvement.

ABPA = allergic bronchopulmonary aspergillosis; ACE = angiotensin-converting enzyme; COPD = chronic obstructive pulmonary disease; GI = gastrointestinal; HF = heart failure.

and nonsteroidal anti-inflammatory drugs are the most common cause of drug-induced asthma and must be avoided if sensitivity to these medications exists, or there is a history of nasal polyps. β-blockers, even topical β-blockers, may exacerbate symptoms in susceptible individuals. Sulfite-containing foods (e.g., processed potatoes, shrimp, dried fruit, beer, wine) should be avoided if patients have a history of sulfite sensitivity. There is no clear evidence regarding the value of HEPA filters, air duct cleaning, or dehumidifiers in the control of asthma. Humidifiers may actually increase allergen levels.

Asthma management uses a step-wise approach based on the severity of symptoms. Asthma is classified as mild-intermittent, mild-persistent, moderate-persistent, or severe-persistent (Table 3).

Regardless of disease severity, all patients are prescribed a short-acting, inhaled β-agonist. This is the drug of choice for reversal of acute symptoms of bronchospasm and is safe, well tolerated, and easy to use. Patients with mild-intermittent asthma do not need daily medication and are treated as needed with quick-relief medication (e.g., a short-acting β-agonist).

Mild-persistent asthma is treated with one long-term controller medication; a low-dose inhaled corticosteroid is preferred. Patients with this level of disease activity are more prone to disease exacerbations and have underlying inflammation. Inhaled corticosteroids reduce bronchial hyperresponsiveness, decrease use of rescue short-acting β-agonists, and control symptoms. A mast cell stabilizer, leukotriene modifier, or sustained-release methylxanthine are alternative long-term controller medications to inhaled corticosteroids.

Treat patients with moderate-persistent asthma with one or two long-term controller medications. Use either low doses of inhaled corticosteroid and a long-acting β-agonist (preferred) or medium doses of a single long-term controller medication. In patients who remain symptomatic while taking medium doses of inhaled corticosteroids, the addition of a long-acting bronchodilator (e.g., theophylline or salmeterol) results in improved lung physiology, decreased use of rescue β-agonists, and reduced symptoms when compared with doubling the dose of inhaled corticosteroid.

Patients with severe-persistent asthma may require at least three daily medications to manage their disease; high doses of an inhaled corticosteroid plus a long-acting bronchodilator and possibly oral corticosteroids. These patients are extremely prone to disease exacerbations and have underlying inflammation. The addition of a leukotriene receptor antagonist can improve FEV_1, decrease daytime symptom scores, and reduce nocturnal awakenings.

Exercise-induced bronchospasm typically begins at the start of exercise and peaks 5-10 minutes after stopping. Several therapeutic options are available for patients with asthma symptoms during exercise, particularly vigorous exercise in cold, dry air. If exercise-induced asthma occurs more than twice a week, use a long-term controller medication. Those who continue to have exercise-induced symptoms can take albuterol, cromolyn sodium, or nedocromil 15 to 30 minutes before exertion. Alternatively, long-term therapy with either a long-acting β-agonist or a leukotriene antagonist can aid in symptom control. Newer evidence suggests that long-term treatment with either salmeterol or montelukast is protective against exercise-induced asthma.

Management of comorbid conditions such as gastroesophageal reflux disease, allergic rhinitis, and chronic sinusitis can result in improved asthma control. Allergy tests, nasal examination, and assessment for gastroesophageal reflux disease should be considered in all asthmatics, particularly those who remain poorly controlled on medications. Patients may need additional medications (i.e., step up to the next level in strength) during an acute upper respiratory infection.

When evaluating a patient for an acute asthma exacerbation, look for certain historical features that identify high risk for a difficult course or complications, including a previous history of intubation, history of intensive care unit admission, history of unscheduled hospital admission, or β-agonist dispensing frequency >1/month. Objective features that raise a red flag include FEV_1 <50% predicted, peak expiratory flow rate (PEFR) <50% predicted, pulse oximetry <95%, $PaCO_2$ >40 mm Hg, PaO_2 <75 mm Hg, theophylline level >12 µg/mL, leukocyte count with >5% eosinophils or a total eosinophil count >1000-1500/µL, respiratory rate >30/min, and heart rate >120/min. These patients may require more intensive monitoring because they are more prone to respiratory compromise.

Follow-Up

For all patients, develop individual self-management plans, taking into consideration the underlying disease severity and the patient's ability to adapt to self-management. For patients with mild disease, provide a simple plan on how to handle exacerbations, including health care contacts in cases of emergency. Patients with moderate-to-severe asthma should keep a daily diary and have a detailed written action plan with specific objective or

Table 3. Classification of Asthma Severity

CLINICAL FEATURES BEFORE TREATMENT*

Step Classification	Symptoms	Nocturnal Symptoms	Lung Function
Step 4 Severe persistent	Continual symptoms; limited physical activity; frequent exacerbations.	Frequent	FEV_1 or PEF <60% predicted PEF variability >30%
Step 3 Moderate persistent	Daily symptoms; daily use of inhaled short-acting β2-agonist; exacerbations may affect activity; exacerbations ≥2 per week; may last days.	>1 per week	FEV_1 or PEF >60%-<80% predicted PEF variability >30%
Step 2 Mild persistent	Symptoms >2 per week but <1 per day; exacerbations may affect activity.	>2 per month	FEV_1 or PEF ≥80% predicted PEF variability 20%-30%
Step 1 Mild intermittent	Symptoms ≤2 per week; asymptomatic and normal PEF between exacerbations; exacerbations brief (a few hours to a few days); intensity may vary.	≤2 per month	FEV_1 or PEF ≥80% predicted PEF variability <20%

*The presence of one of the features of severity is sufficient to place a patient in that category. Assign patient to the most severe grade in which any feature occurs. The characteristics noted in this table are general and may overlap because asthma is highly variable. Furthermore, an individual's classification may change over time.
FEV_1 = forced expiratory volume in 1 second; PEF = peak expiratory flow.

subjective markers for self-directed changes in therapy. Ensure that all patients with persistent moderate-to-severe asthma have a peak flow meter at home and know how to use it. Provide instruction in symptom-based monitoring to patients not using peak flow monitoring.

Book Enhancement

Go to www.acponline.org/essentials/pulmonary-section.html to view flow volume loops, access patient inhaler instructions, an asthma action plan, an occupational asthma algorithm, and review drugs used to treat asthma. In *MKSAP for Students 4*, assess yourself with items 12-21 in the **Pulmonary Medicine** section.

Bibliography

National Asthma Education and Prevention Program. Expert Panel Report 3 (EPR-3): Guidelines for the Diagnosis and Management of Asthma-Summary Report 2007. J Allergy Clin Immunol. 2007;120 (5 Suppl):S94-138. [PMID: 17983880]

Panettieri RA Jr. In the clinic. Asthma. Ann Intern Med. 2007;146:ITC6-1-ITC6-16. [PMID: 17548407]

Shannon JJ, Weiss K, Grant E. Asthma. http://pier.acponline.org/physicians/diseases/d146. [Date accessed: 2008 Jan 11] In: PIER line database]. Philadelphia: American College of Physicians; 2008.

Chapter 77

Chronic Obstructive Pulmonary Disease

Carlos Palacio, MD

Chronic obstructive pulmonary disease (COPD) is characterized by airflow limitation that is not fully reversible. Chronic bronchitis and emphysema are the two predominant conditions included in COPD. Chronic bronchitis is defined as a productive cough for 3 months in each of 2 successive years in a patient in whom other causes of chronic sputum production have been excluded. Emphysema is defined as the presence of permanent enlargement of airspaces distal to the terminal bronchioles with destruction of their walls without obvious fibrosis. Either or both of these conditions may be present in patients. Other conditions characterized by poorly reversible airflow limitation such as bronchiectasis, cystic fibrosis, and bronchiolitis should be differentiated from COPD (Table 1).

Risk factors for COPD include host factors and environmental exposures. Hereditary deficiency of α_1-antitrypsin (AAT) is the best documented genetic factor. Other implicated genes are responsible for the production of enzymes that are involved in the detoxification of cigarette smoke, such as microsomal epoxide hydrolase and glutathione s-transferase. Developmental risk factors (e.g., low birth weight) and childhood illness have a profound effect on lung growth. Important environmental exposures include tobacco smoke, occupational dust, chemical agents, and air pollution.

Cigarette smoke is responsible for the development of bronchial gland hypertrophy and goblet cell metaplasia with inflammatory cell infiltrates. Airway changes include squamous epithelial metaplasia, ciliary loss and dysfunction, and increased proliferation of smooth muscle and connective tissue. In small airways, progressive COPD is associated with an increase in the volume of tissue in the wall and accumulation of inflammatory exudate in the lumen; this inflammation may persist for many years after stopping smoking. Emphysema involves loss of alveolar attachments and elasticity, contributing to small airway collapse during expiration. Peripheral airway obstruction, parenchymal destruction, and pulmonary vascular abnormalities reduce capacity for gas exchange, producing arterial hypoxemia, hypercapnia, and cor pulmonale. Hyperinflation causes respiratory muscle inefficiency and increased work of breathing.

Prevention

Eighty to 90% of the risk of developing COPD is attributable to cigarette smoking. Its effect depends on age of onset, dose, and duration of smoking. An accelerated decline in lung function is the single most important feature of COPD. Smoking cessation slows the accelerated decline in FEV_1 and reduces all-cause mortality. Advise patients not to start smoking and to stop if they have started.

Screening

Screening for airway obstruction in asymptomatic patients is not recommended as there is little evidence that making the diagnosis in this setting is beneficial. α_1-antitrypsin deficiency screening should be done in patients with early-onset COPD and in patients with a strong family history of lung or liver disease.

Diagnosis

Assess the presence of cough, sputum, dyspnea, exercise tolerance and energy level, and inquire about the frequency and severity of exacerbations. A detailed smoking history is essential and a history of exposure to other risk factors should be noted. Self-reported history of COPD, smoking >40 pack-years, age ≥45 years, and maximum laryngeal height ≤4 cm are most predictive of COPD. Laryngeal height is the distance between the top of the thyroid cartilage and the suprasternal notch.

Look for signs of hyperinflation including barrel chest, hyperresonant percussion note, distant breath sounds, and prolonged expiratory time. Pursed-lips breathing, paradoxical chest or abdominal wall movements, and use of accessory muscles are all signs of severe airflow limitation. Cardiac examination may show cor pulmonale (increased intensity of the pulmonic sound, persistently split S_2, and a parasternal lift due to right ventricular hypertrophy). Extra-cardiac signs of cor pulmonale include neck vein distention, liver enlargement, and peripheral edema. Nonspecific radiographic signs of emphysema are flattening of the diaphragms, irregular lung lucency, and reduction or absence of pulmonary vascular markings.

COPD is confirmed by spirometry. The presence of a post-bronchodilator FEV_1 <80% of predicted and an FEV_1/FVC ratio <0.7 confirms the presence of airflow limitation. COPD severity is based on FEV_1 (Table 2). The BODE index for grading severity of COPD consists of the body-mass index (BMI), airflow obstruction, dyspnea, and the 6-minute walk distance; higher BODE scores are associated with a greater risk of death.

Static lung volumes including total lung capacity, residual volume, and functional residual capacity are all increased in advanced COPD. Diffusing capacity (DLco) is reduced, particularly in emphysema. Obtain an oxygen saturation measurement and arterial blood gas measurement if oximetry screen suggests hypoxemia (<94% on room air) or if there is suspicion of hypercapnia.

Table 1. Differential Diagnosis of Chronic Obstructive Pulmonary Disease (COPD)

Disease	Notes
Asthma	Onset typically in childhood, although may occur at any age; history of allergy often present; lability of symptoms with overt wheezing and rapid response to β-agonist bronchodilators are typical. Asthma may be present in about 10% of cases of COPD.
Bronchiectasis	Often excessive sputum production with purulent exacerbations; chest x-ray and CT scan may be diagnostic showing thickened and cystic airways; often a specific inciting event may be recognized, such as pneumonia in childhood.
Cystic fibrosis	Positive sweat-chloride test; onset usually at birth but, in rare cases, may not present until adulthood; cystic fibrosis transmembrane regulator test abnormal in many cases.
Bronchiolitis	Onset often occurs after respiratory tract infection; may be idiopathic or associated with other diseases such as rheumatoid arthritis; poorly responsive to bronchodilators. Postviral bronchiolitis is usually self-limited over a period of up to 3 months. Oral corticosteroids may be helpful in some cases of bronchiolitis.
Upper airway obstruction (e.g., vocal cord paralysis, tumors of the trachea, tracheal stenosis, vocal cord dysfunction)	Symptoms are usually shortness of breath with wheezing or stridor, which may be both inspiratory and expiratory if the obstruction is extrathoracic. Flow-volume curve may show a characteristic expiratory or inspiratory plateau or both. Diagnosis usually requires CT or MRI scan and direct visualization of the affected airway by endoscopy. Upper airway obstruction usually mimics asthma and is more often in the differential diagnosis of asthma; however, patients who have been previously intubated are at risk for subsequent vocal cord paralysis and tracheal stenosis.

CT = computed tomography; MRI = magnetic resonance imaging.

Table 2. Classification and Management of Chronic Obstructive Pulmonary Disease (COPD)*

Stage	Characteristics
0: At risk	• Normal spirometry • Chronic symptoms (cough, sputum production) • Avoidance of risk factors; influenza vaccination
I: Mild	• FEV_1/FVC <70%; FEV_1 ≥80% predicted • With or without chronic symptoms (cough, sputum production) • Add short-acting bronchodilator when needed
II: Moderate	• FEV_1/FVC <70%; 50% ≤FEV_1 <80% predicted • With or without chronic symptoms (cough, sputum production) • Add regular treatment with one or more long-acting bronchodilators; add rehabilitation
III: Severe	• FEV_1/FVC <70%; 30% ≤FEV_1 <50% predicted • With or without chronic symptoms (cough, sputum production) • Add inhaled corticosteroids if repeated exacerbations
IV: Very Severe	• FEV_1/FVC <70%: FEV_1 <30% predicted or FEV_1 <50% predicted plus chronic respiratory failure • Add long-term oxygen if chronic respiratory failure; consider surgical treatments

* Classification based on postbronchodilator FEV_1.

FEV_1 = forced expiratory volume in 1 sec; FVC = forced vital capacity.

Modified from Global Strategy for the Diagnosis, Management, and Prevention of Chronic Obstructive Pulmonary Disease (GOLD). National Heart, Lung, and Blood Institute, World Health Organization. Updated 2005; with permission.

Therapy

Smoking cessation slows the decline in pulmonary function. Pulmonary rehabilitation improves quality of life in patients with moderate to severe symptoms that persist despite optimal management. Exercise improves cardiovascular conditioning and increases ability to perform daily activities, and intensive counseling improves patient compliance and reinforces the proper use of pulmonary medications. Early pulmonary rehabilitation after hospitalization for an exacerbation leads to improved exercise capacity and health status.

In patients with COPD exacerbations, adjunctive non-drug therapies alleviate symptoms of shortness-of-breath and decrease sputum production. The following interventions may be considered: percussion, vibration, and postural drainage to enhance clearance of sputum; relaxation techniques to reduce anxiety from shortness of breath; control of breathing, pursed lips breathing, and diaphragmatic breathing to alleviate shortness of breath.

Surgical interventions, including bullectomy, lung-volume reduction surgery, and lung transplantation may improve symptoms. Lung-volume reduction surgery improves exercise capacity, lung function, dyspnea, and quality of life but does not confer an overall survival advantage. Patients with predominantly upper-lobe emphysema and low baseline exercise capacity may have improved survival.

Drug therapy in patients with COPD is used to alleviate symptoms, improve pulmonary function, and prevent complications. In general, all symptomatic patients should receive a trial of bronchodilator treatment. The approach to managing stable COPD is characterized by a step-wise increase in treatment (Table 2). Inhaled therapy is preferred over systemic agents. Metered-dose inhaler (MDI), with good technique, is as effective as a nebulizer.

Spacers reduce oropharyngeal deposition of drug and decrease subsequent local side effects. Nebulizers may benefit patients who cannot use MDIs because of severe dyspnea, difficulties with coordination, or physical problems such as arthritis.

Three types of bronchodilators are used to treat patients with COPD; β-agonists, anticholinergic agents, and methylxanthines all work by relaxing airway smooth muscle, thereby improving lung ventilation.

Short-acting β₂-adrenergic bronchodilators (e.g., albuterol) act within a few minutes of administration and their effect lasts approximately 4 to 6 hours. Give these as needed for relief of persistent or worsening symptoms and to improve exercise tolerance. Short-acting β-agonists and anticholinergics given by nebulizer are the preferred bronchodilators for hospital treatment of exacerbations of COPD along with oral or intravenous corticosteroids.

The long-acting β₂-agonists (e.g., salmeterol and formoterol) achieve sustained and more predictable improvement in lung function than the short-acting agents. They improve health status, reduce symptoms, decrease the need for rescue medication, and increase the time interval between exacerbations. Long-acting β₂-agonists, which are typically given every 12 hours, can be used as monotherapy or combined with other bronchodilators and inhaled corticosteroids for better control of chronic symptoms.

Vagal stimulation in the lung is mediated via muscarinic receptors. Anticholinergic drugs used to treat COPD include short-acting inhaled agents (e.g., ipratropium) and tiotropium, a long-acting bronchodilator used in stable outpatients. Tiotropium selectively blocks the M3 muscarinic receptor. Short-acting anticholinergics are less potent than long-acting β-agonists or long-acting anticholinergics. Anticholinergics in COPD are especially useful when combined with short-acting or long-acting β-agonists and/or theophylline. Tiotropium should not be combined with short-acting anticholinergics.

Theophylline is a nonspecific phosphodiesterase inhibitor that increases intracellular cyclic AMP within airway smooth muscle and inhibits intracellular calcium release. Theophylline also increases histone deacetylase activity, which may improve the efficacy of corticosteroids. The role of theophylline in COPD exacerbations is controversial; it may be used as an adjunct to aerosol bronchodilators and inhaled corticosteroids. Some patients with COPD may benefit from a trial of theophylline for 1 to 2 months. Maintain serum levels of 8 to12 µg/dL because of the narrow therapeutic window and toxicity. Sustained-release theophylline must be carefully monitored, especially in the elderly. Side effects include nausea, vomiting, and cardiac arrhythmias. Discontinue if symptomatic or objective benefit is not evident within several weeks.

Regular use of inhaled corticosteroids is associated with a reduction in the rate of exacerbations. Consider inhaled corticosteroids in patients whose lung function is less than 50% and those who have frequent exacerbations. Oral corticosteroids are not recommended for long-term maintenance. Use systemic (IV or oral) corticosteroids in acute exacerbations.

Although antibiotics are not generally recommended for regular use in COPD, they are useful in treating exacerbations. Increased sputum volume, purulence, and dyspnea in a patient with stable COPD should prompt consideration of antibiotic treatment. Sputum culture is usually unnecessary. Choose antibiotics according to community patterns of bacterial resistance and factors such as the stage of disease and recent exposure to antibiotics and systemic corticosteroids. Antibiotics are directed at common organisms (*Haemophilus influenzae*, *Streptococcus pneumoniae*, and *Moraxella catarrhalis*). Second- and third-generation cephalosporins, newer macrolides, amoxicillin/clavulanate, or fluoroquinolones may be necessary for patients who do not respond to tetracycline or trimethoprim/sulfamethoxazole or for patients with β-lactamase–producing organisms in the sputum.

Administer annual influenza vaccination to all patients unless contraindicated because of hypersensitivity to egg protein. Administer pneumococcal vaccine to all patients and revaccinate those ≥65 years who were vaccinated before age 65 and more than 5 years previously.

Long-term oxygen therapy improves survival, exercise, sleep, and cognitive performance in advanced hypoxemic COPD. Use oxygen if there is hypoxemia at rest, during exercise, or during sleep. Patients receiving oxygen should have an initial follow-up within 3 months and at least yearly thereafter to determine if oxygen is still needed.

COPD exacerbation is characterized by a change in the patient's baseline dyspnea, cough, and/or sputum production beyond day-to-day variability. Refer patients to the emergency department with a severe exacerbation of COPD (loss of alertness or a combination of two or more of the following parameters: dyspnea at rest, respiratory rate ≥25/min, heart rate ≥110/min, or use of accessory respiratory muscles). Patients with acute or chronic respiratory failure are managed in the intensive care unit for possible assisted mechanical ventilation. After an acute exacerbation, most patients experience transitory or permanent decrease in quality of life and nearly 50% are readmitted more than once in the ensuing 6 months. Therefore, target reducing the number and severity of exacerbations through smoking cessation, preventive vaccination, compliance with maintenance medications, and early attention to mild exacerbations.

Follow-Up

Determine adherence to the medical regimen, response to therapy, and progression of disease. Ensure that patients participate in self-management of their disease by understanding the etiology, management, course, and prognosis. At follow-up, observe patients using inhalers and ensure that inhaler training is reinforced. Monitor pulmonary function periodically to determine need for change in therapy, including possible oxygen therapy.

Book Enhancement

Go to www.acponline.org/essentials/pulmonary-section.html to view flow volume loops, a CT scan of the chest, and an electrocardiogram showing multifocal atrial tachycardia, and to review effects of smoking cessation on lung function, inhaler instructions for patients, and commonly used medications and medication precautions. In *MKSAP for Students 4*, assess yourself with items 22-24 in the **Pulmonary Medicine** section.

Bibliography

Littner MR. Chronic Obstructive Pulmonary Disease. http://pier.acponline .org/physicians/diseases/d153. [Date accessed: 2008 Jan 11] In: PIER [online database]. Philadelphia: American College of Physicians; 2008.

Littner MR. In the clinic. Chronic obstructive pulmonary disease. Ann Intern Med. 2008;148:ITC3-1-ITC3-16. [PMID: 18316750]

Qaseem A, Snow V, Shekelle P, Sherif K, Wilt TJ, Weinberger S, Owens DK; Clinical Efficacy Assessment Subcommittee of the American College of Physicians. Diagnosis and management of stable chronic obstructive pulmonary disease: a clinical practice guideline from the American College of Physicians. Ann Intern Med. 2007;147:633-8. [PMID: 17975186]

Straus SE, McAlister FA, Sackett DL, Deeks JJ. The accuracy of patient history, wheezing, and laryngeal measurements in diagnosing obstructive airway disease. CARE-COAD1 Group. Clinical Assessment of the Reliability of the Examination-Chronic Obstructive Airways Disease. JAMA. 2000;283:1853-7. Erratum in: JAMA 2000;284:181. [PMID: 10770147]

Chapter 78

Obstructive Sleep Apnea

Arlina Ahluwalia, MD

Although more than 70 primary disorders of sleep have been identified, these conditions remain undiagnosed in a large proportion of patients. Within the subgroup of chronic respiratory sleep disorders, obstructive sleep apnea (OSA) is the most common diagnosis. OSA is characterized by recurrent episodes of partial or complete airway obstruction during sleep. Manifestations include limited attention and memory and significantly increased risk of motor vehicle accidents. The pathophysiology of pharyngeal collapse during sleep is not entirely understood. However, patients with OSA have smaller upper airways and substantial decrements in pharyngeal dilator muscle activity during sleep. Recurrent arousals from sleep, in addition to hypoxemia and hypercapnia, constitute the likely physiological mechanism for the characteristic daytime somnolence and sequelae of the disorder. Symptomatic OSA contributes to secondary hypertension, likely related to peripheral vasoconstriction from arousal-prompted sympathetic discharge. In addition, patients with severe OSA accompanied by marked hypoxemia may develop secondary polycythemia and related complications. Hemodynamic consequences include increased left and right ventricular afterload, decreased left ventricular compliance, and increased myocardial oxygen demand; heart failure and stroke are important sequelae of OSA.

Diagnosis

Obtain a sleep history from the patient and bed partner. Specifically address disruptive snoring, witnessed apnea, excessive daytime sleepiness (including while driving), fatigue, nasal congestion, weight gain, morning headaches, and number of hours slept per night (to rule out contributing sleep deprivation). Often patients do not report excessive daytime sleepiness because they accommodate to the symptom complex, so consider using the Epworth Sleepiness Scale (Table 1). This easily-administered, validated questionnaire, though not closely correlated specifically with OSA, is useful in assessing the need for diagnostic testing for sleep disorders.

While prevalence is higher in men, OSA is likely under-diagnosed and under-treated in women. Obesity, the most common risk factor, is associated with an 8-12-fold increased risk of OSA, though thinner, especially Asian, patients may also be affected. Other anatomic features associated with OSA include increased waist-hip ratio, self-reported large neck circumference (e.g., >40 cm [18 inch]), crowded pharynx (due to long, low-lying uvula/soft palate, macroglossia, or enlarged tonsils), nasal obstruction, retrognathia or overbite. Physical examination findings may include systemic hypertension, decreased oxygen saturation, nasal congestion, wheezing, an accentuated P_2 (suggesting pulmonary hypertension), or S_3 (suggesting heart failure).

Obtain a formal polysomnogram to confirm the diagnosis in a patient with a significant number of signs and symptoms of OSA or its complications. This sleep study measures respiratory events and hours of sleep, from which the apnea hypopnea index (AHI) is derived. An AHI of >5 per hour confirms OSA, and a combination of AHI, degree of sleepiness, and presence or absence of cardiovascular problems such as hypertension, stroke, or heart

Table 1. Epworth Sleepiness Scale

How likely are you to doze off or fall asleep in the following situations, in contrast to feeling just tired? This refers to your usual way of life in recent times. Even if you have not done some of these things recently, try to work out how they would have affected you. Use the following scale to choose the most appropriate number in each situation:

0 = would never doze   1 = slight chance of dozing   2 = moderate chance of dozing   3 = high chance of dozing

Situation	Chance of Dozing
Sitting and reading	
Watching TV	
Sitting, inactive in a public place (e.g., a theater or meeting)	
As a passenger in a car for an hour without a break	
Lying down to rest in the afternoon when circumstances permit	
Sitting and talking to someone	
Sitting quietly after a lunch without alcohol	
In a car, while stopped for a few minutes in traffic	
Range of scores is 0-24. Normal total score is <10. A total score ≥10 suggests daytime sleepiness.	(Total Score)

Adapted from Johns MW. A new method for measuring daytime sleepiness: the Epworth sleepiness scale. Sleep. 1991;14:540-5.

failure determines the severity of disease. Use of alternative home respiratory tests, even when interpreted by a certified sleep specialist, may provide less accurate results. Continuous positive airway pressure (CPAP) titration, if indicated, may be conducted in the same session as diagnostic polysomnography.

Consider additional testing to assess possible contributing factors or complications of OSA (Table 2). Order tests of thyroid function to exclude hypothyroidism, screen for acromegaly if clinically suspected, and obtain a complete blood count to assess for polycythemia that may accompany severe OSA. Perform daytime awake pulse oximetry; if a suspected OSA patient demonstrates hypoxemia in this setting, measure arterial blood gases to assess for obesity hypoventilation syndrome. Consider chest radiography or electrocardiography if suspicious for cardiac complications.

The broad differential diagnosis of OSA includes other primary sleep disorders (e.g., central sleep apnea, periodic limb movements of sleep, narcolepsy), medical conditions (e.g., obstructive lung disease, drug use, heart failure), depression, and neurologic disorders (e.g., stroke, movement disorder, seizures) that disturb sleep (Table 3).

Therapy

Treatment of OSA aims to improve daytime sleepiness and cognitive performance and to prevent sequelae of the syndrome.

Table 2. Laboratory and Other Studies for Obstructive Sleep Apnea (OSA)

Test	Notes
Polysomnogram	Considered gold standard test.
Reduced channel polysomnogram (usually includes respiratory monitoring and oximetry)	Sensitivity, 82%-94%; specificity, 82%-100%. Less expensive and less accurate than polysomnogram, but may offer increased access to diagnosis.
Overnight oximetry	Sensitivity, 87%; specificity, 65%; Overnight oximetry is not an accurate test for OSA.
TSH	Yield of 2%-3% in OSA patients; should be obtained in patients with recent weight gain and fatigue.
Complete blood count	Polycythemia can be a complication of severe OSA with accompanying severe hypoxemia.
Chest radiograph	If coexisting heart failure is suspected based on physical exam. Heart failure can be a complication of OSA.
Electrocardiogram	If coexisting heart failure is suspected based on physical exam. Heart failure can be a complication of OSA.
Arterial blood gases	If obesity hypoventilation syndrome is suspected, to look for hypercapnia and hypoxemia.

CT = computed tomography; MRI = magnetic resonance imaging; TSH = thyrotropin-stimulating hormone.

Table 3. Differential Diagnosis of Obstructive Sleep Apnea (OSA)

Disease	Notes
Central sleep apnea	Most commonly seen in patients with heart failure and stroke. Polysomnogram shows an absence of respiratory effort during apnea, distinguishing central from obstructive apnea.
Upper airway resistance syndrome (UARS)	Most commonly seen in loud snorers who complain of excessive sleepiness; sleep study shows a normal AHI <5. Polysomnogram shows that increased respiratory effort is causing frequent EEG interruptions during sleep. Symptoms and treatment are the same as for OSA.
Periodic limb movements of sleep	A neurologic disorder of unknown cause. Frequent episodes of leg kicking during sleep. Most common in patients on dialysis. Polysomnogram shows no evidence of sleep apnea.
Narcolepsy	Severe excessive sleepiness is present; peak age of onset is 15-25 years. Cataplexy (episodes of muscle weakness in response to emotion) is the most specific symptom. Polysomnogram does not show OSA or periodic limb movements, but multiple sleep latency tests show that patients fall asleep quickly and have REM sleep during short naps.
Obstructive or restrictive lung disease	Shortness of breath or cough may disturb sleep. Pulmonary function tests establish the diagnosis and can guide specific therapy.
GERD (see Chapter 17)	Cough or choking may disturb sleep. Acid or burning taste in the throat is helpful but may be absent. A successful empiric trial of treatment may confirm the diagnosis.
Sinusitis	Cough and drainage may disturb sleep. Clinical symptoms of nasal congestion or postnasal drip suggest the diagnosis.
Heart failure (see Chapter 6)	Dyspnea and cough may disturb sleep. Symptoms and exam usually suggest heart disease. Central sleep apnea may be seen in patients with severe heart failure and indicates a worse prognosis.
Epilepsy	Seizures may occur only at night, with or without motor activity. Neurology consultation and EEG testing are best approach.
Sleep deprivation or a short sleep schedule	Inadequate sleeping hours can cause daytime sleepiness; naps are usually refreshing, which is not typical for OSA. Review of sleep schedule is essential, and a trial of longer sleep hours may be helpful.
Hypothyroidism (see Chapter 10)	May have weight gain and fatigue. Only 2%-3% of OSA patients have hypothyroidism. Screen with a TSH test.
Acromegaly	Screen patients with compatible signs and symptoms. Treatment of acromegaly may significantly reduce OSA severity.

AHI = apnea-plus-hypopnea index; EEG = electroencephalogram; REM = rapid eye movement; TSH = thyrotropin stimulating hormone.

Lifestyle changes and CPAP form the cornerstone of therapy; dental devices or upper airway operations may play a role in selected cases.

Crucial lifestyle changes include weight loss (to increase airway size) of at least 10%, avoidance of alcohol/sedatives (to maintain muscle tone of airway dilators) 3-4 hours before bedtime, and lateral sleeping position (to render airway less collapsible). If nasal obstruction or congestion continues after treatment with nasal corticosteroids and decongestants for rhinitis, consider surgical procedures to restore nasal patency.

If moderate-severe OSA persists despite these interventions, nightly CPAP is instituted. This most consistently effective therapy pneumatically splints the entire airway, preventing collapse during sleep. CPAP raises intraluminal airway pressure and increases functional residual capacity. Regular use of CPAP may dramatically improve quality of life by increasing daytime alertness, decreasing hypertension, and eliminating apneic episodes. However, adherence to CPAP is particularly challenging; measures shown to improve compliance include early patient education, follow-up, and establishing a comfortable interface for the CPAP device (nasal mask or nasal pillows). Patients still uncomfortable with CPAP may benefit from a trial of bilevel positive airway pressure (BiPAP), allowing higher inspiratory and lower expiratory pressure settings, or auto-titrating positive pressure devices. The precise role of supplemental oxygen is not yet determined.

Consider oral (dental) appliances or surgical intervention, most commonly uvulopalatopharyngoplasty, as alternative therapies in patients who are unable or unwilling to use CPAP. Resection of enlarged, obstructing tonsils may be beneficial. Oral appliances aim to open the posterior airway space usually by protruding the lower jaw or holding the tongue forward, but eliminate the need for CPAP in only mild-moderate disease. Surgical procedures for OSA, designed to alleviate retropalatal and retroglossal obstruction of the hypoglossal space, have variable success rates depending on complex factors, including BMI, severity of OSA, and individual anatomy.

If CPAP and other non-drug therapies are ineffective, consider a trial of fluoxetine, modafinil, or protriptyline as second-line treatment. These drugs reduce the amount of REM sleep; because REM is often associated with more severe oxygen desaturation, its reduction is associated with an increase in the average oxygen saturation. Antidepressants also increase upper airway muscle tone, but there is no evidence that this increases airway patency. Treatment with these agents is limited due to variable effectiveness and side-effects.

Follow-Up

Arrange follow-up in 1 to 2 months to assess adherence to treatment and change in symptoms, especially daytime sleepiness, and for continued emphasis on weight loss in obese patients. Nonadherence, erroneously titrated CPAP, or coexisting periodic limb movements in sleep may contribute to persistent sleepiness. Perform repeat sleep study if significant lifestyle goals have been attained to assess whether OSA is resolved or if CPAP should be adjusted. Monitor patients with moderate-severe OSA for potentially related cognitive, cardiovascular, or obesity-metabolic conditions.

Book Enhancement

Go to www.acponline.org/essentials/pulmonary-section.html to view a polysomnogram and a video of a patient with sleep apnea. In *MKSAP for Students 4*, assess yourself with item 25 in the **Pulmonary Medicine** section.

Bibliography

Basner RC. Continuous positive airway pressure for obstructive sleep apnea. N Engl J Med. 2007;356:1751-8. [PMID: 17460229]

Claman D. Obstructiv e Sleep Apnea. http://pier.acponline.org/physicians/diseases/d351. [Date accessed: 2008 Jan 30] In: PIER [online database]. Philadelphia: American College of Physicians; 2008.

Guilleminault C, Abad VC. Obstructive sleep apnea syndromes. Med Clin North Am. 2004;88:611-30. [PMID: 15087207]

Chapter 79

Infiltrative and Fibrotic Lung Diseases

Janet N. Myers, MD

The term *diffuse parenchymal lung disease* (DPLD) comprises over 200 distinct disorders that cause infiltration of the gas-exchanging components of the lungs. DPLD is characterized clinically by dyspnea on exertion, cough, and radiographic findings of diffuse pulmonary infiltrates. "Diffuse" suggests widespread involvement of the lungs; however, the process may not affect the lung uniformly and some areas may be spared. Alveolar filling processes are included with DPLD because of the similarity in presentation.

Recent guidelines for the classification of DPLD recommend grouping the disorders into four categories: DPLD of known cause (e.g., drugs, systemic illness such as collagen vascular disease, environmental exposure, infections, or neoplasm); granulomatous DPLD (e.g., sarcoidosis or hypersensitivity pneumonitis); rare DPLD with well-defined features (e.g., lymphangioleiomyomatosis, Langerhans cell histiocytosis, pulmonary alveolar proteinosis, and eosinophilic pneumonia); and idiopathic interstitial pneumonias. The idiopathic interstitial pneumonias are further classified into groups of disorders with distinct clinical and pathologic features. Idiopathic pulmonary fibrosis (IPF) and sarcoidosis are the most common of the chronic DPLDs. Some disorders such as heart failure, chronic aspiration, and acute respiratory distress syndrome may present with the radiographic appearance of DPLD and are considered elsewhere. Key features of selected DPLDs are summarized in Table 1.

Table 1. Distinguishing Features of Selected Diffuse Parenchymal Lung Diseases

Diffuse Parenchymal Lung Diseases with Known Causes	
Pneumoconioses	Asbestosis (pleural plaques on chest x-ray); silicosis ("eggshell" calcification on chest x-ray).
Drug-induced	Two general patterns: chronic form similar to idiopathic pulmonary fibrosis and acute hypersensitivity lung disease with peripheral or tissue eosinophilia.
Infections	Viral, atypical bacteria (e.g., *M. pneumoniae, L. pneumophila, C. pneumoniae*), fungal (*Pneumocystis*), and *Mycobacteria*.
Malignancy	Lymphangitic carcinomatosis (breast, stomach, lung, pancreas, and kidney) associated with insidious onset of cough and dyspnea.
Idiopathic Interstitial Pneumonias	
Idiopathic pulmonary fibrosis	Chronic progressive dyspnea and cough; clubbing is common; x-ray shows basilar infiltrates with fibrosis and honeycombing.
Diffuse interstitial pneumonia or respiratory bronchiolitis with interstitial lung disease	"Smoker's bronchiolitis"; x-ray shows "ground-glass" appearance (hazy opacity indicating filling of alveoli or thickening of the interstitium).
Acute interstitial pneumonia (Hamman-Rich syndrome)	Dense bilateral acute lung injury similar to acute respiratory distress syndrome.
Non-specific interstitial pneumonia	May be responsive to immunomodulating drugs; x-ray shows "ground-glass" without fibrosis.
Cryptogenic organizing pneumonia	May be preceded by a "flu-like" illness; x-ray shows focal areas of consolidation.
Diffuse Parenchymal Lung Diseases Associated with Collagen Vascular Diseases	
Rheumatoid arthritis	Pleural effusions, necrobiotic pulmonary nodules, and interstitial lung disease.
Systemic lupus erythematosus	May present with fever, dyspnea, and hemoptysis or a "shrinking lung" syndrome due to diaphragmatic dysfunction and atelectasis.
Scleroderma/systemic sclerosis	Primary interstitial lung disease and secondary to chronic aspiration; pulmonary hypertension can occur in absence of interstitial disease.
Polymyositis/dermatomyositis	Interstitial lung disease, respiratory muscle weakness, and aspiration.
Granulomatous Diffuse Parenchymal Lung Diseases	
Hypersensitivity pneumonitis	Allergic reaction to inhaled low-molecular-weight antigens; presentation may be acute or chronic.
Sarcoidosis	Cough and dyspnea common but may be asymptomatic. Löfgren's syndrome (fever, erythema nodosa, arthralgia, and hilar lymphadenopathy) has a benign course. Stage I (bilateral hilar adenopathy); Stage II (adenopathy, interstitial lung disease); Stage III (interstitial lung disease); Stage IV (fibrosis).

Evaluation

The process of determining a specific diagnosis from such a broad spectrum of diseases can be daunting. Important points to keep in mind are clinical history and physical findings, tempo of disease progression, and radiographic distribution and pattern of the infiltrate. Depending on these factors, a tentative diagnosis may be confirmed with appropriate diagnostic testing, which may include biopsy.

The patient history should include age, sex, smoking history, current and previous illnesses, immunocompromising conditions including HIV infection, prescription and over-the-counter medications, environmental and occupational exposures, travel, and family history. For example, patients with a history of malignancy may present with DPLD when there is lymphangitic spread. Common causes of pulmonary drug toxicity include antibiotics such as nitrofurantoin, anti-inflammatory drugs such as methotrexate, antiarrhythmics such as amiodarone, or chemotherapeutic drugs such as bleomycin. Environmental exposures, such as asbestos, may be remote or subtle and may not be considered important by the patient. Exposure to low-molecular weight organic antigens from sources such as moldy hay, bird feathers, or mycobacteria found in hot tubs can cause acute or chronic forms of hypersensitivity pneumonitis.

Systemic illnesses may have specific findings that provide clues to the illness. For example, pleuritic chest pain suggests collagen vascular diseases such as systemic lupus erythematosus or rheumatoid arthritis, and hemoptysis suggests an alveolar hemorrhage syndrome due to Goodpasture's syndrome. Some unusual causes of DPLD occur in specific groups. Lymphangioleiomyomatosis, a disorder of smooth muscle proliferation in the lung, primarily affects young women. Other disorders such as respiratory bronchiolitis interstitial lung disease or Langerhans cell histiocytosis are seen predominantly in heavy smokers. Some DPLD may be genetic, as in familial forms of sarcoidosis or interstitial pulmonary fibrosis.

Determining the timing of onset of symptoms or radiographic changes is helpful in diagnosis. Symptoms may be insidious in onset over months to years, as in many of the idiopathic interstitial pneumonias or pneumoconioses. Alternatively, rapidly progressive symptoms of dyspnea and radiographic changes over days to weeks may indicate an acute process such as heart failure, allergy, acute interstitial pneumonia, or drug reaction. Patients with cryptogenic organizing pneumonia may describe an antecedent flu-like illness. A pneumothorax suggests lymphangioleiomyomatosis in a young woman or Langerhans cell histiocytosis in a male smoker.

Physical examination findings are often nonspecific and may include basilar (Velcro-like) crackles. Velcro crackles are common in patients with interstitial lung disease and are frequently heard in patients with IPF, but are rarely present in patients with sarcoidosis. Similarly, clubbing has been described in as many as two-thirds of patients with IPF (Plate 42), but is rare in patients with sarcoidosis. Evidence of right heart failure (jugular venous distention, prominent P_2, right ventricular heave) may be seen in advanced lung disease. The examination should include a careful search for extrapulmonary involvement (e.g., skin, joint, and neurologic findings), suggesting an underlying systemic illness (Table 2).

Laboratory evaluation should include a complete blood count with differential, standard metabolic panel, antinuclear antibody, rheumatoid factor, and urinalysis. Where indicated, additional helpful tests may include extractable nuclear antigen, anti-double-stranded DNA, antineutrophil cytoplasmic antibody (ANCA), anti-glomerular basement (anti-GBM) antibody, electrocardiogram, or echocardiogram (Table 3).

Obtain chest x-ray, CT scan, and high-resolution computed tomography (HRCT). In the appropriate clinical setting, radiographic patterns on HRCT scan may indicate specific diagnoses and provide an assessment of disease activity. For example, "honeycomb" fibrosis, characterized by clusters or rows of cysts <5 mm with shared walls, is typically associated with end-stage, refractory disease, while a "ground-glass" appearance (hazy opacity indicating filling of alveoli or thickening of the interstitium) is associated with active inflammation that may be amenable to therapy. Certain radiographic patterns are suggestive of specific diseases. For example, reticular lower lobe infiltrates with peripheral involvement, traction bronchiectasis and honeycombing suggest IPF (Figure 1); a reverse heart failure pattern suggests chronic eosinophilic pneumonia; diffuse cystic disease suggests lymphangioleiomyomatosis or Langerhans cell histiocytosis; and nodules may indicate metastatic disease or miliary tuberculosis.

Obtain pulmonary function tests (spirometry plus lung volumes) and diffusion capacity for carbon monoxide (DLCO). Patients with DPLD frequently have evidence of restriction with a decreased DLCO. Arterial blood gas abnormalities typically include resting or exercise hypoxemia.

Bronchoalveolar lavage is a procedure where segments of lung are "washed" during bronchoscopy and the fluid collected and analyzed; the procedure is associated with little risk and may help exclude infection. Bronchoalveolar lavage can be diagnostic for lymphangitic carcinomatosis, pulmonary alveolar proteinosis, and pulmonary infiltrates with eosinophilia syndromes. Tissue biopsy with a transbronchial lung biopsy via bronchoscopy, video-assisted thoracoscopic lung biopsy, or open lung biopsy may be necessary to confirm a diagnosis. Surgical lung biopsy carries greater risk, and benefits should be weighed against the potential for harm.

The most common form of DPLD is IPF (also called cryptogenic fibrosing alveolitis), accounting for up to 35% of DPLD cases. A definitive diagnosis requires a biopsy specimen showing evidence of usual interstitial pneumonia (UIP), characterized by patchy collagen fibrosis and scarring in a peripheral pattern with subpleural fibrotic, honeycomb-like changes. Because UIP is not specific for IPF, the diagnosis is one of exclusion. The diagnosis may be made presumptively, in the appropriate clinical setting, such as an older patient with gradually worsening dyspnea, Velcro-like crackles, restrictive pulmonary function tests, diminished DLCO, and a HRCT with reticular subpleural infiltrates and predominantly basilar honeycomb-like fibrosis.

Sarcoidosis, a multisystem disorder of unknown etiology, is the second most common DPLD. The hallmark of sarcoidosis is non-caseating epithelioid cell granulomas in the absence of infection or malignancy. Patients with sarcoidosis are usually younger than

Table 2. Clinical Clues for Causes of Diffuse Parenchymal Lung Disease

Finding	Notes
Age	IPF often >60 years; CVD, sarcoidosis, LAM, LCH usually 20-40 years
Female	LAM and TS almost exclusively
Smoking	Most associated with RB-ILD, DIP, LCH
Exposure	Occupational (e.g., asbestos, silica) and HP (e.g., moldy hay, birds)
Acute onset (days to weeks)	Infection, AIP, AEP, COP, drug-induced ILD, DAH syndrome
Velcro-like crackles	>80% IPF, common in many ILDs
Increased P_2, RV lift, TR murmur	Pulmonary hypertension secondary to advanced ILD or as a specific feature of underlying disease (e.g., scleroderma)
Clubbing	Common in IPF (30%)
Erythema nodosum	Variable association with sarcoidosis, IBD, Behçet's
Maculopapular exanthem	Variable association with sarcoidosis, amyloidosis, Behçet's
Uveitis/conjunctivitis	Variable association with sarcoidosis, Behçet's, AS
Lacrimal/salivary gland enlargement	Variable association with sarcoidosis, Sjögren's syndrome
Adenopathy, hepatosplenomegaly	Variable association with sarcoidosis, amyloidosis
Arthritis	Variable association with CVD, sarcoidosis, Behçet's, AS
Muscle weakness	Polymyositis, dermatomyositis
Neurological abnormalities	Sarcoidosis (cranial nerve deficits), TS (mental retardation)
Response to steroids	COP, LIP good response; IPF, AIP poor response

AIP = acute interstitial pneumonia; AEP = acute eosinophilic pneumonia; AS = ankylosing spondylitis; COP = cryptogenic organizing pneumonia; CVD = collagen vascular disease; DAH = diffuse alveolar hemorrhage; DIP = diffuse interstitial pneumonitis; HP = hypersensitivity pneumonitis; IBD = inflammatory bowel disease; ILD = interstitial lung disease; IPF = idiopathic pulmonary fibrosis; LAM = lymphangioleiomyomatosis; LCH = Langerhans cell histiocytosis; LIP = lymphoid interstitial pneumonia; P_2 = pulmonic component second heart sound; RB-ILD = respiratory bronchiolitis-associated interstitial lung disease; RV = right ventricle; TR = tricuspid regurgitation; TS = tuberous sclerosis. Modified with permission from MKSAP 14, American College of Physicians; 2006.

Table 3. Laboratory Findings in Diffuse Parenchymal Lung Diseases

Finding	Notes
Eosinophilia	Eosinophilic pneumonia, sarcoidosis, systemic vasculitis, drug-induced.
Hemolytic anemia	Collagen vascular disease, sarcoidosis, lymphoma, drug-induced.
Normocytic anemia	Diffuse alveolar hemorrhage syndromes, connective tissue disease, lymphangitic carcinomatosis.
Urinary sediment abnormalities	Systemic vasculitis (collagen vascular disease, Wegener's granulomatosis, Goodpasture's syndrome), drug-induced.
Hypogammaglobulinemia	Lymphocytic interstitial pneumonitis, underlying common variable immunodeficiency.
Serum angiotensin converting enzyme	Non-specific. May be seen in sarcoidosis, hypersensitivity pneumonitis, silicosis, Gaucher's disease.
Anti-nuclear antibody (ANA), rheumatoid factor (RF)	Evaluate for collagen vascular disease. Low-titer ANA and RF may be present in 10%-20% of idiopathic pulmonary fibrosis patients.
Anti-glomerular basement membrane (Anti-GBM) antibody	Diagnostic of Goodpasture's syndrome in patient with alveolar hemorrhage.
Antineutrophil cytoplasmic antibody	Wegener's granulomatosis, Churg-Strauss syndrome, microscopic polyangiitis.
Serum precipitating antibodies	Non-specific. May indicate hypersensitivity pneumonitis.

Modified from Medical Knowledge Self-Assessment Program (MKSAP) 14. Philadelphia: American College of Physicians; 2006.

40 years. Chest radiography commonly demonstrates mediastinal and bilateral hilar lymphadenopathy with or without parenchymal involvement. HRCT may reveal nodular infiltrates in a perilymphatic distribution with a mid-to-upper lung field predominance; in IPF the infiltrates are more peripheral and basilar. Pleural effusions are uncommon. Bronchoscopy with biopsy is helpful in the diagnosis of sarcoidosis.

Therapy

Referral to a pulmonary specialist is strongly recommended. Encourage all patients to stop smoking and provide supportive care, including oxygen, symptomatic treatment for reactive airways or cough, maintenance of nutrition and fitness, and treatment of infections. Wherever possible, suspected causative exposures should be

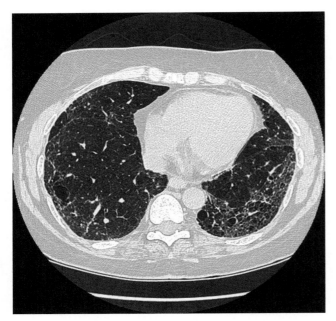

Figure 1 High-resolution thin-section CT scan showing extensive parenchymal involvement with fibrotic and "honeycomb" changes.

eliminated. In these cases, the DPLD may remit. Smoking cessation may result in stabilization or remission of Langerhans cell histiocytosis or respiratory bronchiolitis interstitial lung disease. Patients with DPLD due to collagen vascular disease are treated for the underlying disease. Sarcoidosis will frequently remit spontaneously and the need for treatment is controversial but may include corticosteroids and/or immunosuppressive or cytotoxic drugs.

Immunosuppressive agents and corticosteroids have limited efficacy in the treatment of IPF and side effects often complicate their use. If drug therapy is offered to a patient, it should be started at the initial indication of impairment or decline in lung function before irreversible fibrosis develops. Treatment is discontinued if no improvement is seen, or if significant side effects develop. Patients younger than 60 years may be candidates for lung transplantation and should be referred early to appropriate centers.

Book Enhancement

Go to www.acponline.org/essentials/pulmonary-section.html to access an extensive differential diagnosis, a staging scheme for sarcoidosis, and to view x-rays of interstitial lung disease and digital clubbing. In *MKSAP for Students 4*, assess yourself with items 26-29 in the **Pulmonary Medicine** section.

Bibliography

American Thoracic Society; European Respiratory Society. International Multidisciplinary Consensus Classification of the Idiopathic Interstitial Pneumonias. This joint statement of the American Thoracic Society (ATS) and the European Respiratory Society (ERS) was adopted by the ATS board of directors on June 2001 and by the ERS Executive Committee on June 2001. Am J Respir Crit Care Med. 2002;165:277-304. Erratum in: Am J Respir Crit Care Med. 2002;166:426. [PMID: 11790668]

Ryu JH, Daniels CE, Hartman TE, Yi ES. Diagnosis of interstitial lung diseases. Mayo Clin Proc. 2007;82:976-86. [PMID: 17673067]

Chapter 80

Venous Thromboembolism

Alpesh N. Amin, MD

Pulmonary thromboembolism and deep vein thrombosis are different manifestations of the same disease, often collectively referred to as venous thromboembolism (VTE). An estimated 2 million cases of deep venous thrombosis, 600,000 cases of symptomatic pulmonary embolism, and 300,000 VTE-related deaths occur annually in the United States. The pathophysiology of pulmonary thromboembolism includes formation of deep venous thrombosis and subsequent embolization into the pulmonary arteries. The thrombotic material obstructing blood flow through the pulmonary arteries has several physiologic consequences, including ventilation/perfusion aberrations and relative ischemia of the peripheral lung tissues. The most important clinical effect, however, is an acute increase in pulmonary vascular resistance, which increases the demand on the right ventricle and may lower cardiac output. In its extreme form, this combination of effects can cause right ventricular dysfunction, infarction, and even cardiac arrest. The differential diagnosis of deep venous thrombosis and pulmonary embolism are reviewed in Tables 1 and 2.

Table 1. Differential Diagnosis of Deep Venous Thrombosis (DVT)

Disease	Notes
Venous insufficiency (venous reflux)	Usually due to venous hypertension from such causes as venous reflux or obesity. Obtain ultrasound evaluation of venous reflux.
Superficial thrombophlebitis	Firm, tender, varicose vein. Superficial thrombosis is rarely associated with DVT.
Muscle strain, tear, or trauma	Pain occurring with range of motion more characteristic of orthopedic problem due to trauma. Usually history of leg injury.
Baker's cyst	Frequent pain localized to popliteal region of leg. Seen on ultrasonography.
Cellulitis	Skin erythema and warmth.
Lymphedema	Toe edema is more characteristic of lymphedema than of venous edema. Lymphedema can occur in one or both legs.

Table 2. Differential Diagnosis of Pulmonary Embolism (PE)

Disease	Notes
Acute coronary syndrome (see Chapter 3)	Chest pain associated with specific ECG and echocardiographic changes. Elevated cardiac enzymes help establish diagnosis of infarction but can also be seen with hemodynamically significant pulmonary emboli.
Pericarditis (see Chapter 1)	Substernal chest discomfort that can be sharp, dull, or pressure-like in nature, often relieved with sitting forward. Usually pleuritic. ECG abnormalities are often present, including ST-segment elevation (usually diffuse) or more specifically PR segment depression, also ST-segment depression (less frequent).
Aortic dissection (see Chapter 1)	Substernal chest pain with radiation to the back, mid-scapular region. Often described as "tearing" or "ripping" type pain. Chest x-ray may show a widened mediastinal silhouette, a pleural effusion, or both.
Acute pulmonary edema (see Chapter 6)	Elevated venous pressure, S_3, bilateral crackles and characteristic chest radiography are diagnostic.
Exacerbation of pulmonary hypertension	Persistently split S_2, right sternal heave; tricuspid insufficiency murmur. History of pulmonary hypertension is helpful; however, worsening should prompt consideration of PE as a precipitating factor.
Pleurisy	Sharp, localized chest pain; may be associated with fever; diagnosis of exclusion.
Pneumothorax	Sudden onset of chest pain and dyspnea. Plain chest radiography or CT establishes the diagnosis.
Acute bronchitis or pneumonia	Cough, fever, sputum production. Clinical history, radiographic findings, sputum examination and cultures help differentiate infection from PE.
Exacerbation of asthma and chronic obstructive pulmonary disease	Dyspnea, wheezing and positive response to bronchodilator (asthma). History of these disorders with a compatible course of illness is helpful.
Panic attack	Diagnosis of exclusion; may have a history of somatization.

CT = computed tomography; ECG = electrocardiography

Prevention

Consider VTE prophylaxis for all patients admitted to the hospital, especially medical patients who are immobilized, most surgical patients, and patients who have had major trauma. Prevention techniques include the following:

- Low-dose, subcutaneous unfractionated heparin or low-molecular-weight heparin in high-risk medical patients and in surgical patients except those at highest risk for bleeding
- Warfarin or low-molecular-weight heparin in patients undergoing hip or knee replacement, patients aged >40 years undergoing general surgery for malignancy, and patients with a thrombophilic state
- Fondaparinux (inactivates factor Xa) can also be used for patients undergoing hip and knee replacements
- Pneumatic compression with graduated compression stockings for patients at high risk for bleeding with anticoagulation
- Low-molecular-weight heparin for prophylaxis of VTE in patients with cancer

Screening

Do not routinely screen for deep venous thrombosis in high-risk patients. Noninvasive diagnostic tests are not recommended because they are insensitive and not associated with improved clinical outcomes.

Diagnosis

The diagnosis of VTE begins with a detailed history of risk factors, including current malignancy, past history of VTE, recent immobilization, hospitalization, major surgery, increasing age, obesity, trauma, smoking, acute myocardial infarction, heart failure, coagulopathy, pregnancy, postpartum state, and estrogen therapy.

The most common symptom associated with deep venous thrombosis is calf pain, but many patients are asymptomatic. On physical examination, look for posterior calf tenderness and leg edema. Because signs and symptoms of deep venous thrombosis are nonspecific, clinical prediction rules assist in identifying patients who require further diagnostic testing. Wells' clinical prediction rule is a validated tool for assessing the likelihood of deep venous thrombosis (Table 3); using this tool, a patient's likelihood of deep venous thrombosis is determined to be low, intermediate, or high. Select lower-extremity venous ultrasonography in patients with a high likelihood for deep venous thrombosis. Measure D-dimer levels in patients with a low or intermediate probability of deep venous thrombosis and perform lower-extremity ultrasonography if D-dimer results are positive (Table 4).

The most common symptoms of pulmonary embolism are dyspnea, pleuritic chest pain, cough, and hemoptysis, and the most common physical findings are tachypnea, rales, tachycardia, and S_4 gallop; while these symptoms and signs are relatively sensitive, they lack specificity. Arterial blood gases are frequently obtained, but the distributions of PaO_2 and alveolar-arterial oxygen gradient are similar in patients with and without pulmonary embolism; approximately one of every four patients with pulmonary embolism has a $PaO_2 \geq 80$ mm Hg.

Obtain a chest x-ray on all patients; look for atelectasis, pleural effusion, focal oligemia (lack of vascularity), peripheral wedge-shaped density above the diaphragm, and an enlarged right descending pulmonary artery. An electrocardiogram is often abnormal, but positive findings lack sensitivity and specificity; the most common abnormality is sinus tachycardia. However, rhythm disturbances, right bundle branch block, and a right ventricular strain pattern may be seen in pulmonary embolism.

Estimate the pretest clinical probability of pulmonary embolism based on the initial assessment before further diagnostic imaging (Table 5). Note that post-test probability depends on pretest clinical probability and the result of pulmonary imaging.

Consider the advantages and limitations of each when choosing ventilation/perfusion scanning or CT angiography as the initial pulmonary imaging study (Table 6). Conventional pulmonary angiography remains the reference standard for diagnosing

Table 3. Modified Wells Clinical Score for Deep Venous Thrombosis

Clinical Characteristic	Score
Active cancer (treatment ongoing, within 6 months, or palliative)	1
Paralysis, paresis, or recent plaster immobilization of the lower extremities	1
Recently bedridden >3 days or major surgery ≤12 weeks ago requiring general or regional anesthesia	1
Localized tenderness along the distribution of the deep venous system	1
Entire leg swollen	1
Calf swelling >3 cm larger than asymptomatic side (measured 10 cm below the tibial tuberosity)	1
Pitting edema confined to the symptomatic leg	1
Collateral superficial veins (nonvaricose)	1
Previously documented deep venous thrombosis	1
Alternative diagnosis at least as likely as deep venous thrombosis	−2
Score (Probability of deep venous thrombosis)	**Likelihood Ratio**
>2 (High)	5.2
1 or 2 (Intermediate)	1
<1 (Low)	0.25

Modified from Wells PS, Anderson DR, Bormanis J, Guy F, Mitchell M, Gray L, et al. Value of assessment of pretest probability of deep-vein thrombosis in clinical management. Lancet. 1997;350:1795-8; with permission.

Table 4. Laboratory and Other Studies for Suspected Deep Venous Thrombosis (DVT)

Test	Notes
D-dimer (ELISA)	Sensitivity for proximal DVT, 98%; specificity, 45%. Usually used in combination with ultrasound or clinical scoring.
Duplex Doppler ultrasound	Sensitivity for proximal DVT, 96%; specificity, 94%. Combines Doppler audio measurements of blood flow with visual ultrasound imaging.
Compression ultrasound	Sensitivity for proximal DVT, 94%; specificity, 98%. The compressibility of the proximal veins is assessed with the ultrasound probe.
Venography	Sensitivity, 100%; specificity, 100%. Of limited value if there is poor contrast filling of the deep veins; however, it is the historical "gold standard."
MRV	Sensitivity for proximal DVT, 94%; specificity 95%. MRV is more expensive than ultrasound imaging. Contraindicated for patients with metal devices.

ELISA = enzyme-linked immunosorbent assay; MRV = magnetic resonance venography.

Table 5. Simplified Wells Scoring System for Pulmonary Embolism

Findings	Score*
• Clinical signs/symptoms of deep venous thrombosis (minimum of leg swelling and pain with palpation of the deep veins of the leg)	3.0
• No alternative diagnosis likely or more likely than pulmonary emboli	3.0
• Heart rate >100/min	1.5
• Immobilization or surgery in the past 4 weeks	1.5
• Previous history of deep venous thrombosis or pulmonary emboli	1.5
• Hemoptysis	1.0
• Cancer actively treated within the last 6 months	1.0

* Summed probability scores are as follows: low, <2; moderate, 2-6; high, >6.
Modified from Chunilal SD, Eikelboom JW, Attia J, et al. Does this patient have pulmonary embolism? JAMA. 2003;290:2849-58; with permission.

Table 6. Laboratory and Other Studies for Pulmonary Embolism (PE)

Test	Notes
Plain chest radiograph	Sensitivity, 84%; specificity, 44%. Atelectasis and parenchymal abnormalities are most common (68%), followed by pleural effusion (48%), pleural-based opacity (35%), elevated diaphragm (24%), decreased pulmonary vascularity (21%), prominent central pulmonary artery (15%), cardiomegaly (12%), and pulmonary edema (4%).
12-lead electrocardiogram	Sensitivity, 50%; specificity, 88%. Most common abnormalities are ST segment and T wave changes (49%). P pulmonale, right axis deviation, right bundle branch block and right ventricular hypertrophy occur less frequently. T wave inversions in precordial leads may indicate more severe right ventricular dysfunction.
PaO$_2$ and alveolar-arterial oxygen gradient	Sensitivity, 81%; specificity, 24%. Distributions of PaO$_2$ and alveolar-arterial oxygen gradient are similar in patients with and without pulmonary embolism.
D-dimer (ELISA)	Sensitivity, 80%-100%; specificity, 10%-64%. D-dimer levels <500 ng/mL have a high negative predictive value, useful to exclude PE in patients with low pretest probability or nondiagnostic lung scan. D-dimer measurement is less useful in patients with malignancy, recent surgery or trauma, and liver disease because only a few have D-dimer levels <500 ng/mL.
Ventilation-perfusion lung scan	Normal scan excludes pulmonary embolism. High-probability scan with high pretest clinical probability almost certainly confirms PE. Other scan results should be considered nondiagnostic and indicate need for further testing. Pulmonary embolism is present in 87% of patients with a high-probability scan, 30% of patients with an intermediate-probability and 14% of patients with a low-probability scan. Independent assessment of pretest probability should be combined with lung scan results to improve diagnostic accuracy.
Pulmonary angiography	Pulmonary angiography is considered the gold standard diagnostic test for pulmonary embolism. It is indicated when noninvasive evaluation is nondiagnostic and clinical suspicion is high. Pulmonary angiography is not widely available in community practice, and its accuracy in this setting is unclear.
Contrast-enhanced spiral CT of the chest	Sensitivity (53%-100%) and specificity (81%-100%) of CT are higher for main, lobar and segmental vessel emboli. An advantage of CT is the diagnosis of other pulmonary parenchymal, pleural or cardiovascular processes causing or contributing to symptoms.
Gadolinium-enhanced MR angiography	Sensitivity, 75%-100%; specificity, 95%-100%. MR angiography is expensive and not widely available, but is accurate and does not require iodinated contrast injection. It is also sensitive and specific for diagnosis of DVT and may permit concomitant evaluation and diagnosis of PE and DVT.
Echocardiography	Echocardiography is most useful in the evaluation of acute cardiopulmonary syndromes to help diagnose or exclude pericardial tamponade, aortic dissection, myocardial ischemia or infarction, valvular dysfunction and myocardial rupture.

CT = computed tomography; DVT = deep venous thrombosis; ELISA = enzyme-linked immunosorbent assay; MR = magnetic resonance.

pulmonary embolism but is rarely used because of its invasive nature and risk of contrast-induced nephropathy. In choosing ventilation/perfusion scanning, recognize that a normal ventilation/perfusion scan excludes pulmonary embolism. A high-probability scan in the right clinical setting is diagnostic, but scanning can be nondiagnostic in 40%-70% of patients, requiring additional tests to reach a decision regarding anticoagulation. If the ventilation/perfusion scan is of low or intermediate probability, interpret the results in light of the pretest probability for pulmonary embolism; if pretest probability is high, additional diagnostic tests are required, such as lower extremity ultrasonography or pulmonary angiography.

In choosing CT angiography, recognize that despite its excellent specificity and ability to provide alternative diagnoses, CT angiography may not visualize small subsegmental pulmonary emboli. In patients with a negative CT angiogram but high pretest probability, consider lower-extremity ultrasonography or a strategy combining CT venography and pulmonary angiography to image both areas.

A negative D-dimer test and low clinical probability of deep venous thrombosis or pulmonary embolism helps exclude these diagnoses. A positive D-dimer test does not establish the diagnosis of either deep venous thrombosis or pulmonary embolism.

Therapy

Treatment for VTE includes the use of heparin and warfarin. Intravenous unfractionated heparin or low-molecular-weight heparin therapy is used for VTE in hospitalized patients; low-molecular-weight heparin can be used for outpatient treatment of deep venous thrombosis in selected patients. In most patients, start heparin and warfarin immediately and allow at least 4 to 5 days of therapy on both before stopping heparin (provided that the INR [international normalized ratio] is in the therapeutic range). Continue warfarin for at least 3 months depending on the clinical situation. Adjust the dose of warfarin to achieve an INR of 2 to 3.

Patients without an identifiable risk factor are more likely to have a recurrent venous thrombosis and should be treated for a minimum of 6 months with warfarin. Recent clinical trials indicate that patients with idiopathic deep venous thrombosis may benefit from 2 years or more of oral anticoagulation.

Consider intravenous or catheter-directed thrombolysis with tissue plasminogen activator in selected patients with iliofemoral deep venous thrombosis. Successful thrombolysis may reduce the risk of postphlebitic syndrome. Consider thrombolytic therapy in patients with circulatory shock due to pulmonary embolism and in patients with acute embolism and pulmonary hypertension or right ventricular dysfunction but without arterial hypotension or shock. Rapid clot lysis may lead to hemodynamic improvement

and resolution of right ventricular dysfunction. The most important complication of thrombolytic therapy is bleeding.

Surgical embolectomy for massive pulmonary embolism is indicated if the patient is unstable or if drug therapy has been unsuccessful. Surgical embolectomy requires the immediate availability of cardiopulmonary bypass; the operative mortality ranges from 10%-75%.

Non-drug therapy for deep venous thrombosis is indicated in patients at risk for bleeding or who fail drug therapy. Inferior vena cava filters prevent pulmonary embolism in patients with deep venous thrombosis within the first 2 weeks of filter placement. After 1 year, patients may have higher incidence of postphlebitic syndrome and increased risk of recurrent lower extremity thromboses.

Deep venous thrombosis damages the venous valves in the lower limbs, resulting in chronic venous insufficiency that becomes manifest as lower-extremity edema, discoloration and, in many cases, chronic venous stasis ulcers. All patients with deep venous thrombosis should wear graduated compression stockings to reduce the risk of postphlebitic syndrome, which develops within 2 years in about 50% of patients after a first episode of proximal deep venous thrombosis.

Follow-Up

Once the level of anticoagulation is stable, monitor INR every 4 weeks for the duration of warfarin therapy.

Book Enhancement

Go to www.acponline.org/essentials/pulmonary-section.html to view a high probability ventilation/perfusion lung scan, a pulmonary angiogram, a Baker's cyst, the crescent sign, and to access diagnostic algorithms for nuclear scanning and CT angiography. In *MKSAP for Students 4*, assess yourself with items 30-37 in the **Pulmonary Medicine** section.

Bibliography

Arcasoy S. Pulmonary Embolism. http://pier.acponline.org/physicians/diseases/d361/d361. [Date accessed: 2008 Jan 6] In: PIER [online database]. Philadelphia: American College of Physicians; 2008.

Chunilal SD, Eikelboom JW, Attia J, et al. Does this patient have pulmonary embolism? JAMA. 2003;290:2849-58. [PMID: 14657070]

Mohler E. Deep Vein Thrombosis. http://pier.acponline.org/physicians/diseases/d361/d361. [Date accessed: 2008 Jan 6] In: PIER [online database]. Philadelphia: American College of Physicians; 2008.

Tapson VF. Acute pulmonary embolism. N Engl J Med. 2008;358:1037-52. [PMID: 18322285]

Wells PS, Owen C, Doucette S, et al. Does this patient have deep vein thrombosis? JAMA. 2006;295:199-207. [PMID: 16403932]

Chapter 81

Interpretation of Pulmonary Function Tests

Kevin D. Whittle, MD

Pulmonary function tests are measurements of lung function for diagnosing lung disease and managing patients with known pulmonary disorders. Although pulmonary function tests are very effort-dependent, they are more precise than using symptoms or physical examination findings to gauge the severity of underlying lung disease. Specific indications for pulmonary function tests include assessment of patients at risk for lung disease; evaluation of symptoms such as cough, wheezing, or dyspnea; monitoring the benefits and risks of therapeutic interventions; and assessment of risk before surgery.

The four pulmonary function tests commonly used to measure static lung function are spirometry, lung volumes, flow-volume loops, and diffusing capacity for carbon monoxide (DL_{CO}).

Spirometry can be performed in the office, but measurement of lung volumes, flow-volume loops, and diffusing capacity require a pulmonary function laboratory (Table 1).

Spirometry

Spirometry measures airflow rate and expired volume over time. Spirometry can help differentiate obstructive from restrictive lung disease (Table 2). Results are compared with reference values that are stratified by height, weight, sex, and ethnicity. The most useful measures are the forced vital capacity (FVC), the forced expiratory volume in 1 second (FEV_1), the peak expiratory flow rate (PEFR), and the FEV_1 to FVC ratio. Forced vital capacity is the

Table 1. Pulmonary Function Tests

Test	Notes
Spirometry	FEV_1 and FVC are the main measures. FEV_1/FVC distinguishes obstructive airways disease and restrictive disease. A reduced ratio suggests obstructive airway disease (e.g., asthma, COPD) and a normal ratio suggests restrictive disease (e.g., IPF), if lung volumes are reduced.
Lung volumes	Decreased lung volumes suggest restrictive disease if FEV_1/FVC is normal. Increased lung volumes suggest obstructive airways disease (e.g., COPD) if FEV_1/FVC is decreased. Coexisting restriction and obstruction can occur and is diagnosed with spirometry and lung volumes.
Diffusing capacity (DL_{CO})	Decreased DL_{CO} and restrictive pattern on spirometry suggests intrinsic lung disease (e.g., IPF), whereas normal DL_{CO} accompanied by restrictive pattern on spirometry suggests a non-pulmonary cause of restriction (e.g., severe kyphoscoliosis, morbid obesity). Markedly decreased DL_{CO} and obstructive spirometry pattern suggests emphysema, whereas a normal or mildly decreased DL_{CO} suggests other obstructive airways disease (e.g., COPD).
Flow volume loops	Can identify upper airway obstruction. A characteristic limitation of flow (i.e., a flattening of the loop) during inhalation suggests variable extrathoracic obstruction (e.g., vocal cord dysfunction), while limitation of flow during forced exhalation suggest variable intrathoracic obstruction (e.g., asthma, COPD). Fixed upper airway obstruction (e.g., tracheal tumor) causes flow limitation during both forced inhalation and forced exhalation.
Maximal inspiratory and expiratory pressures	Measurement to detect respiratory muscle weakness.
Pulse oximetry	Screen for oxygen desaturation in patients with dyspnea on exertion or other limitation of exercise. A fall >4% is a significant desaturation.

COPD = chronic obstructive pulmonary disease; FEV_1 = forced expiratory volume in one second; FVC = forced vital capacity; IPF = idiopathic pulmonary fibrosis.

Table 2. Common Causes of Obstructive and Restrictive Lung Disease

Obstructive Lung Disease	Restrictive Lung Disease
Asthma	Chest wall deformities
Bronchiectasis	Interstitial disease
Chronic bronchitis	Neuromuscular disease
Emphysema	Obesity, pregnancy, ascites
Upper airway obstruction	Pain
	Pleural effusion

volume of air held by the lungs, measured from peak inspiration to maximum expiration. Forced expiratory volume in one second is the volume of air exhaled in the first second of the forced vital capacity maneuver. FEV_1/FVC is the percentage of the patient's vital capacity that can be forcibly exhaled in one second. Peak expiratory flow rate is the maximum flow rate generated by the patient during a forced vital capacity maneuver.

Spirometry values >80% of predicted values are categorized as normal. A FEV_1/FVC ratio <70% is indicative of obstructive lung disease. Flow parameters are decreased due either to increased airway resistance or loss of elastic recoil of the lung. Obstructive lung diseases also cause a decrease in vital capacity and an increase in residual lung volume because of air trapping. In patients with obstructive lung disease, FEV_1 is used to gauge the severity of obstruction: mild obstruction, FEV_1< 80% predicted; moderate obstruction, FEV_1 <60% predicted; and severe obstruction, FEV_1 <40% predicted. This staging system is useful in guiding therapy.

If initial spirometry is abnormal and suggests obstructive disease, the test is repeated following administration of an inhaled bronchodilator. A ≥12% increase in either FEV_1 or FVC and an increase ≥200 mL from baseline in either parameter defines a significant response and is compatible with reversible airways obstruction (i.e., asthma). A lack of response to bronchodilators in patients with chronic obstructive pulmonary disease does not preclude a therapeutic trial of bronchodilator therapy.

The methacholine challenge test is used to evaluate reactive airways disease in patients with symptoms suggestive of asthma (e.g., dyspnea, cough) but who have normal spirometry. Spirometry is repeated following inhalation of the cholinergic agent methacholine. A ≥20% decrease in at least two or more flow parameters establishes the diagnosis of asthma. Methacholine challenge is not performed in patients with known obstructive lung disease. Other contraindications include recent myocardial infarction or stroke, aortic or cerebral aneurysm, and uncontrolled hypertension.

An FVC <80% of predictive value is consistent with, but not diagnostic of, restrictive disease. In restrictive lung diseases, flows are decreased in proportion to lung volumes so the FEV_1 is normal or high. Lung volumes are required to confirm the diagnosis of restrictive lung disease.

Forced expiratory flow rate (FEF) is the flow rate of air that can be exhaled in a given time period. It can be measured during the first 25% of a forced vital capacity maneuver ($FEF_{25\%}$) or during the first 50% of a forced vital capacity maneuver ($FEF_{50\%}$); $FEF_{25\%-75\%}$ is the amount of air exhaled from 25%-75% of a forced vital capacity maneuver. $FEF_{25\%-75\%}$ may be more sensitive than FEV_1 for detecting early airway obstruction, but it has a wider range of normal values.

Maximum voluntary ventilation (MVV) measures the maximum amount of air moved in and out of the lungs during a 12-15 second interval. The maximum voluntary ventilation, which is typically 30-40 times FEV_1, is useful in determining the patient's overall respiratory function. MVV may be reduced in obstructive or restrictive lung disease, respiratory muscle weakness, or in frail patients. Although the measurement of MVV is nonspecific and highly effort-dependent, it correlates well with the symptom of dyspnea and decreased exercise capacity.

Preoperative spirometry is generally reserved for patients who are thought to have undiagnosed chronic obstructive pulmonary disease, in determining candidacy for coronary artery bypass graft surgery, and prior to lung resection. In preoperative evaluations, patients with FEV_1 <2 L or FVC <20 mL/kg of ideal body weight are at higher risk for atelectasis and pneumonia following surgical procedures under general anesthesia, especially procedures involving the abdomen or chest.

Lung Volume

Lung volume is usually measured by a dilution technique involving breathing either helium or nitrogen in a closed system. In obstructive lung diseases, the residual volume and total lung capacity are increased due to air trapping. Restrictive lung diseases cause reduced lung volumes due to decreased ability of the lungs to expand. A reduction in total lung capacity defines restrictive lung disease.

Flow Volume Loops

Flow volume loops plot flow (in liters/second) as a function of volume (Figure 1). If the flow volume curve appears normal and FVC is normal, pulmonary function is almost always normal. Patients with obstructive disease have a "scooped out" curve with low flows and a reduced slope. If the slope of the flow volume curve appears normal or increased but FVC is reduced, restriction may be present. Flow volume loops are also useful in assessing upper airway obstruction, which causes a "plateau-ing" of the peak flow. Flow volume loops demonstrating a decrease in both inspiratory and expiratory flow are compatible with fixed obstruction outside of the chest such as tracheal stenosis. An isolated decreased peak inspiratory flow is compatible with obstruction inside the chest, such as tumors or mediastinal mass.

Diffusion Capacity of Carbon Monoxide (DLCO)

The diffusion capacity of carbon monoxide (DLCO) measures the integrity of the alveolar-capillary membrane. Diffusion capacity is reduced in emphysema secondary to loss of pulmonary vasculature and diffusing surface area. Diffusion capacity is also reduced in interstitial lung disease because the disease process results in a physical barrier to gas diffusion; in fact, a low DLCO may be the earliest indicator of parenchymal damage. Diffusion capacity is normal in asthma and bronchitis and in conditions causing restrictive physiology outside the lung (e.g., chest wall deformities, neuromuscular disease, and obesity) because these conditions do not affect the alveolar-capillary membrane.

Other extra-pulmonary conditions can also affect the diffusing capacity. Reduced diffusion can be seen with anemia (fewer red blood cells to transport carbon monoxide), pulmonary embolism (reduced parenchymal blood flow), and pulmonary edema (interstitial edema is a barrier to gas flow). Diffusion can be increased in polycythemia (more red blood cells to transport carbon monoxide), hyperthyroidism (increased pulmonary blood

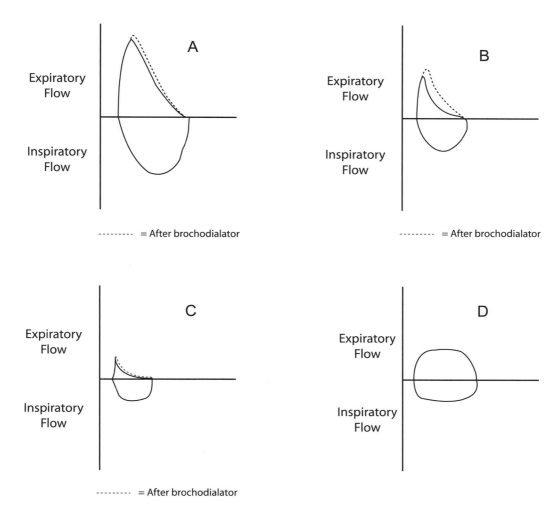

--------- = After brochodialator

--------- = After brochodialator

--------- = After brochodialator

Figure 1 Flow volume loops. Loop A: Flow volume loops plot flow (liters/second) as a function of volume. This is a normal flow volume loop. Following attainment of peak flow, the flow rate declines linearly and proportionally to volume producing a relatively steep and straight slope. Loop B: This flow volume loop shows moderate reduction in airflow as identified by a non-linear decline in flow with decreasing volume. This is recognized as a "scooped out" curve with a reduced slope. Note improvement in airflow following bronchodilator therapy, characteristic of reversible airway disease (i.e., asthma). Loop C: This flow volume loop also shows moderate reduction in airflow as identified by a non-linear decline in flow with decreasing volume with the characteristic "scooped out" curve. Note lack of improvement in airflow following bronchodilator therapy, characteristic of irreversible airway disease (e.g., chronic obstructive pulmonary disease). Loop D: This flow volume loop shows flattening of the loop in both inspiration and expiration characteristic of a fixed upper airway obstruction. This finding is compatible with fixed extra-thoracic obstruction.

flow), left-to-right intracardiac shunts, and early heart failure (increased blood in the lungs).

Book Enhancement

Go to www.acponline.org/essentials/pulmonary-section.html to access tables on severity staging of chronic obstructive pulmonary disease and asthma, and diagnostic criteria for idiopathic pulmonary fibrosis in the absence of a lung biopsy. In *MKSAP for*

Students 4, assess yourself with item 38 in the **Pulmonary Medicine** section.

Bibliography

American Thoracic Society. Lung function testing: selection of reference values and interpretative strategies. Am Rev Respir Dis. 1991;144:1202-18. [PMID: 1952453]

Evans SE, Scanlon PD. Current practice in pulmonary function testing. Mayo Clin Proc. 2003;78:758-63. [PMID: 12934788]

Section XI
Rheumatology

Chapter 82

Approach to Joint Pain

Thomas M. DeFer, MD

Joint pain can be characterized in several overlapping ways that are helpful in formulating a differential diagnosis: specific joints involved, the number and symmetry of involved joints, articular or periarticular, time course, pattern of development, and inflammatory or noninflammatory. The presence or absence of extra-articular manifestations can also provide important diagnostic clues. In some clinical situations the etiology of joint pain can be determined quickly, but in others the patient will need to be seen multiple times before the diagnosis is apparent. This is particularly true in the early stages of systemic conditions that may initially present with only joint pain. Nonspecific rheumatologic tests (e.g., rheumatoid factor, antinuclear antibodies, and erythrocyte sedimentation rate) should be ordered only to confirm a diagnosis suggested by the history and physical examination. Likewise, plain radiographs are indicated only when there is a likelihood that the results will change management. In patients with joint effusion, joint fluid analysis can establish the diagnosis of infection or narrow the differential diagnosis. Table 1 categorizes joint fluid findings and Table 2 summarizes joint fluid characteristics of common forms of arthritis.

Location and Pattern

Particular joint involvement suggests certain diagnoses such as the first metatarsophalangeal joint, gout; the knee, osteoarthritis; and the metacarpophalangeal joints, rheumatoid arthritis. The spondyloarthritides characteristically involve the axial skeleton (i.e., spine, sacroiliac, sternoclavicular, and manubriosternal joints) and large appendicular joints. Ankylosing spondylitis is the most common example of a spondyloarthritis, others include reactive arthritis, psoriatic arthritis, and enteropathic arthritis (associated with inflammatory bowel disease). Joint pain can affect a single joint (monoarticular), two to four joints (oligoarticular), or multiple joints (polyarticular). Common monoarthropathies include gout,

Table 1. Joint Fluid Categories

Characteristic	Normal	Group I* (Noninflammatory)	Group II† (Inflammatory)	Group III‡ (Septic)
Volume (knee)	<3.5 mL	>3.5 mL	>3.5 mL	>3.5 mL
Viscosity	Very high	High	Low	Variable
Color	Clear	Straw	Straw to opalescent	Variable with organisms
Clarity	Transparent	Transparent	Translucent, opaque at times	Opaque
Leukocytes/μL	200	200-2000	2000-100,000	>50,000 (usually >100,000)
Polymorphonuclear cells (%)	<25	<25	>50	>75
Culture	Negative	Negative	Negative	Usually positive

* Examples include osteoarthritis, avascular necrosis, hemochromatosis, sickle cell disease.
† Examples include crystalline arthritis, rheumatoid arthritis, spondyloarthropathy, systemic lupus erythematosus.
‡ Infectious arthritis including staphylococcal, gonococcal, and tuberculosis.

Table 2. Key Synovial Fluid Findings with Some Common Diagnoses

Diagnosis	Gross Appearance	Leukocytes (per μL)	Polymorphonuclear Cells (%)	Crystals	Culture and/or Gram Stain	Other Findings
Bacterial infection	Opaque or cloudy	Often >100,000	>90	None (unless coincidental)	Positive	Bacteria
Crystalline arthritis	Usually cloudy	2000 to 100,000	Often >80	Positive	Negative	—
Osteoarthritis	Clear	<1000	<50	0 or CPPD	Negative	Fibrils
Rheumatoid arthritis	Cloudy	>5000	usually >50	0	Negative	Cytoplasmic inclusions
Fracture	Bloody	Proportional to hematocrit	Up to 70	0	Negative	Fat
Nonfracture, mild trauma	Clear to bloody	<2000	<50	0	Negative	—

CPPD = calcium pyrophosphate dihydrate.

calcium pyrophosphate deposition disease (pseudogout), septic arthritis, and avascular necrosis. The spondyloarthritides are characteristically oligoarticular. Rheumatoid arthritis, systemic lupus erythematosus (SLE), and osteoarthritis are usually polyarticular. Acute gout can occasionally present in a polyarticular manner, which may cause diagnostic confusion. Determine symmetry if more than one joint is involved; rheumatoid arthritis, SLE, and osteoarthritis are typically symmetrical.

Articular and Nonarticular Disorders

Differentiate articular from nonarticular disorders. Articular problems are characterized by internal/deep pain that is exacerbated by active and passive motion and reduced range of motion, and may be accompanied by effusion, synovial thickening, joint deformities/instability, crepitations, clicking, popping, or locking. Periarticular disorders cause more pain with active rather than passive motion, range of motion is often preserved, and tenderness and signs of inflammation are removed from the actual joint. Common periarticular disorders include bursitis, tendinitis, polymyalgia rheumatica, fibromyalgia, and enthesopathies (inflammation of attachment sites of tendons and ligaments to bones). Enthesopathies are characteristic of the spondyloarthritides; the most common are Achilles tendonitis and plantar fasciitis. Dactylitis ("sausage digits") is another classic feature of the spondyloarthritides (particularly psoriatic arthritis and reactive arthritis) caused by synovitis and enthesitis of the fingers and toes (Plate 21).

Time Course and Development

Determine the time course and pattern of development of the joint pain. Some arthropathies present in an acute manner, such as infection, gout, and pseudogout; all patients with acute monoarticular arthritis require an arthrocentesis to establish the diagnosis. Other arthropathies have subacute or chronic presentations, such as osteoarthritis. Occasionally, some chronic arthropathies, such a rheumatoid arthritis, may have an abrupt onset. Ongoing development of joint pain follows three major patterns: additive, migratory, and intermittent. Additive means that new joints become involved while the previous sites remain affected (e.g., osteoarthritis and rheumatoid arthritis). Migratory describes a sequential arthritis of a newly inflamed joint appearing simultaneously with or right after a prior joint's improvement (e.g., gonococcal arthritis). The intermittent pattern occurs when affected joints improve completely and then at a later time the same or different joints become affected in a similar manner (e.g., gout, pseudogout, SLE).

Inflammatory and Noninflammatory Pain

Joint pain is divided into inflammatory and noninflammatory categories. Inflammatory signs (i.e., pain, redness, warmth, and swelling) confined to the joints define true arthritis. Inflammatory arthritides include septic arthritis, gout, pseudogout, rheumatoid arthritis, SLE, and spondyloarthritides. Inflammatory conditions are notable for more severe and prolonged morning stiffness (often an hour or more) and gelling (stiffness after a period of inactivity) that improve with activity. Inflammatory signs are also present in some periarticular conditions such as bursitis, tenosynovitis, and enthesopathies, but are less pronounced. Noninflammatory conditions have less morning stiffness, typically <30 minutes. Osteoarthritis is by far the most common noninflammatory disorder.

Inflammatory arthropathies can be accompanied by systemic symptoms including malaise, fatigue, weight loss, and fever. Laboratory manifestations indicative of inflammation are also seen (e.g., elevated erythrocyte sedimentation rate and C-reactive protein and anemia).

Extra-Articular Manifestations

Focal signs of inflammation or organ dysfunction removed from the joints also have important diagnostic value. Accompanying involvement of the skin, eyes, mucus membranes, central and peripheral nervous system, kidneys, gastrointestinal system, and heart are suggestive of systemic inflammatory diseases. For example, in addition to rheumatoid nodules, the major extra-articular manifestation of rheumatoid arthritis are pulmonary (pleuritis, interstitial lung disease, pulmonary nodules); cardiac (pericarditis, carditis); and ocular (scleritis, episcleritis). SLE can have renal, hematologic, neurologic, and serosal manifestations. Psoriatic arthritis occurs in 5%-8% of patients with psoriasis. Reactive arthritis appears 1-4 weeks after a genitourinary or gastrointestinal infection manifested as urethritis, cervicitis, or diarrhea. Spondylo-arthritis can be associated with ulcerative colitis and Crohn's disease.

Book Enhancement

Go to www.acponline.org/essentials/rheumatology-section.html to view a knee effusion and review how to perform a knee arthrocentesis. In *MKSAP for Students 4*, assess yourself with items 2-4 in the **Rheumatology** section.

Bibliography

American College of Physicians. Medical Knowledge Self-Assessment Program 14. Philadelphia: American College of Physicians; 2006.

Kataria RK, Brent LH. Spondyloarthropathies. Am Fam Physician. 2004;69:2853-60. [PMID: 15222650]

Mies Richie A, Francis ML. Diagnostic approach to polyarticular joint pain. Am Fam Physician. 2003;68:1151-60. Erratum in: Am Fam Physician. 2006;73:1153. Am Fam Physician. 2006;73:776. [PMID: 14524403]

Chapter 83

Approach to Knee and Shoulder Pain

Joseph Rencic, MD

Knee Pain

Osteoarthritis is, by far, the most common cause of chronic knee pain in older persons. Acute knee pain may be due to inflammation (e.g., crystalline arthritis, rheumatoid arthritis), trauma, overuse syndromes, or infection. The knee is the most commonly infected joint, and septic arthritis must be considered in all patients with unilateral knee pain.

Evaluation

Determine location, duration, and precipitating and relieving factors. Ask about locking (meniscal tear) or "popping" sensation (ligamentous rupture). Consider the direction of force on the knee in traumatic knee pain. Joint effusion occurring <2 hours after injury suggests anterior cruciate ligament rupture or tibial fracture.

Inspect the knee for structural changes or swelling both in the standing and supine positions, then palpate for warmth, tenderness, and effusion. Palpate the medial and lateral joint line for medial and lateral collateral ligament injury, the anserine bursa, and popliteal fossa when symptoms are present in those areas. Small effusions may be noted by milking joint fluid into the suprapatellar pouch and then pushing medially on the lateral knee just inferior to the patella with the knee extended. A fluid wave or bulge will be apparent in the medial compartment. Observe the gait and assess range of motion, normally 160° of flexion to full extension. Check for stability of major ligaments by performing stress maneuvers. Ask the patient to squat and walk in the squatting position; if this can be performed, even if painful, the integrity and strength of the joint are intact.

Knee Pain Syndromes

The most common cause of knee pain in patients aged <45 years, especially in women, is the patellofemoral syndrome. The pain is peripatellar and exacerbated by overuse (e.g., running), descending stairs, or prolonged sitting. Diagnosis is confirmed by firmly compressing the patella against the femur and moving it up and down along the groove of the femur, reproducing pain or crepitation. The condition is self-limited; minimizing high-impact activity and nonsteroidal anti-inflammatory drugs (NSAIDs) improve symptoms.

Prepatellar bursitis is associated with anterior knee pain and swelling anterior to the patella and is often caused by trauma or repetitive kneeling. Range of motion is not limited. Infectious prepatellar bursitis can be fairly subtle; always perform a joint aspiration if warmth and erythema are present to rule out infection. Located medially, about 6 cm below the joint line, the pes anserine bursa can also cause pain, which is worse with activity and at night. In general, bursitis treatment includes avoidance of the inciting activity, ice, NSAIDs, and local corticosteroid injection for persistent symptoms.

Iliotibial band syndrome is a common cause of knife-like lateral knee pain that occurs with vigorous flexion-extension activities of the knee (e.g., running). Treat with rest and stretching exercises.

Trauma may result in fracture or ligament tear, which produces a noticeable "popping" sensation in 50% of patients. Typically a large effusion collects rapidly. Obtain x-rays only in patients that fulfill ≥1 of the Ottawa knee rules (Table 1).

Anterior cruciate ligament tears occur with sudden twisting and hyperextension injuries. Collateral ligament tears occur with medial or lateral force without twisting. Posterior cruciate ligament tears occur with trauma to a flexed knee (e.g., dashboard injury). Check for stability of major ligaments by placing the knee in 160° extension and performing medial and lateral stress; normal knees will have minimal give. Flex the knee 20° and place your knee under the patient's knee. Grasp the patient's thigh above the patella with one hand, press down toward your knee to stabilize the thigh, and grasp the proximal tibia with the other hand to pull the tibia forward (Lachman test). A full tear will demonstrate laxity (compared with the other knee) without a firm endpoint (positive likelihood ratio = 25; negative likelihood ratio = 0.1). With the knee in 90° of flexion and the foot resting on the table, check for posterior cruciate rupture by applying posterior force to the leg. Posterior movement of the leg with respect to the thigh, laxity, and lack of a firm endpoint support a diagnosis of posterior cruciate ligament rupture.

Meniscal tears present with pain, locking, and clicking. Tenderness usually localizes to the joint line on the affected side with pain elicited with tibial rotation as the leg is extended. No

---

Table 1. Ottawa Knee Rules

Obtain a knee x-ray following trauma for:

1. Patients aged >55 years
2. Isolated tenderness of the patella
3. Tenderness at the head of the fibula
4. Inability to flex knee to 90°
5. Inability to bear weight immediately after injury or in the emergency department

physical examination maneuver reliably rules in or rules out the diagnosis.

Referred hip pain, or L_5-S_1 root radiculopathy, can cause knee pain, but knee examination will be normal. In chronic pain syndromes, radiographs are unlikely to alter management. The decision to order an MRI should usually be made by a specialist.

Shoulder Pain

Shoulder pain occurs in up to 35% of the general population. It often evolves into a chronic, disabling problem (Table 2). The most common cause is irritation of the subacromial bursa or rotator cuff tendon from mechanical impingement between the humeral head and the coracoacromial arch, which includes the acromion, coracoacromial ligament, and the coracoid process (Figure 1). Chronic overhead activity may contribute to narrowing of this space, which can lead to recurrent microtrauma and chronic local inflammation of rotator cuff tendons.

Evaluation

Determine whether the pain is acute or chronic and a possible mechanism of injury (e.g., trauma, occupational or recreational exposures). Ask for precipitating and relieving factors. Stiffness or loss of motion suggests glenohumeral arthritis or adhesive capsulitis, whereas referred pain is not exacerbated by shoulder movement.

Inspect the shoulder; asymmetry indicates a possible dislocation. Palpate the major anatomical landmarks, including the subacromial space below the tip of the acromion process, the acromioclavicular joint, the biceps tendon groove, the cervical spine, and the scapula. Ask the patient to raise his arms straight above his head (testing flexion and abduction), put both hands on the back of his head (testing external rotation), and put both hands behind his back (testing extension and internal rotation). An ability to perform all these maneuvers, even if painful, indicates normal joint anatomy and muscle strength.

Table 2. Common Causes of Shoulder Pain

Condition	Notes
Rotator cuff tendonitis	Lateral shoulder pain, aggravated by reaching, raising arm overhead, lying on side. Subacromial pain to palpation and with passive/resisted abduction.
Rotator cuff tear	Shoulder weakness, loss of function, tendonitis symptoms, nocturnal pain. Similar to tendonitis examination, plus weakness with abduction and external rotation; positive drop-arm test.
Bicipital tendonitis/rupture	Anterior shoulder pain with lifting, overhead reaching, flexion; reduced pain after rupture. Bicipital groove tenderness; pain with resisted elbow flexion; "Popeye" lump in antecubital fossa following rupture.
Adhesive capsulitis	Progressive decrease in range of motion, more from stiffness than pain. Loss of external rotation, abduction—unable to scratch lower back or fully lift arm straight overhead.
Acromioclavicular syndromes	Anterior shoulder pain, deformity; usually from trauma or overuse. Localized joint tenderness and deformity (osteophytes, separation); pain with adduction.
Glenohumeral arthritis	Gradual onset of anterior pain, stiffness. Anterior joint-line tenderness; decreased range of motion; crepitation.

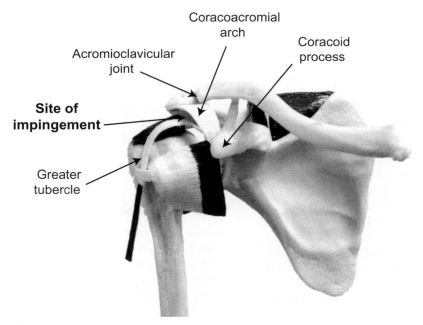

Figure 1 Impingement syndrome.

If the patient cannot perform these maneuvers actively, check passive range of motion; inability to perform passive maneuvers suggests an articular (glenohumeral or capsular), rather than a periarticular, etiology. Perform a neurological exam to rule out a radiculopathy as a cause of referred pain.

Shoulder Pain Syndromes

Patients with rotator cuff tendonitis and subacromial bursitis typically have gradually worsening pain that limits motion, is worse at night, and may extend down the arm but rarely below the elbow.

On exam, raise the arm passively in forward flexion, while depressing the scapula with your other hand. This action pushes the greater tuberosity into the anterior acromion process and will elicit pain when impingement is present ("impingement sign"). The circumduction-adduction shoulder maneuver (Clancy test) is diagnostically helpful (positive likelihood ratio = 19, negative likelihood ratio = 0.05). The patient stands with the head turned to the contralateral shoulder. The affected shoulder is circumducted and adducted across the body to shoulder level with elbow extended and thumb pointing toward the floor. Exert a uniform downward force on the patient's distal forearm/wrist with the patient resisting movement. Anterolateral shoulder pain and/or weakness constitute a positive test.

Pain without weakness is consistent with tendonitis; pain with weakness is consistent with tendon tear. Check internal rotation by having the patient move the thumb up the spine as far as possible, looking for pain or restricted movement.

Severe pain and frank weakness (an inability to maintain the arm at 90° of abduction) suggest complete rupture of the rotator cuff tendon. Magnetic resonance imaging is the most sensitive and specific imaging modality for complete or partial rotator cuff tears, though ultrasound is quite good and more cost-effective.

A trial of an NSAID and rest for 2 weeks is reasonable initial therapy. If no improvement occurs within 4 to 6 weeks, then physical therapy, subacromial corticosteroid injection, or (rarely) surgery may be helpful. Since it is unlikely to change management, imaging plays a limited role in most cases of chronic shoulder pain. If there is no response to conservative therapy in 6 weeks, consultation with a rheumatologist or orthopedist is the appropriate next step.

Other causes of shoulder pain include glenohumeral instability, inflammatory arthropathies (e.g., rheumatoid arthritis), septic arthritis, acromioclavicular degeneration, myofascial pain (e.g., trapezius strain), and referred pain (e.g., cervical radiculopathy). Osteoarthritis of the glenohumeral joint is relatively uncommon.

Book Enhancement

Go to www.acponline.org/essentials/rheumatology-section.html to view normal shoulder and knee anatomy and images illustrating physical examination techniques for the knee and shoulder. In *MKSAP for Students 4*, assess yourself with items 5-8 in the **Rheumatology** section.

Bibliography

Calmbach WL, Hutchens M. Evaluation of patients presenting with knee pain: Part I. History, physical examination, radiographs, and laboratory tests. Am Fam Physician. 2003;68:907-12. [PMID: 13678139]

Calmbach WL, Hutchens M. Evaluation of patients presenting with knee pain: Part II. Differential diagnosis. Am Fam Physician. 2003;68:917-22. [PMID: 13678140]

Matsen FA 3rd. Clinical practice. Rotator-cuff failure. N Engl J Med. 2008; 358:2138-47. [PMID: 18480206]

Solomon DH, Simel DL, Bates DW, Katz JN, Schaffer JL. The rational clinical examination. Does this patient have a torn meniscus or ligament of the knee? Value of the physical examination. JAMA. 2001;286:1610-20. [PMID: 11585485]

Chapter 84

Crystalline Arthritis

Katherine Nickerson, MD

The two most common forms of crystalline arthritis are gout and calcium pyrophosphate deposition disease (CPPD). Gout is caused by the inflammatory reaction to monosodium urate crystal deposition in synovial tissue, bursae, and tendon sheaths. The solubility of urate at physiologic pH is approximately 6.7 mg/dL. If the urate concentration increases above this concentration, urate deposits may develop in these tissues. These deposits develop over time but may be reabsorbed if the plasma level decreases below 6.7 mg/dL. Gout attacks occur when urate crystals are released from pre-existing tissue deposits and are almost always associated with chronically elevated levels of serum uric acid. Gout includes a range of clinical disorders from acute, exquisitely painful, monoarticular arthritis to chronic, crippling, destructive polyarthritis. The risk of developing gout is directly related to the level and duration of elevated uric acid. Uric acid rises with increasing age, weight, and serum creatinine and may be accelerated by secondary factors such as renal insufficiency, alcohol consumption, diuretics, and low doses of aspirin, all of which inhibit renal excretion of uric acid. Hyperuricemia is more often related to under-excretion (90%) than over-production (10%) of uric acid. Acute attacks are frequently triggered by events that precipitously raise or lower serum uric acid level such as dehydration, post-operative fluid shifts, or initiation of uric acid-lowering agents. Gout progresses through three distinct stages: asymptomatic hyperuricemia, which may last several decades; acute intermittent gout; and chronic tophaceous gout (Plate 43), which usually develops only after years of acute intermittent gout. During intercritical periods (the asymptomatic periods between gout attacks), crystals may still be detected in the synovial fluid. Therefore, the presence of crystals in synovial fluid is not always sufficient to provoke an attack.

CPPD is caused by crystallization of calcium pyrophosphate dihydrate in articular tissues. The cause of this crystallization is unknown but is clearly related to aging; a few cases are associated with metabolic abnormalities. While usually asymptomatic, CPPD can cause acute monoarticular or chronic polyarticular arthritis. The acute pseudogout syndrome of CPPD presents with monoarticular or, rarely, polyarticular attacks of arthritis. The knee, wrist, shoulder, and ankle are most commonly affected. Chronic CPPD presents with asymmetric pain, swelling, and morning stiffness involving the shoulders, wrists, metacarpophalangeal joints, or knees.

Prevention

There are no primary prevention measures for gout or CPPD. However, administration of uric acid-lowering drugs to patients receiving chemotherapy for hematological malignancies is recommended to prevent the tumor lysis syndrome (hyperuricemia, hyperphosphatemia, hypocalcemia, hyperkalemia, and acute renal failure). Effective secondary prevention of gout requires decreasing serum urate levels. However, it is not clear that all patients with gouty arthritis need such intervention.

Screening

Do not screen for asymptomatic hyperuricemia. Potential reactions to uric acid-lowering drugs may outweigh treatment benefits, and hypersensitivity reactions to allopurinol can be fatal.

Diagnosis

Perform arthrocentesis in the case of acute monoarticular arthritis to rule out infection (Table 1). A definitive diagnosis of gout is made by demonstrating negatively birefringent monosodium urate crystals within synovial fluid leukocytes or in a suspected tophus. If joint fluid cannot be obtained, clinical criteria can be used. Rapid onset, intense inflammation, complete resolution between attacks, involvement of the first metatarsophalangeal joint (podagra), and radiographs demonstrating subcortical erosions are distinguishing features of gout.

The diagnosis of CPPD is made by finding positively birefringent rhomboid intracellular crystals in the synovial fluid. Radiographs can reveal chondrocalcinosis, linear calcifications along the articular and fibrocartilage (Figure 1), degenerative changes, and osteophytes. Screen patients younger than 50 years old with CPPD for associated metabolic conditions (e.g., hemochromatosis, hyperparathyroidism, hypothyroidism, gout, hypomagnesemia, hypophosphatasia, familial hypocalciuric hypercalcemia, acromegaly, and ochronosis).

Therapy

Advise patients with gout to avoid alcohol, which increases uric acid production and may impair renal uric acid secretion. High-purine foods such as organ meats, red meat, scallops, anchovies, and sardines should also be avoided. However, dietary interventions are rarely adequate to reverse hyperuricemia and prevent attacks of gout.

Effective treatment of acute attacks of gout involves high-dose therapy with nonselective or cyclooxygenase-2 selective nonsteroidal anti-inflammatory drugs (NSAIDs), corticosteroids, or colchicine. The choice of agents for acute gout depends on patient characteristics and on the presence or absence of concomitant

Table 1. Differential Diagnosis of Gout

Disease	Notes
Calcium pyrophosphate deposition disease (CPPD)	Multiple presentations, including osteoarthritis and gout-like inflammation, or may be asymptomatic. Cartilage calcification, especially in fibrocartilage of knee meniscus, symphysis pubis, glenoid and acetabular labrum, and triangular cartilage of wrist are pathognomonic. Osteoarthritis in unusual places (wrist, elbow, metacarpophalangeal joints, or shoulder) without a history of trauma suggests CPPD. Defined by finding calcium pyrophosphate dihydrate crystals in synovial fluid and by chondrocalcinosis on radiography.
Gout	History of acute attacks of monoarthritis with joint erythema. Bony enlargement of joints may be present. Tophi typically present in disease greater than 5-10 years. Radiographs often show large erosions with overhanging edges and occasionally soft tissue calcification of tophi. If gout is suspected, examine joint fluid for monourate sodium crystals. Gout and CPPD may coexist.
Osteoarthritis (see Chapter 85)	Bony enlargement, no acute signs of inflammation; patient may have acute exacerbation of joint symptoms, especially after use. Radiographs may show focal joint-space loss within the joint, bony repair with osteophytes, subchondral sclerosis.
Psoriatic arthritis	Joint distribution and appearance similar to reactive arthritis. Predilection for distal interphalangeal joints of fingers, often with concomitant nail changes. Elevated uric acid levels proportional to skin involvement.
Reactive arthritis	Inflammatory oligoarthritis, weight-bearing joints most often affected, may have tendon insertion inflammation. Extraarticular manifestations include conjunctivitis, urethritis, stomatitis, and psoriaform skin changes. Patient usually has had infection with an appropriate organism (*Salmonella, Shigella, Yersinia, Campylobacter,* or *Chlamydia* species within the 3 weeks before onset of initial attack.
Rheumatoid arthritis (RA) (see Chapter 87)	Symmetrical polyarthritis that preferentially affects small joints of hands and feet. About 30% have subcutaneous rheumatoid nodules. Radiographic changes include soft-tissue swelling, diffuse joint-space narrowing, marginal erosions of small joints, and symmetrical multiple joint involvement; no osteophytes. Acute RA sometimes mimics gout. The greater the number of joints involved, the more likely that RA is the diagnosis.
Septic arthritis (see Chapter 88)	Fever, arthritis, great tenderness. Up to one half of patients have concomitant RA. The source (skin, lungs) is often evident. Usually occurs in previously abnormal joints. Gout and septic arthritis may coexist.

disease (Table 2). NSAIDs are effective but must be avoided in older individuals, patients with renal insufficiency, heart failure, peptic ulcer disease, and in those on concurrent anticoagulation or other interacting drugs. In these situations, intraarticular or systemic corticosteroids are used. High-dose oral colchicine has a variable response rate and is almost invariably associated with severe diarrhea; therefore, this route of administration should rarely be used and is contraindicated in the presence of renal or liver disease. Intravenous colchicine has been removed from the U.S. market.

Management or prevention of recurrent gout and chronic tophaceous gout requires drug therapy to decrease and maintain serum uric acid levels between 5 and 6 mg/dL. The xanthine oxidase inhibitor allopurinol is most effective but must be given lifelong and is associated with a 1%-2% incidence of allergic reactions which can be severe and life-threatening. Initiate therapy after the resolution of an acute attack, usually with concomitant low-dose colchicine, which is then continued for approximately 6 months to prevent acute attacks. Uricosuric agents (e.g., probenecid, sulfinpyrazone) are sometimes used but are less effective at lowering the uric acid, are not effective in patients with a creatinine clearance of less than 40 mL/min, and should only be used in patients who secrete <600 mg of uric acid daily.

Treatment of CPPD is symptomatic. There is no agent that successfully reverses deposition or formation of calcium pyrophosphate. Joint fluid aspiration, NSAIDs, and intraarticular steroids are useful in managing an acute attack. Colchicine may be used, as it is in gout, as prophylaxis.

Book Enhancement

Go to www.acponline.org/essentials/rheumatology-section.html to view common locations of gout involvement and to view a tophus and its uric acid crystals using polarized microscopy. In *MKSAP for Students 4*, assess yourself with items 9-11 in the **Rheumatology** section.

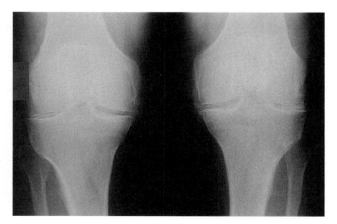

Figure 1 Linear calcification of the menisci and articular cartilage characteristic of calcium pyrophosphate deposition disease.

Table 2. Drug Treatment of Gout

Agent	Notes
ACUTE GOUT	
Nonsteroidal anti-inflammatory drugs (NSAIDs)	Blocks formation of inflammatory prostaglandins and has analgesic effects. Effective within 12-24 hours of onset. The NSAID used is less important than the rapidity with which the NSAID is started. Any NSAID *except* aspirin is appropriate. Start at high dose, then taper rapidly over several days.
Colchicine (oral)	Colchicine decreases L-selectin expression by polymorphonuclear neutrophils, making them less able to adhere to vascular endothelium and egress into tissues. Nausea, vomiting, and diarrhea are dose related. Bone marrow suppression can be life threatening if maximum doses are exceeded. Myopathy and neuropathy can occur at any dose. Modify dose according to renal function. Avoid in dialysis patients because not removed by dialysis.
Colchicine (intravenous)	Can cause severe myelosuppression, renal failure, and death if given improperly. Removed from US market in 2008.
Corticosteroids (oral)	Suppress inflammation by several mechanisms. Useful when NSAIDs are contraindicated (e.g., those with renal insufficiency). Contraindicated in active peptic ulcer disease. May interfere with control of diabetes.
Corticosteroids (intra-articular)	Especially useful if only one joint is inflamed and patient has contraindications to other agents. Rule out infectious etiology before injecting.
CHRONIC GOUT	
Allopurinol	Xanthine oxidase inhibitor. Inhibits uric acid synthesis. Dose is increased over 2-3 weeks to minimize acute gout attacks that may occur with abrupt fluctuations in uric acid levels. Initial dose is modified according to creatinine clearance. Target uric acid levels ≤6.0 mg/dL.
Probenecid, sulfinpyrazone	Uricosuric. Effective in long-term treatment of chronic gout if sodium urate levels are maintained below 6 mg/dL. Not effective in renal insufficiency.

Bibliography

Kalunian K. Calcium Pyrophosphate Deposition Disease. http://pier.acponline.org/physicians/diseases/d357. [Date accessed: 2008 Feb 7] In PIER [online database]. Philadelphia: American College of Physicians; 2008.

Keith MP, Gilliland WR. Updates in the management of gout. Am J Med. 2007;120:221-4. [PMID: 17349440]

Teal GP, Fuchs HA. Gout. http://pier.acponline.org/physicians/diseases/d160. [Date accessed: 2008 Feb 7] In: PIER [online database]. Philadelphia: American College of Physicians; 2008.

Chapter 85

Osteoarthritis

Amanda Cooper, MD

Osteoarthritis is characterized by the breakdown of articular cartilage, subchondral bone alterations, meniscal degeneration, and bone repair (osteophytes) with minimal synovial inflammatory response. Loss of articular cartilage causes pain and loss of joint mobility. Osteoarthritis can involve any joint but most often affects the spine, hand, foot, hip, and knee. Osteoarthritis increases markedly with age and causes a significant burden of lost time at work and early retirement. After age 50 men are more likely to be affected by hip osteoarthritis, whereas women are more likely to develop hand, knee, and foot osteoarthritis. There is a familial tendency, indicating at least a partial genetic effect.

Prevention

Obesity and repetitive joint strain may be modified to decrease the risk of developing osteoarthritis. Counsel patients to lose weight if their body mass index is >25. For each additional pound of body weight, the force across the knee increases by 2-3 lb, thus increasing the risk of cartilage damage. Avoiding repetitive knee bending and heavy lifting helps reduce excessive loading of the knee and may reduce osteoarthritis. Advise athletes to follow graduated training schedules to build up muscle strength, which helps improve joint stability and avoid intrinsic damage.

Diagnosis

Osteoarthritis pain is a poorly localized, deep, aching sensation. Initially, there is pain with joint use and then, as the disease progresses, pain at rest. Stiffness lasts <30 minutes. Examination findings include tenderness, swelling, crepitus, bony enlargement or deformity, restricted motion, pain with passive movement, and joint instability. Bony enlargement of the distal interphalangeal joints (Heberden's nodes) and proximal interphalangeal joints (Bouchard's nodes) are particularly characteristic of osteoarthritis (Plate 44). Osteoarthritis of the first carpometacarpal joint is very common and it often coexists with osteoarthritis of the distal interphalangeal joints and proximal interphalangeal joints, but it may be an isolated finding. It causes pain at base of the thumb and bony enlargement producing a squared appearance to the base of the hand. Crepitus and pain may be elicited with passive circular motion of the joint ("grind test"). Laboratory tests are not helpful for diagnosis. Radiographs are most helpful in diagnosing osteoarthritis in the hip but only help confirm osteoarthritis in the knee and have lower sensitivity and specificity than physical exam for osteoarthritis of the hand. Osteophytes, subchondral sclerosis,

and joint space narrowing seen on radiographs are indicative of osteoarthritis (Figure 1). Joint aspiration should be considered if there is an effusion present and the diagnosis is in question or a concomitant infection is suspected. Synovial fluid is typically clear, with <2000 leukocytes/μL (Table 1).

Therapy

In overweight patients with hip or knee disease, weight loss combined with exercise has been shown to be superior to either alone. Strengthening muscles around the involved joint is of high importance in reducing pain. A low-impact exercise program is recommended and can also promote weight loss and increased muscle strength. Specifically, quadriceps-strengthening exercises are prescribed for knee osteoarthritis because it can reduce pain and improve physical function. Patients with medial knee compartment osteoarthritis may benefit from heel inserts of 5 to 10 degrees that help relieve the pressure on the medial compartment. Use of a cane in the hand contralateral to the painful joint may help by unloading forces on the knee or hip, and knee taping improves knee alignment thus improving pain. Referral to physical or occupational therapy for active and passive range of motion exercises, instruction, or joint protection education may be helpful.

Consider pharmacologic agents when conservative measures fail to relieve pain and improve function. Recommend acetaminophen as initial drug therapy for osteoarthritis in doses no greater than

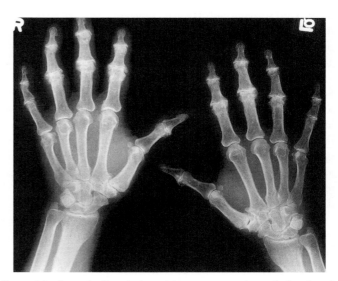

Figure 1 Radiograph of hands shows joint space narrowing and sclerosis and osteophyte formation. Prominent involvement of proximal interphalangeal joints and distal interphalangeal joints is indicative of osteoarthritis.

315

Table 1. Differential Diagnosis of Osteoarthritis

Disease	Notes
Hemochromatosis	Secondary OA due to iron overload, predominantly men aged 40 to 60. OA in the second and third MCP joints with hook-like osteophytes are characteristic. Rare in premenopausal women.
CPPD (see Chapter 84)	Chondrocalcinosis in knees, triangular fibrocartilage of the wrist and symphysis pubis; attacks of pseudogout; OA in the second and third MCPs. Calcium pyrophosphate dihydrate crystals may be identified in synovial fluid.
Rheumatoid arthritis (see Chapter 87)	Synovial (soft tissue swelling), not bony, enlargement of the PIP and MCP joints; rarely involves the DIP joints; inflammatory signs (fatigue, prolonged stiffness); rheumatoid nodules; inflammatory synovial fluid; marginal erosions and juxta-articular osteopenia seen on radiographs.
Psoriatic arthritis	Synovial and entheseal swelling present; may involve DIPs; dactylitis (sausage digits) present; erosions and periostitis seen on x-ray films.
Trochanteric bursitis	Pain and tenderness over the greater trochanter; pain may radiate down lateral aspect of thigh; hip range of motion is normal.
Anserine bursitis (see Chapter 83)	Pain and tenderness over the anteromedial aspect of the lower leg below the joint line of the knee. May be a confounding cause of knee pain in patients with knee OA.
Osteonecrosis	Joint pain out of proportion to radiographic changes. Risk factors: high-dose corticosteroids, ethanol abuse, systemic lupus erythematosus, hemoglobinopathies. Usually involves hip or knee. Diagnosis confirmed by magnetic resonance imaging.
Gout (see Chapter 84)	History of acute attacks of mono-arthritis with joint erythema. Bony enlargement of joints may be present. Tophi may be present on examination. X-ray films show large erosions with overhanging edges. If gout is suspected, fluid from the involved joint(s) should be examined for crystals. Chronic tophaceous gout may involve the DIP and PIP joints and first MTP causing deformities and bony enlargement akin to OA.

CPPD = calcium pyrophosphate deposition disease; DIP = distal interphalangeal; MCP = metacarpophalangeal; OA = osteoarthritis; PIP = proximal interphalangeal; RA = rheumatoid arthritis.

4000 mg/day. Acetaminophen is an effective, safe, and relatively inexpensive treatment. Patients with inadequate response can be started on nonsteroidal anti-inflammatory drugs (NSAIDs), preferably at the lowest effective dose to limit side effects such as gastritis or renal insufficiency. Cylcooxygenase-2 (COX-2) inhibitors are not more effective than NSAIDs but are less likely to cause gastrointestinal tract ulceration, are significantly more expensive, and are associated with an increased risk of adverse cardiovascular events. Concomitant use of a proton pump inhibitor with a NSAID should be considered in patients at increased risk for gastrointestinal bleeding (e.g., age > 65 years, history of peptic ulcer disease, gastrointestinal bleeding, or anticoagulant use).

Glucosamine sulfate is the building block of proteoglycans, the ground substance of articular cartilage. However, two recent meta-analyses show symptom improvement with glucosamine is similar to placebo. Substance P has been implicated in the pathogenesis of pain. Topical capsaicin depletes substance P and may be used in addition to or as an alternative to systemic medications. For full efficacy, it should be applied three times a day for three weeks. Narcotic analgesics or tramadol may play an additional role in patients whose pain is not well controlled or who have a contraindication to NSAIDs. Tramadol is a centrally acting synthetic opioid agonist that has comparable efficacy to NSAIDS in treating osteoarthritis hip and knee pain. Significant abuse has not been identified with tramadol, although nausea, constipation, and drowsiness may limit its use.

Pain unresponsive to systemic medications may respond to local therapy. Intra-articular corticosteroid injections are particularly effective in relieving pain from an acute exacerbation of osteoarthritis. Whenever joint fluid is aspirated, a sample should also be sent for analysis to rule out infection or crystal-induced arthritis. Never administer intra-articular corticosteroids when infection is suspected. The benefit from intra-articular steroids is variable; statistically significant pain relief has only been documented to 1 week after injection. Do not inject corticosteroids more frequently than every 4 months due to the risk of tendon rupture. Intra-articular hyaluronan may be beneficial, but the effect is small compared with placebo.

Consider total joint arthroplasty for patients who do not adequately respond to non-surgical methods. Replacement of the damaged joint restores normal biomechanics and often results in dramatic improvements in quality of life. Arthroscopic lavage with or without debridement is not beneficial. Joint fusion is an option that may successfully alleviate osteoarthritis pain; it is typically reserved for joints not critical for mobility, such as the spine and small joints of the hand and foot. While meniscal tears are almost universally present in knee osteoarthritis, they are not necessarily a cause of increased symptoms and surgery is not routinely recommended unless significant knee locking or loss of knee extension is present.

Book Enhancement

Go to www.acponline.org/essentials/rheumatology-section.html to view a knee x-ray, hand x-rays, clinical photographs of typical osteoarthritis findings, location of the anserine and trochanteric bursas, and a figure showing the most common locations of osteoarthritis. In *MKSAP for Students 4*, assess yourself with items 12-18 in the **Rheumatology** section.

Bibliography

Hugenberg ST, Flaspohler L. Osteoarthritis. http://pier.acponline.org/physicians/diseases/d206. [Date accessed: 2008 Feb 7] In: PIER [online database]. Philadelphia: American College of Physicians; 2008.

Hunter DJ. In the clinic. Osteoarthritis. Ann Intern Med. 2007;147:ITC8-1-ITC8-16. [PMID: 17679702]

Chapter 86

Polymyositis and Dermatomyositis

Kevin M. McKown, MD

Polymyositis and dermatomyositis are autoimmune inflammatory disorders that affect muscle, among other tissues, and typically have a subacute onset of symmetrical proximal weakness. They are associated with significant morbidity and mortality and always need to be considered in a patient with proximal weakness. Other causes of proximal weakness must be considered, especially medications (Table 1).

The cause of polymyositis and dermatomyositis is unknown, but is thought to be triggered by environmental factors (e.g., viral infection) in genetically susceptible individuals. Dermatomyositis, and less frequently polymyositis, may also occur as paraneoplastic phenomenon. There is evidence that at least some myositis-specific autoantibodies may play a role in disease pathogenesis. Involved muscles demonstrate muscle fiber necrosis, regeneration, and inflammatory infiltrates; however, there are histopathologic differences between polymyositis and dermatomyositis that are thought to reflect differences in their pathophysiology. The lymphocytic infiltration in polymyositis is predominantly composed of CD8+ T cells within muscle fascicles. In dermatomyositis inflammation occurs predominantly around the muscle fascicles, and in the interfascicular and perivascular areas. In dermatomyositis the terminal C5b-9 membrane attack complex can be found in vessel walls and muscle damage may be due to infarction of small blood vessels supplying the muscle.

Diagnosis

Proximal weakness is suggested by difficulty in rising from a chair, walking, and raising the arms or head. Pharyngeal and respiratory involvement is associated with higher mortality and is suggested by difficulty swallowing, nasal regurgitation, and dyspnea. Symptoms such as dysesthesia, numbness, tremor, stiffness, focal or asymmetrical neurological findings, or distal weakness suggest peripheral nerve, spinal cord, or brain disorders rather than muscle disease. Interstitial lung disease, cardiomyopathy, arthritis, photosensitive rashes, and malignancy are associated with polymyositis and dermatomyositis.

Look for weakness raising the arms against resistance or when arising from a chair along with relative sparing of distal strength (e.g., grip strength). Oculomotor muscles are spared, sensation and reflexes are normal, and significant muscle tenderness is unusual, as is muscle atrophy. Look for scaly, purplish papules and plaques located on the extensor surfaces of the metacarpophalangeal and interphalangeal joints (Gottron's papules) and an edematous, heliotrope (dusky purple) discoloration of the upper eyelids and periorbital tissues. Both of these rashes are diagnostic for dermatomyositis (Plate 45). Look for signs of malignancy (e.g., weight loss, ascites, breast mass, change in bowels, cough, or shortness of breath), dry crackles (interstitial lung disease), heart failure (cardiomyopathy), and arthritis.

Table 1. Differential Diagnosis of Dermatomyositis and Polymyositis

Disease	Notes
Hypothyroidism (see Chapter 10)	Weakness, stiffness, CK elevation. Screen with TSH.
Diabetes (see Chapter 8)	Fatigue, generalized muscle weakness. Diabetes causes neuropathies and plexopathies.
Drug- and alcohol-induced muscle disease	Can cause weakness, pain, and elevated CK. Consider statins, fibric acid derivatives, organophosphate poisoning.
Inclusion body myositis	Has a combination of proximal and distal weakness and is asymmetric. More common than polymyositis in older people; does not respond well to corticosteroids and immunosuppressants. Biopsy is essential to make the diagnosis.
Infections	Viruses often cause pain and may cause frank myositis. HIV can cause myositis. Consider bacterial, *Trichinella*, and other parasitic infections.
SLE, scleroderma, Sjögren's syndrome, amyloidosis, vasculitis, rheumatoid arthritis	May mimic myositis, have an element of myositis, or coexist independently of polymyositis. When two or more connective tissue diseases are present, the patient is said to have an overlap syndrome. When the combined disease is associated with high titers of anti-RNP antibodies, it is classified as mixed connective tissue disease.
Critical illness neuromyopathy	Profound generalized weakness following prolonged therapeutic paralysis in an intensive care unit. Electromyographic studies indicate combinations of muscle and nerve dysfunction.
Rhabdomyolysis	Acute muscle necrosis with myoglobinuria leading to renal failure. Caused by drugs, alcohol, trauma, seizures, and muscle disease. CK is usually >10,000 U/L.

CK = creatine kinase; HIV = human immunodeficiency virus; RNP = ribonucleoprotein; SLE = systemic lupus erythematosus; TSH = thyrotropin stimulating hormone.

Table 2. Laboratory and Other Studies for Dermatomyositis and Polymyositis

Test	Notes
CK	One of the diagnostic criteria. Levels are 10 to 50 times normal. Myocardial muscle isoforms may be elevated. Exclude hypothyroidism, alcohol, medications, exercise, cardiac disorders, and muscular dystrophy as alternative causes for an elevated CK.
Aldolase, AST, ALT, LDH	May also be elevated in muscle disease but proportionately less than CK. Elevated AST, ALT, and LDH may mistakenly suggest liver dysfunction.
Electromyography	One of the diagnostic criteria. It supports the diagnosis of a muscle disorder or, alternatively, a neuropathic or spinal cord disorder.
Anti-Jo-1 antibody	20%-25% of adult cases have these antibodies. Those who are positive are more likely to have interstitial lung disease and higher mortality rates.
Anti-RNP antibodies	In the presence of myositis and another connective tissue disease, usually SLE and scleroderma, defines mixed connective tissue disease.
Anti-MI-2 antibody	Seen in dermatomyositis with V-sign and shawl-sign rashes; good response to therapy. Seen in 5%-10%.
ANA and rheumatoid factor	Positive in a fraction of patients with polymyositis but have no predictive value.
Muscle MRI	Helps to localize inflammation and indicate site of biopsy. It may be corroborative when the diagnosis cannot be confirmed by other criteria. Conversely, a negative MRI of a weak muscle makes polymyositis unlikely.
Muscle biopsy	A positive muscle biopsy is the definitive criterion for inflammation.
Chest x-ray	Interstitial lung disease may be present before, at, or long after onset of muscle disease and can follow a variable course.
Pulmonary function studies	Respiratory dysfunction in polymyositis and dermatomyositis can be caused by respiratory muscle weakness or more often by interstitial lung disease.

ALT = alanine aminotransferase; ANA = antinuclear antibody; AST = aspartate aminotransferase; CK = creatine kinase; CT = computed tomography; LDH = lactic dehydrogenase; MRI = magnetic resonance imaging.

Serum creatine kinase, aldolase, and aspartate aminotransferase (AST) are usually elevated to at least twice the normal level. Other causes of elevated creatine kinase need to be considered, including drugs (e.g., statins) and hypothyroidism. Obtain a muscle biopsy in all patients with unexplained proximal muscle weakness and an elevated creatine kinase level. Biopsy is the most definitive test to classify a myopathy as polymyositis, muscular dystrophy, inclusion body myositis, or another less common disease. Inflammatory infiltrates of lymphocytes invading nonnecrotic muscle cells, or interstitial and perivascular areas, will be seen in about 80% of cases of polymyositis or dermatomyositis. A clinically weak muscle that has not been damaged by electromyography should be chosen for biopsy. MRI is sometimes done to select the biopsy site, as muscle involvement can be patchy. Sometimes MRI or electromyographic studies are done to provide further evidence of a myopathy, especially if a biopsy cannot be obtained or the results are non-diagnostic. Myositis-specific autoantibodies may help predict manifestations such as interstitial lung disease, as well as responsiveness to therapy and mortality (Table 2).

Malignancies are increased in adults with dermatomyositis and in adults age >45 years with polymyositis. Many experts recommend upper and lower endoscopy and chest, abdominal, and pelvic imaging studies in these patients. For other patients, obtain age and gender-appropriate cancer screening tests.

Therapy

Therapy consists of prednisone and immunosuppressive agents. Prednisone is typically started at doses of 1 mg/kg/day and tapered as the patient responds. Methotrexate or azathioprine is used with prednisone to improve the response rate and to act as steroid-sparing agents.

Follow-Up

Serum creatine kinase and muscle strength are followed to assess response to treatment. Treatment-induced toxicities are monitored with serial complete blood counts, liver aminotransferase levels, and blood glucose. Patients need to be observed for infection and receive calcium, vitamin D, and a bisphosphonate when on high-dose or long-term corticosteroids. Patients also need to be monitored for the development of cardiac or pulmonary manifestations, malignancy, and the development of other autoimmune disease.

Book Enhancement

Go to www.acponline.org/essentials/rheumatology-section.html to view examples of a heliotrope rash, Gottron's sign, and macular erythema and to access a list of drugs that can cause myositis. In *MKSAP for Students 4*, assess yourself with items 19-20 in the **Rheumatology** section.

Bibliography

Dalakas MC, Hohlfeld R. Polymyositis and dermatomyositis. Lancet. 2003;362:971-82. [PMID: 14511932]

Olsen NJ, Freeman DL. Dermatomyositis and Polymyositis. http://pier.acponline.org/physicians/diseases/d285. [Date accessed: 2008 Jan 10] In: PIER [online database]. Philadelphia: American College of Physicians; 2008.

Chapter 87

Rheumatoid Arthritis

Kathryn A. Naus, MD
Seth Mark Berney, MD

Rheumatoid arthritis is a chronic, systemic, inflammatory disorder of unknown etiology primarily involving the joints and affecting 1%-1.5% of the population worldwide. The incidence rises during adulthood and peaks in individuals aged 40-60 years. The ratio of female-to-male patients ranges from approximately 2:1 to 4:1. The hallmark features of rheumatoid arthritis are symmetric polyarthritis (synovitis) affecting the fingers, hands, wrists, and feet, and the formation of the rheumatoid factor. In addition, patients may experience constitutional symptoms (e.g., weight loss, low-grade fever, and malaise), develop rheumatoid nodules, and involvement of multiple organs. Chronic rheumatoid arthritis commonly results in joint deformity, significant decline in functional status, and premature death.

Though the precise etiology is unknown, there have been multiple factors associated with its development including: genetic susceptibility, infections (e.g., atypical bacteria, Epstein-Barr virus, and retroviruses), hormonal factors, trauma, cigarette smoking, and autoantibodies. The role of the mediators of inflammation, cytokines, growth factors, chemokines, adhesion molecules, and matrix metalloproteinases has not been clearly defined in the pathogenesis of rheumatoid arthritis. These substances appear to be involved in attracting and activating immune cells and contributing to the activation, proliferation and phenotypic transformation of synoviocytes into pannus. Pannus behaves similar to a locally invasive tumor by invading and eroding articular cartilage, subchondral bone, tendons, and ligaments. Edema of the synovium and periarticular structures contributes to stiffness in rheumatoid arthritis by interfering with the usual biomechanics of the joint.

Screening

There are no screening tests for rheumatoid arthritis. Rheumatoid factor is present in 75%-80% of patients but is also found in multiple infections, malignancies, autoimmune diseases, and 10% of the normal population. Therefore, rheumatoid factor should only be measured if there is objective evidence suggesting rheumatoid arthritis.

Diagnosis

The initial presentation of rheumatoid arthritis may be insidious or acute. Patients usually experience morning stiffness lasting >1 hour, joint pain and swelling, and difficulty performing activities of daily living. Symmetric joint involvement is typical and most commonly involves the metacarpophalangeal joints, proximal interphalangeal joints (Plate 46), wrists, elbows, knees, foot metatarsophalangeal, and proximal interphalangeal joints and the cervical spine while sparing the distal interphalangeal joints and the lumbosacral spine. The presence of cervical spine subluxation (C_1-C_2) can cause spinal instability and cord impingement, and is a general anesthetic risk.

A patient has rheumatoid arthritis if four of the seven criteria listed in Table 1 are present for at least 6 weeks, distinguishing it from viral infection. Because patients frequently do not understand the distinction between their joints "feeling swollen" and the presence of synovitis, the synovitis must be observed by a physician. Extra-articular manifestations of rheumatoid arthritis are associated with excessive mortality and include rheumatoid nodules and pulmonary, ocular, cardiac, and neurological involvement. Rheumatoid nodules are pathognomonic for rheumatoid arthritis and are associated with more severe disease. Nodules occur in 30% of patients and are commonly on the extensor surfaces of the forearms. Rheumatoid nodules may be clinically indistinguishable from gouty tophi and are best distinguished by aspiration and analysis of the aspirate under polarizing microscopy. Tophi consist of monosodium urate crystals and rheumatoid

Table 1. Clinical Criteria for Rheumatoid Arthritis

Criterion	Definition
Morning stiffness	Morning stiffness in and around the joints >1 hour before maximal improvement.
Arthritis of three or more joint areas*	Synovitis in at least three of the following joints: PIP, MCP, wrists, elbows, knees, ankles, and MTP.
Arthritis of hand joints*	Synovitis in at least one wrist, MCP, or PIP joint.
Symmetric arthritis*	Simultaneous and symmetrical involvement of the same joint areas; bilateral involvement of PIP, MCP, or MTP joints is acceptable without absolute symmetry.
Rheumatoid nodules*	Subcutaneous nodules over bony prominences or extensor surfaces, or in juxta-articular regions.
Serum rheumatoid factor	Positive result.
Radiographic changes	Must include erosions or unequivocal bony decalcification localized in or most marked adjacent to the involved joints.

* Must be observed by a physician. MCP = metacarpophalangeal; PIP = proximal interphalangeal; MTP = metatarsophalangeal.

nodules of cholesterol crystals. Pulmonary involvement occurs in 20%-25% of cases and includes pleuritis, pleural effusions, interstitial fibrosis, nodular lung disease, bronchiolitis, and arteritis with pulmonary hypertension. The most common ocular involvement is keratoconjunctivitis sicca (dry eyes), which affects approximately 30% of rheumatoid arthritis patients. Pericarditis is the most common cardiac manifestation. Severe rheumatoid arthritis is associated with accelerated atherosclerosis and premature death due to coronary artery disease. Felty's syndrome is defined by the presence of rheumatoid arthritis, neutropenia, and splenomegaly, and occurs in approximately 1% of patients.

Differential diagnosis includes the spondyloarthropathies (e.g., ankylosing spondylitis, reactive arthritis, psoriatic arthritis), viral (e.g., Epstein-Barr virus, parvovirus-B19, HIV, hepatitis C) and bacterial (e.g., endocarditis, gonococcus, Lyme disease) infections, metabolic disease (e.g., gout, calcium pyrophosphate deposition disease, hemochromatosis), connective tissue disease (e.g., systemic lupus, erythematosus, scleroderma, dermatomyositis/polymyositis), sarcoidosis, amyloidosis, and malignancy (Table 2). Osteoarthritis is characterized by bony joint enlargement, which is easily distinguished from synovitis (which it rarely causes).

Patients with active rheumatoid arthritis often have a normocytic anemia, thrombocytosis, and an elevated erythrocyte sedimentation rate and C-reactive protein, which typically parallel the joint inflammation. Rheumatoid factor, an antibody directed against the Fc fragment of IgG, is present in the sera of more than 75% of patients. An antibody against filaggrin anti-cyclic citrullinated peptide (anti-CCP) is highly specific for rheumatoid arthritis. The earliest x-ray abnormalities include soft-tissue swelling, uniform joint-space narrowing, and juxta-articular demineralization occurring in the wrists or feet. Marginal erosions, found at the attachment of the synovium to the bone, are seen initially at the head of the fifth metatarsal bone or ulnar styloid.

Drug Therapy

The goal of treatment is to suppress the inflammation and preserve joint structure and function. Early aggressive use of disease modifying anti-rheumatic drugs (DMARDs) and biologic response modifiers (BRMs) alone or in combination is most effective in achieving the treatment goal. DMARDs include methotrexate, sulfasalazine, leflunomide, hydroxychloroquine, and minocycline.

Table 2. Differential Diagnosis of Rheumatoid Arthritis (RA)

Disease	Notes
Ankylosing spondylitis (AS)	Inflammatory disorder of the axial skeleton; may have peripheral involvement; apical pulmonary fibrosis; back pain. Differs from RA because AS uncommonly has peripheral involvement and usually involves the lumbar spine.
Calcium pyrophosphate deposition disease (CPPD) (see Chapter 84)	Deposition of calcium pyrophosphate crystals in and around joints; may be monoarticular or acute oligoarticular with hot and red joint; may be chronic polyarticular in 5%; most commonly in wrist, MCP joint, shoulder, knee. Arthrocentesis: weakly positive birefringent crystals. X-ray: chondrocalcinosis. CPPD can have a pseudo-RA pattern.
Gout (see Chapter 84)	Deposition of monosodium urate crystals in tissues of and around joints; initial attack is monoarticular, most commonly the first MTP joint; chronic form may have symmetric involvement of small joints of the hands and feet with tophi and have a pseudo-RA pattern. Definitive diagnosis is synovial fluid or tophi with strongly negative birefringent crystals on polarized microscopy. Gout is extremely uncommon in premenopausal women with normal renal function.
Infective endocarditis (see Chapter 54)	Large proximal joints; fever with leukocytosis; heart murmur. Obtain blood cultures in all patients with fever and polyarthritis. RF is frequently positive.
Lyme disease	Caused by *Borrelia burgdorferi*; Early: erythema migrans rash and cardiac abnormalities; Late: intermittent monoarthritis or oligoarthritis that may become chronic. Rash and either tick exposure or travel to an endemic area are important for the diagnosis. Confirm positive ELISA test with Western blot.
Osteoarthritis (see Chapter 85)	Degeneration of articular cartilage with involvement of DIP joints, PIP joints, first CMC joints, the cervical and lumbar spine, hips, knees, and first MTP joints; pain with use; osteophytes with joint-space narrowing on x-ray. Normal laboratory studies. Little soft tissue swelling and minimal morning stiffness.
Psoriatic arthritis (see Chapter 82)	Multiple presentations: monoarthritis, oligoarthritis (asymmetric), polyarthritis (symmetric), arthritis mutilans, axial disease. Common involvement of DIP, fusiform swelling of digits, and skin and nail changes consistent with psoriasis. Can have pseudo-RA pattern but tends to be RF negative.
Peripheral arthritis associated with inflammatory bowel disease	Associated arthritis in up to 20% of cases; usually nondestructive and commonly in the lower extremities; often reflects activity of bowel disease; may be indistinguishable from AS.
Reactive arthritis (Reiter's syndrome) (see Chapter 82)	Can be precipitated by gastroenteritis or a genitourinary infection; urethritis, conjunctivitis, and arthritis; heel pain with enthesitis; keratoderma blennorrhagicum on palms or soles; circinate balanitis on penis. Differs from RA in that it is oligoarticular and asymmetric.
Septic joint (see Chapter 88)	Usually monoarticular but may be oligoarticular; large joints; hot, red, and swollen joints with a limited range of motion; may be migratory; joint aspiration is essential; RA patients may have septic joints as well.
SLE (see Chapter 89)	Clinically indistinguishable from RA; however, the arthritis in SLE is non-nodular and nonerosive.
Viral arthritis	Epstein-Barr virus, adenovirus, parvovirus B19, rubella, HIV, hepatitis B and C (potentially all viruses); morning stiffness with symmetric involvement of hands and wrists; may be RF-positive (thus is a pseudo-RA pattern); viral exanthem. Resolves in 4-6 weeks in most cases (except for parvovirus).

ANA = antinuclear antibody; CMC = carpometacarpal; DIP = distal interphalangeal; ELISA = enzyme-linked immunosorbent assay; HIV = human immunodeficiency virus; MCP = metacarpophalangeal; MTP = metatarsophalangeal; PIP = proximal interphalangeal; RF = rheumatoid factor; SLE = systemic lupus erythematosus.

Biologic response modifiers include etanercept, adalimumab, infliximab, and, more recently, rituximab and abatacept. These medications require screening for a latent tuberculosis infection prior to starting therapy because of the risk of reactivation.

Most of the life-threatening conditions are treated with DMARDs, BRMs, high-dose corticosteroids, and/or immunosuppressants (azathioprine, cyclosporine, and cyclophosphamide). The regular use of alcohol and hepatitis B or C infection are contraindications to the use of methotrexate or leflunomide.

Follow-Up

The strategy recommended by the American College of Rheumatology for monitoring methotrexate or leflunomide toxicity is to screen the patient for hepatitis A, B, and C and to measure serial serum aspartate or alanine aminotransferase levels (AST or ALT) and albumin, creatinine, and complete blood counts every 4-8 weeks.

Book Enhancement

Go to www.acponline.org/essentials/rheumatology-section.html to view a spectrum of hand changes in patients with rheumatoid arthritis, a rheumatoid nodule, hand x-ray, and a patient with Sjögren's syndrome and to access a table listing the radiographic manifestations of rheumatoid arthritis and rheumatoid arthritis articular and extra-articular manifestations. In *MKSAP for Students 4*, assess yourself with items 21-22 in the **Rheumatology** section.

Bibliography

Khurana R, Berney SM. Clinical aspects of rheumatoid arthritis. Pathophysiology. 2005;12:153-65. [PMID: 16125918]

O'Dell JR, Cannella AR. Rheumatoid Arthritis. http://pier.acponline .org/physicians/diseases/d205. [Date accessed: 2008 Jan 11] In: PIER [online database]. Philadelphia: American College of Physicians; 2008.

Chapter 88

Septic Arthritis

J. Michael Finley, DO

Approximately 80% of joint infections are monoarticular; acute monoarthritis, particularly in large joints such as the knee, should prompt consideration of septic arthritis. Many pathogens can cause septic arthritis; however, bacteria are the most significant and nongonococcal infections are the most serious. Bacterial arthritis is usually acquired hematogenously, although infection may also result from direct inoculation of bacteria into the joint space following surgery, trauma, arthrocentesis, or from contiguous infection from soft tissue or bone. Because the synovium lacks a basement membrane, bacteria easily access the joint space where they deposit on the synovial membrane and incite a swift inflammatory response. Within days cytokines and proteases can cause cartilage degradation and bone loss. Misdiagnosis of septic arthritis as rheumatoid arthritis or gouty flare not only delays treatment but results in poor functional outcome and even loss of life.

Prevention

Pre-existing arthritis, especially rheumatoid arthritis, and total joint replacement predispose to septic arthritis. Skin and wound infections are frequent sources of bacteria that seed diseased and prosthetic joints, resulting in septic arthritis. Treat all skin infections and wound infections promptly and vigorously in patients predisposed to septic arthritis. Prophylactic antibiotics given before an invasive procedure that leads to bacteremia (e.g., dental work, endoscopy, cystoscopy) may reduce the rate of prosthetic joint infections.

Diagnosis

Monoarthritis should prompt a thorough history, physical examination, and an arthrocentesis for synovial fluid analysis. Consider septic arthritis when a patient with rheumatoid arthritis has a monoarticular flare and in patients with acute gouty arthritis. Large joints are the most frequently affected, but any joint can be involved. Septic arthritis may affect the axial skeleton, including the sternoclavicular and sacroiliac joints and symphysis pubis. Clues such as fever, joint pain, joint swelling, and recent trauma can be helpful but may be absent, particularly in the elderly with multiple co-morbidities. Examine all joints for redness, warmth, swelling, and limitation of movement. Distinguish joint involvement from other causes of pain around a joint such as bursitis, tendonitis, or referred pain. Septic arthritis usually results from bacteremia; look for wound, skin, urinary tract and intra-abdominal infections, and pneumonia as potential sources. Table 1 summarizes a differential diagnosis for septic arthritis.

Obtain joint fluid in all cases of suspected septic arthritis and send for culture, Gram stain, polarized microscopy for crystals, and cell count and differential (Table 2). In most patients, the synovial fluid leukocyte count is approximately 50,000/μL, 90% of which are neutrophils. Confirm the diagnosis of nongonococcal septic arthritis by the isolation of microorganisms from the synovial fluid. *Staphylococcus aureus* and *Streptococcus pneumoniae* are the most common causative organisms. Culture the blood and any extra-articular sites of possible infection to establish a microbiologic diagnosis.

Migratory arthralgia or arthritis settling in one inflamed joint and the presence of tenosynovitis (wrist or ankle) and/or typical dermatitis (Plate 36) in a sexually active young adult raises the suspicion of disseminated gonococcal infection. Confirm the diagnosis by the isolation of the microorganism from the synovial fluid, blood, skin pustule, urethra, cervix, rectum, or throat.

Maintain a high index of suspicion for prosthetic joint infection because common symptoms and signs of infection, other than pain, may be absent. Failure to diagnose infection may lead to excess morbidity, implant removal, and death. *Staphylococcus epidermidis* is much more common in prosthetic joint infections than in native joint infections.

Hospitalize patients with septic arthritis or suspected septic arthritis to confirm the diagnosis, initiate prompt intravenous antibiotic therapy, and monitor closely the response to treatment. Management is directed toward drainage of the purulent joint space, preservation of joint integrity and function, and prompt initiation of intravenous antibiotics to ensure the best possible outcome.

Therapy

Use repeated needle aspiration to drain purulent joint fluid as completely as possible; arthroscopic drainage may be necessary when needle aspirates fail. Surgery may be indicated in suspected infection of a prosthetic joint for diagnosis and therapy when a patient reports pain in a previously painless and functioning joint prosthesis.

Because of increasing prevalence of community-associated methicillin-resistant *Staphylococcus aureus* infections, many experts recommend initiating vancomycin and ceftazidime or a quinolone if the Gram stain is positive for gram-positive cocci or if the Gram stain is negative and the risk for *N. gonorrhoeae* infection is low. If the Gram stain shows gram-negative cocci or the risk

Table 1. Differential Diagnosis of Septic Arthritis

Disease	Notes
Crystal-induced synovitis (see Chapter 84)	In gout, the first metatarsophalangeal joint is the most frequently affected joint, and monosodium urate crystals are present in the synovial fluid. In pseudogout, the knee or the wrist is the most common site of acute synovitis, and calcium pyrophosphate dihydrate crystals are present in the synovial fluid. Consider the possibility of the coexistence of crystal-induced arthritis and septic arthritis.
Rheumatoid arthritis (RA) (see Chapter 87)	RA is usually a symmetric polyarthritis affecting large and small joints associated with a positive rheumatoid factor in 80% of cases. It rarely presents as a monoarthritis. RA flares may be monoarticular and present as pseudoseptic arthritis. Synovial fluid analysis including Gram stain and culture will usually distinguish RA flare from septic arthritis.
Systemic lupus erythematosus (see Chapter 89)	Acute arthritis, especially monoarthritis, in an immunosuppressed SLE patient requires a diligent work-up to rule out septic arthritis. The search should also include opportunistic infections in addition to the common pathogens.
Reactive arthritis	Can be precipitated by gastroenteritis or a genitourinary infection; urethritis, conjunctivitis, and arthritis; heel pain with enthesitis; keratoderma blennorrhagicum on palms or soles; circinate balanitis on penis. Upon initial presentation initiating antibiotic therapy is very reasonable until culture results are known and the diagnosis of reactive arthritis can be substantiated.
Sickle cell disease (see Chapter 40)	Acute joint pain is seen with sickle cell's painful crisis. Arthralgia is common but frank arthritis can be encountered. In the event of an acute inflammatory arthritis, septic arthritis, bone infarction, and osteomyelitis must be considered. In addition to arthrocentesis, joint and bone imaging may be helpful in establishing a diagnosis.
Hemarthrosis	Blood in a joint may lead to an intense inflammatory reaction that mimics septic arthritis. The source of the blood may be from trauma, hemophilia, over anticoagulation, or other bleeding disorders (e.g., thrombocytopenia, severe liver disease, acquired clotting factor deficiency).
Other infectious arthritis	Although subacute or chronic in many cases, infectious arthritis can be caused by fungi, viruses, parasites, tuberculosis, and Lyme disease.

Table 2. Laboratory and Other Studies for Septic Arthritis

Test	Notes
WBC count	The lack of leukocytosis does not rule out septic arthritis.
Synovial fluid Gram stain	The rate of finding gram-positive cocci by Gram-stained smear varies between 50% and 75%. They are more easily seen than gram-negative organisms. The rate of finding gram-negative bacilli by Gram-stained smear is only 50%. From 70%-90% of synovial fluids show positive culture results in cases of septic arthritis not due to *N. gonorrhoeae*. Less than 50% of synovial fluids are positive for *N. gonorrhoeae* arthritis. In the remaining cases, the diagnosis is established by culturing *N. gonorrhoeae* at an extra-articular site, such as blood, skin pustule, urethral/cervical, or rectal or throat swab.
Synovial fluid WBC count	The leukocyte counts of the synovial fluids in septic arthritis vary considerably. Most would fall into the moderately (10,000-50,000 cells/µL) to highly (50,000->100,000 cells/µL) inflammatory ranges.
Synovial fluid culture	Gram-positive organisms account for 75%-80% of all infection. *S. aureus* accounts for 50% of all cases; streptococci, 25%; gram-negative, 20%; and others (including *S. epidermidis* and *H. influenzae*), 5%.
Blood culture	Culture blood and extra-articular sites of possible infection to establish microbiologic diagnosis.
X-rays and MRI	Changes seen on x-ray of joint and bone damage due to infection are relatively late findings. In acute septic arthritis, soft tissue fullness and joint effusions are often the only initial x-ray findings. MRI of the affected joint is especially useful in detecting avascular necrosis, soft tissue masses, and collections of fluid not appreciated by other imaging modalities.

MRI = magnetic resonance imaging; WBC = white blood cell.

for *N. gonorrhoeae* infection is high, ceftriaxone is an appropriate first choice; also treat empirically for concurrent *Chlamydia* infection. Ceftazidime is recommended for infection with gram-negative bacilli. If *Pseudomonas* infection is possible (e.g., intravenous drug user), gentamicin is added to ceftazidime. As culture results become available the antibiotic choice can be narrowed. Duration of treatment is based on the initial response to antibiotic treatment, the specific microorganism, and patient characteristics. Shorten the duration of antibiotic administration to 2 weeks or less when the microorganism is exquisitely sensitive to the drug used, such as *N. gonorrhoeae*, and the patient responds promptly. Administer antibiotics for 4 weeks or longer for virulent microorganisms such as *S. aureus* or difficult-to-treat pathogens such as *P. aeruginosa*. Consider chronic suppressive antibiotic treatment of infected prosthesis without removal only under certain circumstances, such as the prosthesis not being loose or the patient being a poor surgical candidate.

Follow-Up

Use serial examination of synovial fluid to help monitor the response to therapy. Serial synovial fluid specimens usually show a decrease in total leukocyte count, conversion to negative culture result, and a decrease in the amount of fluid reaccumulation that parallel other clinical signs of response. Pain on range of motion should decrease, and function of the joint should improve or be regained.

Book Enhancement

Go to www.acponline.org/essentials/rheumatology-section.html to review the steps in knee arthrocentesis, to view a knee effusion and an x-ray of septic hip arthritis, and to access a table on synovial fluid findings. In *MKSAP for Students 4*, assess yourself with items 23-28 in the **Rheumatology** section.

Bibliography

Ho G. Septic Arthritis. http://pier.acponline.org/physicians/diseases/d923/d923.html. [Date accessed: 2008 Feb 7] In: PIER [online database]. Philadelphia: American College of Physicians; 2008.

Margaretten ME, Kohlwes J, Moore D, Bent S. Does this adult patient have septic arthritis? JAMA. 2007;297:1478-88. [PMID: 17405973]

Chapter 89

Systemic Lupus Erythematosus

Nicole Cotter, MD
Seth Mark Berney, MD

Systemic lupus erythematosus (SLE) is an autoimmune disease characterized by immune complex deposition, autoantibody formation, and organ inflammation. SLE affects women nine times more commonly than men, and most patients are diagnosed in their third or fourth decades. Some races are more commonly affected (e.g., African Americans, Asians, Hispanics). Although the etiology is unknown it appears multifactorial. There is a genetic association with 25%-50% concordance rates in monozygotic twins and 5% concordance in dizygotic twins and non-twin siblings. Environmental influences (e.g., ultraviolet light), infections, and hormones likely contribute to SLE development. Although multiple immunological abnormalities have been identified in SLE, most lupus experts are unsure whether these cause or result from the disease. SLE commonly involves the blood components, central and peripheral nervous systems, heart, joints, kidneys, lungs, serosa and skin. The most characteristic laboratory finding is the antinuclear antibody (ANA).

Screening

Screening for SLE in asymptomatic patients or in patients with atypical symptoms is not indicated. Antinuclear antibodies are found in 95%-99% of all SLE patients but lack specificity. They are also found in patients with viral and bacterial infections, other autoimmune diseases, malignancies, cirrhosis, and 10% of the normal population.

Diagnosis

To diagnose SLE, a patient must have a supportive history, physical examination, and laboratory data. A patient is classified as having SLE if four of the eleven American College of Rheumatology criteria (mnemonic: SOAP BRAIN MD) are confirmed by a physician. These eleven criteria are discussed below and summarized in Table 1.

Serositis includes pleuritis, pericarditis, and peritonitis. Patients may report pleuritic chest pain or positional pain consistent with pericarditis and must have chest radiographic, electrocardiographic, or echocardiographic findings consistent with serositis.

Oral ulcers are painless and usually seen on the hard palate or nasal mucosa.

Arthritis is clinically indistinguishable from rheumatoid arthritis but does not cause nodules or erosions. Some patients may develop ulnar deviation, boutonniere, and swan-neck deformities (Jaccoud's arthritis).

Table 1. SOAP BRAIN MD Mnemonic for SLE Criteria

Serositis	**B**lood dyscrasias	**M**alar rash
Oral ulcers	**R**enal	**D**iscoid rash
Arthritis	**A**NA	
Photosensitive rash	**I**mmunologic	
	Neurologic	

Any rash caused or worsened by ultraviolet light exposure is a *photosensitive rash*. Patients will develop this rash in tanning beds and in direct sunlight, and because clouds do not block ultraviolet radiation, they will also develop the rash when it is cloudy.

The *blood dyscrasias* include leukopenia, lymphopenia, thrombocytopenia, or a Coomb's positive (autoimmune) hemolytic anemia with reticulocytosis. The presence of any of these documented on two separate occasions fulfills the criterion for diagnosis. The cytopenias are generally secondary to peripheral destruction, not marrow suppression.

Renal disease is very common in SLE. A patient satisfies this criterion by having >500 mg of urine protein in a 24-hour collection, >10 red blood cells per high power field, red blood cell or leukocyte casts in a sterile urine (by culture), or by kidney biopsy.

The *ANA* criterion is titer >1:80.

The *immunologic* criterion includes the very specific but insensitive antibodies: anti-double stranded DNA (DsDNA) and anti-smith (anti-Sm). The other immunologic abnormality is antiphospholipid antibodies, which may be detected by a positive test for the SLE anticoagulant, a false-positive RPR or VDRL, or a positive anticardiolipin antibody assay. The presence of any of these fulfills this criterion.

Although the *neurologic* criterion includes only seizure and psychosis, a variety of neurological and psychiatric manifestations may be seen including cerebritis, cranial and peripheral neuropathies, transverse myelitis, mood disorders (e.g., depression), and acute confusional state.

Malar rash (butterfly rash) is a maculopapular or erythematous rash that usually involves the cheeks and the bridge of the nose but spares the nasolabial folds (Plate 14).

Discoid lesions occur as discrete plaques on face, ears, scalp and extremities that may leave scars on healing. Many patients have discoid lupus without any systemic manifestations of SLE and negative or low ANA titers. Such patients do have an increased risk of developing SLE.

Fever, fatigue, weight loss, alopecia, arthralgia, and nausea are also common symptoms.

SLE is also associated with Raynaud's phenomenon (fingers or toes become white then blue when cold and red when warmed) and secondary Sjögren's syndrome, which causes dry mucous membranes (mouth, nose, eyes, vagina).

A patient suspected of having SLE needs a thorough physical examination to identify which organs are involved, with emphasis on the classification criteria. Nonspecific findings such as fever, tachycardia, and lymphadenopathy commonly occur but must not automatically be attributed to SLE. The most common cause of fever in SLE is infection. Closely inspect nasal and oral mucus membranes for painless ulcerations. Dentures should be removed to inspect the hard palate. Discoid rashes occur commonly in the external ear, on the forearms and scalp, and may cause alopecia. Funduscopic exam may reveal grayish-white fluffy exudates (cytoid bodies or cotton-wool spots), indicating focal retinal infarctions. Pleuritis and pericarditis may be detected by auscultating a friction rub or identifying signs of an effusion. Hepatosplenomegaly may be seen in SLE. Intestinal perforation (resulting from corticosteroids, vasculitis, or infection) must also be considered as a cause of abdominal pain. On musculoskeletal exam, patients may have joint tenderness or synovitis. Neurological deficits, seizures, or confusion indicate central nervous system infection, ischemia, or brain or spinal cord inflammation (cerebritis or transverse myelitis), or the more subtle neuropsychiatric lupus. Sensory or motor symptoms may be due to peripheral neuropathy, muscle inflammation, or ischemia (e.g., vasculitis).

In active SLE, the circulating immune complexes activate complement causing their consumption, resulting in the decrease of C3, C4, and the total hemolytic complement (CH50 or CH100). Serial C3, C4, CH50, or CH100 measurements may help determine whether SLE is becoming more active or responding to therapy. Additionally, the level of Ds-DNA may reflect the disease activity: the higher the Ds-DNA titer, the more active is the disease.

The differential diagnosis of SLE is broad, including viral and bacterial infections, malignancies, other autoimmune diseases, cirrhosis, and hypothyroidism (Table 2). Extensive laboratory investigation is commonly necessary to establish a diagnosis of SLE in a patient presenting with a multisystem disease.

Therapy

SLE may flare as a result of physical or emotional stress, including infection, trauma, and ultraviolet radiation exposure. Thus, patients should try to avoid stress, stay rested, and maintain good nutrition. To minimize the risk of SLE exacerbation by solar radiation, patients should wear a hat and protective clothing to cover as much skin as possible, and use sunscreen with an SPF of 15 or higher. Patients with SLE are at increased risk of premature atherosclerosis and steroid-induced osteoporosis and should eat a low-fat, low-cholesterol diet, avoid cigarettes, exercise, and take calcium and vitamin D supplementation. It was previously thought that oral contraceptives or pregnancy always caused SLE flares. However, recent data have contradicted this belief, and now oral contraceptives and pregnancy are considered acceptable for most patients.

Drug therapy for SLE depends on the manifestations for a particular patient. Arthralgias, arthritis, myalgias, fever, and mild serositis may improve on nonsteroidal anti-inflammatory drugs or

Table 2. Differential Diagnosis of Systemic Lupus Erythematosus (SLE)

Disease	Notes
Chronic fatigue syndrome; fibromyalgia	Eleven or more characteristic tender points (in fibromyalgia), with chronic pain above and below the waist. About 30% of patients with SLE may also have fibromyalgia; most patients with SLE have chronic fatigue syndrome.
Rheumatoid arthritis (see Chapter 87)	Symmetric polyarthritis, very similar to SLE, but deforming arthritis and erosions are more common. Patients with SLE can have a positive rheumatoid factor.
Drug-induced lupus	Fever, serositis, arthritis. Minocycline, hydralazine, procainamide, and isoniazid are the major drugs that cause drug-induced lupus.
Hepatitis C (essential mixed cryoglobulinemia)	Palpable purpura, nephritis, neuropathy. Although mild elevation of transaminase levels are found in 30% of patients with SLE, elevated transaminases should lead to a search for hepatitis B and C.
Wegener's granulomatosus (see Chapter 90)	Sinus disease, lung nodules, renal disease. ANCA is usually positive.
Polyarteritis nodosa (see Chapter 90)	Vasculitis, renal disease, mononeuritis multiplex. Biopsy shows medium-vessel vasculitis.
Parvovirus (fifth disease)	Can cause a symmetric polyarthritis, usually self-limited. May be associated with "slapped cheeks" disease in the local school system.
Serum sickness	Can mimic SLE with fever, rash, and complement consumption.
Thrombotic thrombocytopenic purpura (see Chapter 41)	May mimic SLE; fever, CNS changes, thrombocytopenia, and renal failure. Finding schistocytes on the peripheral smear is a major clue.
Malignancy	Positive ANA, anemia, high ESR, polyarthritis, pleural effusions, fever, and other symptoms can occur.
HIV/AIDS (see Chapter 50)	Can lead to production of antiphospholipid antibodies and a positive Coombs' test, and can cause thrombocytopenia. Some patients with SLE will have false-positive ELISAs for HIV. Western blot confirmation of HIV is essential.

AIDS = acquired immunodeficiency syndrome; ANA = antinuclear antibody; ANCA = antinuclear cytoplasmic antibody; CNS = central nervous system; ELISA = enzyme-linked immunosorbent assay; ESR = erythrocyte sedimentation rate; HIV = human immunodeficiency virus.

require methotrexate, hydroxychloroquine, or, occasionally, low-dose corticosteroids. The skin manifestations of SLE may respond to antimalarials, methotrexate, or topical or intralesional corticosteroids. Systemic corticosteroids are reserved for moderate-to-severe SLE. For severe manifestations (nephritis, pneumonitis, pericarditis, cerebritis, vasculitis, and severe cytopenias), high-dose corticosteroids or pulse methylprednisolone and other immunosuppressive agents (azathioprine, mycophenolate, and cyclophosphamide) or biologic therapy (rituximab) may be required. However, prior to or simultaneous with initiation of systemic corticosteroids or other immunosuppressive or biologic therapy, a purified protein derivative (PPD) must be placed to establish whether the patient is at risk for reactivation tuberculosis. For patients who require high doses of corticosteroids for long periods of time, immunosuppressive drugs may be used as steroid-sparing agents. Vaccination against pneumococcus, *Haemophilus influenzae*, influenza, and possibly meningococcus is indicated because these patients appear to have functional asplenia.

Follow-Up

Patients need regular follow-up to detect disease flares. A complete blood count, creatinine, C3 and C4, and urinalysis with culture and sensitivity at routine follow-up visits should be performed to screen patients for anemia, leukopenia, thrombocytopenia, or evidence of nephritis. Lifestyle modifications and pharmacological therapies to reduce cardiovascular risk factors must be instituted, because cardiovascular disease is the major cause of death in SLE patients.

Book Enhancement

Go to www.acponline.org/essentials/rheumatology-section.html to view images of discoid lupus, subacute cutaneus lupus, and an aphthous ulcer, to access tables on autoantibodies associated with SLE and antinuclear antibody associations with non-SLE conditions, and to access additional information about lupus nephritis. In *MKSAP for Students 4*, assess yourself with items 29-31 in the **Rheumatology** section.

Bibliography

Dall'Era M, Davis JC. Systemic lupus erythematosus: how to manage, when to refer. Postgrad Med. 2003;114:31-7, 40. [PMID: 14650091]

D'Cruz DP. Systemic lupus erythematosus. BMJ. 2006;332:890-4. [PMID: 16613963]

Chapter 90

Vasculitis

Patrick C. Alguire, MD

Vasculitis is an inflammation of blood vessels that causes stenosis, obstruction, or attenuation with subsequent tissue ischemia, aneurysms, or hemorrhage. This condition may be secondary to an underlying process or occur as a primary disease of unknown cause. Primary vasculitides may be categorized based on the size of the blood vessel that is predominantly involved (small, medium, and large vessel), the pattern of organ involvement, and the histopathology. Systemic vasculitis is often a diagnosis of exclusion in patients with multisystem disease. Clinical clues often point to the diagnosis, especially if there are skin, renal, or large vessel signs. The diagnosis of vasculitis requires biopsy of an affected site or arteriography if medium-sized or large vessels are involved.

A vasculitis of particular relevance to general internal medicine is giant cell arteritis (temporal arteritis) because the disorder is relatively common (prevalence 1.5%), is found exclusively in the elderly, and is frequently in the differential diagnosis of perplexing geriatric symptoms (it rarely occurs in those <50 years old). Giant cell arteritis causes localized inflammation in the smaller branches of the external carotid artery. Involvement of the ophthalmic artery can cause blindness. The release of inflammatory cytokines contributes to the prominent constitutional symptoms of malaise, fever, and weight loss associated with this disorder; it is frequently associated with anemia of inflammation.

Diagnosis

Consider a diagnosis of vasculitis in patients with systemic symptoms and single- or multiple-organ dysfunction. Exclude infectious, hematologic, drug-related, and other organ-specific processes that can mimic vasculitis. Ask specifically about previous thrombotic events, cocaine abuse, endocarditis, hepatitis, and HIV infection. Look for recent invasive arterial procedures (e.g., cardiac catheterization) because cholesterol emboli can mimic vasculitis. Use of vasoconstrictive drugs (e.g., phenylpropanolamine, ephedra alkaloids) can also mimic vasculitis (Table 1). The most common symptoms of giant cell arteritis are headache, jaw claudication, visual complaints, and an association with polymyalgia rheumatica (PMR), though most patients with PMR do not have giant cell arteritis. While insensitive, the presence of jaw claudication and diplopia are the most predictive symptoms, with positive likelihood ratios between 3 and 4. Polymyalgia rheumatica is characterized by aching and morning stiffness in the proximal muscles of the shoulder and hip girdle and may develop in patients with giant cell arteritis or as a primary condition.

On physical examination, look for the more common features of vasculitis: rashes (Plate 47), nail bed infarcts, or digital tuft ulcers; pulse asymmetries or bruits or aortic regurgitation; muscle weakness or tenderness; nasal, oral, or genital ulcers; and sinusitis. The presence of temporal artery beading, prominence, or enlargement is the most predictive physical finding (positive likelihood ratios >4) for giant cell arteritis, whereas the presence of synovitis makes the diagnosis much less likely.

Obtain the following tests in all patients with suspected vasculitis: complete blood count, serum creatinine level, aminotransferase levels, and erythrocyte sedimentation rate or C-reactive protein. Obtain a urinalysis and assess for erythrocytes, erythrocyte casts, and mixed cellular casts. Urinalysis is essential because glomerulonephritis is common in many systemic vasculitides and is clinically silent until uremia develops. In suspected Wegener's granulomatosis, the presence of c-ANCA (cytoplasmic antineutrophil cytoplasmic antibody) with enzyme immunoassay specificity for proteinase 3 provides strong support for the diagnosis. In suspected microscopic polyangiitis and Churg-Strauss syndrome, the combination of p-ANCA (perinuclear antineutrophil cytoplasmic antibody) and antibodies to myeloperoxidase is strong circumstantial evidence. Ultimately, it is the clinical pattern of disease and confirmatory biopsy that makes the diagnosis of vasculitis (Table 2). Giant cell arteritis is associated with an elevated erythrocyte sedimentation rate, but this finding is nonspecific, whereas a sedimentation rate less than 50 mm/h makes the diagnosis very unlikely (negative likelihood ratio 0.35). On temporal artery biopsy, giant cell arteritis is associated with panmural mononuclear cell infiltration that may be granulomatous with histiocytes and giant cells, confirming the diagnosis.

Therapy

Angioplasty or bypass procedures may be needed in patients with large vessel vasculitis and critical ischemia. Aortic root reconstruction or valve replacement may be indicated in patients with large vessel vasculitis and severe aortic involvement.

Drug therapy depends on the specific type of vasculitis and the degree of end-organ involvement (Table 2). In patients with a strong clinical suspicion for giant cell arteritis, immediate initiation of prednisone is indicated to prevent blindness. Treatment should not be delayed until biopsy is obtained or results are returned. Corticosteroid therapy, 40-60 mg/d, rapidly relieves cranial and systemic symptoms of giant cell arteritis, and then is usually gradually tapered. Most patients require 2 years of therapy, although more than 4 years may be required in some patients.

Table 1. Differential Diagnosis of Vasculitis

Disease	Notes
Infection (see Chapter 54)	Heart murmur, rash, and musculoskeletal symptoms can occur in infective endocarditis, sterile emboli, cardiac myxoma, and antiphospholipid antibody syndrome.
Drug toxicity/poisoning	May produce vasospasm resulting in symptoms due to ischemia. Check for cocaine, amphetamines, ephedra alkaloids, phenylpropanolamine.
Coagulopathy (see Chapters 41 and 42)	Occlusive diseases (disseminated intravascular coagulation, antiphospholipid antibody syndrome, thrombotic thrombocytopenic purpura) can produce ischemic symptoms.
Atrial myxoma	Classic triad: embolism, intracardiac obstruction leading to heart failure, and constitutional symptoms (fatigue, weight loss, fever). Skin lesions can be identical to those seen in leukocytoclastic vasculitis. Atrial myxomas are rare, but they are the most common primary intracardiac tumor.
Multiple cholesterol emboli	Associated with severe atherosclerosis. Embolization may occur after abdominal trauma, aortic surgery, or angiography. Look for livedo reticularis, petechiae and purpuric lesions, and localized skin necrosis.
Congenital collagen disorders (Ehlers-Danlos syndrome, Marfan syndrome)	Marfan: tall stature, scoliosis, arachnodactyly, pectus excavatum, high-arched palate, subluxation of the lens, mitral valve prolapse, dilatation of ascending aorta. Ehlers-Danlos: easy bruising, distensible skin, arterial aneurysms/rupture, enteric/uterine rupture, spontaneous pneumothorax, hernias, history of poor wound healing. Not all patients have all features of disease. No associated systemic symptoms (e.g., fever, malaise).
Fibromuscular dysplasia (see Chapter 37)	More common in females than males. Stenoses are more common than aneurysms. Renal arteries are the most commonly involved vessels. No associated systemic symptoms (e.g., fever, malaise).

Table 2. Categorization and Therapy of Vasculitides

Disease	Notes
Giant cell (temporal) arteritis	Granulomatous arteritis of the aorta and its major branches; commonly affects the temporal artery. Cardinal symptoms are headaches, scalp tenderness, jaw claudication, carotidynia, and fever. Ocular symptoms, including blindness, may occur in 5%-30% of cases. Usually occurs in patients >50 years. Treated initially with prednisone 50-60 mg/d.
Takayasu's arteritis	Chronic, granulomatous inflammatory disease primarily of the aorta and its main branches. Affects women during their reproductive years. Cardinal symptom is claudication associated with pulse deficits, bruits, or asymmetric blood pressures. Treated with prednisone 1 mg/kg; methotrexate is added to resistant cases. Percutaneous transluminal angioplasty for fixed vascular lesions causing ischemia.
Polyarteritis nodosa	Nongranulomatous necrotizing vasculitis of medium or small arteries without glomerulonephritis. Key features: renal disease, hypertension, gastrointestinal pain, peripheral neuropathy, and skin lesions. Vasculitis can also cause testicular pain, cardiac disease, and strokes. May be related to hepatitis B. Treated with corticosteroids and cyclophosphamide for life-threatening disease. If secondary to viral hepatitis, anti-viral treatment is indicated.
Wegener's granulomatosis	Necrotizing granulomatous inflammation of small- to medium-sized vessels. Predilection for the upper and lower respiratory tracts and kidneys. Associated with positive c-ANCA; the antibody-targeted antigen is usually proteinase 3. Treated with corticosteroids and cyclophosphamide. Relapse is common.
Churg-Strauss syndrome	Granulomatous inflammation of small- to medium-sized vessels with key features of asthma and eosinophilia. Pulmonary involvement with transient, patchy, alveolar infiltrates is common. Renal disease occurs in about 50% of cases. Can be confused with Wegener's granulomatosis, which usually lacks asthma. Prednisone 1 mg/kg/d is effective; cyclophosphamide is added for resistant or life-threatening disease.
Microscopic polyangiitis	Nongranulomatous, necrotizing inflammation of small vessels with or without medium-vessel involvement. Commonly affects the lungs and kidneys. Distinguished from polyarteritis nodosa by the presence of pulmonary capillaritis or glomerulonephritis. Can be confused with the pulmonary-renal presentation of Wegener's granulomatosis, but distinguished by lack of otolaryngologic features. Combination therapy with cyclophosphamide and prednisone 1 mg/kg/d is initial treatment.
Henoch-Schönlein purpura	Vasculitis of small vessels that typically involves the skin, gut, and kidneys (nephritis). Fever and arthralgias/arthritis are common. Gut involvement is less common in adults than in children. Biopsy shows predominantly IgA immune-complex deposition. Often initiated by an upper respiratory infection. Corticosteroids have no proven benefit.
Essential cryoglobulinemic vasculitis	Small-vessel inflammation characterized by the presence of cryoglobulins. Skin and kidneys are often involved. Most often due to hepatitis C infection. Treat hepatitis C; avoid corticosteroids.
Leukocytoclastic vasculitis	Vasculitis of small vessels that most commonly affects the skin (Plate 47). Can result from many conditions, including autoimmune disease (e.g., systemic lupus erythematosus, rheumatoid arthritis), infection (viral, especially hepatitis viruses), malignancy, and medications. Treatment depends upon cause.

Follow-Up

Arrange follow-up (every 1 to 4 weeks) for patients with vasculitis to evaluate disease activity and monitor for medication toxicity. Although laboratory studies are not definitive markers of disease activity, most diseases can be monitored with the erythrocyte sedimentation rate and C-reactive protein level and urinalysis.

Book Enhancement

Go to www.acponline.org/essentials/rheumatology-section.html to access a table of recommended tests and to view examples of cutaneous infarction, livedo reticularis, giant cell arteritis, and an angiogram of a patient with Takayasu's arteritis. In *MKSAP for Students 4*, assess yourself with items 32-35 in the **Rheumatology** section.

Bibliography

Shaw ML, Hoffman GS. Vasculitis. http://pier.acponline.org/physicians/diseases/ d321. [Date accessed: 2008 Jan 17] In: PIER [online database]. Philadelphia: American College of Physicians; 2008.

Smetana GW, Shmerling RH. Does this patient have temporal arteritis? JAMA. 2002;287:92-101. [PMID: 11754714]

Index

Basilar artery, 245
Basilar skull fracture, 242
BCR-ABL gene, 162
Behavioral counseling, 117
Behavorial therapy, 105
Behçet's disease, 184
Benign familial hypocalciuric hypercalcemia, 226
Benign growth, 130-131
Beta cell failure, 37
Beta-2-adrenergic bronchodilator, 288
Beta-2-microglobulin, 165
Beta-agonist, 283, 288
Beta-agonist inhaler, 113
Beta-blocker
    in acute coronary syndrome, 13
    for angina, 9
    in bradyarrhythmia, 15-16
    for cirrhosis, 85
    in heart failure, 26, 27
    for hypertension, 138, 139
    in mitral stenosis, 31
    syncope and, 102
    in thyroid disorder, 46
    for ventricular tachycardia, 22
Beta-thalassemia, 145
Bezold-Jarisch reflex, 100
Bias in screening, 96
Bicarbonate, 218
Bicipital tendonitis, 310
Bile acid, 62
Biliary colic
    pancreatitis vs, 67
    peptic ulcer vs, 72
Biliary disease, 64-66
    diagnosis of, 64-65
    dyspepsia vs, 74
    follow-up for, 65-66
    prevention of, 64
    treatment of, 65
Biliary obstruction, 83
Biliary pain, 57
Bilirubin, 144
Biologic response modifier, 321
Biopsy
    in polymyositis and dermatomyositis, 318
    for skin cancer, 268
Bisoprolol, 27
Bisphosphonate
    for multiple myeloma, 166
    osteoporosis and, 53
Bladder, 181
Bleeding
    abdominal pain with, 57
    abnormal uterine, 126
    gastrointestinal, 76-79
        in inflammatory bowel disease, 87
    thrombocytopenic purpura and, 156
Bleeding disorder
    antibodies to clotting factors in, 151
    approach to patient with, 149
    disseminated intravascular coagulopathy as, 151
    hemophilia as, 150
    liver disease causing, 150
    vitamin K deficiency and, 150-151
    Von Willebrand disease as, 149-150
Bleeding time, 150
Blood culture
    in infective endocarditis, 200
    in septic arthritis, 323
Blood disorder, 143-169. *See also* Hematologic disorder

Blood dyscrasias, 325
Blood gases
    arterial, 291
    in delirium, 233
    for pulmonary embolism, 299
Blood loss, 147
Blood pressure
    hypertension, 137-140
    in sickle cell anemia, 154
Blood smear
    in immune thrombocytopenic purpura, 156
    in multiple myeloma, 165
Blood test, 102
Blood transfusion, 153
Blood urea nitrogen, 233
Blood vessel, 328-330
BODE index, 286
Body mass index, 118
Body temperature, 171
Bone
    in multiple myeloma, 165
    osteomyelitis of, 203-205
    osteoporosis and, 52-54
Bone marrow, 155
Bone marrow aspiration
    in immune thrombocytopenic purpura, 156
    in multiple myeloma, 155
Bone metastasis, 264
Bone mineral metabolism, 214
Bordetella pertussis, 113
Borrelia burgdorferi, 241
Bortezomide, 166
Bowel
    inflammatory disease of, 87-89
    irritable, 59-60
    obstruction of, 58
Bowel habits, 257
Bowen's disease, 269
Brachytherapy, 263
Bradyarrhythmia, 15-16
Bradycardia, 101
Brain, 237-238
BRCA gene mutation, 253
Breast cancer, 253-255
Bronchiectasis, 286
Bronchiolitis, 286
Bronchiolitis obliterans, 198
Bronchitis, 114, 178
    nonasthmatic eosinophilic, 114
    pulmonary embolism vs, 297
Bronchoalveolar lavage, 294
Bronchodilator
    for asthma, 283
    for chronic obstructive pulmonary disease, 288
Bronchogenic carcinoma, 198
Bruit, 244
Bumetanide, 27
Bupropion, 105
    in smoking cessation, 117
Bursitis, 309
Butterfly rash, 325
Bypass surgery, 14

C

CAGE questionnaire, 107
Calcitonin, 53, 54
Calcium
    in chronic kidney disease, 213, 214
    metabolism of, 225-226
    in multiple myeloma, 165

osteoporosis and, 52
Calcium antagonist, 139
Calcium channel blocker
    for angina, 9
    for hypertension, 138
    in mitral stenosis, 31
    for tachycardia, 18
Calcium pyrophosphate deposition, 312-314
Calculus
    biliary, 64-66
    renal, 59
Calymmatobacterium granulomatis, 184
Campylobacter jejuni, 61
c-ANCA, 328
Cancer, 253-272
    breast, 253-255
    bronchogenic, 198
    cervical, 265-267
    colon, 256-258
    dyspepsia vs, 74
    hypercalcemia and, 225-226
    infective endocarditis vs, 202
    low back pain with, 110
    lung, 259-261
    pain management of, 271-272
    peptic ulcer vs, 72
    prostate, 262-264
    rectal, 257
    screening for, 96-97
    skin, 268-270
    thrombophilia and, 158
    weight loss with, 121
Candesartan, 27
Candida albicans, 130
Candidiasis, 187
Capsulitis, 310
Captopril, 27
Carbohydrate intolerance, 62
Carbon monoxide, diffusing capacity of, 282, 302-303
Carcinoid syndrome, 50
Carcinoma, 126
Cardiac transplantation, 26
Cardiogenic shock, 175
Cardiomyopathy, hypertrophic, 28, 29, 100
Cardiovascular disorder
    acute coronary syndrome as, 11-14
    chest pain in, 3-6
    chronic stable angina as, 7-10
    in diabetes mellitus, 37
    dyspnea in, 275-277
    heart failure as, 24-27
    hypertension and, 138
    infective endocarditis, 200-202
    low back pain with, 110
    in sickle cell anemia, 152
    supraventricular arrhythmia as, 15-19
    syncope in, 100
    valvular heart disease as, 28-33
    venous thromboembolism and, 298
    ventricular arrhythmia as, 20-23
    weight loss with, 121
Cardiovascular system
    in chronic obstructive pulmonary disease, 286
    hyperkalemia and, 223
    in sickle cell anemia, 154
Cardioversion
    in aortic stenosis, 30
    in arrhythmia, 18
    in ventricular tachycardia, 22
Carotid bruit, 244
Carotid massage, 18

Thrombotic endocarditis, 202
Thrombotic thrombocytopenic purpura, 155
Thrombotic thrombocytopenic purpura-
    hemolytic uremic syndrome, 156-157
Thyroid disorder, 44-47
    diagnosis of, 44-45
    hypercalcemia and, 226
    hypertension in, 137
    hyponatremia and, 221
    obesity as, 119
    screening for, 44
    treatment of, 45-47
Thyroid peroxidase antibody, 45
Thyroid storm, 45
Thyroidectomy, 45
Thyroid-stimulating hormone, 47
    in anemia, 144
    in hyperthyroidism, 44
    in hypothyroidism, 45
    in sleep apnea, 291
    weight loss and, 122
Thyrotoxicosis, 44
    diagnosis of, 46
    follow-up of, 47
    pheochromocytoma vs, 50
    treatment of, 46
Thyroxine, 45
Tigecycline, 129
Tilt table testing, 101, 102
Tinea, 269
Tinea infection, 129-130
Tiotropium, 288
Tirofiban, 13
Tobacco, 24
Tolerance, 272
Tophaceous gout, 313
Tophus, 319-320
Torsades de pointes, 22
Torsemide, 27
Torsion
    ovarian, 58
    testicular, 59
Total incontinence, 135
Total joint arthroplasty, 316
Toxic exposure, 83
Toxic megacolon, 58, 59
Toxicity, 329
Toxin
    altered mental state from, 231
    thrombocytopenia and, 155
Toxoplasmosis, 187, 188
Tramadol, 316
Transdermal opioid patch, 272
Transferrin receptor, 144
Transfusion, 153
Transient ischemic attack, 244
Transjugular intrahepatic portosystemic stent
    shunt, 85
Transplantation, cardiac, in heart failure, 26
Transthoracic echocardiography
    in heart failure, 26
    in mitral stenosis, 31
Traube's sign, 30
Trauma
    acute kidney, 209-212
    to knee, 309
    thrombophilia after, 158
Treponema pallidum, 184
Triad, 57
Tricuspid regurgitation, 29
Tricyclic antidepressant, 105
Triglyceride

in hyperlipidemia, 42
in pancreatitis, 68
screening for, 41
Trimethoprim-sulfamethoxazole
    for cellulitis, 129
    for urinary tract infection, 181-182
TTP-HUS, 156-157
Tuberculosis, 193-195
    meningitis and, 241
Tubing, 191
Tubule, renal
    obstruction of, 210
    water metabolism and, 220
Tumor
    adrenal, 48-49
    ovarian, 124
    pheochromocytoma, 50-51
    pituitary, 124
    tuberculosis vs, 194

U

Ulcer
    duodenal, 73
    leg, 153
    oral, in lupus, 325
    peptic, 57, 72-73
        cholecystitis vs, 65
Ulcerative colitis, 62, 87-89
Ulcer-like dyspepsia, 74
Ultrasonography
    in acute kidney injury, 211
    in biliary disease, 64, 65
    breast, 254
    in chronic kidney disease, 213
    in cirrhosis, 84
    for venous thromboembolism, 299
Upper abdominal pain, 57-58
Upper airway cough syndrome, 114
Upper airway obstruction, 286
Upper airway resistance syndrome, 291
Upper respiratory infection, 177-179
Urate, 312
Urge incontinence, 135
Urgency, 138
Uric acid, 312
Uricosuric agent, 313
Urinalysis
    in acute kidney injury, 211
    in chronic kidney disease, 213
    hypertension and, 138
    for infection, 180-181
Urinary incontinence, 135-136
Urinary obstruction, 59
Urinary tract infection, 180-182
    catheter-related, 189
Urinary tract obstruction, 210
Urine
    in hyponatremia, 220-221
    in parenchymal lung disease, 295
Urine protein, 165
Urine protein electrophoresis, 144
Ursodeoxycholic acid, 65
Urticaria, 131
    opioids causing, 272
US Preventive Services Task Force, 107
US Public Health Service
    on drug use, 109
    on smoking cessation, 117
Uterine bleeding, 126

V

Vaccination, 326
Vaccine
    hepatitis, 80, 98, 99
    human papilloma virus, 98, 265
    influenza, 98, 288
    measles, mumps, rubella, 98
    meningococcal, 99
    pertussis, 98
    pneumococcal, 98
    in sickle cell anemia, 154
    tetanus and diphtheria, 98
    varicella, 99
Vaginitis, 181
Valacyclovir, 185
Valsalva maneuver, 18
Valsartan, 27
Valvular heart disease
    acute coronary syndrome vs, 13
    angina with, 8
    aortic insufficiency, 30
    aortic stenosis as, 28-30
    dyspnea and, 276
    mitral regurgitation, 31-32
    mitral stenosis, 31
    mitral valve prolapse, 32
    murmurs in, 28
    prevention of, 28
    screening for, 28
Vancomycin
    for cellulitis, 129
    for *Clostridium difficile*, 191
    for meningitis, 242
Varenicline, 117
Varicella vaccine, 99
Varicella zoster virus, 130
Varices, 85
Vascular dementia, 237
Vascular disorder
    in diabetes mellitus, 37
    neurologic, 231
Vascular occlusion, 67
Vasculitic mononeuropathy, 248
Vasculitis, 317
Vasodilator
    for aortic insufficiency, 30
    in mitral regurgitation, 32
Vasopressin, 176
Vasopressor, 175
Vasovagal syncope, 100, 101
Velcro crackles, 294
Venlafaxine, 105
Venography, 299
Venous insufficiency, 297
Venous pressure, central, shock and, 175
Venous thromboembolism, 158-160
    in sickle cell anemia, 153
Venous thrombosis, 297
Ventilation/perfusion scan, 298, 299, 300
Ventilator-related infection, 190, 191
Ventricular arrhythmia
    diagnosis of, 20-22
    hyperkalemia and, 223
    prevention of, 20
    screening of, 20
    therapy of, 22-23
Ventricular obstruction, 101
Ventricular tachycardia, 22
Verruca vulgaris, 131
Vertebral artery, 245

Color Plates

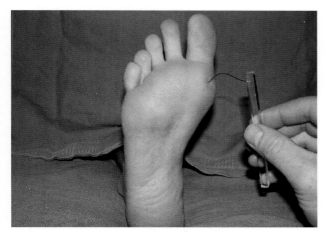

Plate 1 Testing for sensory neuropathy with a 5.07/10g monofilament.

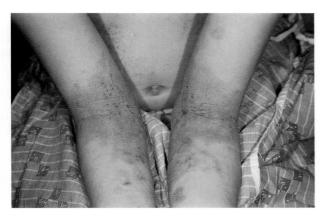

Plate 2 Subacute eczema of the flexural folds showing erythema with crusts typical of atopic dermatitis.

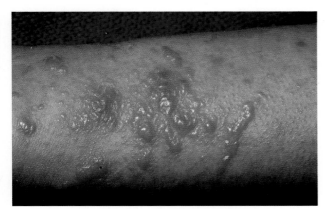

Plate 3 Discretely grouped red vesicles and bullae in a linear distribution characteristic of contact dermatitis due to poison ivy.

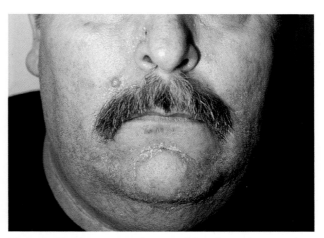

Plate 4 Erythematous plaques with a dry scale occurring in the beard area and nasolabial folds characteristic of seborrheic dermatitis.

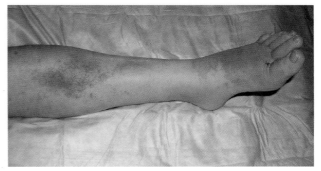

Plate 5 Lower leg cellulitis characterized by well-demarcated areas of erythema. Physical examination would reveal warmth and tenderness as well.

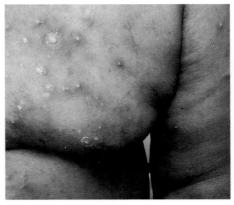

Plate 6 Multiple papules and pustules around the hair follicles is diagnostic of folliculitis. Extension of the infection can lead to furuncle formation.

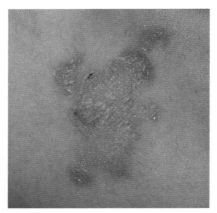

Plate 7 Superficial skin infection characterized by erosions with golden-yellow crusts typical of impetigo caused by *Staphylococcus aureus* and *Streptococcal pyogenes.*

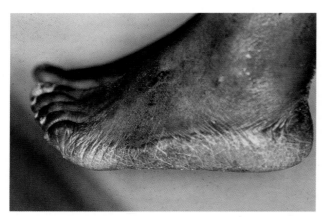

Plate 8 Well-demarcated erythema, papules, fine scales, and hyperkeratosis confined to the lateral foot, heel, and sole characteristic of "moccasin"-type tinea pedis.

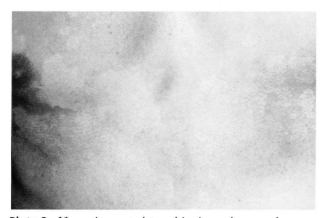

Plate 9 Hypopigmented-to-white irregular macules on the chest characteristic of tinea versicolor caused by the yeast *Malassezia furfur.*

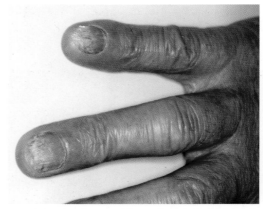

Plate 10 Distal subungual hyperkeratosis (thickening) and onycholysis (nail separation) involving most of the nails characteristic of onychomycosis.

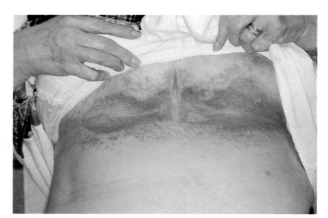

Plate 11 Bright red papules, vesicles, pustules, and patches with satellite papules in the intertriginous area beneath the breasts characteristic of candidiasis.

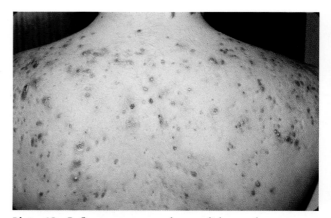

Plate 12 Inflammatory papules, nodules, and cysts located on the back typical of severe papulonodular inflammatory acne.

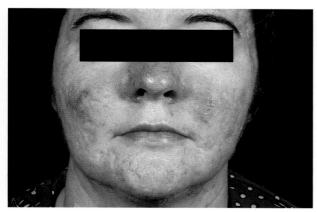

Plate 13 Papules, pustules, and dilated blood vessels involving the central face, including the nasolabial folds, typical of rosacea.

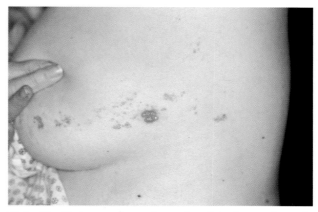

Plate 16 Pink-to-red papules and vesicles in a unilateral dermatomal distribution characteristic of herpes zoster virus infection.

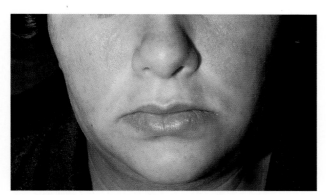

Plate 14 Erythematous plaques with fine scale involving the bridge of the nose and malar areas with sparing of the nasolabial folds under the nose and lower lip characteristic of systemic lupus erythematosus.

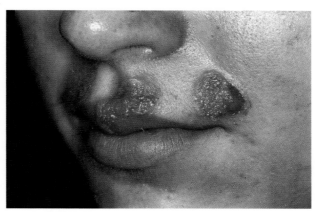

Plate 17 Oral mucosa is involved in primary herpes simplex virus infection and is characterized by painful vesicles that slough to form erosions. Recurrent lesions are similar to primary infection but may occur at any mucocutaneous site.

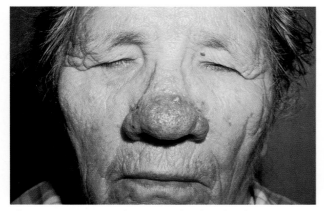

Plate 15 Patient with rosacea that has developed centrally located papules and pustules, hyperplastic sebaceous glands, and enlargement of the nose, known as *rhinophyma*.

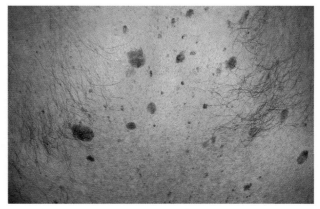

Plate 18 Brown-to-tan sharply demarcated warty- or waxy-like papules, plaques, and nodules characteristic of seborrheic keratosis.

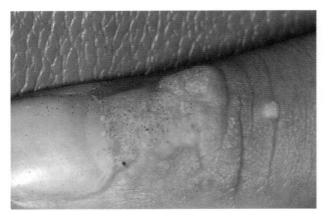

Plate 19 Verruca vulgaris (warts) lesions are recognized as firm hyperkeratotic papules with a rough cleft surface.

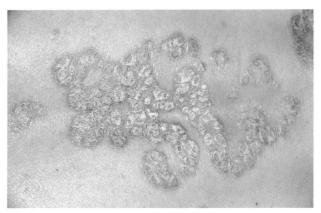

Plate 20 Silvery-white scale on top of papules and polymorphous plaques characteristic of plaque psoriasis.

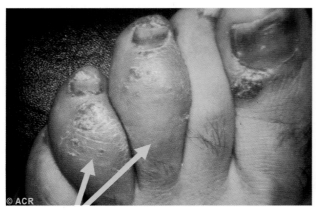

Plate 21 Small-joint polyarthritis with typical psoriatic skin lesions and nail pitting characteristic of psoriatic arthritis. (Courtesy of the American College of Rheumatology.)

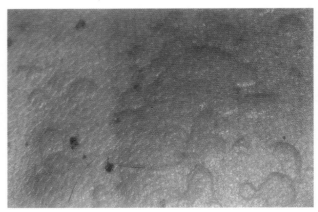

Plate 22 Urticaria is recognized by the transient appearance of pruritic papules and plaques. Urticaria may be acute, recurrent, or chronic.

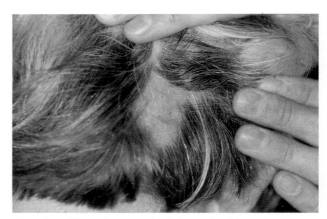

Plate 23 Alopecia areata is characterized by a sharply outlined portion of the scalp without erythema, scaling, atrophy, or scarring.

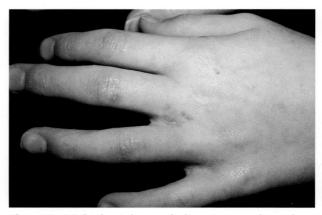

Plate 24 Multiple pink-to-red glistening papules and erosions associated with diffuse scaling, predominantly in the finger webs characteristic of scabies.

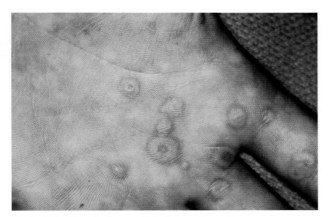

Plate 25 Classic "target" lesions of erythema multiforme consisting of flat, dull red macules that expand in a concentric ring configuration.

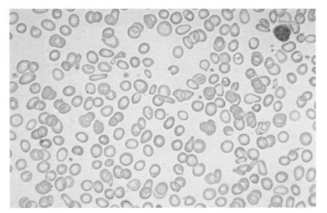

Plate 28 Erythrocyte hypochromia, anisocytosis, and "pencil cells" characteristic of iron deficiency anemia.

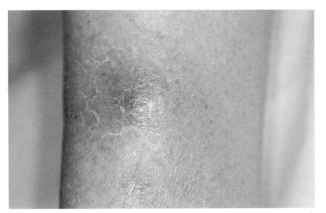

Plate 26 Tender, pink-to-dusky-red subcutaneous deep nodule located on the anterior leg characteristic of erythema nodosum.

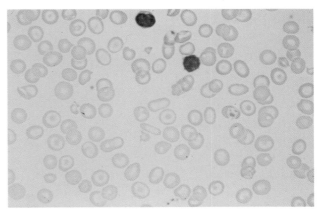

Plate 29 Erythrocyte hypochromia and target cells characteristic of thalassemia trait.

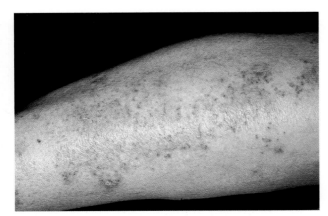

Plate 27 Asteatotic eczema is characterized by redness and a "tile-like" pattern on dry skin (xerosis) with evidence of trauma due to scratching. It typically occurs during midwinter in northern climates.

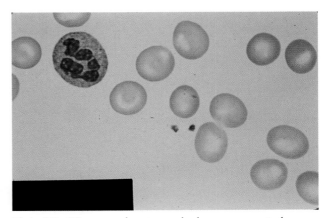

Plate 30 Macro-ovalocytes and a hypersegmented polymorphonuclear leukocyte characteristic of megaloblastic anemia.

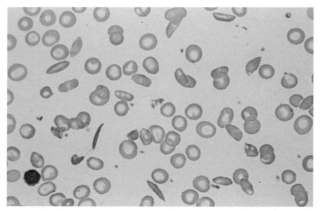

Plate 31 Erythrocyte anisocytosis and poikilocytosis with several sickle cells.

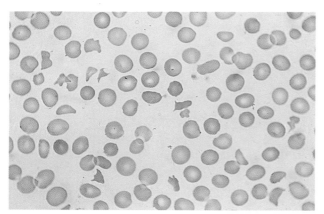

Plate 32 Marked anisocytosis and poikilocytosis with prominent schistocytes.

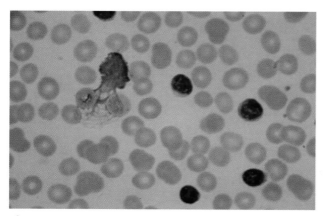

Plate 33 Increased number of mature lymphocytes and two "smudge" cells on peripheral smear (*center and bottom*) characteristic of chronic lymphocytic leukemia.

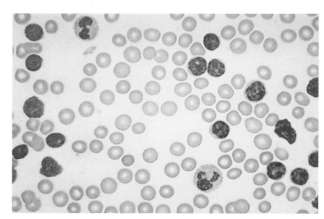

Plate 34 Increased number of granulocytic cells in all phases of development on the peripheral blood smear characteristic of chronic myeloid leukemia.

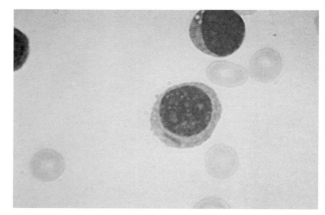

Plate 35 Peripheral blood smear showing an immature granulocyte with a rod-shaped inclusion body (Auer rod) characteristic of acute myeloid leukemia.

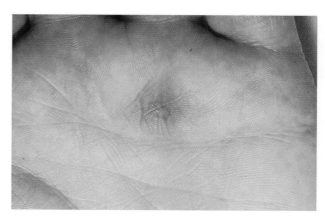

Plate 36 Lesions of disseminated gonorrhea are painful purple-to-red papules with a central pustule that may become necrotic. Petechial lesions or hemorrhagic bullae may also develop.

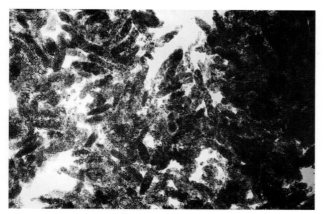

Plate 37 Muddy-brown granular casts consistent with renal injury secondary to tubular necrosis.

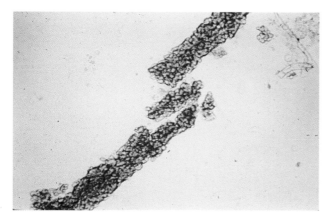

Plate 38 Red blood cell cast consistent with glomerulonephritis.

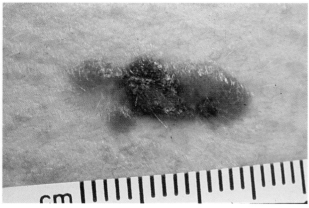

Plate 39 Malignant melanoma with characteristic asymmetrical shape, irregular borders, and variegated coloration.

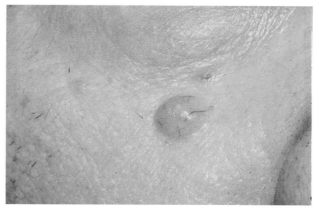

Plate 40 Nodular basal cell carcinoma with characteristic pearly translucent papule with telangiectasia.

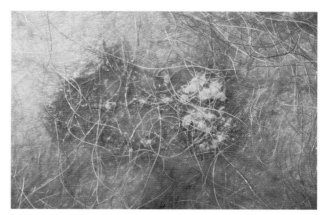

Plate 41 Well-demarcated erythematous scaling plaque in a sun-exposed area characteristic of squamous cell carcinoma.

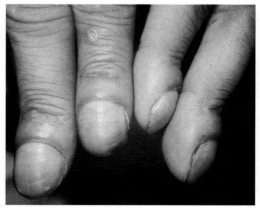

Plate 42 Example of clubbing, a painless enlargement of the connective tissues of the terminal digits. The angle of the nail to the digit is >190°.

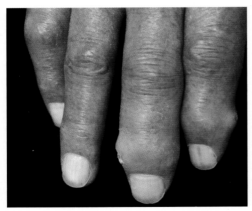

Plate 43 Milky-colored nodules characteristic of chronic tophaceous gout. Aspiration of the nodules shows sheets of monosodium urate crystals that are negatively birefringent and needle shaped.

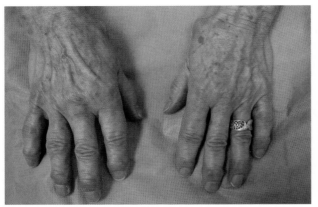

Plate 44 Heberden's nodes in osteoarthritis are bony spurs at the dorsolateral and medial aspects of the distal interphalangeal joints.

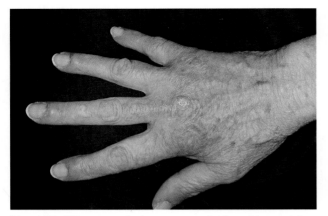

Plate 45 Discrete red plaques over the knuckles and fingers (Gottron's papules) and a dusky purple (heliotrope) rash on the eyelids are characteristic of dermatomyositis.

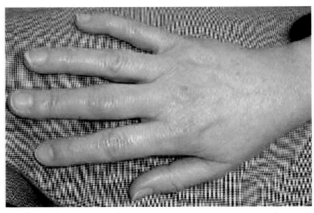

Plate 46 Typical fusiform swelling of the proximal interphalangeal joints with sparing of the distal interphalangeal joints characteristic of rheumatoid arthritis.

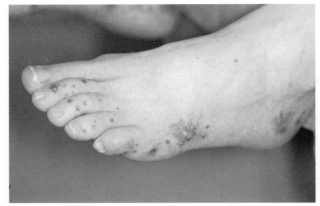

Plate 47 The hallmark of leukocytoclastic vasculitis is palpable purpura: bright red macules and papules and occasionally hemorrhagic bullae confined to the lower leg and foot.

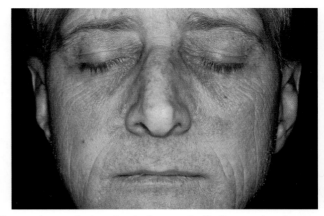